# PAINFUL CERVICAL TRAUMA

*Diagnosis and Rehabilitative Treatment of*

*Neuromusculoskeletal Injuries*

# PAINFUL CERVICAL TRAUMA

*Diagnosis and Rehabilitative Treatment of Neuromusculoskeletal Injuries*

*Edited by*

## C. DAVID TOLLISON, Ph.D.

*Pain Therapy Centers*
*Greenville Hospital System*
*Greenville, South Carolina*

*Associate Clinical Professor*
*Department of Anesthesiology*
*Medical College of Georgia*
*Augusta, Georgia*

## JOHN R. SATTERTHWAITE, M.D.

*Consulting Anesthesiologist*
*Pain Therapy Centers*
*Greenville General Hospital*
*Greenville, South Carolina*

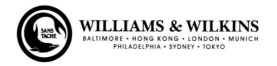

**WILLIAMS & WILKINS**
BALTIMORE · HONG KONG · LONDON · MUNICH
PHILADELPHIA · SYDNEY · TOKYO

*Editor:* John P. Butler
*Managing Editor:* Linda Napora
*Copy Editor:* Megan Westerfeld
*Designer:* Dan Pfisterer
*Illustration Planner:* Lorraine Wrzosek
*Production Coordinator:* Adèle Boyd

Copyright © 1992
Williams & Wilkins
428 East Preston Street
Baltimore, Maryland 21202, USA

Accurate indications, adverse reactions, and dosage schedules for drugs are provided in this book, but it is possible that they may change. The reader is urged to review the package information data of the manufacturers of the medications mentioned.

*Printed in the United States of America*

**Library of Congress Cataloging-in-Publication Data**

Painful cervical trauma: diagnosis and rehabilitative treatment of
   neuromusculoskeletal injuries / edited by C. David Tollison, John R. Satterthwaite.
      p.   cm.
   Includes bibliographical references.
   Includes index.
   ISBN 0-683-08337-6
   1. Vertebrae, Cervical—Wounds and injuries.   2. Neck pain.
   I. Tollison, C. David, 1949-    .  II. Satterthwaite, John R. [DNLM: 1. Cervical
   Vertebrae—injuries.   2. Pain.   3. Spinal Injuries—diagnosis.   4. Spinal
   Injuries—therapy.]
   RD521.P35 1991
   617.5′3044—dc20
   DLC
   for Library of Congress                                          90-12892
                                                                       CIP

                                                          91  92  93  94
                                              1  2  3  4  5  6  7  8  9  10

*This book is dedicated
with the highest honor,
love, and respect
to our fathers*

*Wade A. Tollison
1915–1967*

*Walter V. Satterthwaite
1923–1990*

# PREFACE

Traumatic injury to the neck is one of the most common causes of chronic pain, disability, and litigation in healthcare today. In fact, because cervical pain occurs so commonly in our society and carries such a vast array of implications, we have coined the graphic term "pain in the neck" when routinely referring to the anguish commonly created by our interactions with certain persons, situations, and events. Why? Because, "pain in the neck" is personally meaningful to such a large percentage of our population. Within any given month approximately 10% of the population will report a significant episode of severe neck pain, often with radicular components (1). In epidemiologic studies, a history of a stiff and painful neck, with or without arm pain, has been found in 50 to 75% of all individuals (2). Cervical trauma, a leading cause of chronic neck pain, is increasing in frequency as our society engages in more recreational pursuits and spends more travel time in automobiles. Football, swimming and diving, skiing, racquetball, and other sports and recreational injuries are increasing in number, and automobile accidents, a leading cause of cervical trauma, continue increasing in frequency. In fact, of all the conditions causing pain and subsequent disability in man, traumatic pain and dysfunction in the cervical region is exceeded only by the torture of low back pain (3).

Further compounding the problem is the frequency of litigation in cervical trauma injuries, particularly in cases involving automobile accidents. Anglo-Saxon law dictates compensation from liable parties for certain personal injuries received, and controversy has long raged over the question of whether such compensation functions to the general detriment of appropriate medical care. Regardless, the legal system is adversarial and often involves the carrier and attorney for the patient's group insurance policy, the carrier and attorney for the medical portion of the patient's automobile insurance policy, and the carrier and attorney for the suspected liable individual's insurance policy. In such cases, treating physicians and health professionals often find themselves poorly prepared to be thrust in the middle of opposing pressures regarding the patient's injuries, treatment, and prognosis, and ignorant of the legal system mandate of depositions and court appearances.

As if the rising incidence of both trauma and litigation were not enough, consider the complexity of the cervical region. The human neck is evolutionally an exceedingly complex structure with multiple osseous, ligamentous, muscular, vascular, and neural components, all of which are capable of generating pain. Furthermore, the biomechanics are such that the neck is responsible for the support and motion of a weighted "ball" weighing 10 pounds or more, which is capable of exerting extreme forces on the cervical structures. As such, the neck can be affected by significant as well as relatively insignificant trauma, in conjunction with subsequent, preceding, or unrelated processes such as degenerative osteoarthritis, inflammatory diseases of muscles and ligaments, vascular insufficiency, and neural compression syndromes, to mention only a few. However, considering all cases of neck pain, musculoskeletal and neuromuscular extension/flexion trauma, or "whiplash" injuries, remain the most common culprit.

Equally important, in a social sense, the neck acts as a fulcrum from which our eyes, ears, nose, mouth, and head function to interact with our environment. Neck mobility and comfort are essential for the full appreciation of the world around us. More than we realize, the neck is essential for common activities such as turning, nodding, smiling, and shaking hands. Any disruption in its normal function is noticeably limiting and may quickly be experienced as painful.

To further complicate the situation, pathologic processes in other areas of the body, such as the shoulder, diaphragm, heart, or jaw, may cause pain that is referred to the neck. Thus, one may see the complaint of neck pain in patients suffering acromioclavicular joint disease, diaphragmatic irritation, hypertension and myocardial infarction, temporomandibular joint syndrome, and other medical conditions. Accurate differential diagnosis is critical to determine the appropriate medical treatment and clinical outcome.

Finally, even the most minor discomfort in the neck, particularly that resulting from cervical trauma, has the potential to be influenced by psychological factors. It is well established that psychological factors may precipitate complaints of pain, exacerbate existing discomfort, and/or result as a consequence of chronic discomfort and alteration in lifestyle (4). If litigation is involved, the potential for psychological influence may be increased. Regardless, the accurate assessment and management of psychological factors in chronic pain resulting from cervical trauma is germane to comprehensive clinical treatment.

Fortunately, 70% of individuals seeking medical intervention for acute cervical pain are either free from discomfort or significantly improved within one month, and the majority of the remaining 30% obtain symptomatic relief with the passage of time and therapeutic interventions (1). However, given the prevalence of this disorder, a large number of victims graduate to a diagnosis of intractable cervical pain that defies traditional medical care.

This book specifically and comprehensively outlines the current treatment of cervical neuromusculoskeletal injuries and pain as determined by the editorial contributions of a carefully selected interdisciplinary group of noted clinical and research authorities. The text is divided into four sections. The first section addresses the current state of Diagnostic Foundations. This section will highlight functional anatomy as well as specifics of the medical history and physical examination of the painful cervical region. Additional chapters will include numerous foundational diagnostic studies and techniques, and the section will conclude with a critically important chapter on differential diagnosis. A particularly interesting two-part chapter in this section includes a comprehensive discussion of clinical radiographic imaging techniques.

Section II is a detailed and practical presentation of therapeutic techniques. Included in this section is an array of interdisciplinary nonsurgical interventions, from conventional modalities to more innovative techniques. Practical step-by-step application and delivery of the numerous interventions is stressed, including three chapters on pharmacologic treatment. The section concludes with a chapter on the comprehensive "pain program" approach to the highly complex and intractable cervical pain syndrome that does not respond to alternative treatment techniques.

Section III outlines specific treatment strategies for a variety of selected painful cervical disorders. This section begins with the principles of emergency management of cervical injuries and indications for surgical intervention. Treatment specifics for a variety of selected diagnoses and disorders follow, including a detailed chapter on the treatment of extension/flexion or "whiplash" injuries. Consistent with the comprehensive scope of the text, the section concludes with a chapter on cognitive deficits commonly encountered but frequently undiagnosed in the treatment of cervical and head trauma.

The fourth section of the text is a unique attempt to address those medical-legal issues frequently involved in cervical injuries. Specifically, this section educates physicians and health professionals in two anxiety-provoking responsibilities of frequent uncertainty: disability and impairment determination, and legal depositions and court appearances. Authored by noted clinical and legal authorities, this section outlines information required in performing disability impairment determinations and educates health professionals in both the defense and claimant's counsel questioning of the physician.

This text is intended for those health professionals who routinely accept the responsibilities of diagnosing and treating individuals suffering painful cervical trauma, as well as those individuals who serve as conduits and evaluators of information involved in mediating legal disputes arising from neck injuries. Consequently, a variety of individuals will find the text valuable, including orthopaedic and neurological surgeons, emergency room physicians, neurologists, pain management specialists, rheumatologists, family and internal medicine specialists, physiatrists and physical therapists, psychologists and psychiatrists, radiologists, nurses, attorneys, chiropractors, insurance claim adjusters, and accident reconstructionists.

### REFERENCES

1. Aryanpur J, Ducker TB: Differential diagnosis and management of cervical spine pain. In Tollison CD (ed): *Handbook of Chronic Pain Management*. Baltimore, Williams & Wilkins, 1989.

2. Lawrence J: Disc degeneration, its frequency and relationship to symptoms. *Ann Rheumatol Dis* 28:121, 1969.

3. McCulloch JA: Differential diagnosis of low back pain. In Tollison CD (ed): *Handbook of Chronic Pain Management*. Baltimore, Williams & Wilkins, 1989.

4. Tollison CD, Kriegel ML: Interdisciplinary rehabilitation: An overview. In Tollison CD, Kriegel ML (eds): *Interdisciplinary Rehabilitation of Low Back Pain*. Baltimore, Williams & Wilkins, 1989

# ACKNOWLEDGMENTS

Anyone who has labored intently in the preparation of a medical reference text quickly learns that countless individuals contribute, both directly and indirectly, to the final product. Although it would be impossible to recognize the important contributions of each individual who influenced this project, we shall identify a limited number of people who provided valued assistance. We hereby extend our sincere appreciation to these and numerous unnamed others who provided guidance and support.

First, we would like to extend our appreciation to the contributing authors. Forty-eight authors contributed their time, talents, and considerable expertise to this book. Each is a highly regarded authority with multiple demands on his/her time and attention; yet each cheerfully cooperated with the numerous requests inherent in such a project and, as best we can determine, each continues to remain on speaking terms with us. Our sincere thanks to each one of you.

We would also like to extend our appreciation to Williams & Wilkins. The Executive Editor, John P. Butler, and his associates exhibited a great deal of patience and confidence and provided much support throughout this project.

We owe a signifcant debt of gratitude to our medical colleagues and to the staff of the Pain Therapy Center of Greenville. Meg Kessler, Melinda Davis, and Sharon Ellis not only kept us organized and on task, but also assumed much of the operational responsibilities for guiding this project through completion.

We would particularly like to express our appreciation to our respective families for their encouragement and support. The first editor extends gratitude to his wife, Linda, and children, Courtney and David. The second editor extends appreciation to his wife, Sharon, and children, Jennifer and Joel.

Finally, we would be remiss without acknowledging the thousands of patients in pain who have allowed us to learn from them.

*C. David Tollison, Ph.D.*
*John R. Satterthwaite, M.D.*

# CONTRIBUTORS

ELSAYED ABDEL-MOTY, Ph.D.
*Research Assistant Professor*
*Department of Industrial Engineering*
*College of Engineering, University of Miami*
*Research Assistant Professor*
*Department of Neurological Surgery*
*University of Miami School of Medicine*
*Miami Beach, Florida*

JOHN ARYANPUR, M.D.
*Department of Neurosurgery*
*The Johns Hopkins University School of Medicine*
*Baltimore, Maryland*

STEVEN G. ASHMAN, D.D.S.
*Clinical Associate Professor*
*Department of Oral and Maxillofacial Surgery*
*Baltimore College of Dental Surgery*
*University of Maryland*
  *School of Dentistry*
*Baltimore, Maryland*

J. HAMPTON ATKINSON, Jr. M.D.
*Associate Adjunct Professor*
*Department of Psychiatry*
*University of California San Diego, School of*
  *Medicine*
*La Jolla, California*

KIM J. BURCHIEL, M.D.
*Professor and Head*
*Division of Neurosurgery*
*Oregon Health Sciences University*
*Portland, Oregon*

JEROME BUXBAUM, D.D.S., F.A.G.D.
*Clinical Professor*
*Department of Physiology*
*Baltimore College of Dental Surgery*
*University of Maryland School of Dentistry*
*Baltimore, Maryland*

JOHN R. CASSIDY, M.D.
*Neurological Associates*
*Sarasota, Florida*
*Formerly Department of Neurological Surgery*
*The Johns Hopkins University School of Medicine*
*Baltimore, Maryland*

ARMINIUS CASSVAN, M.D.
*Chief, Rehabilitation Medicine and Electrodiagnostic*
  *Center*
*Franklin Hospital Medical Center*
*Director, Department of Rehabilitation Medicine*
*Hempstead General Hospital Medical Center*
*Associate Professor of Clinical Rehabilitation*
  *Medicine*
*State University of New York at Stony Brook*
*Stony Brook, New York*

DONALD S. CICCONE, Ph.D.
*Associate Director, Pain Management Services*
*Kessler Institute*
*East Orange, New Jersey*
*Assistant Professor, Department of Physical Medicine*
  *and Rehabilitation*
*University of Medicine and Dentistry, New Jersey*
  *Medical School*
*Newark, New Jersey*

BENJAMIN L. CRUE, Jr., M.D., F.A.C.S.
*Emeritus Clinical Professor of Neurological Surgery*
*University of Southern California School of Medicine*
*Los Angeles, California*
*Medical Director*
*Durango Pain Rehabilitation Center and Regional*
  *Rehabilitation Center*
*La Plata Community Hospital*
*Durango, Colorado*

SEYMOUR DIAMOND, M.D.
*Director, Diamond Headache Clinic and the*
  *Inpatient Headache Unit*
*Louis A. Weiss Memorial Hospital*
*Chicago, Illinois*
*Adjunct Professor of Pharmacology*
*The Chicago Medical School*
*North Chicago, Illinois*

ALAN S. EXLER, D.D.S.
*Clinical Assistant Professor*
*Department of Oral and Maxillofacial Surgery*
*Baltimore College of Dental Surgery*
*University of Maryland*
  *School of Dentistry*
*Baltimore, Maryland*

AVITAL FAST, M.D.
*Director*
*Department of Rehabilitation Medicine*
*St. Vincent's Hospital and Medical Center of New*
  *York*
*New York, New York*

GERALD M. FINKEL
*Finkel, Georgaklis, Goldberg & Sheftman, P.A.*
*Columbia, South Carolina*

PRESTON BLAINE FITZGERALD, D.C.
*Board Eligible Chiropractic Orthopedist*
*Director, Fitzgerald Neck & Back Center*
*Manning, South Carolina*

FREDERICK G. FREITAG, D.O.
*Associate Director, Diamond Headache Clinic*
*Chicago, Illinois*
*Visiting Lecturer, Department of Family Medicine*
*Chicago College of Osteopathic Medicine*
*Chicago, Illinois*

LAWRENCE W. FRIEDMAN, M.D., F.A.C.A.,
  F.I.C.A.
*Chairman, Physiatrist-In-Chief*
*Department of Physical Medicine and Rehabilitation*
*Nassau County Medical Center*
*East Meadow, New York*
*Professor of Rehabilitation Medicine*
*Health Sciences Center*
*State University of New York at Stony Brook*
*Stony Brook, New York*

R. MICHAEL GALLAGHER, D.O.
*Associate Director*
*Diamond Headache Clinic*
*Chicago, Illinois*
*Clinical Associate Professor*
*University of Medicine and Dentistry of New Jersey*
*School of Osteopathic Medicine*
*Stratford, New Jersey*
*Clinical Associate Professor*
*Philadelphia College of Osteopathic Medicine*
*Philadelphia, Pennsylvania*

ROY C. GRZESIAK, Ph.D.
*Assistant Professor*
*Department of Anesthesiology*
*Co-Director, Pain Management Center*
*University of Medicine and Dentistry*
*New Jersey Medical School*
*Newark, New Jersey*

WILLIAM N. HARSHA, M.D., J.D.
*Oklahoma Spine Pain Management Clinic*
*Oklahoma City, Oklahoma*

DONALD W. HINNANT, Ph.D.
*Program Director*
*Pain Therapy Centers*
*Greenville Hospital System*
*Greenville, South Carolina*

H. DENNIS KADE, Ph.D.
*Center for Psychological Services*
*Riverside Regional Medical Center*
*Newport News, Virginia*

TAREK M. KHALIL, Ph.D., P.E.
*Professor and Chairman*
*Department of Industrial Engineering*
*College of Engineering, University of Miami*
*Chief, Ergonomics Division*
*Comprehensive Pain and Rehabilitation Center*
*University of Miami School of Medicine*
*Miami Beach, Florida*

HANS KRAUS, M.D.
*New York, New York*

PAUL LEUNG, Ph.D.
*Division of Rehabilitation Education*
*University of Illinois*
*Champaign, Illinois*
*Formerly Director*
*Division of Rehabilitation Counseling*
*University of North Carolina at Chapel Hill*
*Chapel Hill, North Carolina*

EDGAR L. MARIN, M.D.
*Associate Chairman*
*Department of Physical Medicine and Rehabilitation*
*Assistant Professor of Rehabilitation Medicine*
*State University of New York at Stony Brook*
*Stony Brook, New York*

GLENN A. McCAIN, M.D., F.R.C.P.C.
*Associate Professor of Medicine*
*Rheumatic Diseases Unit*
*University Hospital*
*University of Western Ontario*
*London, Ontario, Canada*

RALPH C. McCULLOUGH II
*Finkel, Georgaklis, Goldberg & Sheftman, P.A.*
*Columbia, South Carolina*

JACINTA M. McELLIGOTT, M.D.
*Assistant Professor of Physical Medicine and*
  *Rehabilitation*
*Associate Director of Work Evaluation Program*
*Department of Physical Medicine and Rehabilitation*
*East Carolina University School of Medicine*
*Greenville, North Carolina*


RICHARD B. NORTH, M.D.
*Department of Neurological Surgery*
*The Johns Hopkins University School of Medicine*
*Baltimore, Maryland*


PATRICIA A. PADULA, D.P.M., F.A.C.F.O.
*Consultant Attending in Biomechanics and Podiatry*
*Department of Physical Medicine and Rehabilitation*
*Professor of Orthopedic Sciences*
*New York College of Podiatric Medicine*
*New York, New York*


WINSTON C.V. PARRIS, M.D.
*Associate Professor of Anesthesiology*
*Director, Pain Control Center*
*Vanderbilt University Hospital*
*Nashville, Tennessee*


R. HARRISON PLEDGER, Jr.
*Attorney at Law*
*McLean, Virginia*


BARRY A. REICH, Ph.D.
*Director, Comprehensive Pain Program*
*Nassau Pain and Stress Center*
*Mineola, New York*


HUBERT L. ROSOMOFF, M.D., D.Med.Sc.
*Medical Director*
*Comprehensive Pain and Rehabilitation Center*
*Professor and Chairman*
*Department of Neurological Surgery*
*University of Miami School of Medicine*
*Miami, Florida*


RENEÉ S. ROSOMOFF, B.S.N., M.B.A.,
  C.R.C., C.I.R., C.R.R.N.
*Programs Director*
*Comprehensive Pain and Rehabilitation Center*
*Adjunct Instructor*
*Department of Neurological Surgery*
*University of Miami School of Medicine*
*Miami, Florida*


JOHN R. SATTERTHWAITE, M.D.
*Consulting Anesthesiologist*
*Pain Therapy Centers*
*Greenville General Hospital*
*Greenville, South Carolina*


DANIEL SHAPIRO, M.D.
*Assistant Clinical Professor of Physical Medicine and*
  *Rehabilitation*
*State University of New York*
*Chief, Department of Physical Medicine and*
  *Rehabilitation*
*Long Island Jewish Medical Center*
*New Hyde Park, New York*


MARK A. SLATER, Ph.D.
*Assistant Professor*
*Department of Psychiatry*
*University of California, San Diego*
*Director, Pain Management Program*
*San Diego VA Medical Center*
*San Diego, California*


WILLIAM I. SMULYAN, M.D.
*Baltimore, Maryland*


GLEN D. SOLOMON, M.D., F.A.C.P.
*Section on Headache,*
*Department of Internal Medicine*
*Cleveland Clinic Foundation*
*Cleveland, Ohio*


RAJKA J. SORIC, M.D., M.Sc., F.R.C.P.C.
*Department of Rehabilitative Medicine*
*Mount Sinai Hospital*
*Assistant Professor*
*Department of Rehabilitation Medicine*
*University of Toronto*
*Toronto, Ontario, Canada*


ROBERT W. TEASELL, M.D., F.R.C.P.C.
*Assistant Professor of Medicine*
*Chief, Physical Medicine and Rehabilitation*
*University Hospital*
*University of Western Ontario*
*London, Ontario, Canada*


C. DAVID TOLLISON, Ph.D.
*Senior Vice President and Director*
*Pain Therapy Centers*
*Greenville General Hospital*
*Greenville, South Carolina*

SANFORD H. VERNICK, M.D., Ph.D.
*Associate Professor of Physical Medicine and*
  *Rehabilitation*
*Director of the Chronic Pain Clinic*
*Director of the Residency Training Program*
*East Carolina University School of Medicine*
*Greenville, North Carolina*

R. GEOFFREY WILBER, M.D.
*Assistant Professor of Orthopaedics*
*Case Western Reserve University*
*School of Medicine*
*Cleveland, Ohio*

FREDERICK WOLFE, M.D.
*Clinical Professor of Medicine*
*University of Kansas School of Medicine*
*Director, Arthritis Center*
*Wichita, Kansas*

JUNG YOO, M.D.
*Instructor in Orthopaedics*
*Case Western Reserve University*
*School of Medicine*
*Cleveland, Ohio*

ALAN E. ZIMMER, M.D.
*Director of Neuroradiology*
*Associate Professor of Clinical Radiology*
*University of Medicine and Dentistry*
*New Jersey Medical School*
*Newark, New Jersey*

# CONTENTS

# SECTION II
## THERAPEUTIC TECHNIQUES

# SECTION III
## TREATMENT OF SELECTED DISORDERS

## *SECTION IV*

## MEDICAL-LEGAL ISSUES

# DIAGNOSTIC FOUNDATIONS

*1*

# FUNCTIONAL ANATOMY
# OF THE CERVICAL SPINE

*William N. Harsha*

In the axial skeleton, the spine (cervical, dorsal, lumbar, sacral, and coccygeal) is the main support, both for its own soft tissues and for the appendicular (head, arms, and legs) components of the body. The basic structures are the bony vertebrae, intervertebral discs, spinal cord, ligaments, capsules, muscles, tendons, and the surrounding subcutaneous tissue and dermis (skin).

## SPINAL COLUMN

The spinal column is made up of the articulated cervical, dorsal (thoracic), lumbar, sacral, and coccygeal vertebrae. Between each vertebra is an inter-vertebral disc. Each disc has its own capsule, frequently intimately combined with adjacent ligaments. In effect, the ligaments completely surrounding the vertebral bodies support or hold the vertebrae together in a flexible, yet stable, column. Posterior to each vertebra are bilateral pedicles, which are rigid posts that make up the lateral aspect of the spinal canal and the base for the paired facet joints. The laminae fuse in their midposterior aspect and continue posteriorly to form the spinous process. The laminae form the posterior aspect of the spinal canal, and the posterior edge of the vertebral body forms an anterior aspect.

## SPINAL CORD AND NERVE ROOTS

The spinal cord starts from the brain at the skull and goes inferiorly (caudad) through the spinal canal to the tip of the last coccygeal element. The spinal cord gradually diminishes en masse until it reaches L2. There it terminates as the lumbar, sacral, and coccygeal nerve roots that exit in their respective neuroforamina and proceed to their destination in peripheral soft tissues. The distal (caudal) spinal cord is held in place by a dense extension of the dura, called the ligamentum terminale, which terminates within the spinal canal at the last sacrococcygeal segment.

At each level from the first cervical to the last coccygeal vertebral element, there are a pair of foraminae (holes) through which right and left nerve roots leave the spinal cord, passing posteriorly to their respective intervertebral disc out the foramen (which is really a short bony canal) and into adjacent soft tissues.

## TRANSVERSE PROCESS AND RIBS

Extending from the neck vertebrae at the base of the pedicle and pointing laterally are the bony transverse processes. The above-mentioned nerve roots pass anteriorly to these processes, which, in the cervical and lumbar spine, can be 1–1.5 inches long. In the dorsal spine, they are short and have paired joints that articulate with the ribs. Transverse processes are absent in the sacral and coccygeal segments.

## INTERVERTEBRAL DISCS

Intervertebral discs lie between the vertebrae, and are named and numbered for the lower vertebral body (i.e., the C2 disc lies between the C1 and C2 vertebrae). The highest (cephalad) disc lies between C1 and C2 and the last functional disc lies between L5 and S1, if there are no congenital variations.

The intervertebral disc acts as a shock absorber and participates in the smooth motion of its vertebral motion segment (adjacent vertebral bodies with posterior facets that glide over each other like shingles and their adjacent ligaments, joint capsules, and muscles).

The intervertebral disc is composed of two indistinct parts that meld with each other. The inner component is the nucleus pulposus, a gelatinous substance in its normal state, containing a moderate amount of water and functioning as an enclosed hydraulic system. The outer component of the disc is made of concentric fibrous rings that contain the nucleus pulposus and firmly attach to the vertebral body above and below (cephalad and caudad). The fibers of this annulus fibrosis are woven in intricate geometric patterns that allow motion and prevent the nucleus pulposus from extruding when under pressure (loaded).

Progressive degeneration of the intervertebral disc begins in the third decade of life, resulting in gradual weakening of the annulus and dehydration with chemical changes in the nucleus pulposus. The annulus is thinner at the posterolateral corners, because it is not supported there by the posterior longitudinal ligament. It is at this weaker point that fissuring with age occurs in the annulus, allowing movement of the nuclear material posteriorly. If there is sufficient nuclear displacement posteriorly through these fissures, a bulge in the posterior aspect of the annulus may occur and the overlying nerve root may be tented over the bulge. This defines a protruded intervertebral disc. If a hole occurs in the annulus, an extruded intervertebral disc is defined.

## LIGAMENTS

Each vertebral body is surrounded by dense interlacing fibers called ligaments. Their function is to hold the elements in place and to prevent excessive motion. Where greater support is necessary, they become thickened bands, such as the anterior and posterior longitudinal ligaments.

Between the spinous processes at each level occur the very dense interspinous ligaments called the ligamentum flavum, which continue anteriorly and span the proximal and distal (cephalad and caudad) edges of the lamina. Between the spinous processes the spinal canal is covered by the contiguous surfaces of these several ligaments combined with the laterally placed facet capsules.

## THE NERVOUS SYSTEM

The primary function of the spinal (vertebral) column is support, while the spinal cord contained within its spinal canal functions as a conduit carrying messages from the brain to specific muscle groups. These messages direct muscular activity so that muscles will move and/or support the spine as the brain directs. The spinal cord is capable of independently ordering movement, often in concert with the brain.

The brain and spinal cord have many other functions not discussed in this section, such as transmission of (afferant) messages from the distal points of the body (such as pain, proprioception, hot/cold, position, and vibration) to the brain via the nerve roots and spinal cord.

## SPINAL CORD

The spinal cord in the average adult is 1.5 feet long. It is largest in diameter in the cervical area (0.5 to 0.75 inch), tapering to 0.25 inch at the conus medullaris, where the cord ends. Although the cord usually terminates at L2, it may end anywhere between D12 and L3. Functionally, the spinal cord may be considered as an electrical conduit from the brain to the peripheral nerves, although admittedly this is oversimplification.

If a segment of the spinal cord is cut or crushed and becomes nonfunctional, spinal shock ensues, in which the muscles informed by that segment become flaccidly paralyzed and appropriate reflexes are absent. The shock state will pass, usually in 24–72 hr. After this period, permanent loss of motor and sensory function can be assessed. Recovery is sequential, noted as an increase in reflexes with or without spasticity, followed by a phase during which reflex responses gradually subordinate to outside stimulation and voluntary function is restored to the degree that is possible. The amount of residual spasticity and increased reflex activity varies, being greater in cervical cord injuries than in those in the lumbar region.

## MENINGES

The spinal cord is covered by three layers. The innermost, a delicate fibroelastic membrane called the pia mater, is attached to the cord itself. Where the cord ends in the lumbar area, the pia mater goes on to form the ligamentum terminale. The second (middle) membrane, the arachnoid mater, is connected to the pia by many spider-like (thus its name) fibers and also attached to the outer (dural) layer. It is through this layer that the spinal fluid circulates. The outer layer is the dura mater, a tube of tough connective tissue that loosely surrounds the spinal cord. It extends from the foramen magnum in the skull to the second or third sacral vertebra, and then continues as the posterior longitudinal ligament. The dura further extends over each nerve root and blends with movable soft tissue in the neuroforaminal area. As a result, the dura mater is partially suspended in the epidural space and partly supported by the epidural connective tissue and vessels.

Subdural spaces—potential or minimal spaces between the smooth inner surface of the dura and the adjacent arachnoid membrane—are of little clinical importance.

## NERVE ROOTS

Spinal nerve roots are made up of a series of nerve fibers that exit the functional area of the spinal cord and meld together to form the dorsal and ventral roots, then continue laterally to exit their respective neural foramina. It is important to remember that the spinal cord is shorter than the vertebral column. This results in spinal cord segments that are considerably shorter than their corresponding vertebra. As one goes down the spinal canal there is an increasing discrepancy between a given spinal cord segment and its nerve root and the corresponding vertebra where the nerve root exits the vertebral column. In the cervical and dorsal areas, the nerve root proceeds almost directly lateral from the spinal cord to its neural foramen. However, in the lumbar area the L5 nerve root, for example, leaves the spinal cord at about the L1 vertebral level and proceeds at an angle distally for several inches before exiting the L5–S1 neuroforamen.

This anatomic situation has great clinical and legal importance, particularly in the diagnosis of neck or low back problems. The cervical nerves start in the high cervical area, passing directly laterally to their neuroforamina. Moving distally, the nerves become obliquely placed, proceeding through the dorsal spine and becoming oriented in the lower dorsal or upper lumbar area. Thus, alteration or loss of nerve function is always more distal in the body than is reflected by the level of spinal cord damage.

Functionally, the nerve roots carry impulses originating in the brain via the spinal cord and along pathways known as dermatomes. Dermatomes are supplied by a single spinal segment and provide sensation in areas of skin supplied by that segment. Specific groups or parts of muscle masses likewise are supplied by specific spinal segments called myotomes.

The nerve root also transmits impulses that activate reflexes. Typically muscle stretch reflexes result in contraction of that muscle. Complete interruption of the nerve, nerve root, or spinal cord causes loss of the reflex. Stretching or pressure on a nerve root (such as tenting of a nerve root over a protruded intervertebral disc) or compression of a nerve (seen in nerve compression syndromes) will diminish the reflex, approaching loss of the reflex. In these cases comparison of the diminished reflex with that of the opposite side of the body is important.

## THE MUSCLES

The complex nature of the spinal musculature is embryonic in origin. The muscles embryonically are segmental, running from one vertebra to the next. Fusion between segments then forms a longer muscle. Tangential splitting results in a number of superimposed layers. Unlike muscles in the extremities, all but the shortest and deepest lying muscles of the neck and back have multiple origins and insertions into bone.

In most muscles of the neck and back, bundles of any one origin fan out to blend with muscle bundles that arise one or two segments above and below. The melded muscle bundles form new muscles that have successive insertions in the vertebral column. This complexity has its origin in part during that phase of fetal development in which the vertebral segments divide and move proximally and distally to fuse with the adjacent halves.

Understanding the complexity of the muscles of the neck and back is important in the comprehension of continuing muscle function below spinal cord functional loss levels. Also, the multiple innervation is helpful in rehabilitation of back injury patients.

## PATHOPHYSIOLOGY OF A PAINFUL NECK

There are three discriminators, or three areas, in evaluation of neck pain: (a) duration, (b) location, and (c) anatomic localization.

Duration of neck pain is related to capacity for spontaneous repair. What is the pathophysiology of soft tissue repair?

1. Strong connective tissue has a limited blood supply and few cells, and thus repair is slow.
2. Where blood is not available, nutrition is obtained by means of extravascular diffusion. Diffusion is enhanced by motion and delayed by inactivity.
3. Animal models have shown that activity speeds the slow repair process and organizes the tissue. Spontaneous repair with inactivity allows random collagen alignment and the potential for segmental shortening as a result of collagenous cross-linking. Guided activity has been demonstrated to align collagen and enhance tissue compliance, thus avoiding contractures due to cross-linking and random fiber orientation.

Since clinical studies demonstrate no advantage to prolonged inactivity, in all patient evaluations the duration of pain complaints before initiation of treatment should be identified in order to determine capacity for spontaneous repair. Neck pain can be described as acute, subacute, or chronic. The *acute phase* has a duration of 1 week to 10 days with the possibility of rapid repair associated with good blood supply. The *subacute phase* of neck pain has a duration of 1 week to 3 months, with a lesser potential for spontaneous repair. Cases of recurrent pain and repeat injury most often belong to this category. In the *chronic phase* of neck pain there is a limited opportunity for spontaneous repair. In the presence of subacutely painful tissue clinical function may be maintained over 3 months.

The location (distribution) of pain supplies information on the type and amount of structural damage if specific anatomic localization of the damage has not been made. Pain associated with cervical radiculopathy has a specific relationship to the peripheral nerves. Such pain usually is in the shoulder and arm, and radiates into the hand. Imaging studies may correlate the pain with specific lesions.

Pain without radiculopathy cannot be located anatomically. Anatomists have shown overlapping innervations spanning at least three vertebral levels, in which the nerves to the intervertebral tendons that go to the facet joints and posterior structures have branches from each level that span three levels in the back. The amount of noxious stimuli broadens the distribution of pain in the body, as well as its intensity, in a mechanism known as "referred pain." The distribution of referred pain ordinarily follows a typical nondermatomal pattern.

Pain distribution can be documented and followed by changes in pain drawings. Pain and function are the only discriminators of severity. Pain location is much more important in the subacute phase. Pain related to disuse (the deconditioning syndrome) rather than to the structural site of injury is an important factor in the chronic phase.

The concept of myofasciitis, tender points, and the role of neural reflexes and their etiology are well substantiated in the myofascial pain syndrome. The role of various therapeutic modalities—heat, cold, ultrasound, electrotherapy, and massage—in the treatment of these problems, and the role of acupuncture, acupressure, and injection therapies to myofascial trigger points, should be understood.

Another important concept is the role of the facet joints in the painful motion segment. Different sorts of deterioration have been demonstrated in a variety of studies. The issue of fringe impingement with synovial tab hypertrophies versus fibrillated or torn articular cartilage may explain much in the locking up of the facets. The pain response to these pathologies may induce a reflex sensory or autonomic nerve response.

Finally, the role of the intervertebral disc in neck and back pain must be considered also. At the present time, discography gives the only insight to the symptomatic disc.

## EVALUATION OF BACK AND NECK PAIN

The bottom line of evaluation of back and neck pain seems to be that activity enhances repair and delay is not justified. The central concerns of evaluation are: (*a*) the efficacy of treatment must be compared with the natural history of the problem; (*b*) the possibility of further damage and/or deconditioning in addition to the original injury must be considered in relation to the intensity of the pain complaint; and (*c*) deconditioning must be treated as part of the rehabilitation program.

Physicians need to remember the placebo effect. Fully one third of all treatments the physician orders are fairly promptly effective for an indefinite period. Another third are therapeutically effective for a short time (3 months or so) and then become ineffective. Another third of treatments do not effect a change in patients' symptoms.

## MOTOR IMPAIRMENT

A thorough search for subtle signs of a distal upper motor neuron lesion is imperative in any patient who has an apparently isolated nerve root lesion, particularly in the cervical region. In contrast to a complete peripheral nerve lesion, in which motor function is completely destroyed in the distribution of that nerve, a complete nerve root lesion may cause partial—although sometimes severe—paresis but not usually total paralysis of the various muscles innervated by that nerve root. This is because each muscle is innervated by multiple nerve roots arising from more than one spinal level.

The diaphragm is predominantly innervated by C3 and C4; therefore, a lesion high in the spinal cord threatens respiratory function. Shoulder abduction is a good test for C5 lesions. In the presence of normal function of the deltoid muscles, weak elbow flexors, predominantly the biceps muscles, suggest a C6 lesion. The elbow and wrist extensors are served primarily by the triceps brachia and extensor carpi radialis and ulnaris muscles, which are innervated by C7, which also contributes to the function of the pronator teres. Lesions at C8 predominantly affect the intrinsic muscles of the hand, which are also innervated by T1.

Abdominal muscles can be tested for lesions affecting the thoracic nerves. Hip flexors and abductors and the quadriceps muscle are innervated by L2 and L3; L4 and L5 innervate the ankle dorsiflexors and great toe extensors, while plantar flexors are innervated by S1.

## SENSORY IMPAIRMENT

Sensory examination often provides the most significant information in localizing spinal cord lesions. However, if the results of the examination are normal, the patient's symptoms may be the most important clue. The segmental distribution may be most useful in diagnosis when both nerve root and spinal cord are involved, as seen in a dumbbell tremor or a neuroma.

The sensory dermatomal pattern provides a useful guide. The C1 root has no significant sensory component; thus a lesion high in the spinal cord has its most proximal effect on C2, which is the posterior part of the scalp. Since the descending spinal tract of the trigeminal nerve (V) extends into the upper cervical cord, lesions at this level may produce changes in pain and temperature sensations over the temple and forehead, possibly with a diminished corneal reflex. Segments C6–8 and T1 innervate the arm and hand, and the deltoid muscle is supplied by C5. The thumb is a good marker for C6, the index and middle fingers for C7, and the ring finger for C8. T1 innervates the medial upper arm and adjacent axilla. The nipple line is innervated by T4 and an area over the umbilicus by T10.

Electromyographic and nerve conduction velocities may be slightly to moderately decreased. Needle examination demonstrates abnormal insertional changes in a specific nerve root or plexus. When nerve roots are involved, the paraspinal muscles are particularly affected, often bilaterally pointing to the root level. These findings may suggest a present concomitant interspinal lesion. Myelography is normal but cerebrospinal fluid pressure may be elevated.

## HEAD AND NECK INJURIES

Head and neck injuries are commonly associated, so the treating physician must consider the head and neck as a unit when evaluating and treating a patient who has sustained multiple trauma. In assessing cervical spine injuries, *head injuries must always be included.* Conversely, when an unconscious or semiconscious patient is seen in an emergency facility with a head injury, an associated spine injury should always be considered. The head must be stabilized in respect to the cervical spine before looking for fracture or dislocation; moving the patient prior to such stabilization might induce a catastrophic situation. Evaluation of the cranial nerves can be rapidly and systematically done by simply remembering the normal functions. It is difficult, of course, to do an adequate evaluation of cranial nerves in a comatose patient.

In a study reviewing 300 cervical spinal injuries, autopsy findings in 48 cases indicated that only three had total cord disruption (1). Most patients with evidence of total cord lesions had incomplete contusions indicating sparing of neural tissue. In addition, some patients had significant quadriparesis with anterior cord syndromes but had a microscopically normal spinal cord without evidence of gross cord disruption. These findings indicate that ischemia and direct neural compression may play a role in the recovery from an incomplete spinal cord injury. Patients who had unilateral facet dislocations had an impairment of major radicular feeder vessels of the spinal cord, associated with central cord necrosis. This would imply that early reduction of spinal fractures would lessen the chance of necrosis.

## FLEXION INJURIES OF CERVICAL SPINE

Anterior subluxation, bilateral interfacet dislocation, wedge fracture, clay shoveler's fracture, and teardrop fracture are classified as flexion injuries. These injuries usually result from blows to the back of the head or forceful deceleration, as experienced in motor vehicle accidents.

*Anterior subluxation* results from the least amount of flexion force that causes a radiographically recognizable injury. The lesion disrupts the posterior longitudinal ligament, interspinal ligament, and interfacet joint capsule. Because the anterior longitudinal ligament and disc space are relatively intact, the injury is not unstable. A patient with this injury has severe neck pain and spasm at the time of injury. Recovery is usually uneventful but, if the lesion is not discovered on initial evaluation, progressive anterior subluxation may develop. If this occurs despite adequate conservative treatment, stabilization is indicated, usually by spinal fusion, either posterior or anterior.

*Bilateral facet dislocation* results from complete disruption of the posterior ligamentous complex; the disc space, and usually the anterior longitudinal ligaments, are also disrupted. The superior facets pass upward and over the inferior facets at the joint, which always causes anterior dislocation of the upper vertebral body by at least a distance of one half the anterior-posterior diameter of the vertebral body. The extensive ligamentous disruption of these injuries is associated with a high incidence of cord damage. In this injury, transportation or manipulation of the patient's head at the site of the accident in a manner that will allow further flexion without splintage may allow significant damage to the spinal cord.

Flexion trauma often results in a *wedge fracture* of the vertebral body without ligamentous disruption. X-rays reveal a loss of vertebral height anteriorly and widening of the paraspinal soft tissue shadows. Such injuries are stable and rarely associated with neurologic injuries, and often can be treated conservatively with halo bracing, only occasionally requiring spinal fusion. (Halo bracing involves fixing the skull using four pins inserted into the skull and attached to a metal halo, which is then fixed to a torso cast or brace via rigid metal bars to produce static and very stable traction or fixation of cervical spine.)

Another relatively minor injury resulting from flexion trauma is the *clay shoveler's fracture*. This injury involves the spinous processes of C6, C7, or T1, and results from flexion of the head and neck against the tense posterior cervical muscles.

A severe cervical injury is the *teardrop fracture*. The fracture occurs in such a way that the anterior inferior corner of the involved vertebral body has the shape of a teardrop. The anterior, posterior, and longitudinal ligaments, as well as the disc space and posterior ligament complexes, are totally disrupted. In addition, facet joints are bilaterally subluxed. This injury is totally unstable and is usually associated with severe neurologic dysfunction.

## EXTENSION INJURIES OF CERVICAL SPINE

Hyperextension cervical spine injury with a normal radiographic appearance, fracture dislocation of the posterior arch of the atlas, extension teardrop fracture, and hangman's fracture are examples of the extension type of cervical spine injury.

High forceful *hyperextension* of the cervical spine usually results from a forward fall with a blow to the anterior part of the head, such as in diving or football accidents. If the spinal canal was previously narrowed as a result of chronic degenerative arthritis, the hyperextension may be sufficient to compress the spinal cord, even in the absence of actual fracture dislocation. This type of injury frequently causes selective damage to the central part of the spinal cord. Treatment is immobilization of the spine and careful observation for additional evidence of spinal cord compression. Anterior or posterior surgical decompression may be necessary.

Hyperextension combined with compressive forces may cause *fracture or dislocation.* The injury frequently fractures the lateral vertebral masses, pedicles, and laminae. In addition, the posterior ligamentous complex and disc spaces are disrupted, so the injury is unstable. Even though the injury involved hyperextension, the vertebra is subluxed anteriorly. Although severe hyperextension may fracture the posterior arch of the atlas (C1) or the region between the occiput and the arch of axis (C2), this injury is stable and does not cause neurologic dysfunction.

Similarly, hyperextension may lead to avulsion of the anterior inferior corner of C2, resulting in an *extension teardrop fracture.* This injury is stable in flexion but unstable in extension because of disruption of the anterior and longitudinal ligaments.

Violent hyperextension may result in bilateral fracture of the pedicles at C2 with anterior dislocaton of C2 and C3. This injury is produced by hanging and is known as a *hangman's fracture*. If there is no spinal cord compression, a hangman's fracture can also be treated by a halo body plaster jacket.

## EXTENSION-ROTATION INJURIES

The combination of forcible extension and rotation may produce a fracture of the lateral masses known as a *pillar fracture*. This is a stable injury that responds to conservative treatment by halo bracing.

## COMPRESSION INJURY

The Jefferson fracture of C1 and the Birch fracture of the lower cervical vertebra are compression fractures. Such injuries are uncommon because vertical compression must be applied at a time when the spine is perfectly straight. This results from vertical blows to the head that may occur during motor vehicle accidents, diving, sports injuries, and the like. Falling objects can also cause compression trauma.

The Jefferson (Birch) *fracture* of C1 was first described by Jefferson in 1920 (2). A compressive force causes bilateral fracture of the anterior and posterior arches of C1 with disruption of the transverse atlantal ligament and resulting subluxation of C1 and C2. Special odontoid x-ray views are necessary to exclude this fracture, which is unstable and variably associated with neurologic abnormalities. External immobilization with halo bracing is frequently successful.

A *Birch fracture* of the lower cervical vertebrae results from an explosion of compressed disc material into the vertebral body, with resultant comminution of the vertebral body. This fracture may impinge on the ventral aspect of the spinal cord, leading to neurologic deficits. Because the posterior longitudinal ligamentous complex is intact, the injury is usually stable.

### REFERENCE

1. Murphy MJ, Ogden JA, Southwick WD: Spinal stabilization in acute spinal injuries. *Surg Clin North Am* 69(5):1035–1047, 1980.
2. Jefferson, G: Fracture of atlas vertebra: report of four cases and a review of those previously recorded. *Br. J Surg* 7:407–422, 1920.

## 2

# BIOMECHANICS OF CERVICAL TRAUMA

*Lawrence W. Friedmann, Edgar L. Marin, and Patricia A. Padula*

To understand how trauma may affect the structure and function of the cervical spine, one needs to understand the basic biomechanical factors involved. These biomechanical factors include the strength of the structures, deformability, amount and center of mass, range of movement, the direction and amount of force, the resistance to force, gravity, time of application of force, position of structures when force is applied, frequency of force application, and the number and time of rest periods. Since the parameters are interrelated, no one factor completely describes the cause of injury. One must describe the totality of movements caused by the application of force.

Abnormal forces can cause subluxations, dislocations, fractures, strains, and/or sprains. The biomechanical mechanisms that are involved determine the type and severity of the injury. The two major categories of abnormal forces are linear forces and shear stress. Linear forces are pressure, compression, and tension. Most of these forces act in a concurrent system. That is, those forces acting on the body are applied to the body from different angles to differing body parts, producing a complex multiaxial movement. Shear stress is a force directed against a structure at an angle that causes one part of the structure to slide over another. The amount of shear represents the intensity of the force.

In analyzing force and position,there are static measurements and dynamic assessment. Dynamic factors include acceleration, momentum, friction, velocity, the changing positions of rotational axes, and the resistance and support offered by soft tissues. Dynamic factors are kinematics.

In a rigid body any motion in which all the coordinates of motion of some fixed point in the body are parallel describes the plane of motion of that point. This type of motion has three degrees of freedom, two of sliding and one of rotation. In cervical flexion, for instance, a vertebral point is moving in a plane. At every instant during the motion there is a point somewhere within that body that does not move.

The axis of the motion may change its location and its orientation across the total range of motion that is available. Motion between the vertebrae takes place at the fibrocartilaginous intervertebral disc and at the zygapophyseal joints formed by the inferior facets of the superior vertebra and superior facets of the inferior vertebra. Movement is governed by the compliance of the disc and the slope of the articulating facets. All spinal motions require free gliding of their articular facets. While the motion between any two vertebrae is quite minimal, the motions are additive.

The inferior surfaces of the cervical vertebral bodies are concave. The superior bodies are convex in their anteroposterior and lateral aspects to allow overlapping during motion. The inferior articular surfaces of the atlas have a medial and inferior slant that forces the atlas to move inward toward the odontoid to allow rotary movement of the head. Excessive anteroposterior movement is prevented by the anterior and posterior rings and ligaments. The atlas and odontoid serve as a pivot for the cranium and both are highly vulnerable to injury. If the odontoid fractures, which is very common in head and neck injuries, the atlas becomes unstable and can readily

10

cause the freed peg to compress or lacerate the medulla (1).

Axial load is carried by the vertebral facets and the vertebral body. The cancellous core and the cortical shell of the vertebral body each provide approximately 50% of the vertebral strength up to the age of 40 years. Strength diminishes after the age of 40. Bone strength appears to be directly related to mineral content, and a small loss of osseous tissue has a profound effect on bone strength. Trauma to the neck of postmenopausal women over age 40 causes a high incidence of compression fractures for this reason.

The nucleus is highly resistant to compression. It distributes the majority of the axial compression forces. It transmits forces horizontally to the annulus. The amount of force increases when the spine is flexed. Displacement of the nucleus occurs during normal motion. Extrusion of disc material occurs most often as the result of disc or annular degeneration and abnormal distribution of forces on the disc (2).

In the cervical region flexion, extension, rotation, lateral flexion, and circumduction are the basic movements. Movements of the head on the neck are generally confined to the occiput-atlas-axis complex, which has separate movements from those of the trunk. The cervical spine is most flexible in flexion and rotation. The latter occurs most freely in the upper cervical area and is progressively restricted moving down through the cervical area. There is a wide variance in opinion as to the location of the center of motion and the range of motion in this particular area.

Stability is provided to the C1–C2 joint by paravertebral ligaments and muscular attachments. When weakening of these supports occurs, such as found in rheumatoid arthritis, a dangerous state of instability arises.

The superior articular facets of C1 are shallow. The head can nod with a hinge motion on these facets. There is no rotary or lateral motion between the cranium and the first cervical vertebra. The head and first cervical vertebra rotate as a unit around the pivot of the odontoid process. The articular processes permit the sliding motion between the atlas and the axis. The remaining cervical vertebrae are similar to the dorsal vertebrae. The cervical spinal cord is extremely vulnerable to injury. It needs sufficient space in the spinal canal so that it can be suspended without direct contact with the surrounding vertebral walls.

The C1–2 joint is an unusual joint in that the inner anterior arch of C1 has a small facet that is separated from the odontoid process of C2 only by a small synovial cavity. The osseous and ligamentous complex of this area allows great rotation and some flexion and extension. The anterior arch of C1 normally remains 1 mm from the odontoid in flexion and extension. A widening of this space to greater than 3 mm usually indicates that damage to the transverse ligament has taken place.

Rotation of C2 on C3 is limited by a mechanical blocking mechanism that protects the vertebral artery against excessive torsion. The anterior tip of the superior articular process of C3 impinges on the lateral margin of the foramen transversarium of C2. This blocking mechanism is found in the subjacent vertical vertebrae.

The interspinous and supraspinous ligaments attach along the spinous processes from the occiput to the dorsal spine and serve as a check rein to prevent overflexion of the head. They become increasingly tight as the neck flexes forward.

In cervical flexion, the spinal cord goes from a relaxed state to a tense state. This tension is transmitted throughout the entire cord. Extension causes the spinal cord and its roots to slacken. The free space of the canal is decreased by three factors during extension: posterior bulging of the intervertebral disc, folding of the relaxed annulus and posterior longitudinal ligament, and anterior bulging of the ligamentum flavum. This is crucial in hyperextension trauma since the spinal cord is often thereby compressed.

If the neck is not erect at the moment of trauma, then other factors are added. During rotation, the ipsilateral anterior roots relax and the dorsal roots become stretched. In lateral flexion, the intervertebral facets narrow in height ipsilaterally and widen contralaterally.

## ACUTE TRAUMA

Injuries to the neck produce a broad spectrum of disabling conditions ranging from minor neck discomfort to quadriplegia, and even death. Acute neck pain does not rank as the major loss of time from work that is seen in acute low back pain, but still must be considered a significant problem.

## STRAIN AND SPRAIN

Simple uncomplicated musculoligamentous neck sprain is the most common of all neck injuries. The majority of cases follow automobile collision from the rear, sports injury, or employment injuries. Muscular strain in the cervical area can be extremely complex. The large number of small muscles in the region have different functions in different head positions. It is an area quite subject to strain. It may be difficult to distinguish between sprain, strain, and nerve root involvement. Differentiation cannot always be obtained from the history.

Muscle spasm may follow overuse of muscles of the neck, or can be the product of a force against a contracting muscle. Any violent motion may cause strain, sprain, subluxation, dislocation, and/or fracture. When strain occurs as a separate entity, active function as well as passive stretching of the involved muscle will be painful. In minor injuries diagnosis is not so critical. Muscular spasm that follows the injury is universal and is of little diagnostic significance. Tenderness within the muscle itself or its attachment may give a clue. If the strain is relatively mild, the treatment should be conservative. Local rest, heat, and reduction of activities are important.

Whereas a strain is caused by overuse of a muscle, a sprain is caused by forcing a joint through an abnormal range of motion. The ligament designed to prevent this motion is damaged. Sprain of the neck is a very common injury and may be of any degree. Mild injury may be of little significance and may require but little treatment. The moderate injury, in which there has been some loss of ligament strength, will require protection primarily from the type of force that caused the injury. Much more complicated is a severe injury in which there is a complete loss of integrity of the ligaments. If this ligament loses its function, the motion that it is designed to prevent is unrestricted. The motions that ordinarily are controlled by this ligament are then transferred to other areas of the lever system.

The ligamentous injury may allow subluxation. The posterior interspinous ligament restricts flexion of the neck. The anterior longitudinal ligaments prevent anterior separation of the bodies of the vertebrae and so hyperextension. There is usually some combination of ligament damage because when one ligament tears, the force is shifted to another ligament and may damage it as well. The process may continue until there is a complete disruption of all the supporting ligaments and complete dislocation of one vertebra on another.

In extension injury, the anterior longitudinal ligament tightens throughout the cervical spine and serves to prevent separation of the anterior margins of the cervical vertebrae. The neck moves into extension and the spinous processes tend to impinge. As the force continues the lever changes from a first degree with the fulcrum at the cervical articulation to a second degree with the fulcrum at the tip of the spinous process. As this force is applied, the cervical posterior elements are forced together.

Neck sprain, while a misnomer, describes a clinical condition involving nonradiating discomfort or pain of the neck area associated with a concomitant loss of neck motion. While the clinical syndrome may present as a headache, most often the pain is located in the middle to lower part of the back of the neck.

A history of injury is rarely obtained, but the pain may start after a night's rest or a simple turning of the head. The source of pain is most commonly believed to be the ligaments about the cervical spine and/or the surrounding muscles. The actual pain may also be produced by small annular tears without disc herniation or by the joint facets. The pain associated with the neck sprain is often a dull, aching pain that is exacerbated by neck motion. The pain is usually abated by rest or immobilization.

A moderate-degree sprain involves tearing of the ligament. The symptoms can be severe. The patient holds the head in extension because of muscle spasm and resists any attempts to flex it because of the pain at the site of injury. If the patient can rotate the atlanto-occipital joint (i.e., nod the head) without pain, one may assume the injury is below C2.

If there is a sharply localized tenderness over the spinous process or ligament, injection of this area with a long-acting anesthetic and/or a corticoid preparation may give substantial relief. If there is complete separation of the ligament, instability is severe. A portion of the ligament may be torn off a single spinous process while the main body of the ligament remains intact. This is a much less serious injury than that occurring when the ligament itself is torn in two.

If the ligament is ruptured either in its substance or off one of the processes, the symptoms will be quite severe, with sharply localized pain. A defect may be felt in the ligament, particularly if the head is forced into flexion. Further flexion will be forcibly resisted. The patient will feel that the head is insecure and will hold the neck quite rigid. Painful spasm supervenes and the head is pulled into hyperextension. Radiographs made with the head and neck in flexion may reveal unusually wide separation of the spinous processes.

The C5–6 interspace is the apex of the normal

cervical lordosis and serves as the point of maximal functional activity. When a severe axial compression force is applied to an extended neck, C5 dislocates anteriorly. The inferior C5 facet overrides the superior C6 facet and becomes locked, compressing the spinal cord. This is one reason why the neck of a patient suffering a severe head blow should never be flexed or extended.

## SUBLUXATION, DISLOCATION, AND FRACTURE

In the more severe flexion injuries of the neck, the cervical disk is compressed. The vertebral bodies are forced together in front and apart posteriorly. Excessive motion occurs at the apopyseal articulation. If the interspinous ligament gives way while the body remains intact, the tension on the laminal, articular, and posterior longitudinal ligaments will separate the articulation and rupture the ligaments. A subluxation of the cervical vertebrae will occur.

As flexion is continued, there is a shearing force that causes the superior articulations to displace forward over the ones below. If some of the ligaments are left intact, a great deal of stability is still present in the spine. The articular process of the vertebra above slips in front of the superior articular process of the vertebra below. This dislocation locks in the unreduced position.

Subluxation followed by spontaneous reduction probably occurs quite frequently in flexion injuries of the neck. One of the reasons why the neck should be carefully protected against repetition of flexion forces is to prevent a complete dislocation from occurring with a subsequent injury.

In bilateral dislocation, the head is characteristically held thrust forward in hyperextension. The spinous process of the vertebra below is prominent. The patient is usually extremely apprehensive and will resist any attempt to move his head in any direction. This injury has serious potential for cord and root damage. A careful examination should be done for the presence of a neurologic deficit before any attempt at radiography or reduction is made. The neck should be prevented from movement until *after* radiography has ruled out fracture or dislocation.

The flexion and shearing force that causes the dislocation may continue with destruction of the remaining ligamentous support. With this injury there is instability such that the neck will frequently fall back into a correct position. Physical and radiographic examination including computer-aided tomography, may be entirely negative. This injury is often seen in football players following tackling. The dislocation may have been reduced without cord damage only to have cord damage occur because the injury was not recognized.

As this dislocation occurs, the posterior part of the neural arch may disrupt. The fracture may take place at the pars interarticularus or the laminae. This protects the cord since the shearing action of the posterior portion of the ring is prevented as the ring expands. This accounts for the case of complete dislocation of the vertebra forward with no neurologic symptoms. Such cases serve to emphasize the importance of careful handling of the cervical injury.

Isolated fractures following trauma occur at all levels of the cervical spine. The most frequent fractures are at C6 and C7 and the least frequent at C4. The four common types of vertebral body fractures are anterior marginal fractures from anterior/posterior forces, comminuted fractures from axial forces, and lateral wedge and uncinate process fractures from lateral stress.

Vertical compression or flexion compression damage is sometimes seen but extension injuries are more common. Spinous process fractures usually occur at C6 or C7 after acute flexion or a blow to the flexed neck, producing ligamentous avulsion. There is an immediate hot pain in the area of the spinous process that is increased by flexion. Any injury to C6–C7 is difficult to view on radiographs because of overlapping structures. Tomography may be helpful.

A much more frequent injury appears to be fracture of the odontoid from the body of C2. There is much leeway for the cord and it is less likely to be impinged. The patient usually realizes that the injury is serious. Definitive diagnosis is made by radiologic study (3).

As the flexion force is increased, the spinous process may separate. The bodies are forced together and a fracture may occur. A fracture of the cervical body is more frequent than a complete tear of the posterior longitudinal ligaments. A fracture is not always accompanied by a dislocation. The body may compress anteriorly as much as 75% while the posterior part maintains its normal height.

## INJURIES OF THE CERVICAL SPINE IN THE ATHLETE

In the athlete, the cervical spine is the most vulnerable part of the spinal column. Simple uncomplicated musculoligamentous neck sprain is the most common injury and is usually comprised of minor ligamentous capsular or tendinous tears and muscle injury by overstretch. The tissues are fundamentally intact, although injured. The symptoms are cervical spine pain, headache, occipital pain, limitation of movement of the cervical spine, pain in the shoulder, arm, and forearm, and transient paresthesia. The initial symptoms are mild and appear slowly, days after a traumatic event, gradually becoming progressive and increasing in intensity. They are persistent in duration.

The signs are limitation of movement, appearance of being in pain, and active cervical spine motion that is more diminished than passive cervical spine motion. Tenderness of the spinous processes of the cervical vertebra and muscle spasm about the shoulders, neck, scalp, forearm, and hands is found. There are no signs of spinal cord involvement, subluxation, nerve root compression, or organic disorder. Loss of range of motion, swelling, deformity, and guarding are present. Full range of passive movement is very limited. There is a straight cervical spine secondary to muscle spasm.

The scalenus anticus syndrome has become less frequently diagnosed as more specific diagnoses such as cervical ribs, cervical herniated disc, and various vascular conditions are made. Symptomatology arises because of the occlusion of the artery or vein and/or pressure on the brachial plexus caused by pressure from the anterior scalene muscle. Certain anatomic characteristics make this more frequent, particularly the presence of a cervical rib. The symptoms are usually of the lower roots of the plexus, with pain along the ulnar distribution particularly whenever the arm is above the head. This position is common in many sports. A blow at the base of the neck over a cervical rib may well cause the sharp accentuation or initiation of the neurologic and vascular symptoms of cervical rib. Recognition of the possibility of a cervical rib will permit adequate diagnosis and treatment.

Another and more common condition in the cervical area may give the athlete and the physician a good deal of uneasiness. This is the presence of an audible and palpable click or snap of the neck on certain rotations. The cause of this popping or snapping is varied. It may be due to irregularity of the articulation but much more commonly it is due to forceful snapping of a tendon over a bony prominence. The athlete has an impulse to "pop" the neck, which seems to provide great relief. Treatment for this condition is to prevent the snapping. One must make sure that no underlying pathologic condition is present, such as irregularity of the articular facet, tenosynovitis of the tendon, or muscle spasm that tends to roll the tendon across the bony prominence. A fairly extensive regimen of physical therapy should be instituted.

Damage to the elements of the brachial plexus with evidence of nerve involvement that lasts more than a few hours demands very careful study with an attempt to delineate the exact root or trunk involved. Frequently, there will be a generalized involvement of the arm with diffuse numbness and a feeling of heaviness that gradually recovers. Injury to the posterior cord affecting the use of the triceps, for example, may easily be overlooked since the arm will readily fall into extension by gravity. Several days may pass before the physician realizes that a loss of function is actually present.

Disturbances in the cervical plexus usually arise from muscular spasm in one or more of the six muscle bundles that have attachments on the occiput, atlas, or axis. Unequal tension or fibrotic changes within the paravertebral muscles can readily influence the delicate nerve fibers and vascular flow.

The vertebral arteries are frequently compressed by the overlying muscles in the suboccipital triangle. In fact, the vertebral artery has been completely occluded by turning the head backward and to the opposite side during postmortem studies. Neurologic disturbances may result from muscular and fibrotic changes along with cranial nerve pathways that exit from the skull and pass between and under the suboccipital fasciculi. Five of the cranial nerves are thus vulnerable: the facial, glossopharyngeal, vagus, spinal accessory, and hypoglossal (4). Circulatory impairment of major and minor nerves of the neck also may alter the function of those cranial nerves that do not exit from the skull proper—the olfactory, optic, oculomotor, trochlear, trigeminal, abducens, and auditory.

Some athletes have repeated episodes of pain in the neck caused by a twist of the head, with nerve root symptoms in the arm that are accompanied by no observable pathology in the neck. These may be interpreted as resulting from impingement of the nerve due either to hypermobility of a joint or to narrowing of the nerve root canal so that the nerve is pinched by a motion that ordinarily would leave it amply free.

Adhesions about the nerve root prevent it from

moving normally during joint motion. Excessive and sometimes normal motions may then cause traction on the nerve during an unguarded motion. These biomechanical conditions require careful study to determine whether or not athletic participation should be permitted.

Excessive compression forces on the neck commonly lead to facet jamming and fixation, isolated or multiple fractures of the atlantal ring, and/or vertical, oblique, or comminuted fractures of the lower cervical body.

Excessive anterior bending forces may produce hyperflexion sprain of the posterior ligaments, compressive wedging of the anterior annulus and vertebral body, anterior subluxation, anterior bilateral or unilateral dislocation with locked facets, and spinous process avulsion. Abnormal widening of a spinous interspace on a lateral film after hyperflexion injury should make one suspicious of rupture of the posterior ligaments. The effects of posterior bending movements include sprain of anterior ligaments, wedging of posterior annulus and vertebral body, posterior subluxation, compression of the posterior arch and associated structures, posterior bilateral or unilateral dislocation, spinous process fracture, and traumatic spondylolisthesis.

Excessive shear forces may create disruption of either the anterior or posterior ligaments with subluxation. If the injury is more severe, anterior or posterior dislocation and/or fracture of the dens may occur. In a still more severe form, compression fracture of the anterior ring of the axis will take place.

The effects of excessive lateral bending include lateral dislocation fracture of the odontoid process, lateral compression of the annulus, and wedging of the vertebral body with brachial plexus trauma.

Distraction force applied to the anterior longitudinal ligament may result in avulsion of a fragment of the body. If the ligament maintains its integrity, there may be a fracture at the spinous process. When the force is arrested, the neck returns to its normal position and there are relatively few symptoms since the normal position of the neck puts no strain on the anterior longitudinal ligaments. Usually the athlete knows that the neck has been injured, and examination will reveal that pain and tenderness are anterior and that the symptoms are aggravated by extension of the neck.

If the injury is mild, no particular treatment is indicated except a cervical collar holding the neck in extension. If the injury is moderate, the neck

should be placed in flexion rather than extension. The motion to be prevented by the brace is extension rather than flexion. If the injury is severe, and there has been tearing of the anterior longitudinal ligament, the symptoms will be more extreme and protection must be prolonged. The other danger is repetition of the force that caused the original injury. Riding in a car or participating in a body contact sport should be ruled out without protection of the neck.

## CERVICAL ACCELERATION/ DECELERATION INJURIES

Whiplash injuries such as those sustained in motor vehicle accidents are referred to as cervical acceleration/deceleration syndrome. The cervical injury is due to indirect trauma from acceleration/deceleration forces. If the head does not strike anything, the injury is produced solely by inertial forces. The body is moving as a whole at the same speed as the automobile. If the stopped automobile is struck from the rear, the unrestrained head is flipped backward and then rebounds forward.

An overwhelming percentage of acute neck injuries are the result of rear-end automobile accidents. It is appropriate to review the factors concerning automobile accidents that influence the development of a significant acute neck injury. These include the wearing of seat belts and/or shoulder harnesses, the use of head or neck restraints, the sitting location of the injured individual, the speed of the car when hit, and the age, sex, and size of the occupants.

The driver stopped at a light or a stop sign is usually relaxed and unaware of the impending collision. The sudden acceleration of the struck vehicle pushes the back of the car seat against the driver's torso. This pushes the driver's torso forward while the head remains where it was, causing hyperextension of the neck. This occurs within the first quarter second after impact. If no head rest is present, the driver's head is hyperextended past the limit of the stretch of the soft tissues of the neck. In the recoil forward action that occurs when the car stops accelerating, the head is thrown forward. This forward flexion of the head is usually limited by the chin striking the chest and does not usually cause significant injury.

Usually the driver is unaware that he or she has been injured. The individual suffers little discomfort at the scene of the accident and often does not wish to go to the hospital. Twelve to 14 hours after the accident, the patient begins to feel stiffness in the neck. The pain at the base of the neck increases and is made worse by head and neck movements. Soon, any movements of the head or the neck cause excruciating pain. It should be emphasized that the pain pattern is of little value in determining the site of the lesion.

The anterior cervical muscles are often tender to the touch. The patient may have pain on mouth opening or chewing, hoarseness, or difficulty swallowing. Often the patient has already had some radiating pain from the back of the neck into one or both shoulders or arms and up to the base of the skull. Pain may also radiate into the intrascapular region and chest as well as into the vertex of the skull.

The sternocleidomastoid muscles, the scalenes, and the longus colli muscles may be mildly injured or torn. Muscle tears of the longus colli muscles might involve injury to the sympathetic trunk unilaterally or bilaterally, resulting in Horner's syndrome, nausea, or dizziness.

Hyperextension may injure the esophagus, resulting in temporary dysphasia, and the larynx, causing hoarseness. Tears in the anterior longitudinal ligament may cause hematoma formation with resultant cervical radiculitis. During the impact the mouth opens since the jaw lags behind the skull movement. This may result in injury to the temporomandibular joint, causing pain on chewing and limiting mouth opening.

In elderly people with preexisting cervical spondylosis, the sagittal diameter of the spinal canal is compromised at each disc level and a severe hyperextension injury can result in spinal cord compression, resulting in paralysis or central spinal cord syndrome.

Patients receiving a whiplash injury of the neck can also suffer from a cerebral concussion. If the head is thrown forward and then strikes the steering wheel or windshield, a head injury can occur. Also, mechanical deformation of the brain occurs during the acceleration/deceleration phase of the injury and a concussion can occur without the head actually striking anything. This can account for transient loss of consciousness as well as postconcussion symptoms of headache, photophobia, mild transient confusion, tinnitus, fatigue, and transient difficulty with concentration.

The high cervical spine is the most vulnerable area in whiplash injuries. Flexion and extension injury to the atlanto-occipital joint or high neck sprain or strain is more common than injury at the C4–5, C5–6, or C6–7 level. In very severe rear-end automobile collisions, severing of the spinal cord and decapitation have occurred at both the atlanto-occipital and the atlantoaxial joints.

The onset of symptoms occurs earlier in atlanto-occipital trauma than in trauma of the lower neck. Dizziness, occipital headaches radiating over the head to the retro-orbital area, blurred vision, lacrimation, impaired balance caused by reflex sympathetic stimulation, and pain and stiffness exaggerated by any motion or sudden jarring may occur. The patient may turn the whole body instead of turning the neck.

In C4 through T1 injuries, symptoms are referred to the shoulders, chest, and upper extremities. Simple nodding is performed hesitantly and with pain. Manual traction increases pain and the result of the compression test is negative. The anterior-posterior distraction test (one supportive hand is placed behind the neck and pushes the neck forward while the other hand forces either the chin or the forehead gently backward) is positive.

Back-seat passengers have pain higher up in the neck from such injuries than do front-seat passengers because of the height of the seat. Back-seat passengers are likely to be thrown forward after the initial extreme hyperextension. Radiologic studies can be negative. More comprehensive investigation is usually required.

The symptom of headache requires careful analysis and thought. Vertebral artery irritation may be present from subluxation of the atlanto-occipital joint. Edema, swelling, vasospasm, and increased pain are present. Irritation of the upper two cervical nerves causes occipital pain. Any of these may be the source of the patient's headache.

If the automobile is struck from the front or hits a relatively immovable object, the head is thrown forward. The first movement is that of translation, which produces shearing forces at the base of the neck because bending is greatest at that point. Posterior neck and occipital pain accompanied by upper back pain is common.

## CHRONIC TRAUMA

Vertebral dislocation is usually the secondary effect of a pathologic process such as rheumatoid arthritis and various other conditions. The severity of neurologic involvement varies considerably from case to case depending on the progress of the disease.

Symmetrical facets glide with the production of little friction. Alterations of the direction of the facets most commonly occur in the lower cervical region. If these facets deviate in their direction of movement, the unparallel articulating surfaces will rub against one another. Rubbing of the processes and facets over a period of time, even in the absence of injury, will cause thickening of the subcortical bone of the facet, which is referred to as "marginal sclerosis." This hardening process is usually followed by hypertrophy or exostosis, which appears as an irregular articular surface in the radiographs. The interarticular spaces gradually become narrowed and then obliterated on films.

Chronic strain often comes from postural faults that cause persistent muscular fatigue. Constant-posture jobs such as those of the secretary who leans over the desk, or the taxi driver or truck driver who sits all day and maintains a poor posture, are examples. The taxi or truck driver also may be driving over rough streets, resulting in the application of vertical compression forces to the spine repeatedly during the day. The frequency of these compression forces is also a factor, with 5 Hz the worst frequency. The dentist who bends over the patient in a twisted position and rotates back and forth to get instruments will also have chronic cervical trauma.

Many occupations require that the arms and head be positioned for prolonged periods more anterior to the trunk than is comfortable. This positioning changes the length-tension relationship of the anterior, lateral, and posterior cervical musculature. These changes in muscle length may eventually be permanent.

When the head is positioned anterior to the center of gravity, it tilts downward. To compensate for downward vision in this position, the posterior cervical muscles contract in order to hold the head vertical. This adapted position allows the eyes a horizontal field of vision. The muscles thus exert a backward bending force on the occiput. These postural adaptations cause structural stress of the cervical spine, contributing to the development of early degenerative changes. Forces from altered posture lead to the formation of traction spurs, which may encroach upon nerve roots, resulting in painful radiculopathies.

In the United States and in other parts of the world, particularly Scandinavian countries and Australia, there has been an increasing prevalence of cervicobrachial disorders in workers that have come to be known as cumulative trauma disorders, repetition strain injury, or overuse syndromes. Most cases occur in modern manufacturing industries and in offices, and predominantly among women. The introduction of mechanized and automated processes in industry has made the physical workload lighter, but has resulted in an increased rate and regularity of physical movement under load that frequently concentrates the stresses locally.

This work is often performed seated and under time stress. These tasks are characterized by repetitive motion of the head, arms, and visual control, and simultaneously demand accuracy and precision. This repetitive, chronic microtrauma of muscles, ligaments, and joints in the cervical area eventually causes pain and triggers the body's responses to overuse (osteoarthritis, tendonitis, chronic myositis, fibrosis, etc.). Chronic muscle fatigue stretches the muscle fibers, the perimysium, and the ligaments and tendons. The patient "hangs" on the soft tissues. As they stretch, additional stresses may be placed on the joints. Inflammation may arise from this stress.

Repeated microtrauma is a form of chronic trauma. The basic principles are that injury occurs not only from a suprathreshold force, which causes damage even with one incident, but also from lesser forces repeated often. The effects are cumulative and depend on the number of repetitions; the rise and fall times and patterns of pressure application; peak force levels; duration of force; quantity, duration, and spacing of rest intervals; the vascular supply; and cell nutrient demand.

## TRAUMA TO THE ABNORMAL CERVICAL SPINE

### CERVICAL DISC HERNIATIONS

Cervical disc herniations occur mostly in the fourth decade of life. The most common areas of disc herniation are C6–7 and C5–6. In contrast to the lower lumbar spine, the cervical spine encloses the spinal cord. A patient with a weak annulus fibrosis who sustains a cervical injury could develop myelopathy if the herniated disc is large enough to eliminate the spinal reserve capacity and compress the cord.

### DEGENERATIVE DISEASE

The elasticity of tissues decreases with an increase in age. The range of motion in the cervical spine also decreases. In both cases, the potential for injury is increased because the neck is less resilient. The strength of the neck musculature also diminishes with age. Over the adult life span, the cervical range of motion is reduced by an average of nearly 40%, the cervical muscle reflexes slow by 23%, and voluntary strength capability diminishes by 25% (5).

Degenerative disease, or spondylosis, is the most common cause of neck pain. The patient tends to be about a decade older than the patient with a prolapsed disc, and predominantly male. In a working population over the age of 50, over 3% of the people will have neck pain and stiffness. Of this group, some 25–40% will have at least one episode of brachialgia, or arm pain, associated with their neck stiffness.

Degenerative joint disease (osteoarthritis) is very common. It is reported that 75% of subjects in their seventh decade displayed some degenerative changes in the cervical spine. Cervical degenerative disc disease has more recently been called *cervical spondylosis.* It causes disc space narrowing, osteophytosis, foraminal narrowing, and degenerative changes of the facets (6). These degenerative changes can reduce the size of the spinal canal, leaving less space than necessary for the cord to function. In individuals with cervical spondylosis, the sagittal diameter of the spinal canal is compromised at each disc level and a severe hyperextension injury can cause spinal cord compression, resulting in central cord syndrome (7).

In the cervical spine, most of the motion in flexion-extension is in the central region, between C5 and C6 (8). There may be some causal relationship between this observation and the incidence of cervical spondylosis at that interspace. Some investigators have observed that a compensatory increase in motion occurs in cervical spine segments adjacent to interspaces, with reduced motion due to either degeneration or posttraumatic changes (9).

Among the inflammatory arthropathies, *rheumatoid arthritis* is the most common. Cervical spine involvement secondary to the inflammatory changes of rheumatoid arthritis (synovitis) includes atlanto-axial dislocation, upward migration of the odontoid, and subaxial instability. Obviously, a whiplash injury in a patient with C1–2 dislocation can be fatal. Patients with rheumatoid arthritis of the cervical spine generally have much more severe rheumatoid disease than those with rheumatoid arthritis of other areas, and their prognosis is usually worse.

Rheumatoid arthritis, a chronic inflammatory disease with broad immunologic, environmental, and autoimmune underlying mechanisms, has a prevalence rate from 0.3 to 1.5% in the United States. The prevalence increases with advancing age up to the seventh decade. Virtually all tissues of the body may be involved in varying magnitudes. The tissues most involved are articular and periarticular. The cervical spine, particularly the upper portion, is the second commonly involved area in the body.

When rheumatoid arthritis is severe in the neck, the ligaments of the odontoid weaken. This predisposes to subluxation. The symptoms are cervical spine, neck, temple, and retropharyngeal pain, paresthesia, hyperesthesia and hypesthesia or anesthesia, vertigo, loss of consciousness, drop attacks, and transient blindness. The clinical symptoms reflect the pathologic process in the cervical spine and, most severely, at the occiput-atlas-axis complex (2).

Signs of upper and lower motor neuron myelopathic symptoms may occur as a result of compression of the spinal cord. Weakness of the arms and legs, disturbance in gait, loss of sensory perception at the level at which the nerve roots or the spinal cord is compressed, nystagmus, radiologic evidence of gross subluxation, hyperactive deep tendon reflexes, atrophy of muscles, quadriparesis or quadriplegia, or death may ensue.

*Ankylosing spondylitis* is an inflammatory disease attacking the joints of the axial skeleton, the nonsynovial cartilaginous synchondrosis of the intravertebral spaces, the diarthrodial synovial joints, and the sacroiliac joints. It has a striking predilection for the cartilaginous joints and often affects the cervical spine. The disease has a major genetic component.

The average age of onset is 15–40 years, with characteristic features of back discomfort, insidious onset, duration longer than 3 months, and association with morning stiffness that improves with exercise. About 25% of the patients have peripheral arthritis but not with the inflammatory intensity seen in rheumatoid arthritis. There is a gradual onset of pain and aching in the lower back and both buttocks. Morning stiffness that improves with exercise is found in 15–25% of the patients with ankylosing spondylitis. There is diminished motion in the entire spine, and chest expansion is reduced to less than 1 inch. Patients with ankylosing spondylitis should stop smoking completely because of the risk of developing pulmonary disease.

Frank osteitis of underlying adjacent subchondral bone exists, and fibrosis of the joint capsule and annulus occurs. Therefore, a fracture of the rigid segments of the spine can be sustained from a relatively minor fall. The patient has an inability to utilize movements of the neck to extend the field of vision or to allow more effective use of other senses. Patients adopt odd postures to put the head in a useful position. These measures are seldom adequate. A halo apparatus or spinal fusion between the second cervical and the second thoracic vertebrae may improve the situation.

Focal points of tenderness exist at the heels, sternum, iliac crest, and ischial tuberosity. Peripheral joints may be swollen. The Schober's test may be positive, forward flexion is limited, and sacroiliac joint tenderness and pain may coexist. The majority of patients with ankylosing spondylitis may expect a good prognosis and a good life-style. The disease progresses to severe and total ankylosis in relatively few patients.

## PREVENTION

### MOTOR VEHICLE ACCIDENTS

There are several basic safety precautions that can reduce "whiplash" flexion-extension injuries under otherwise identical circumstances. First are the seat belts and/or shoulder harnesses. Next are the head restraints. Air bags are useful in frontal collisions. Finally, there is the spring of the seatback: The stiffer the spring the safer the seat.

The influence of seat belts on acute neck injuries is dependent on other factors, the most important of which is the presence or absence of a head restraint. If a head restraint is present, the use of a seat belt alone results in fewer neck injuries. The combining of a seat belt with a shoulder strap reduces the incidence of acute neck injuries with or without a head restraint. By restraining the motion of the chest with a shoulder strap, there is a decrease in the amount of inertial forces exerted on the cervical spine.

Head restraints limit the possible amount of extension that is allowed in the case of rear-end collision. However, there have been a number of studies that have shown that the use of head restraints in the rear seat of an automobile would not significantly reduce neck injuries. Head restraints should be adjusted so the center is at or above the level of the ears. This is about the center of gravity of the skull. If it is below the center of gravity, it serves as a fulcrum and accentuates the injury. Unfortunately, most drivers do not bother to adjust the position.

Weisel et al. have shown that 75% of head restraints that are adjustable are in the lowest possible position, which is inappropriate for the protection of the vehicle occupants (9). A visual survey of drivers in 4983 moving domestic passenger cars with adjustable head restraints in the Los Angeles and Washington, D.C. metropolitan areas indicated that in Los Angeles 74% of the male drivers and 57% of the female drivers had head restraints that were not in proper position. The proper positioning of head restraints would undoubtedly increase their protective value significantly.

The number of injuries to the rear-seat passenger and the vehicle driver are essentially the same. There is general agreement that whiplash neck injury is more frequent among front-seat passengers than among rear-seat passengers. The individual most frequently injured is the front-seat passenger (9).

Several foreign and American made carmakers install air bags as standard equipment. Since their use is fairly new, as yet there are insufficient hard data to verify their effectiveness in preventing neck or other injuries. The combined use of seat belts, shoulder straps, and head restraints is known to significantly reduce the number of acute neck injuries (9).

## SPORTS

Classically, the role of hyperflexion has been emphasized in cervical spine trauma, whether the injury was due to football, diving, or rugby. However, recent laboratory and clinical observations indicate that in the majority of instances athletically induced cervical spine trauma results from axial loading of the spine, which is a segmented column (2).

In axial loading injuries to the cervical spine, the neck is slightly flexed and normal lordosis is eliminated. Assuming the head, neck, and trunk components to be in motion, rapid deceleration of the head occurs when it strikes another object, such as another player, a lake bottom, or a trampoline. This results in the cervical spine being compressed by the force of the oncoming trunk. When maximum vertical compression is reached, the straightened cervical spine fails in a flexion mode and fracture, subluxation, or unilateral or bilateral facet dislocation can occur (10).

Among the contact sports, football has the highest number of players who sustain cervical trauma. When the use of football helmets was enforced, a decrement in the number of cervical injuries was anticipated. This did not occur because players started to use their helmet-encased heads as battering rams, thus exposing their cervical spines to injury. The tackling technique where the top of the helmet is used for initial contact (spearing) places the cervical spine at risk of catastrophic injury (10).

In the mid-1970s, spearing became an infraction and head-first tackling and blocking were disallowed. Since then, there has been a marked reduction in the incidence of catastrophic cervical spine injuries. We expect that improvement in designing of sports equipment, enforcement of rules to protect the players, and education of athletes that protective equipment does not make them invulnerable will make a significant improvement in the safety of these sports.

## INDUSTRY

Physical job demands vary according to the specific assignments or tasks to be performed by the employee, and may vary despite identical job titles. Certain occupations require dynamic muscular activity in which the muscles contract and relax rhythmically. Examples of dynamic tasks are walking, climbing, loading boxes, and pushing a cart. Rhythmic neck motions occur when a worker looks to an in-box to obtain work, does the task, and then turns the head toward the out-box.

Other types of work require static muscle activity, which supports a given weight without movement but with steady consumption of energy. This requires a sustained effort with muscles being maintained at a constant length and contraction. Examples of static tasks are holding the neck and head in a forward posture while sitting, laterally overflexing the neck to hold a telephone receiver, and holding the head steady to look at a computer terminal. There are, of course, tasks that require a combination of dynamic and static muscular activities (9).

When a particular job demands excessive static activity, overfatigue and strain are more likely to occur. These two factors contribute to the discomfort and stiffness of the neck and upper shoulders of individuals performing sedentary, desk-type tasks. Undertakings that require dynamic muscular effort can be carried out for a more prolonged period of time without the same degree of fatigue. However, the joint consequences are worse for dynamic movements.

A partial explanation for the muscular difference may be the blood circulation during each type of activity. During static muscular effort, the blood flow into the muscle and other soft tissue is decreased. This leads to a diminished supply of oxygen and a buildup of waste products. The accumulation of certain elements such as carbon dioxide and particularly lactic acid gives rise to a painful state of fatigue. In dynamic muscular activities, there is a period of muscle relaxation. This allows a blood flow increase that replenishes the oxygen supply and energy-producing substances and at the same time eliminates the waste products (9).

At the present time, most available jobs are in the service and information categories. Individuals in such jobs perform their tasks in a desk-sitting, computer-adapted environment, making them prone to chronic neck trauma and consequent pain. Employers should be encouraged to evaluate equipment design and work environment to minimize and prevent musculoskeletal problems in the neck and upper shoulder areas.

## REFERENCES

1. Bland JH: *Disorders of the Cervical Spine: Diagnosis and Medical Management.* Philadelphia, WB Saunders, 1987.
2. Cailliet R: *Neck and Arm Pain.* Philadelphia, FA Davis, 1974.
3. O'Donoghue DH: *Treatment of Injuries to Athletes,* ed 4. Philadelphia, WB Saunders, 1984.
4. West HG: Vertebral artery considerations in cervical trauma. *ACA Journal of Chiropractic* Dec 18–19, 1968.
5. Foreman SM, Croft AC: *Whiplash Injuries—The Cervical Acceleration/Deceleration Syndrome.* Baltimore, Williams & Wilkins, 1988.
6. Friedenberg ZB, Miller WT: Degenerative disc disease of the cervical spine—a comparative study of asymptomatic and symptomatic patients. *J Bone Joint Surg [Am]* 45:1171–1178, 1963.
7. Schott CH, Dohan FC: Neck injury to women in auto accidents. *JAMA* 206:2689, 1986.
8. White A, Panjabi M: *Clinical Biomechanics of the Spine.* Philadelphia, JB Lippincott Co, 1978.
9. Wiesel SW, Feffer HL, Rothman RH: *Neck Pain.* Charlottesville, VA, The Michie Co, 1986.
10. Torg JS, Vegso JJ, Sennett B: The National Football Head and Neck Injury Registry: 14-Year Report on Cervical Quadriplegia (1971–1984), *Clin Sports Med* 6:61–72, 1987.

# 3

# DIAGNOSTIC METHODS AND THERAPEUTIC TECHNIQUES

*R. Geoffrey Wilber and Jung Yoo*

## DIAGNOSTIC FOUNDATION

### FUNCTIONAL ANATOMY

Cervical spine trauma is unfortunately a frequently encountered malady in our highly motorized society. Injury can range from mild muscular strain to fracture-dislocation leading to paralysis. The most severe trauma results from high-speed injury such as automobile accidents, falls, or contact sports. However, even minor trauma to the cervical region frequently can cause painful cervical conditions. The type and extent of injuries are the result of many variables, including direction and magnitude of the applied force and the anatomy of the cervical spine. Although individual anatomic variation is frequently seen, certain aspects of the cervical spine remain fairly constant, and it can be divided into two distinct functional units.

The upper cervical spine consists of the atlas (C1) and the axis (C2). The unique anatomy of these two vertebral segments and their articulations, the occipitoatlantal and atlantoaxial joints, permit about one half of the total movement found in the cervical spine (Fig. 3.1). Embryologic development of the atlas and axis incorporates the centrum of the atlas into the axis as a part of the odontoid process. The unique construction of the occipitoatlantal facet articulation provides for minimal rotation, yet accounts for approximately 40° of sagittal motion. Conversely, the atlantoaxial articulation accounts for minimal sagittal motion but provides about half of the rotation associated with the entire cervical spine. Sagittal

motion is prevented by the confinement of the odontoid process between the anterior arch of the atlas and its transverse ligament. This ligament attaches to a prominent tubercle on each side of the inner wall of the atlas, and the spinal cord lies directly behind it. Thus a competent transverse ligament is the first and most important defense against odontoid process impingement on the spinal cord at this level. In a normal individual this ligament is very strong, and the odontoid process generally fails before the transverse ligament in an acute flexion injury. Acute transverse ligament rupture is seen more commonly with Jefferson fractures, in which bursting of the ring of the atlas occurs as a result of axial loading of the skull on the ring of the atlas.

The lower cervical vertebrae, the third through seventh, are very similar to one another in size and shape (Fig. 3.2). Articulations between these vertebrae have very little bony stability. The integrity of their association depends heavily upon the intervertebral discs and ligaments that link these segments together. This arrangement provides a stable yet mobile connection between the segments. Experimental work has shown that these lower segments can move along all three axes. Flexion and extension range from 8° to 17°, lateral bending from 4° to 11°, and rotation from 8° to 12° at each articulation (1). Although movement of a single articulation is small, the additive effect of multiple mobile segments allows a large functional arc of movement.

The most important ligaments that provide stability to the cervical spine are the interspinous, lig-

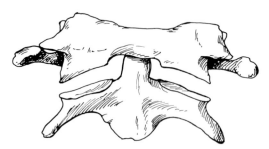

**Figure 3.1.** Anterior view of the C1–2 articulation. Fifty percent of cervical spine motion occurs between the occiput and C2.

amentum flavum, posterior longitudinal, and anterior longitudinal ligaments. As their name implies, the interspinous ligaments link the spinous processes of adjacent segments. The ligamentum flavum is also segmentally arranged and connects the laminae of each adjacent segment of the cervical spine. The anterior longitudinal ligament is located anterior to the vertebral body and is closely adherent to the outer layer of the annulus fibrosus of the intervertebral discs. It extends from the anterior ring of the atlas down the entire spinal column. The anterior atlanto-occipital ligament is proximally continuous with it and provides anterior stability to cranial articulations. The posterior longitudinal ligament is located directly posterior to the vertebral body and extends from the posterior surface of the anterior ring of the atlas down the entire extent of the spine. The integrity of the posterior elements (i.e., vertebral arches) depends on the integrity of the facet joints, the interspinous ligaments, and the ligamentum flavum.

The intervertebral discs found in the skeletal system are unique structures. They link the vertebral bodies and provide stability and movement at each level via two cartilaginous endplates. The main component of the disc can be divided into the outer annulus fibrosis and inner nucleus pulposus. The annulus fibrosis is composed of abundant type I collagen that is layered multidirectionally, giving inherent strength to the disc and preventing extrusion of the much more compliant nucleus pulposus. The nucleus is thought to be a remnant of embryonic notochord and contains viable chondrocytes that produce abundant proteoglycans. Water makes up about 80% of the weight of the nucleus pulposus, a result of proteoglycan's unique ability to attract and retain water molecules (2). Because of this high water content, the nucleus is highly compliant and serves as an excellent shock absorber for the spine.

## BIOMECHANICS OF CERVICAL TRAUMA

Although direct cervical trauma is occasionally seen (as in a penetrating injury such as a gunshot wound), most injury to this area is the result of force indirectly applied to the spine. The most common mechanisms of injury to the cervical region are flexion and extension forces applied to the cervical skeletal system. These are generally indirect forces applied to the cervical spine as a result of the force created by a sudden movement of the head. The position of the head and cervical spine at the time along with the direction of the applied force will determine the center of rotation (the fulcrum) of the injury. The individual anatomy as well as the direction and magnitude of the force will determine the severity and type of injury sustained. In general, force applied to the cervical spine is not a pure unidirectional force but also may have a component of rotation and shear as well as compression and distraction. Severy et al. showed that extension injury is the mechanism of most rear-end collision injuries. As the car is struck from the rear, the body accelerates forward in relation to the head, tilting the head posteriorly and resulting in extension of the cervical musculature and spine (3).

A variety of injuries resulting from acceleration-extension injury have been described, but frank fracture and/or dislocation of the cervical spine from this mechanism is relatively rare. Soft tissue injuries such as tearing of the sternocleidomastoid, strap muscles, and longus colli may, however, occur. MacNab also noted damage to the apophyseal joint in some cases, resulting in mismatching of surfaces, although radiographic findings were negative (4).

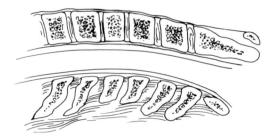

**Figure 3.2.** Lateral view of the cervical spine showing orientation of anterior and posterior longitudinal ligaments as well as the posterior ligamentous structures.

Flexion-deceleration injury to the neck is most commonly caused by sudden deceleration of a motor vehicle hitting a solid object in front. Injuries seen from this mechanism differ markedly in their severity and include fracture and dislocation of the cervical spine. Lesser injuries such as the clay shoveler's fracture (avulsion of the spinous process of C6 or C7, typically), partial tearing of muscles, and traction of the greater occipital nerves also occur (5).

Axially directed forces cause injuries such as the Jefferson fracture, in which the base of the skull directly impinges on the ring of the atlas, as seen frequently in diving accidents. Here force is directly applied to the top of the head and indirectly transmitted to the upper cervical spine. Axial forces can sometimes be transmitted to the lower cervical spine, leading to compression or burst fractures.

In many cases there is extreme flexion and extension of the head on the cervical spine. Many factors determine where the fulcrum of the sagittal motion will occur. If the fulcrum is at the atlantoaxial junction then odontoid fracture may occur. A wide variety of injuries can occur if the fulcrum is in the lower cervical spine segments. Even at a specific segment of the cervical spine, the center of rotation can vary in an anterior or posterior direction. The variations in the point of fulcrum, and in the direction and magnitude of the applied force, may lead to a wide range of injury patterns such as burst fracture, compression fracture, and bilateral facet dislocation, subluxation, or fracture. An example is the teardrop fracture, a sagittal fracture of the midportion of the body of the vertebra (generally C5) with compression anteriorly and a fragment retropulsed from the posterior portion of the body, which results from a combination of axial load and flexion.

Rotational or lateral forces, most commonly applied in conjunction with sagittal force, can lead to many asymmetrical injury patterns, such as unilateral facet dislocation or traumatic atlantoaxial rotatory subluxation. Rarely, a distraction force may be applied to the cervical spine. The most frequently seen fracture from this mechanism of injury is the hangman's fracture, which was first described in association with judicial hanging. The fracture of the pedicles of the axis results in listhesis of the body of the axis and frequently traction of the cord itself.

It is important to remember that the forces are directed not just to the bone and ligaments but to the musculofascial structures as well. Since most of these tissues are peripherally located, they are sometimes the first structures to resist extremes of motion, and are frequently injured. The presence of these soft tissue symptoms may point to underlying major structural damage that may be ignored because of a normal radiograph.

## MEDICAL HISTORY AND PHYSICAL EXAMINATION

The medical history and physical examination are the proper starting point of any medical evaluation. Cervical trauma evaluation is no different. How the history is taken and the physical examination is performed depend upon the setting in which the physician encounters the patient.

In an acute traumatic situation, cervical trauma may only be inferred since the patient may be uncooperative as a result of head injury, shock, alcohol, or intoxicative drugs. In these situations cervical trauma is assumed to exist until proven otherwise by further studies. Thus it is imperative that the cervical spine be immobilized and protected while further medical evaluation proceeds.

Even in situations in which a patient is uncooperative, a history can be taken from witnesses or rescuers at the accident scene. An initial physical examination can be done to a limited extent. Head and facial injury are indicative of increased likelihood of cervical spine trauma (6). Generalized muscle tone and various reflexes can be noted even in an unconscious patient.

The patient who is awake and cooperative can give a more accurate history, and the physical examination is more useful as a diagnostic aid. Any complaint of cervical pain requires immediate immobilization before any other evaluation proceeds. The patient's complaints should be carefully noted—localization of spinal pain; radicular symptoms such as pain, hypesthesia, or paresthesia; and any history of immediate paralysis, even though it may be currently resolved.

The initial physical examination is very important in establishing a baseline, since any worsening neurologic examination may necessitate earlier surgical or medical intervention. Initial sensory and motor examinations require testing of each dermatome for touch, pain, temperature, and proprioception; motor strength grading of major muscle groups; and the presence of normal sphincter tone (Tables 3.1 and 3.2). Testing different sensory modalities is especially important

**Table 3.1.**
**Sensory Levels**

| Levels | Sensory Region |
|--------|----------------|
| C5 | Lateral arm |
| C6 | Lateral forearm, thumb pulp |
| C7 | Middle finger pulp |
| C8 | Small finger pulp |
| T1 | Medial arm |

**Table 3.2.**
**Motor Neurologic Levels**

| Levels | Muscles |
|--------|---------|
| C5 | Biceps, deltoid |
| C6 | Extensor carpi radialis longus and brevis |
| C7 | Triceps, flexor carpi radialis |
|    | Finger extensors |
| C8 | Finger flexors |
| T1 | Interossei |

**Table 3.3.**
**Reflex Chart**

| Reflex | Neurologic Level |
|--------|------------------|
| Biceps | C5 |
| Brachioradial | C6 |
| Triceps | C7 |
| Cremasteric | T12, L1 |
| Patellar tendon | L4 |
| Tibialis posticus | L5 |
| Achilles | S1 |
| Anal | S2, S3, S4 |

in cases of spinal cord injury. This may differentiate types of incomplete cord injuries and indicate eventual prognosis for recovery. The normal reflex text requires intact sensory as well as motor pathways and is an important part of the evaluation of spinal neurologic function. Reflexes tested should include the biceps (C5), triceps (C6), cremasteric (L1), patellar tendon (L2–4), Achilles tendon (S1), and bulbocavernosus reflex (S2–3) (Table 3.3).

Patients are usually seen in less urgent situations, after the initial traumatic event, with complaints of pain or other symptoms that will not resolve. The mechanics of injury, localization, duration, time course of symptoms, and compensatory and legal actions are all factors in determi-

nation of eventual level of recovery and are integral to the history.

The physical exam should note the area of pain, presence of muscular spasm, and neurologic integrity. Radicular symptoms may suggest impingement of the nerve root from lateral disc herniation. Lower extremity spasticity or weakness, or an isolated complaint of bowel or bladder dysfunction, may be present and may be secondary to spinal cord impingement and compromise. Localized pain in the cervical spine and paraspinal musculature may suggest musculotendinous strain, disruption of the vertebral anatomy such as avulsion fractures of a spinous process, or herniated nucleus pulposus. Thus a thorough and systematic physical examination is imperative.

## CLINICAL RADIOGRAPHIC EXAMINATION

Radiographic evaluations are indispensable diagnostic tools in the evaluation of any patient with the complaint of cervical pain. The armamentarium available to the clinician includes the roentgenogram, tomography, computed tomography (CT) scanning, myelogram, and magnetic resonance (MR) imaging. There is disagreement as to which radiographic projections should be ordered as a routine cervical spine series. Any patient complaining of cervical pain following trauma as well as any unconscious patient should have radiographic evaluations before discontinuing cervical immobilization. Most clinicians obtain the cross-table lateral, anteroposterior, and odontoid views as a first screening examination. Other views such as the pillar or oblique views should also be obtained if the clinician is not fully convinced that no cervical spine pathology is present. In many instances, facet dislocations, subluxations, and fractures can only be found in these projections (7).

It is imperative that all seven cervical vertebrae be seen in the lateral projection. Many serious fractures of the cervical spine have been missed as a result of inadequate and incomplete lateral cervical spine radiographs (8). If all seven vertebrae are not seen on a lateral projection, then a Swimmer's view should be obtained. These projections are indispensable in evaluating for a gross alignment of bony architecture. Even if segmental alignment is intact, swelling in the prevertebral soft tissue is indicative of major spine trauma.

A lateral projection with flexion and extension of the cervical spine can provide information on the dynamic stability of the cervical spine, including the atlantoaxial junction. The test should never be performed on an unconscious patient nor done with force; otherwise serious neurologic sequelae may result. A conscious, cooperative patient should be able to voluntarily flex and extend the cervical spine and will protect himself before injuring the spinal cord. Any abnormal distance between spinous processes, dynamic listhesis, and increasing space between the anterior arch of the atlas and the odontoid should be noted.

In the anteroposterior view, alignment of the spinous processes and the integrity of the vertebral bodies should be noted. Malalignment of the spinous processes may be secondary to unilateral dislocation of the facet joint. This diagnosis may be confirmed on an oblique projection, noting disruption of the normal "shingling" appearance of the facet joints. The anteroposterior open-mouth odontoid view is helpful in diagnosing both odontoid and Jefferson fractures. If the borders of the lateral masses of the atlas are separated and extend beyond the edge of the axis, then a Jefferson fracture is suspected. A CT scan may be needed to confirm this diagnosis in subtle cases, since radiographs frequently will not project any fracture lines. Transverse ligament rupture, which places the spinal cord at great risk, can also be suggested by a combined overhang distance of greater than 7 mm (8).

Tomography is rarely used in assessing cervical trauma. Occasional diagnostic problems in evaluating for a nondisplaced odontoid fracture or facet fracture may require tomography. With tomography not only are fracture lines seen more clearly, but also any presence of sclerosis or rounding of bony structures may assist the clinician in diagnosing acute versus chronic injury.

CT scanning, and more importantly CT scanning following myelography, has become an important radiologic tool in evaluation of patients with cervical spine pain. CT scanning provides an accurate representation of the cross-sectional view of the spine segments. It is indispensable in evaluating spinal canal compromise, structural integrity of the bony ring surrounding the canal, and integrity of the facet articulations. Furthermore, a CT scan following myelography is helpful in detecting a herniated disc or extradural hematoma, which can be missed with other radiographic techniques.

Although MR imaging has been in clinical use for only a short time, it has become an important diagnostic tool in evaluating patients with cervical spine complaints. This technique provides information on the spinal cord, discs, and soft tissues that other radiologic studies cannot provide. It can be helpful in detecting herniated discs, rupture and hemorrhage of musculotendinous regions, and intracord pathology as well. However, most MR scanners are not accessible in trauma situations. Exclusion of ferromagnetic substances in the testing environment currently prevents MR examination of the patient with cervical spine immobilization or who is on a respirator. With the increasing use of MR-compatible halo rings and tong traction, this scanning technique is becoming more frequently used, especially as a late diagnostic aid to continuing pathology following injury.

## ELECTRODIAGNOSTIC STUDIES

Unlike their use in peripheral nerve lesions, electrodiagnostic studies are not usually conclusive in evaluating cervical spine injuries. Although not routinely used, electromyography (EMG) can be helpful in localizing single or multiple nerve root lesions following cervical trauma. This is especially true in a long-standing nerve root lesion resulting in muscle fibrillation. Nerve conduction tests may also help the physician detect peripheral nerve lesions that may mimic radiculopathy.

## PSYCHOLOGICAL STUDIES

Pain is a subjective response to a physical phenomenon. Therefore an individual's psychological makeup largely determines his response to noxious physical stimuli. Although much of the interpretation of a patient's complaint lies in the realm of the art of medicine, certain psychological tests have been shown to be helpful in evaluating these patients. The Minnesota Multiphasic Personality Inventory (MMPI) and the Cornell Medical Index (CMI) have been used to predict surgical outcome of spine patients. Those patients who score high on Hysteria and Hypochondriasis measures have been shown to have poor surgical outcomes (10). These tests may aid the clinician in evaluating those patients who have marginal observable pathology but serious subjective complaints. This in conjunction with psychological evaluation may help in treating these patients.

Frequently the patient who has been experiencing chronic pain following cervical therapy may develop some emotional component to his perception of pain. Many times these patients are dismissed as being hypochondriacal. Complete and proper evaluation of all patients is essential lest real pathology be overlooked.

## ASSOCIATED CONDITIONS AND DIFFERENTIAL DIAGNOSIS

Preexisting medical conditions will frequently dictate the severity and type of cervical injury. A patient with marked spondylosis may sustain severe cord injury without fracture. This occurs with cervical spine hyperextension as a result of impingement on the spinal cord by the posterior osteophytes. The injury pattern may be that of the central cord syndrome, wherein the upper extremity is more involved than the lower extremity, or frequently even that of complete cord injury. Also at risk is the patient with a congenitally narrow spinal canal. Many authors have shown that patients with complete cord injury tended to have congenital stenosis as a preexisting condition (11). Any fusion of the segments of the cervical spine puts at risk those segments above and below the fusion because of the longer lever arm present when force is applied. Patients with ankylosing spondylitis are at risk not only because of the presence of a long lever arm, but also because severe hemorrhage can occur following cervical fracture, which may result in cervical cord ischemia. Patients with preexisting spondylosis or herniated discs may experience worsening of their symptoms or reaggravation after even a relatively minor trauma. These conditions, although not cord threatening, may cause much discomfort to the patient.

If the patient's complaint is much more severe than suggested by the mechanism of injury, trauma may only be an incidental event. The most commonly found pathologies in the cervical spine other than arthrosis and disc herniations are neoplasms, infection, and inflammatory disease. Almost all types of neoplasms, both malignant and benign, have been described in the cervical spine. In elderly patients, metastatic disease is common, the most frequent primary tumors being lung, prostate, kidney, breast, and thyroid carcinomas. The most common primary bone tumor of the cervical spine is multiple myeloma, which frequently can affect multiple segments of the cervical spine with severe osseous destruction. Vertebral osteomyelitis unfortunately is increasing as a result of intravenous drug use. The patient may

not have any other signs of infection, such as chills or fevers, making diagnosis difficult until radiographic changes are seen. The sedimentation rate is almost always elevated in the case of vertebral osteomyelitis and should be determined routinely. Rarely, inflammatory disease such as rheumatoid arthritis may present clinically as cervical spine pain and should be suspected, especially if other joint complaints are present.

## THERAPEUTIC TECHNIQUES

Most patients with cervical pain do not require surgical intervention. Even those patients who may present with herniated discs with mild radiculopathy usually benefit from conservative treatment. The goals of any cervical spine therapy should be:

1. Improve muscle strength and balance
2. Relieve muscular spasm
3. Reestablish normal muscle flexibility
4. Relieve stresses (postural and occupational)
5. Prevent recurrence

## PHYSICAL MEDICINE MODALITIES

Most physical therapy modalities are directed toward reestablishing normal muscular function about the cervical spine and relieving painful muscle spasm. Reestablishment of normal muscular function about the neck requires proper muscle flexibility and strength. Normal muscular flexibility and strength also require pain-free movement of spinal segments.

Prior to any range-of-motion and strengthening program, the patient's muscle spasm should be relieved. With the presence of the muscle spasm, the patient may experience increasing pain upon exertion during the rehabilitation phase of recovery. Massages and heat have been used through the ages as remedies for treating a variety of musculoskeletal conditions and remain effective in treating patients with painful cervical pathology.

Massage can be defined as a passive manipulation of soft tissue used to relieve muscle spasm. The mechanism of the benefit of massage is not understood, but relief of tension, stretching of musculature, inhibitory tactile stimulation, and possible improvement of circulation all have been postulated.

Cold therapy, although routinely used in the treatment of extremity problems to reduce acute swelling, is rarely useful or helpful in cervical pathologic conditions. The beneficial effect of heat also is not completely understood; it may increase tissue perfusion and serve as tactile stimulation inhibiting pain pathways. It is well accepted that heat will decrease muscle spasm and increase muscle flexibility. Other passive therapies, such as ultrasound and transepidermal nerve stimulation, can be helpful adjuncts to heat and massage, although reasons for their effectiveness are not clear.

Once muscle spasm is relieved, the patient can progress to the range-of-motion and muscular strengthening phase of rehabilitation. Limited range of motion of any segment of the cervical spine will increase the stresses on the other more normal segments, leading to further aggravation of neck pain. Gentle active, and rarely passive, range-of-motion exercises will improve overall mobility of the segments and reduce pain at ranges of motion required for the activities of daily living. Any passive manipulation of the cervical spine must be done gently and by an experienced clinician; otherwise more harm than good may be done to the patient.

Strengthening of cervical musculature can be achieved most safely and effectively through autoresistive exercise. The neck should remain in a neutral position as the head is pressed against interlaced hands in flexion, extension, and lateral bend. This isometric exercise will strengthen the musculature with minimal potential for reinjury.

## CERVICAL TRACTION AND ORTHOTICS

The cervical collar is the most frequently used orthotic device in treatment of painful neck syndromes. Unfortunately it is often used with little thought to overall patient management. An important aspect of cervical collar use is a plan to eliminate the need for it.

A soft cervical collar is generally used in the acute situation where unstable injury to the cervical spine has been ruled out. It is used to relieve muscular spasm and provide additional support during the acute healing phase of the soft tissue. It also provides mild traction of the cervical spine and may decrease joint reaction forces. Once spasm and acute pain have subsided, the soft collar should be discontinued. Prolonged use may lead to further weakening of the musculature and greater chance for reaggravation.

Cervical traction is accomplished generally using a halter traction device with chin and occipital support. Generally, a pulley system provides an axial force of about 10–20 pounds. Traction can accommodate variations in the patient's position and is employed in a variety of painful cervical conditions. It is used to relieve muscular spasm, decrease nerve root irritability, lessen joint reaction force, and increase joint flexibility. An old theory of sucking the herniated disc back into the confines of the annulus fibrosus is most likely invalid. The true efficacy of cervical traction for any of the above conditions is not known.

If the patient's condition is improved by the traction then he may be slowly weaned, with shorter duration of traction daily. If there is no change in clinical condition, both duration and weight can be increased. Weight should be increased by 3–5 pounds, to a maximum of 25–30 pounds, and duration by 5 minutes daily. If the patient's condition worsens, traction can be discontinued or weight and duration can be lessened by one half of the original amounts (12).

Cervical traction therapy should not be used in cases of inflammatory arthritis or preexisting neoplastic lesion of the cervical spine. Patients with acute whiplash injury also may experience worsening of symptoms with cervical halter traction and generally should be treated with a soft cervical collar that provides some gentle distraction. Cervical halter traction has also increased symptoms of temporomandibular arthritis in some patients. It must be remembered that cervical traction is not a complete therapeutic modality for any neck injury and should be used as an adjunct to physical therapy and rehabilitation.

## MANIPULATION AND MOBILIZATION

Manipulation and mobilization are therapeutic techniques that employ passive movement to joints. Manipulation of the cervical spine is a therapeutic maneuver performed by a clinician causing a single localized movement of a joint; mobilization is repetitive passive movement that attempts to restore full motion of a joint. The essential goal of manipulation and mobilization is to increase the painless arc of motion of any joint involved.

Numerous health professions utilize manipulation in the treatment of spine problems, and each has its own theory to explain why it may be effective. For example, chiropractors claim that malalignment of spinal joints is the cause of spine discomfort, and attempt to "realign" the spine with, usually, vigorous manipulation. Although many patients are helped by these types of chiropractic manipulations, it seems unlikely that the bony-ligamentous relationship of the axial skeleton can be changed permanently by the manipulation (13).

Other mechanical theories suggest that there are synovial menisci found in the facet joints of the cervical spine and these may be occasionally deranged, resulting in locking of the joint. An analogy to a meniscal tear in the knee with joint locking shows that the joint can be manipulated to position the torn meniscus in proper alignment to allow more free range of motion. Another mechanical theory is that the arthritic facet joint is separated and stretched during manipulation, decreasing the joint reaction force and pain. No studies substantiating the long-term benefits of manipulation are available.

## NERVE BLOCKS AND TRIGGER POINT AND FACET JOINT INJECTIONS

Selective nerve block with local anesthetic agents can help localize the etiology of the patient's pain as well as serving as a temporizing measure. In some cases neurolytic agents such as alcohol and phenol can be used to permanently damage the nerve, hoping for more permanent relief of pain. However, these neurolytic agents may cause further aggravation of symptoms and are not routinely employed (14). Selected branches of the brachial plexus, greater occipital nerve, and spinal accessory nerves are the most common peripheral nerves injected in patients who have associated cervical spine problems. These injections may help the clinician differentiate between a nerve root entrapment and a peripheral nerve root lesion.

The efficacy of trigger point injections is not well documented. Generally, a trigger point is described as a soft tissue or soft tissue attachment with hyperirritability. If these are in muscle tissue, then they may be described as "hard fibrotic" areas. Local anesthetic agents are used to inject these trigger points. The duration of symptom relief is thought to be rather short (15).

Facet joint injections are frequently used in lumbar spine pathology but rarely used in the cervical spine. Although lumbar facet joints are much larger and easier to penetrate accurately, it has been shown that the local anesthetic agent and steroid are not always confined to the facet joint when these joints are injected percutaneously in the lumbar spine. Some of the symptomatic relief is thought to occur as a result of the anesthetic effect on the nerve tissue from the extravasated anesthetic agents. Certainly the dangers of inaccurate injection of a cervical facet joint preclude the routine use of this technique.

## BIOFEEDBACK AND RELAXATION THERAPIES

It is well known that patients who are under much mental stress maintain increased tone in the extension musculature of their spines. Patients who have sustained acute injury to the neck may experience much anxiety since these conditions tend to be rather persistent and many patients wonder if they will ever be well again. Relaxation therapies are designed to help alleviate some of these physical responses to anxiety. They are generally employed as a part of the therapeutic management of a patient rather than as an isolated therapy.

There are a variety of relaxation techniques and most are simple and nonvigorous. Patients may be taught as simple a maneuver as breathing exercises that employ deep, rhythmic respiration. More complex maneuvers, such as alternating muscle tensing-relaxation exercises as well as gentle shaking and swinging exercises, have been employed as relaxation techniques. It should be remembered that a gentle, attentive clinician will put patients at greater ease and help them relax as well.

Biofeedback is another method by which the patient is taught to relieve stress. The patient who is stressed may have visceral reactions such as tachycardia, palpitation, and sweating associated with sympathetic stimulation. Those visceral responses can coexist with spasm and pain of the cervical musculature. The patient, with the help of a therapist, learns to recognize these visceral and somatic reactions to stress. This can be done with technical aids such as skin temperature, sweat, and pulse monitors or EMG. Once the patient learns to recognize the stress reaction, then a variety of relaxation techniques are used to alleviate symptoms. Biofeedback and relaxation therapy can be helpful adjuncts to overall pain management.

## MEDICATIONS

It seems the number of medications used in treating patients with spine pain has been constantly increasing. Most commonly used medications can be categorized as follows:

1. Nonsteroidal anti-inflammatory drugs (NSAIDs)
2. Acetaminophen
3. Narcotic medications
4. Antispasmodic medications
5. Psychotropic medications

Numerous new NSAIDs have come into the marketplace. Their mechanism of action is thought to be inhibition of prostaglandin production, with modulation of both pain and inflammation. These medications are usually the first ones given to the patient for relief of symptoms. NSAIDs are effective in obtaining relief in most patients with mild musculoskeletal pain, but they are not without side effects. Many patients experience mild gastrointestinal discomfort. (NSAIDs should generally be taken with food.) Persistent gastrointestinal discomfort or evidence of bleeding requires stopping of the medication. The long-term effects of NSAIDs are not known. There is some experimental evidence to suggest that cartilage proteoglycan metabolism is adversely affected by NSAIDs.

The only available nonopiate analgesic other than NSAIDs is acetaminophen. The mechanism of acetaminophen in pain relief is not known. A central nervous system effect has been postulated as one mechanism. Acetaminophen has no effect on prostaglandin metabolism and thus has much fewer gastrointestinal side effects than NSAIDs. However, since acetaminophen does not modulate the inflammatory process as do NSAIDs, it may be less effective in the posttraumatic cervical spine.

Narcotic medications are used in patients who are in severe pain. Codeine and propoxyphene are mild narcotic analgesics and can be used without great potential for addiction if given for a short period of time. These medications are available commercially in combination with salicylate or acetaminophen. Although injectable demerol is a highly efficacious pain-relieving medication, the oral form appears to be less effective. It may actually be weaker than codeine and propoxyphene. Oxycodone also appears to be a highly efficacious pain-relieving medication, but it appears to have a much higher addictive potential as well. Patients who have been on oxycodone for a period of time can have withdrawal symptoms on cessation of intake. It should be avoided in any situation in which the potential for development of chronic pain exists.

Antispasmodic medications are commonly used with NSAIDs or narcotics in treating patients with neck pain following trauma. The most commonly used antispasmodics include cyclobenzaprine (Flexeril), methocarbamol (Robaxin), carisoprodol (Soma), and diazepam (Valium). The mechanism of action of these antispasmodic medications appears to be depression of central nervous system activity and not activity at the neuromuscular junction. Patients with muscular spasm following trauma can receive a fair amount of relief with these medications. However, since they are central nervous system depressants, they can cause drowsiness and may make operating machinery or driving hazardous. Diazepam also has an anxiolytic effect and can be useful in treating some anxiety associated with injury, as well as spasm. It does have an addictive potential and should be used only over a short period of time.

Occasionally patients develop some depression in association with chronic pain following their cervical trauma. Drugs such as amitriptyline (Elavil) not only have an antidepressant effect but also are effective in treating chronic pain as well. The mechanism of their pain-relieving effect is not known.

## ERGONOMIC CONSIDERATIONS AND INTERVENTION

The evaluation of a patient's occupation becomes a major consideration in treating cervical spine problems. This may begin at the time of initial assessment. Patients may initially be in too much discomfort to work. Work situations may have to be assessed for potential aggravation of the patient's condition. A simple modification of the height of a desk or workbench may result in lessening of the patient's symptoms. Patients may also be educated as to good posture and potential injurious maneuvers.

## TREATMENT OF SELECTED DISORDERS

The spectrum of injuries to the cervical spine certainly can be large. However, such injuries can be grouped into categories. The severity of injuries may range from soft tissue trauma, such as whiplash injuries, to severe trauma, including fractures and dislocations of the spine.

## EMERGENCY MANAGEMENT OF STABLE AND UNSTABLE INJURIES

Since cervical spine integrity is important in protecting neural structures, any fracture or dislocation may lead to immediate or late neural trauma.

Any instability of the spine can lead to worsening neurologic injury. The spine should be protected with immobilization in any trauma situation.

The cervical spine can be immobilized in a variety of ways. The soft cervical collar does not immobilize the spine adequately and has no place in trauma situations. Immediate adequate immobilization before radiographic confirmation of fracture or dislocation can be obtained with a stiff Philadelphia collar or sandbags at the sides of the head. The head is then taped to a bed or board.

If the patient has a radiographically confirmed fracture or dislocation, halo or tong traction may be indicated. A halo vest and ring provides the most stable external support for the cervical spine. This allows for early mobilization and easier care of the patient.

The clinician must perform a meticulous neurologic examination in all cases of cervical injury. Some minimal sacral sensory or motor function may occasionally be spared in the patient who appears to have sustained a complete cord lesion. This then is by definition an incomplete cord lesion, which gives a better prognosis. Any worsening neurologic exam must be investigated as soon as medically possible. Early surgical intervention may be required to prevent further damage to the spinal cord.

Any subluxations or dislocations of the facet joint can be initially treated with skeletal traction and may be reduced by closed methods. Even the patient with structural compromise of the spinal canal and cord does not require immediate surgical intervention unless his symptoms worsen. A penetrating injury, especially a gunshot wound, generally does not require surgical intervention and should be treated with immobilization.

Other medical conditions can arise from an acute spinal cord lesion. The patient with spinal cord injury may experience respiratory distress even if his initial motor level is C5 or below. Although diaphragmatic breathing is still intact, the lack of intercostal breathing compromises respiratory function. These patients may require ventilator assistance for a period of time. Most are successful in becoming ventilator independent. Other serious consequences of a spinal cord injury are hypotension and gastric ulceration (17). Stress ulcers can be common, especially if high-dose steroids are given, and prophylaxis may be needed. The role of corticosteroids has been widely debated in spinal cord trauma treatment. At present, no clear benefit of steroid use is seen and generally steroids should not be employed. Spinal shock with hypotension and associated bra-dycardia are common but other causes of hypotension should be ruled out.

Unstable injury to the cervical spine should undergo further evaluation in the hospital after placement in traction or after immobilization. Fracture patterns and canal compromise can subsequently be evaluated by CT, myelogram, tomography, and MR imaging.

## INDICATIONS FOR SURGICAL INTERVENTION

The indications for surgical intervention after cervical trauma can be divided into three categories: emergent, subacute, and late. The need for emergent surgical treatment of cervical spine trauma is rare. Those patients who are found to have progressing neural compromise as a result of bony or disc impingement on the neural elements may require surgical decompression. It is imperative that medical conditions such as hypoxia and hypotension be corrected first to ensure optimal cord recovery and safer surgery.

In subacute and late situations, the two main indications for surgical intervention are instability and neural compression. Bony injury generally tends to heal, whereas ligamentous injury does not. Those patients who have acute rupture of the transverse ligament will require atlantoaxial cervical fusion to prevent odontoid impingement on the cord. The patient who has sustained a dislocation as a result of a posterior ligamentous injury may or may not obtain stability and may require posterior fusion with wiring.

Many clinicians believe that the high rate of nonunion and instability following a displaced type II odontoid fracture (fracture at the base of the odontoid) is unacceptable and so recommend fusion of C1 and C2 (18). Recently, direct odontoid fixation with screws has been performed with a high success rate. This is an attractive option since it preserves all motion segments. A type III odontoid fracture (fracture extending into the body of C2) has a very high rate of union and is generally treated conservatively with a halo device. Any nonunion of the odontoid will require surgical stabilization (19).

Facet subluxation or dislocation, as well as rotatory subluxation of the atlantoaxial articulation, may require surgical intervention if the condition is not resolved with skeletal traction. If rotatory subluxation of the atlantoaxial articulation cannot be reduced, the motion segment is fused in its dislocated or subluxated position. Surgical reduction is not recommended (20). Failed skeletal traction treatment for unilateral or bilateral facet dislocations of the lower cervical spine should indicate open reduction and posterior fusion of the involved segment.

Neural decompression is the second reason for surgical intervention. The patient may have involvement of the cord or specific nerve roots. Late decompression of the neural canal has been shown to improve some patients who have sustained cord damage. Those who have incomplete spinal cord injury have seen marked improvement of their neurologic status after decompression. The majority of patients who sustain a complete cord lesion are able to obtain function at one or two nerve root levels after decompression (21). Since impingement is present in the anterior portion of the spinal canal from retropulsed material or posterior vertebral body osteophytes, decompression is performed anteriorly with strut grafting with iliac bones. Posterior decompression through laminectomy may make the spine unstable and lead to worsening of neurologic symptoms. This should not be done unless definite posterior impingement is seen.

Occasionally the patient may develop very painful degeneration of a cervical segment following trauma without clinical instability or neural compromise (22). This usually calls for conservative therapy, but may occasionally require fusion of the level. Most cases of cervical trauma do not require surgical intervention.

## MANAGEMENT OF MYOFASCIAL PAIN AND WHIPLASH INJURIES

Most trauma to the neck results in no radiographically evident injury to the cervical spine, but there may be considerable disturbance of the muscles, fascia, and ligaments. These injuries commonly present with pain either immediately or, more frequently, a few hours or days after the injury, when edema and inflammation of the muscle and fascial tissues is maximal. Patients can present with occipital headaches or shoulder pain associated with neck pain. The response of muscle to damage may be painful spasm, resulting in loss of cervical lordosis in the lateral cervical spine radiograph. Mild muscle spasm can be treated with rest and restriction of activity. Symptomatic treatment such as heat may also relieve spasms over time. Severe spasm may require a soft cervical collar and muscle relaxants. The passive protection afforded by the cervical collar can prevent further injury to the neck. Prolonged use of the cervical collar may result in further weakening of the cervical mus-

culature and psychological dependence on the collar. The collar should be removed when the patient is making symptomatic recovery.

Patients should be made aware that the prognosis for overall recovery from these types of injuries is good. It is important that patients take an active role in their own care. Attempts to relieve cervical muscle spasm with heat, ultrasound, massage, and gentle movements are encouraged. When muscle spasm subsides, the patient can participate in strengthening exercises for the cervical spine.

With conservative management, MacNab has found that the prognosis is generally good for these patients (4). Various studies have found a 12–45% incidence of persistent pain and discomfort 12 months following cervical trauma (5, 12). Most of the radicular pain seems to disappear, although the patient may complain of intermittent neckache and stiffness. Dunn and Blazar suggested that transcutaneous nerve stimulation can help in cases of persistent pain (5). If the patient has no relief of symptoms after prolonged therapy and rest, then surgically correctable lesions must be ruled out. Late development of cervical spine instability has been described, and repeat flexion-extension cervical spine films should be obtained (23).

## HEAD AND NECK PAIN

The patient whose neck has been injured frequently complains of the variety of symptoms for which a clear etiology is not well defined. Patients generally complain of neck pain either immediately or a few hours following the injury. This may be due to immediate muscle damage and hemorrhage or to inflammation and edema. Occipital headaches have been frequently described, as well as radiation of pain down the arms, shoulders, and spine. Frequently patients describe blurred vision, eye pain, and dizziness associated with neck pain. The etiology of these symptoms is not clear. Even with the common complaint of radiating pain, actual nerve entrapment or damage is rare.

Generally, symptomatic relief is obtained with use of relaxation techniques, mild analgesics, and physical therapy to relieve muscle spasms. Aggravation of temporomandibular conditions has been described following cervical trauma and may contribute to headaches and facial pain. Bite plates have been used to relieve these symptoms. Most of these symptoms are self-limited, and assurance may be the most important advice given to the patient.

## DEGENERATIVE DISC, CERVICAL JOINT PAIN, AND NEURAL LESIONS

It is well documented that acute cervical trauma can cause herniation of the disc with resulting nerve root compression or, rarely, myelopathy. Conservative therapy with a cervical collar and traction, avoidance of the extended position, and administration of NSAIDs may provide symptomatic relief. After acute symptoms subside, isometric neck strengthening is initiated. With conservative measures, improvement can be expected in 80–85% of patients with disc herniation. If a patient does not respond to conservative therapy and shows symptoms of radiculopathy, then surgical intervention may be considered. The diagnosis of a herniated disc can be confirmed by myelogram combined with CT and by MR imaging.

The surgical treatment of a herniated cervical disc is generally anterior disc excision and anterior interbody fusion with bone grafting. The posterior approach with laminectomy and foramenotomy has also been used, although retraction of the spinal cord to visualize the foramen is required. Postoperatively the patient is protected with a semirigid cervical immobilizer, such as a two-poster brace, for about 6 weeks to obtain a stable interbody fusion. Isometric strengthening and range-of-motion exercises are started after brace removal. Loss of neck motion is minimal because of a compensatory increase of motion at the unfused levels.

Whether or not cervical trauma can initiate degeneration of a disc is a subject of debate. In a 10-year follow-up study of patients with neck pain, Gore et al. found that there was a greater incidence of patients with cervical disc degeneration who were injured compared to the incidence in the uninjured population (22). The initial treatment of patients with cervical disc degeneration, which on plain radiographs presents as disc space narrowing and osteophyte formation, is conservative. Those patients who fail with conservative measures such as physical therapy and NSAIDs may be candidates for surgical intervention. Documention of discogenic pain is difficult. Myelography may show no evidence of nerve compression and MR imaging may show decreased signal intensity. Discography can be a valuable tool in evaluating these patients. If the patient has reproduction of his symptoms with injection of the disc, then disc excision and interbody fusion should relieve the symptoms.

The evaluation of cervical joint pain is difficult.

The treatment of these problems is generally nonsurgical. Physical therapy to increase the range of motion of all segments of the cervical spine and isometric muscle strengthening exercises for better control are the mainstay of treatment. Occasionally a patient may require halter traction or a cervical collar to relieve locking and spasm thought to be associated with this condition. Some clinicians recommend manipulation to relieve the joint locking, but no literature exists to prove or disprove its efficacy.

### REFERENCES

1. White AA III, Panjabi MM: The basic kinematics of the human spine. *Spine* 3:12, 1978.
2. Parke WW, Schiff DCM: The applied anatomy of the intervertebral disc. *Orthop Clin North Am* 2:309, 1971.
3. Severy DM, Mathewson JH, Bechtol CO: Controlled automobile rear end collisions, an investigation of related engineering and medical phenomena. *Can Serv Med J* 11:727, 1955.
4. MacNab I: The whiplash syndrome. *Orthop Clin North Am* 2:389, 1971.
5. Dunn EJ, Blazar S: Soft tissue injuries of the lower cervical spine. *Instr Course Lect* 36:499, 1987.
6. Bohlman HH: Acute fracture and dislocations of the cervical spine. *J Bone Joint Surg [Am]* 61:1119, 1979.
7. Alker, G: Radiographic evaluation of patients with cervical spine injury. *Instr Course Lect* 36:473, 1987.
8. Evans DK: Dislocations at the cervicothoracic junction. *J Bone Joint Surg [Br]* 65:124, 1983.
9. White AA III, Panjabi MM: *Clinical Biomechanics of the Spine.* Philadelphia, JB Lippincott, 1978, p 203.
10. Wiltse LL, Rocchio PD: Pre-operative psychological tests as predictors of success of chemonucleolysis in the treatment of the low back syndrome. *J Bone Joint Surg [Am]* 57:4, 1975.
11. Eismont FJ, Clifford S, Goldberg M, Green B: Cervical saggital spinal canal size in spine injury. *Spine* 9:663, 1984.
12. Grieve GP: *Common Vertebral Joint Problems.* New York, Churchill Livingstone, 1988, p 566.
13. Gile LGF: Lumbosacral and cervical zygapophyseal joint inclusions. *Man Med* 2:89, 1986.
14. Black RG, Bonica JJ: Analgesic blocks. *Postgrad Med* 53:105, 1973.
15. Mehta M: *Intractable Pain.* London, Saunders, 1973, p 147.
16. Pierce DS: The halo orthosis in the treatment of cervical spine injury. *Instr Course Lect* 36:495, 1987.
17. Bohlman HH: Complications of treatment of fractures and dislocations of the cervical spine. In *Complications in Orthopaedic Surgery.* Philadelphia, JB Lippincott Co, 1986, p 681.
18. Anderson LD, D'Alonzo PT: Fractures of the odontoid process of the axis. *J Bone Joint Surg [Am]* 56:1663, 1974.
19. Schatzher J, Rorabeck CH, Waddell JP: Fractures of the dens. *J Bone Joint Surg [Br]* 53:392, 1971.
20. Fielding JW: Injuries to the upper cervical spine. *Instr Course Lect* 36:483, 1987.
21. Bohlman HH: Late anterior decompression of spinal cord injuries. A preliminary report of 36 cases. *J Bone Joint Surg [Am]* 57:1025, 1975.
22. Gore DR, Sepic SB, Gardner GM, Murray MP: Neck pain, a long term follow up of 205 patients. *Spine* 12:1, 1987.
23. Herkowitz HN, Rothman RH: Subacute instability of the cervical spine. *Spine* 9:348, 1984.

## 4

# RADIOLOGIC IMAGING
# OF THE CERVICAL SPINE

*Alan E. Zimmer*

Like Atlas supporting the globe, the first cervical vertebra, which bears his name, supports a 14-pound head, or about the weight of a bowling ball (J. Hansen, University of Rochester School of Medicine, personal communication), precariously perched upon six other ⅝ths-inch thick vertebral bodies and intervertebral discs, braced by a musculature and ligaments of variable strength. There is thus little wonder that with such an unstable situation the cervical spine is subject to frequent injury. Neck pain, a frequent sequela of trauma and other etiologies, can be so distressing that we use without further thought a metaphor depicting how annoying a person or thing can be: a "pain in the neck."

When a body part hurts, the physician turns to the radiologist for assistance, so great has the impact of radiologic imaging been on diagnosis. In few areas of the body is radiologic technique so crucial in permitting a precise diagnosis as in the cervical spine. (The reader is referred to a forthcoming series of articles in *Pain Management* and related publications for detailed technical aspects of radiologic examination of the cervical spine, including anteroposterior open-mouth views of the C1–2 region, techniques to maximize satisfactory visualization of the technically more demanding study of the cervicothoracic junction, and additional aspects of computed tomographic and magnetic resonance imaging.)

The initial radiographic examination of the patient with a suspected neck injury often centers on excluding a fracture of C7 before moving the patient. Where a high level of suspicion of fracture persists after apparently normal routine views, I

believe there is merit in using the clinical radiologic algorithm advocated by Wales et al. for evaluating the acutely injured cervical spine (1). They emphasized the portable supine horizontal lateral, the full AP view, the AP open-mouth view, the odontoid view, and also oblique views, including the 60° oblique view, which further avoids the need of even lifting the head for the commonly performed, and in my opinion less satisfactory, 45° view. They use a 30–40° pillar view. They do not use the oblique or pillar views as emergent views.

One must not forget that transverse fractures through the cervical spine with a significant lateral dislocation may only be seen on the anteroposterior (AP) projection, as is dramatically shown in Rogers and Lee's case (2). The lateral view of the cervical spine showed no evidence of displacement, but the AP projection showed a complete transection of the cervical spine (Fig. 4.1). However, the six views of the cervical spine recommended by earlier authors (stereoscopic lateral, AP, open-mouth, and obliques) may no longer be necessary in this age of thin-section computed tomography (CT) with multiplanar reformations. Of course, one must suspect the fracture before CT is done. Short cuts in performing CT with thicker sections without multiplanar reformations may lead to missed fractures.

There still seems to be some need for clinical judgment. Mirvis et al. (3) reported that the American College of Surgery recommends lateral cervical radiographs for all patients with blunt trauma. However, these authors noted that 34% (138) of those blunt trauma patients studied ra-

33

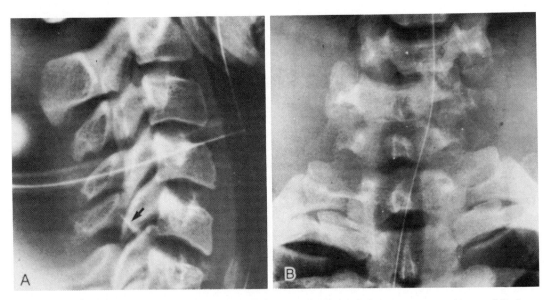

**Figure 4.1.**    Gross lateral dislocation of C5 upon C6. *A*, Lateral radiograph demonstrates no evidence of displacement. The alignment of the vertebral bodies is normal. The only suggestion of abnormality is an increased distance between the spinous processes of C5 and C6 and a small bony fragment overlying the inferior margin of the articular mass of C5 *(arrow)*. *B*, Dislocation is obvious on AP radiograph. The fifth cervical vertebra is displaced approximately 50% of its width to the left of the sixth cervical vertebra. It is wise to always obtain both an AP and a lateral view of the cervical spine. (From Rogers LF, Lee C: In Dalinka MK, Kaye JJ (eds): *Radiology in Emergency Medicine.* New York, Churchill Livingstone, Inc, 1984, pp 276–277.)

diographically at their emergency facility in Maryland were mentally alert and without symptoms. Six of their patients had CT to clarify questionable x-ray findings. Only one of these (less than 1% of 138 asymptomatic patients) showed a nondisplaced fracture of the transverse process of C7, at a cost of $59,202.

Although space limitations preclude details on techniques to study the cervicothoracic junction in difficult patients, one such example should be shown here (Fig. 4.2). The cervicothoracic junction warrants particular attention. Of 397 patients with cervical spine injury studied by Nichols et al. (4) recorded in the Spinal Injury Registry of St. Joseph's Hospital and Medical Center and Barrow's Neurological Institute in Phoenix from January 1980 through June 1985, 37 (9%) had cervicothoracic injury. Nine of the 37 (24%) were obtunded and had negative neurologic examinations. Neck pain was present in 7 (19%), 8 (22%) had neurologic deficits only, 13 (35%) had pain and deficit, and 9 (19%) had no pain or deficits. Of those with symptoms referable to the cervicothoracic junction, 35% had fractures, 47% had soft tissue swelling, and 18% had widened bony spaces. One of their normal control group

showed evidence of past facet injury (4). In addition to this report, a 7% incidence of cervicothoracic trauma was found by Miller et al. (5). As with the examples shown in this chapter, dislocations at the cervicothoracic junction are not rare; Evans reported a 3% incidence in his cases (6).

## NEED FOR COMPUTED TOMOGRAPHY IN PROBLEM SITUATIONS

The necessity of a swift resolution of the problematic cervicothoracic junction as well as that of the craniocervical junction in the seriously injured, comatose, or uncooperative patient without straining radiologic resources and personnel has resulted in a pragmatic approach of thin-section computed tomography (CT) of the areas in question (Fig. 4.3). Thin-section conventional and pluridirectional tomography is useful but frequently entails turning a patient with a potentially unstable spine fracture. In the past 10 years, CT has evolved as the most accurate way of detecting the presence and full extent of cervical spine fractures (7–16).

Acheson et al. (16) reported that, although there was a high index of suspicion on the plain film interpretation as well as a large percentage of false positives, many fractures that they found on CT were not suggested, even in retrospect, on the plain radiographs. Of the 136 fractures ultimately identified in their patients, CT detected 135 (99%), whereas only 64 (47%) were seen or suspected on the initial screening radiographs. The plain films actually suggested a fracture in the vertebra that was subsequently confirmed or detected in an adjacent vertebra by CT. The authors also concluded that if an adequately exposed and positioned plain film series of the cervical spine is normal, it is unlikely that a fracture will be revealed by CT. (The term "CT" generally replaced

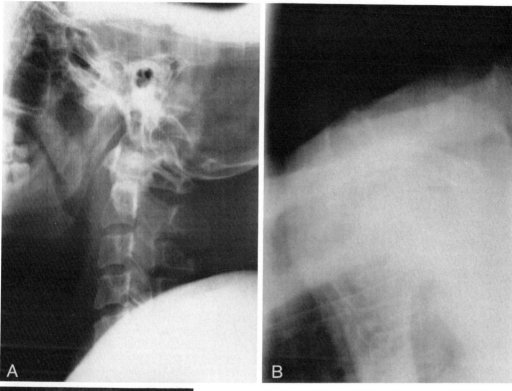

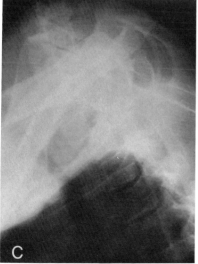

**Figure 4.2.**   Use of the grid cassette in the Bucky tray in radiographic evaluation of the cervicothoracic junction in large patients. *A,* Supine lateral projection reveals vertebrae down to C5. *B,* Conventional Swimmer's view with a grid cassette without "coning" results in an image that is dark enough but lacking in detail. *C,* The cleanup of x-ray scatter with a grid cassette in the Bucky tray is good with and even without collimation.

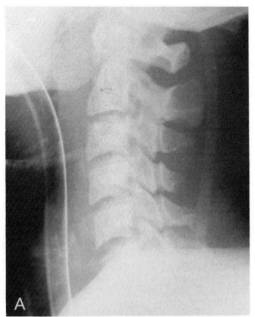

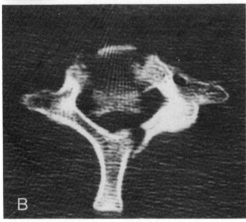

**Figure 4.3.**   Use of CT to see lower cervical spine. *A*, Lateral projection radiograph reveals spine only down to C6. *B*, Retropulsed C7 fracture produced cord compression. Note comminuted fracture of the body and left lamina with lateral displacement of the left neural arch.

in 1975 the now-archaic "CAT scan," which stood for computerized axial tomography or computer assisted tomography). While conventional radiographs fail to detect a surprising number of fractures, they retain their value as a screening tool and as a guide to selective CT imaging.

In CT, a sharply collimated fan-shaped beam of x-rays is rotated around a body part. The divergent x-ray beam strikes an array of curved detectors in an arc (third-generation CT scanners) or a circle (fourth-generation scanners), and each detector that receives a portion of the x-ray beam that has passed through the patient generates an electrical pulse proportional to the intensity of the beam. A series of numerical values is generated by each detector as the x-ray tube and detectors move in a circle about the patient.

A series of slices with thicknesses ranging from 10 mm down to as little as 1 mm on present-day scanners is produced. The block of tissue studied in a 10-mm thick slice might measure $0.1 \times 0.1 \times 10$ mm. This volume element, or *voxel*, has a numerical value of the average attenuation value of all tissues within its thickness. The computer calculates what the attenuation values must be for each voxel within the x-ray slices by a technique known as fast Fourier transform or by "back-projection." These values are then converted to CT numbers (Hounsfield units) and represented in a $64 \times 64$ or $512 \times 512$ matrix of rows and columns. Each box in the matrix—called a picure element, or *pixel*— measures 0.1 to 0.3 mm square.

Each pixel's numerical value is assigned a shade of gray ranging from black to white according to its number of Hounsfield units. If an axial slice measuring 5 or 10 mm encompasses intervertebral disc, compact bone in the endplate of the vertebral centrum, and a portion of spongy bone and bone marrow in the voxels, *partial volume averaging* of the tissue results in an appearance of the pixel on the scan that is dense or white, like bone; the intervertebral disc has "disappeared," having been averaged out with the denser, compact bone, which has a density of approximately 400 Hounsfield units (HU), compared with disc, which has a density of about 40 HU. Similarly, a fracture passing parallel or obliquely to the plane of section may be obscured by partial volume averaging in a thick slice, whereas multiple thin slices with small individual voxels may permit detection of the fracture (Fig. 4.4). The quintessential example of this is the basal skull fracture, which will invariably be missed or averaged out with 10-mm thick sections but will usually be displayed in incredible detail with 1.5-mm thick sections targeted for maximum bone detail.

The original Hounsfield units of $\pm 512$ were changed to the "new" Hounsfield units ranging from $+1024$ HU for white to $-1024$ HU for black. This range proved inadequate, especially for studying compact bone, and all manufacturers now use an extended scale of approximately 4000 HU ($-1024$ to $+3072$ HU). The extended scale and techniques of high-resolution "targeting" for maximum bone detail now permit exquisite bone detail that could never have been imagined in the past. A variety of "soft tissue algorithms" have been developed that can "borrow" data from adjacent pixels and produce a smoothing of the image. Filter functions, such as the "bone algorithm," cause an edge enhancement by inverting (i.e., increasing or decreasing) the numerical value adjacent to the edges of abruptly changing tissue densities. Other algorithms offer a compromise intermediate between the overly smoothed soft tissue and edge-enhanced bone algorithms.

CT slice thicknesses on high-end scanners vary with the manufacturer, ranging from 1 to 10 mm. The medium and low-end scanners tend to offer less flexibility. As CT slice thickness increases, a

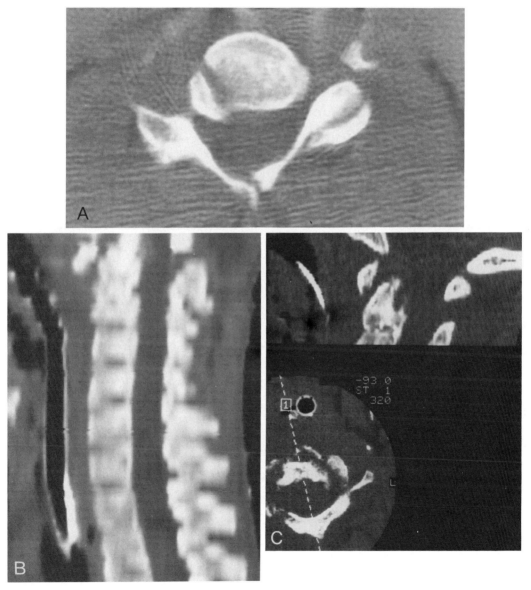

**Figure 4.4.** Partial volume averaging in CT of the spine. *A*, Partial volume averaging of tilted endplate simulates fracture. *B*, Sagittal reformations show blurring of bone and discs by volume averaging. *C*, Sagittal reformations in a patient with osteomyelitis of the dens and atlas employing 1.5-mm thick axial slices targeted for maximum bone detail.

proportionally greater number of x-ray photons are absorbed by the detectors, increasing and improving the signal-to-noise ratio. This results in less grainy and more pleasing images and is perfectly suited for body parts in which very little change takes place between slices—for example, in the abdomen or cerebral hemispheres. If 1.5-mm thick slices are used to study soft tissues, the signal-to-noise ratio will drop to 1.5:10, or about one seventh of that in the 10-mm thick slice, resulting in a grainy image comparable to the appearance of "snow" on a television picture with a weak signal, both of which are suffering from photon starvation. For bone imaging this is not a problem and requires no increase in milliampere-seconds (mAs) by the technician to obtain satisfactory bone detail. Indeed, the cervical spine is better studied for bone with the relatively low mAs settings employed for rapid "dynamic" scanning, by means of which all of the slices are rapidly obtained and the images subsequently constructed or batch processed from the raw data. The lower mAs settings result in less radiation to the patients, despite the more numerous slices, than is received with the more conventionally used 3- or 5-mm thicknesses at higher mAs settings.

A more important reason for using thin slices to study the cervical spine concerns the necessity of obtaining coronal and sagittal images from the axial images by a process called multiplanar reformations (MPRs). These are commonly incorrectly referred to as "reconstructions." Twenty or 30 slices are obtained each consisting of 512 X 512, or about one-quarter million, voxels. The computer is then instructed to select a plane of voxels in this three-dimensional array in the coronal, sagittal, or an oblique plane. The computer will then disregard all voxels outside the plane selected and a new plane will be *reformatted* from the previously constructed axial images. When the slices are 3 or 5 mm thick, the reformatted images will appear box-like and indistinct; in practice, 3-mm thick slices are barely acceptable and 5-mm slices are no longer so. Dynamic scanning with 1.5- or 2-mm thick slices at low mAs settings with a bone algorithm will rival conventional AP or lateral tomograms. The dramatic difference in quality between thin- and thick-section reformatted images is demonstrated in Figure 4.4.

The MPRs are obtained after the examination has been completed and usually after the patient has been taken off the table. Obviously, if the patient moves in the slightest, the reformations will show distressing step-like artifacts on the corresponding line of data that may render the MPRs of little value. It must be remembered that when MPRs are anticipated, the number of axial slices should be kept to under 45 to limit radiation, tube heating, and length of study. Thus, one or two cervical vertebrae may be studied in great detail with 1.5-mm thick slices while the entire cervical spine is studied with contiguous 3-mm thick slices.

Some CT scanners and software permit curvilinear reformations that can produce impressive reformations parallel to the cervical lordosis as well as through vertebral bodies and adjacent pedicles. The major companies now bundle the three-dimensional technology with their software, and a number of independent manufacturers sell the software or free-standing hardware for this purpose. In my experience these images are most helpful for the maxillofacial surgeon in planning reconstructive surgery, or to the neurosurgeon or orthopaedic surgeon in handling injuries to the spine. Several of these companies will also produce images of this type off-line from CT and MRI data transferred to them by modem, and wire the reformatted images back to the sender. However, physicians treating serious trauma cases do not have the luxury of waiting to make decisions.

## A BRIEF NOTE ABOUT MAGNETIC RESONANCE IMAGING

Magnetic resonance (MR) imaging, formerly known as nuclear magnetic resonance (NMR), came upon the scene as a practical imaging modality just 10 years after CT. It is based on the physical properties of hydrogen atoms in water and lipids in the body. The spinning hydrogen nuclei in water and lipids behave, as do all charged particles in motion, as ultramicroscopic magnets. When the body is placed in a powerful magnetic field, the mobile protons or hydrogen nuclei align themselves in a north-south fashion. These nuclei are caused to tip over 90° by the application of a radiowave at the frequency at which the protons are wobbling, or precessing, in the magnetic field, followed by a 180° radio frequency pulse. The protons are energized and unstable and give back this energy as they return to equilibrium, resulting in the emission of radio frequency signal. This process is repeated for each line of data in each image slice.

The radio signal is received by a system of body and surface coils and the data are processed so as to produce the MR image. The chemical composition of each tissue and fluid causes it to behave in a specific manner. The time between the applied radio wave and the signal received (the TE, or echo time) is selected by the technician, as is the repetition time (TR) during which the signal from each line of data and each slice is processed by the computer. The physical characteristics of the tissue determine the signal's appearance. With a short TE and short TR (STE/STR), or so-called $T_1$-weighted sequence, cerebrospinal fluid and tissues with a high water content will be black and lipids will give an intense signal and be bright. With a long TE and long TR (LTE/LTR), a so-called $T_2$-weighted sequence, cerebrospinal fluid is white and lipids are gray. Subacute hemorrhages will appear bright on $T_1$- and $T_2$-weighted images. Chronic subdural hematomas, edematous tissues, contused spinal cord, and certain tumors will have an intense $T_2$ signal and appear hypointense or isointense on $T_1$-weighted images. With a short TE and long TR (STE/LTR), a hybrid or so-called proton density scan is obtained. The $T_1$-weighted images give beautiful anatomic studies, often with no trace of disease, whereas the proton density and $T_2$-weighted scans are the sensitivity studies that usually reveal much about the pathology.

Space limitation necessitates curtailing discussion of inversion recovery sequences, gradient images, fat suppression (useful for differentiating extradural clot from fat), and the important consideration of cerebrospinal fluid pulsation artifacts. The latter may cause spatial mismatching, especially on $T_2$-weighted images, and produce serious image degradation as well as false bright signals in the spinal cord and dark signals in the fluid simulating vascular malformations.

## INCIDENCE OF CERVICAL TRAUMA

In a retrospective and prospective study of 1000 vertebral injuries seen from 1981 through 1986 at the Trauma Center of Allegheny General Hospital, Daffner noted 65% of the injuries were cervical compared to 19% thoracic and 16% lumbar. Of the 646 cervical injuries, 511 were the result of flexion, 124 of extension, and 11 of rotation injuries, with no shearing injuries as he had observed at the thoracolumbar junction in 12 cases. Isolated fractures of spinous processes or transverse processes were not included in his series (17).

## MECHANISMS OF INJURIES TO THE CERVICAL SPINE

Man's upright posture with his relatively heavy head subjects the cervical spine to forces and stresses for which it was not optimally designed. Decelerating and to a lesser extent accelerating injuries may lead to hyperflexion and hyperextension, each of which can cause injuries to bones and joints, resulting in a variety of hyperflexion and hyperextension fractures/dislocations. Simultaneous injuries to the face, top of the head, and back of the head produce superimposed axial loading forces resulting in hyperflexion-compression fractures, bursting fractures, and hyperextension-compression fractures. In impaction or compression fractures (axial loading fractures) two vertebrae are pushed together during flexion or extension. When this occurs in flexion in its simplest form, it produces an anterior wedge-shaped fracture of the vertebral body with preservation of the posterior aspect of the vertebral body, vertebral arch, and posterior ligaments (17,18).

## FLEXION INJURIES

Although during marked physiologic flexion a small amount of motion occurs in the upper cervical spine, most flexion takes place between C5 and C7, as though around an axle running from side to side. The inferior articular facets from C5 to T1 slide forward on the superior facets of the vertebrae below. The articular facets remain parallel to each other (Figs. 4.5A and 4.7). The spinous processes separate with slight stretching of the interspinous ligaments. The young, healthy intervertebral discs are resilient cushions that compress like springs, changing shape to accommodate the contour in flexion and thereby minimize the strain on the facetal joints. Physiologic dislocation of C2 on C3 may be seen normally in children. A line drawn from the anterior cortex of the spinous process of C1 to the same point on C3 will pass within 2 mm of the corresponding cortex of C2 (Fig. 4.6). When C2 appears dislocated on C3 and the cortex of the C2 spinous process is further than 2 mm from Swischuk's line, a pathologic dislocation or hangman's fracture may be present (see below) (19).

With the inevitable aging of the intervertebral structures starting insidiously in adolescence, the discs undergo drying and degeneration and there

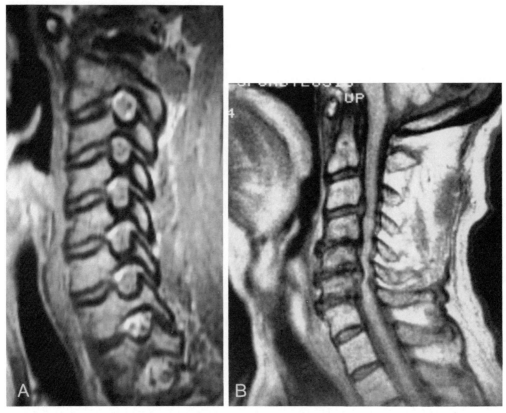

**Figure 4.5.** Compact bone of the vertebrae gives no MR signal. The marrow, nerve roots, and spinal contents do produce useful signals. *A*, Oblique spin density of the cervical spine demonstrating the foramina, facets, and nerve roots. *B*, Sagittal inversion recovery image demonstrating advanced spondylosis deformans with chronic compression of the cervical cord by the spondylotic ridging. (Courtesy of Siemens Medical Systems.)

**Figure 4.6.** Example of Swischuk's posterior cervical line demonstrating physiologic displacement of C2 on C3 in flexion. Note the line touches the lamina of C2 in flexion. When the posterior arch of C2 projects more than 2 mm behind the posterior cervical line, a hangman's fracture of C2 may be present.

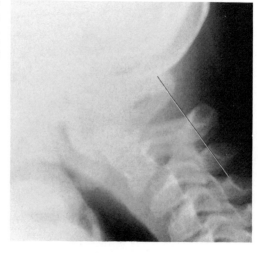

is less disc mobility. With a forceful traumatic flexion, there is forward slipping and tilting of the facets with stretching or tearing of the facetal ligaments and capsule, and tearing and avulsion of the interspinous ligaments occurs. This produces a V-shaped widening of the facets indicative of a *hyperflexion sprain,* or self-reducing hyperflexion dislocation (20) (Fig. 4.7). In mild apophyseal joint injuries, the distraction of the facetal joints may result in hyperflexion sprain with stretching and some tearing of ligaments. When injuries are more severe, either a partial or complete rupture of the ligaments occurs, with frank unilateral (UID) or bilateral (BID) interfacetal dislocations (Figs. 4.8, 4.9, and 4.10). Dislocation of the facetal joints is associated with complete disruption of normal contact between articular surfaces (18, 20). Subluxation is a partial dislocation. Since physiologic subluxation occurs in flexion, use of the term should be reserved for partial dislocations shown by imaging of the joint in the neutral or postreduction position. The instability resulting from such injuries may be apparent only on flexion-extension films. The patient should be advised to perform these movements to avoid dislocating the facetal joints or causing neurologic damage.

The notion of an imaginary transverse axle passing through the cervical canal between the anterior and posterior elements helps to understand the pathogenesis of flexion injuries. The forward tipping of the vertebral bodies produces compression of the endplates with anterior wedging of the vertebral body, with no apparent injury to the posterior arch or posterior ligaments on conventional films and no neurologic deficit. This is referred to as a simple flexion injury. However, MR imaging and thin-section CT with multiplanar reformations may show evidence of more subtle soft tissue injuries that frequently escape detection on plain films. As the hyperflexion-compressive forces increase a fragment of bone often avulses from the anteroinferior endplate of the vertebral body. With still greater compressive forces, vertebral bursting occurs with a so-called *teardrop fracture* anteriorly and retropulsion of the vertebral body; this results in cord compression, often with devastating neurologic deficit. Posttraumatic syringomyelia may result from such injuries (Figs. 4.11 and 4.12).

When the flexion is produced by or associated with a fall on the head, with the vertex of the head striking a windshield or other object, or with a heavy object falling on the head, the axial loading injury results in compression, bursting, or impaction fractures. Flexion injuries may therefore be classified as simple, burst, distraction, dislocation, and combined (17).

Hyperflexion-compression injuries produce typical wedge-shaped fractures of a vertebral body, typically C5 or C6. The type of fracture in practice represents a point in a continuum or spectrum of injuries in flexion, axial loading, and extension injuries. We may therefore see combinations of flexion + rotation, flexion + compression, and extension + rotation as well as pure axial loading injuries (18).

Hyperextension, producing a so-called whiplash injury, followed by hyperflexion also may cause retropulsion of the involved vertebral body. This type of injury can result in cord compression, often with devastating neurologic deficit.

Distraction of the spinous processes may exhibit varying degrees of rupture of the nuchal ligament and of the interspinous ligaments. The separation of the spinous process is usually obvious on lateral projections but may be suspected on AP roentgenograms when the interspinous distance (ISD) is greater than 1.5 times that between the vertebrae above or below the vertebra in question. Naidich et al. have shown this to be indicative of an anterior cervical dislocation and a hyperflexion injury in a series of studies with no false positives or negatives (21) (Fig. 4.9). The disruption of the interspinous ligaments and the associated soft-tissue injury may also show an increased signal on MR imaging.

Although distraction fractures of the spinous process are more likely to occur as isolated fractures secondary to a sudden pull of the trapezius and rhomboid muscles, as the name *clay shoveler's fracture* suggests, this fracture may be associated with other injuries. The clay shoveler's fracture is most common at T1 and next most common at C7 and T2. It may also result from forceful pulling ("root puller's fracture") (18). Typically cervicothoracic, it does not have to be limited to the cervicothoracic junction (Fig. 4.13).

Hyperextension-compression injuries of the spinous processes may also cause them to fracture. Less commonly, direct injury may fracture one or more spinous processes. Other isolated fractures include fractures of the transverse process.

In the post–flexion injury resting state, signs of a more significant injury may be relatively subtle.

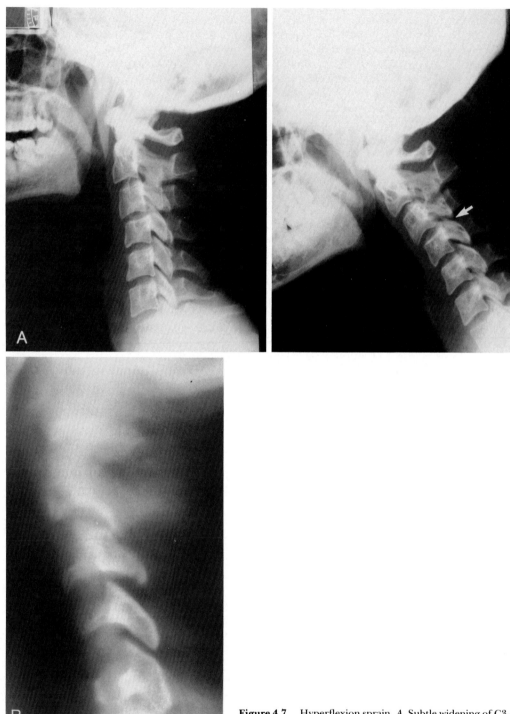

**Figure 4.7.**  Hyperflexion sprain. *A*, Subtle widening of C3–4 facet joint in flexion *(arrow)*. *B*, Confirmation on polytome.

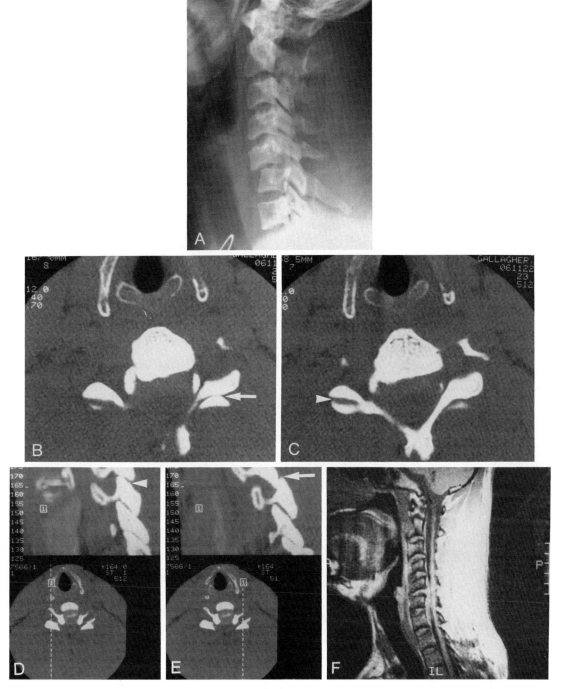

**Figure 4.8.** Hyperflexion injury. *A,* Note forward subluxation of C5 on C6, widening of the interspinous distance, widened right facetal joint, and locked left facets. *B,* Axial CT shows the unilateral interfacetal dislocation on the left *(arrow). C,* Axial CT showing the widened facetal joint (hyperflexion sprain) *(arrowhead). D,* Sagittal MPR through the right side demonstrating the hyperflexion sprain with slight subluxation and widening of the C5–6 facetal joint on the right *(arrowhead). E,* Sagittal MPR on the left demonstrating the locked C5–6 facets *(arrow). F,* Slightly to the right note the herniated nucleus pulposis with epidural methemoglobin-containing subacute hematoma.

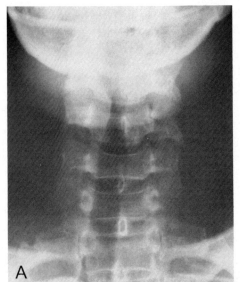

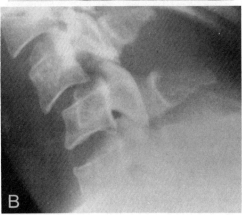

**Figure 4.9.** Demonstration of increased interspinous distance (ISD) secondary to hyperflexion injury with a unilateral interfacetal dislocation. *A*, The ISD at C5–6 is more than 1.5 times the ISDs at C4–5 and C6–7. *B*, In a different patient with a similar injury, note the sagittal T$_1$-weighted image demonstrates an extruded disc at C6–7. Widening of the interspinous distance is present.

In one such case a teenage cyclist collided with a moving auto and struck his posterior vertex with his neck in flexion. On the plain films he appeared only to have sustained a "simple" wedge fracture of the body of C5. With hyperflexion, the spine pivoted forward and downward in an arc while the vertebral body at the fulcrum of the forces tilted forward and backward, avulsing the anteroinferior aspect of the body. A chip fracture of the anteroinferior aspect of the vertebral body resulted in C4, and a fracture of C5 was seen on the axial

CT. Although the intervertebral disc is usually resistant to simple flexion injuries, as observed by Roaf (22), the injury was more severe than originally suspected and was seen to have resulted in disc herniation at C4–5. (Although it has long been held that cervical disc herniations result from injury to previously degenerated discs, our experience with MR imaging has shown disc herniation to occur in young healthy discs.)

As the upper cervical spine rotated forward, the C4 vertebra pivoted downward and backward, with disruption of the apophyseal capsule and the posterior portion of the C4–5 disc. The deforming forces at the moment of impact resulted in a momentary dislocation of the apophyseal joints, distraction injury to the interspinous ligaments, and retropulsion of the body of C5, with cord contusion and paraparesis. As the severity of the axial compression increases, the body of the vertebra may burst with comminution and explosive separation of the fragments under the combined axial and flexion forces. With a mechanism similar to that described above, a fragment of the anterior aspect of the vertebral body is displaced anteriorly.

Pure axial loading fractures may cause the bursting fracture of the atlas known as the *Jefferson fracture,* which is described in some detail below. With the head rigidly erect, an axial compressive force applied to the vertex may cause bursting at the end of the vector—for example, at C5. Such a bursting fracture causes vertebral shattering with anterior and posterior displacement of fragments and upward movement of the disc into the inferior endplate above. As with hyperflexion-compression fractures, the retropulsed fragment may severely injure the cord (Figs. 4.3*B* and 4.11).

## EXTENSION INJURIES

Extension injuries may result in fractures that may be categorized as simple, distraction, and dislocation types. When hyperextension occurs high in the cervical spine, it may result in the hangman's fracture or traumatic spondylolisthesis of C2 (described in detail below). Lower in the cervical spine, hyperextension may in mild cases cause a hyperextension sprain with disruption of the anterior ligaments with injury to the disc bond. In severe cases a disruption of the disc bond and facetal ligaments occurs with retrolisthesis, and devastating cord injury may occur. The mech-

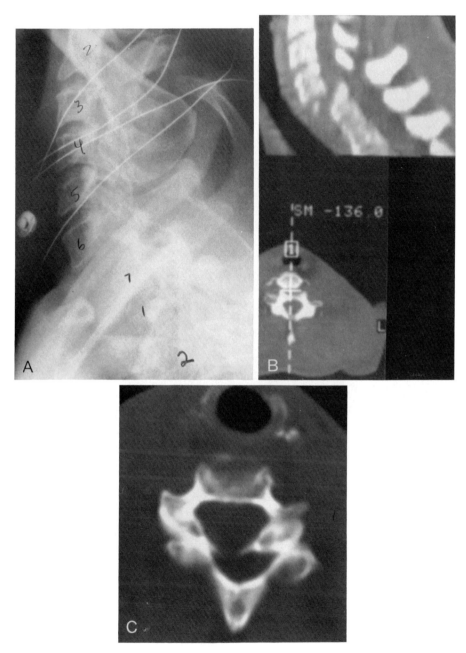

**Figure 4.10.** Example of Boynton and Kalb's double lumen sign of spinal dislocation. *A,* Forward subluxation of C6–7 seen on Swimmer's view due to bilateral interfacetal dislocation. *B,* Sagittal MPR shows the severity of the AP narrowing of the canal. *C,* The double lumen and double vertebral body signs.

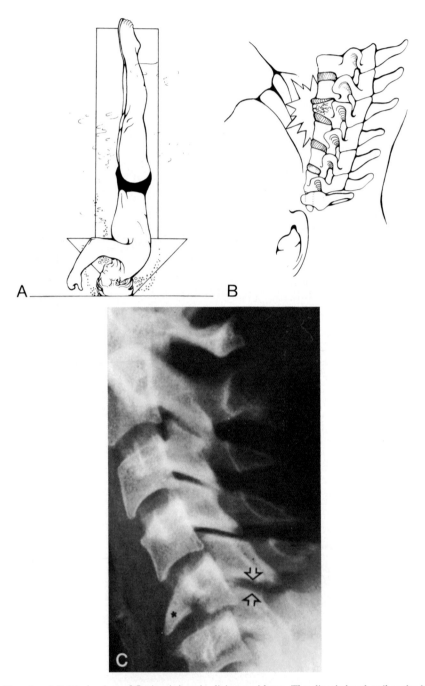

**Figure 4.11.** *A and B,* Mechanism of flexion injury in diving accidents. The diver's head strikes the bottom with resultant forced flexion and increase in axial load. This mechanism characteristically produces a teardrop fracture, usually at C5. *C,* Teardrop fracture of C5 from a diving accident. There is posterior dislocation of C5 on C6. Note the teardrop fragment (*). As further evidence of flexion injury, there is widening of the facet joints of C5–6 *(open arrows).* There is also widening of the interspinous space. (From Daffner RH: *Imaging of Vertebral Trauma.* Rockville, MD, Aspen Publishers Inc, 1988.)

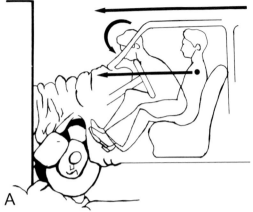

**Figure 4.12.** *A*, Mechanism of flexion injury in an unrestrained motor vehicle driver. On impact, the victim pitches forward. The chest is impaled on the steering column. The knees strike the dashboard. This mechanism is sufficient to produce flexion injuries in the lumbar vertebrae. In addition, if the head pitches forward, flexion injury may result as contact is made with the windshield. (From Daffner RH: *Imaging of Vertebrae Trauma*. Rockville, MD, Aspen Publishers, Inc, 1988.) *B*, Hyperflexion injury sustained by a 20-year-old male in a motor vehicle accident. Again we see a burst and tear-drop fracture of C5 with retropulsion of the body of C5, and C4–5 and C5–6 hyperflexion sprains. The character of the injury is virtually identical to that sustained by a diver.

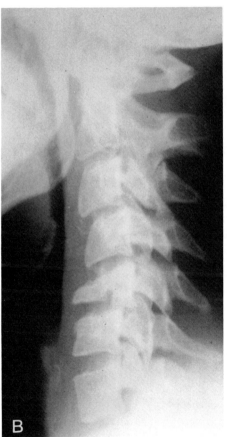

anism and the appearance of a widened interspace and the vertebral retrolisthesis are shown in Figure 4.14.

In severe hyperextension injuries the transverse axis around which extension occurs shifts posteriorly, which is frequently associated with forward movement of the vertebrae above this axis. This results in anterior dislocation of the body and of the inferior facets bilaterally, resulting in locked facets (BID). Severe neurologic injury may result. In patients with ankylosing spondylitis in whom fusion of the apophyseal joints is present secondary to this form of arthritis, a hyperextension injury may result in a so-called banana fracture.

Among the clues to be sought as an indicator of

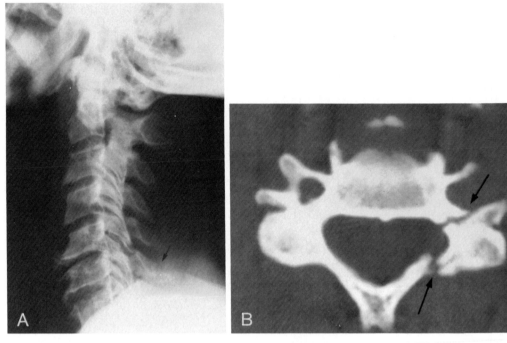

**Figure 4.13.**    *A*, A clay shoveler's fracture at C6 *(arrow)*. *B*, In the same patient, associated fractures through the left pedicle and lamina of C5 on the left *(arrows)* produce a "floating pillar."

a more severe injury, one should carefully inspect the prevertebral soft tissues. A prevertebral hematoma is a frequent and important indicator occurring as a result of disruption of the anterior longitudinal ligament and fractures involving the anterior surface of the cervical vertebral bodies and anterior arch of C1. This was shown by Penning in 18 of 30 hospitalized cervical injury patients in whom there was widening of the prevertebral soft tissue space as a result of hematoma (23). Penning suggested the following upper limits of normal: 10 mm at C1, 5 mm at C2, 7 mm at C3 and C4, and 20 mm from C5 down. He pointed out that a hangman's fracture without an anterior fracture had normal prevertebral soft tissues whereas an anterior avulsion chip fracture with disruption of the anterior longitudinal ligament was associated with a noticeable soft tissue swelling.

Templeton et al. found that the absolute measurements of the retropharyngeal soft tissues suggested by Penning included too many false positives and false negatives (24). These authors found a Gaussian distribution of 2–10 mm of prevertebral soft tissue space in the normal cervical spine, peaking at 4 or 5 mm. Use of greater than 5 mm would produce 65% false positives and use of

greater than 7 mm gave 5% false positives at C2 and 23% at all levels. A value of 0.3 times the diameter of the C5 body produced 55% false positives. Templeton et al. concluded that at C2, C3, or C4 a space of 7–10 mm indicates a possible abnormality and a space of greater than 10 mm definitely requires additional investigation.

Whalen and Woodruff brought attention to the cervical prevertebral fat stripe, noting that it could be an aid in evaluating the prevertebral soft tissue space (25). These authors found that the prevertebral fat stripe allowed for detection and localization of cervical fractures, masses, and inflammatory conditions and helped to elucidate confusing normal densities. Williams et al., who emphasized the essentiality of the lateral film of the cervical spine, also suggested the usefulness of the prevertebral fat stripe (26). Like Templeton, we have rarely been able to identify it in abnormal cases. We have tended to rely mainly on widening of the retropharyngeal soft tissue space. Because of the high sensitivity of MR imaging we have been able to delineate the prevertebral fat stripe by virtue of its short, bright appearance on $T_1$-weighted sagittal images where it was not apparent on plain films. Fat loses much of its signal on $T_2$-weighted images, whereas methemoglobin in a subacute hematoma will be bright in all sequences. Chemical shift imaging for fat suppression should improve its visualization further by decreasing the signal from fat while retaining that from subacute hematoma in a $T_1$-weighted study.

## PILLAR FRACTURES

The most common site of cervical fracture is the vertebral arch. Fifty percent of all patients in the Duke series of 400 patients had vertebral arch fractures (27). Many of these patients had other fractures as well. Thirty percent of all arch fractures were at C6, whereas C3 was the most protected (only 8% of fractures were at this level). Of the vertebral arch fractures, 21% involved the pillar as compared with 13% each involving the pedicle, lamina, and spinous process and only 2% involving the transverse process. The most common *isolated* fracture of the vertebral arch involved the articular pillar in 8% of the Duke patient population. These fractures were of three types. Simple

compression fracture of the pillar was the most common, followed by compression-distraction and displaced pillar fractures in which there were avulsion, comminution, or oblique displacement of the fragments. When pillar views were obtained and pillar fractures were recognized, 77% of these patients reported having sustained neck injuries for the most part between 3 months and 14 years prior to this more detailed examination. *All of these patients had normal routine views.* The study's skilled technologist took 45 minutes to obtain *13 views* (27).

Abel observed increasing gross pillar deformity with age, increasing from no abnormality in subjects under 1 year of age to a 51% incidence of pillar compression fractures in those over 60 years of age. His natural conclusion, therefore, was that these pillar deformities are acquired (28). The apparent frequency of this finding prompted Vines to study these pillars in detail. He found a 2-mm discrepancy in pillar height to be significant and observed unilateral compression of the articular

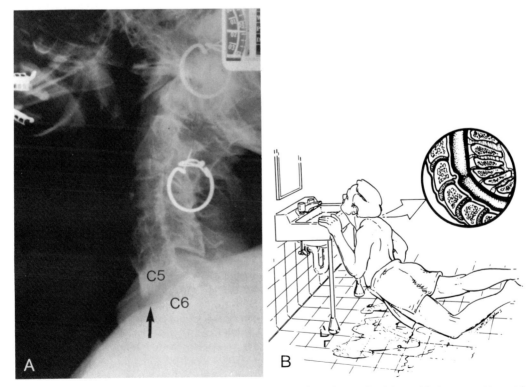

**Figure 4.14.** Hyperextension injuries. *A,* Distraction-type extension injury at C5–6 in an elderly woman. Note widening of the C5–6 disc space *(arrow).* The patient became quadriplegic and died of respiratory arrest. *B,* One mechanism of distraction-type hyperextension injury. (From Daffner DH: *Imaging of Vertebral Trauma.* Rockville, MD. Aspen Publishers, Inc, 1988.)

pillar to be common and unrelated to age or degenerative changes. He concluded that such compression could not be used as a criterion of recent trauma (29). Fortunately, with contemporary radionuclide pharmaceuticals and conventional and single-photon emission CT bone scanning it is possible to detect an increased uptake in relatively recent fractures. Consistently satisfactory pillar views are readily obtained by gray-scale digital subtraction angiographic imaging.

Since 99% of cervical fractures are detected by CT at this time, I do not believe that we can justify time-consuming detailed studies as a routine approach. It is not feasible to obtain contiguous 1.5-mm thick CT sections of the entire spine for each patient. The trend in most institutions, including ours, is to perform CT of the cranioatlantoaxial and of the cervicothoracic regions and of any area of suspected fracture or facetal dislocation. I am sure we and others are missing pillar fractures when we neglect to obtain pillar views or screen the entire spine with contiguous 3- or 4-mm thick CT sections.

## CRANIOATLANTOAXIAL INJURIES

In Daffner's series (17), while more than three quarters of the fatalities that occurred among 646 cervical injuries involved the cranioatlantoaxial region, of those who survived their neck injuries 2.17% sustained fractures of C1 and 18.27% had fractures of C2. In a postmortem radiologic study of 146 traffic accident fatalities reported by Alker et al. (30), 42% of cases had radiologically demonstrable head injuries and 21% had cervical injuries. Of 31 cervical fractures, half involved the atlanto-occipital region (8 cases) or C1 (7 cases) and one third involved C2 (10 cases). Thus 80% of the neck injuries were cranioatlantoaxial fractures and/or dislocations. Associated chest and abdominal injuries may have been considered to be the cause of death. Cervical spine injuries therefore may not have been suspected as the cause of death when radiologic examination of the cervical spine was not carried out pre- or postmortem (30). In view of the greater risk of death with cranioatlantoaxial injuries, I believe that these injuries are more common than suggested in this series.

These figures tend to reflect our own experience at the State Trauma Center. The need for a meticulous technique in studying the craniovertebral complex is apparent in view of these considerations. Indeed, suspicion of fractures or dislocations or dis-

placements at C1–2 have prompted additional CT and lateral flexion-extension views.

## ATLANTO-OCCIPITAL DISLOCATIONS

Atlanto-occipital dislocation or dissociation (AOD) is a condition following trauma characterized by a complete disruption of the ligaments that bind the atlas and dens to the base of the skull, namely, the anterior and posterior atlanto-occipital ligaments or membranes, the transverse, alar, tectorial, and apical dental ligaments, and the atlanto-occipital articular capsules. Once separated from the atlas, the skull commonly dislocates anteriorly, causing a usually lethal shearing compression of the cervicomedullary junction. The unfortunate individual may die immediately, as we noted in one such 8-year-old boy struck by a car who was dead on arrival. The craniocervical disruption and anterior AOD were quite striking.

True occipitoatlantoid dislocations have been reported by Dally (31) and Englander (32) with a clinical picture similar to that of atlantoaxial dislocation except that the transverse process of C1 could be palpated behind the mastoid instead of anterior to it. Sullivan (33) observed that the occipitoatlantoid joints are more horizontal in children than in adults, which may explain the greater frequency of dislocations in children.

The criteria for the roentgenographic diagnosis of this condition were clarified by Powers et al. (34). In the normal individual the distance from the basion (B), or anterior margin of the foramen magnum, to the midposterior arch of the atlas (C) is equal to or less than the distance from the opisthion (O), or posterior margin of the foramen magnum, to the anterior arch of C1 (A). The ratio BC/OA is therefore normally less than or equal to 1. When an anterior AOD is present, BC/OA is greater than 1 (Fig. 4.15A). In an alternative measurement (Lee's method), lines are drawn from the basion to the posterior arch of C2 (DD = descending limb) and from the posterior inferior cortex of C2 up to the opisthion (AA = ascending limb). Line DD normally passes within 5 mm of the dens and line AA passes near the posterior laminar line. With anterior AOD, line DD passes closer to or through the tip of the dens (35) (Fig. 4.15B).

I am personally not fond of ratios and lines requiring measurement. Frequently, however, the opisthion is difficult to identify on nontomographic studies. Recognizing that the basion lies

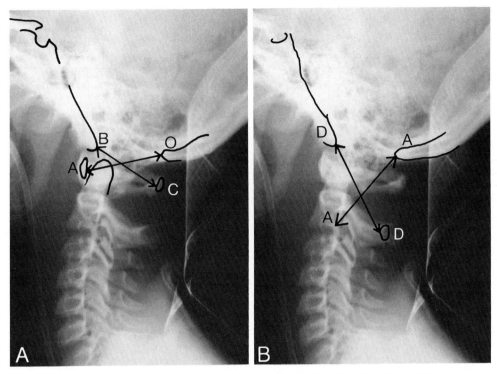

**Figure 4.15.** *A*, Powers ratio in child with anterior atlanto-occipital dislocation. The distance *BC* from the basion to the anterior surface of the posterior arch of the atlas is equal to or less than the distance *OA* from the opisthion to the anterior arch of C1. Therefore, the ratio BC/OA is normally equal to or slightly less than 1. In this child, the Powers ratio is slightly greater than 1. *B*, Lee's method on tomogram of same case. Lines are drawn from the basion to the posterior arch of C2 (*DD* = the descending limb) and from the posterior inferior cortex of C2 up to the opisthion (*AA* = the ascending limb). Line DD normally passes within 5 mm of the dens, and AA passes near the posterior laminar line. With anterior atlanto-occipital displacement, line DD passes closer to or through the tip of the dens. The opisthion is often hard to see.

4–5 mm above the tip of the dens and is bound to the basion by the apical ligament, the aforementioned disruption of the atlanto-occipital ligaments and membranes invariably results in an anterior location of the basion with regard to the tip of the dens. It has been my practice, therefore, to construct a line parallel to the posterior surface of the dens and body of C2 passing through the tip of the dens and extrapolated through the base of the skull. This basiepistropheal-apical line invariably intersects the basion or passes within 2 mm posterior to it. The line generally intersects the base of C2 between the midpoint and junction of the middle and posterior thirds (see Fig. 4.16 for examples of this line). Although others have recognized a fairly constant relationship between the basion and the tip of the odontoid process (36, 37), there has been no quantification of atlanto-occipital alignment. The value of the basiepistro-

pheal-apical line has recently been detailed and confirmed (38). It must be noted that in posterior AODs, the Powers ratio is less than 1. Since a Powers ratio of less than 1 may be normal, the posterior AOD is therefore disregarded. Lee's method is also imprecise since the opisthion may not be seen well enough to be detected.

Gammal and Brooks noted that on an upright, neutral-position lateral view, a line drawn along the plane of the clivus will normally point to the top of the odontoid process (39). I have found this to work only with the patient's neck in 20–30° of extension. Use of the basiepistropheal-apical line makes posterior AOD readily recognizable regardless of the degree of flexion of the neck and, since the advent of MR imaging, suggests that it may not be quite so rare (see below).

There have been a number of case reports of anterior AOD with brief or prolonged survival

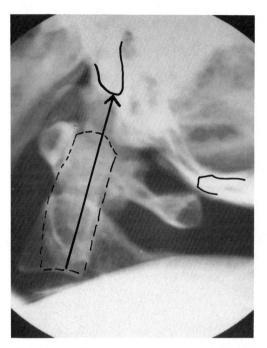

**Figure 4.16.** The author's method of evaluating the cranioatlantoaxial alignment. A line passing parallel to the posterior surface of C2 through the tip of the dens intersects or passes within a few millimeters behind the basion.

(17). Since these injuries are usually fatal, the condition may not be seriously considered and may be overlooked, as in the case in Figure 4.17. A 7-year-old boy injured in a motor vehicle accident sustained an anterior AOD that is obvious in retrospect but was not initially suspected by the general radiologist. The axial CT was deceptive since the forward displacement of the occiput on the atlas can only be ascertained by comparative measurements of the distance of basion and of the dens to the bottom of the frame on the axial CT images. (A warning is in order here to those who rely only on axial CT imaging of the cranioatlantoaxial junction. Axial CT, especially with thin slices alone, will frequently fail to suggest AOD. Thin-section CT with multiplanar reformation in the midline and through the atlanto-occipital joints would be diagnostic, as would midline conventional tomograms and sagittal MR images. The condition has been recognized on base views of the skull and on laminagraphy.) Slight technical underexposure of the lateral projection of the cervical spine and rotation of the head to one side frequently obscures the clivus and anterior lip of

the foramen magnum, further increasing the risk of not making the correct diagnosis early.

Although pure posterior AODs have traditionally been considered to be rare and usually fatal (40–43), the ease of visualizing the atlanto-occipital junction on MR imaging and the use of the basiepistropheal-apical line have made this displacement more readily appreciated (Fig. 4.18). In such cases the anterior and posterior atlanto-occipital ligaments are stretched or partially torn or an occult fracture of the tip of the dens (os odontoideum), increased ligamentous laxity secondary to inflammation, or other anomaly may be present.

I believe that posterior AODs are virtually a physical impossibility in the presence of an intact dens and atlas. Patzakis et al. reported a case with recovery in whom he showed an anterior arch of C1 behind the dens with a chip fracture of C2 anteriorly and superiorly (41). Tomograms showed no fracture of the dens. According to the x-ray, the apical ligament apparently was disrupted and the author would have us believe that the arch of C1 jumped the dens. Haralson and Boyd's (42) and Sassard et al.'s (43) cases were equally startling. Thin-section CT with multiplanar reformations and MR imaging were not available at that time and might have shed additional light on the cases these authors described.

## JEFFERSON FRACTURE

Sir Geoffrey Jefferson (1920) described four cases of fracture of the atlas vertebra and analyzed 42 previously recorded cases (44). He observed that the common cause was a fall on the head. The downward and outward movement of the occipital condyles into the lateral masses of C1 and the upward-outward thrust of the lateral masses produced a combined outward vector spreading the atlas outward and laterally, causing a separation of the lateral masses of C1 (Figs. 4.19 and 4.20). If the head hits the ground or a stationary object while inclined to one side, the force passes in greater proportion through one lateral mass but frequently produces a tension fracture of the arch elsewhere.

Fracture of the atlas was once thought to be frequently fatal, but Jefferson himself noted a recovery rate of 45.7% and cord injury in only 50% of the cases he studied. Except for Astley Cooper's case in 1922 of a 3-year-old boy (45), Jefferson fractures have been extremely rare in preteen-

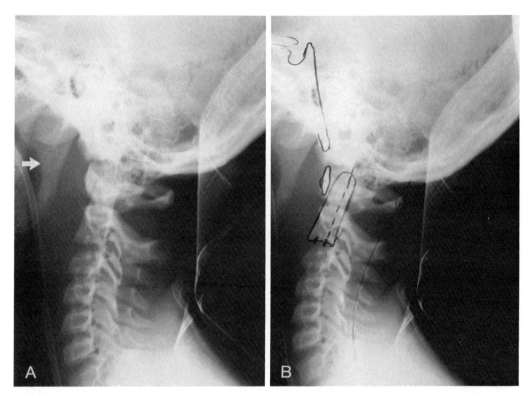

**Figure 4.17.**    Radiographs of a 9-year-old boy with neck pain and quadriparesis following a motor vehicle accident. *A*, Supine lateral projection shows a subtle and initially missed anterior atlanto-occipital dislocation. Note the prevertebral soft tissue swelling *(arrow)*. *B*, Use of the author's line in this case.

agers. Suss et al. attribute this to the fact that children weigh less and have a more plastic and absorbent skull and more flexible neck and that the synchondroses of C1 may serve as an elastic buffer (46). Referring to Jefferson's schematic (Fig. 4.19*A*), the lesser wedge of children's occipital condyles suggests a possible additional explanation for the relative rarity of Jefferson fractures in children.

In 21 (or half) of Jefferson's cases there were isolated fractures of the atlas, and 25 were complicated by multiple fractures, atlantodental subluxations, or rotary atlantoaxial dislocation. Computed tomography is singularly well suited for displaying atlas fractures, and the incidence of multiple fractures demonstrated by CT indicates that they occur more frequently than was originally suspected. It has long been known that fractures of the posterior arch are readily detected on conventional roentgenograms whereas fractures of the anterior arch, lateral masses, and occipital condyles are picked up with greater frequency on CT.

Jefferson's work almost completely eliminated hyperextension of the neck as a cause of atlas fractures resulting from crushing between the occipital bone and posterior arch of C2. While sudden severe hyperextension of the neck could theoretically produce these fractures, in practice most of Jefferson's cases occurred without extension or actually in flexion. Similarly there was no convincing evidence of neck extension having caused the dens to fracture the anterior arch of C1. With a history of recent injury by a blow to or fall upon the head, rigidity of the neck, limitation of head movement, and perhaps hypesthesia or neuralgia in the territory of the first or second cervical nerves, which may be injured as well, a fracture of the atlas should always be considered. Good lateral radiographic technique, preferably with sharp stereoscopic lateral views, will frequently indicate the presence of this injury and suggest the need for CT.

Although Clark et al. found that in 62 of 137 patients plain films gave a full diagnosis and no additional information was afforded by other stud-

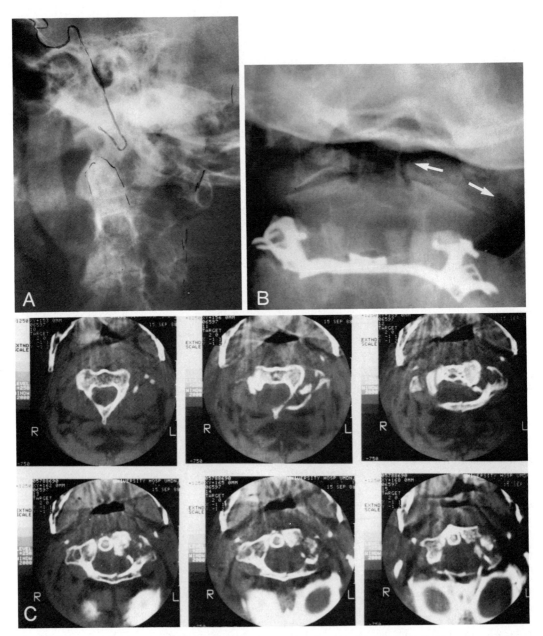

**Figure 4.18.**    Posterior atlanto-occipital dislocation. *A*, Lateral projection of the craniocervical junction of a 92-year-old man following a fall. A posterior occipitoatlantoaxial displacement is evident. *B*, The AP open-mouth view shows a "fat lateral mass" on the left, the equivalent of Smoker and Dolan's fat C2 in the lateral projection. *C*, Axial CT explains the posterior AOD, showing a comminuted and distracted fracture of the lateral mass of C1 on the left. A fracture of the atlas on the right is obscured. Type II rotary fixation is present on the left and the cranium and posterior arch of the atlas are displaced posteriorly—in essence an inclined Jefferson fracture.

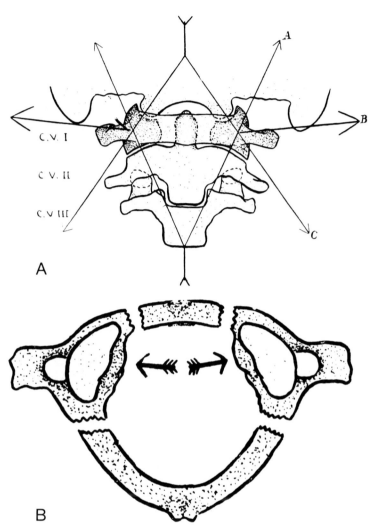

**Figure 4.19.** The Jefferson fracture. *A*, Jefferson's schematic representation of the forces, *A* and *C*, through the occipital condyles to the atlas, axis, and vertebral column. Note that the resultant (*B*) of these forces is more or less horizontal and "spreads" the atlas laterally. *B*, Axial view of the atlas to show the result of spreading on the bony arch which yields at its weak points. (From Jefferson G: Fracture of the atlas vertebra. *Br J Surg* 7:407–422, 1920.)

ies, they thought that plain films should be used to direct further diagnostic evaluations (47). In an equal number of cases additional studies complemented the plain films, and in 11 of 137 the plain films were deemed negative. These authors also found that pluridirectional tomograms were of particular value in evaluating the facets. Clark et al. (47), Keene et al. (48), Kershner et al. (49), Stern et al. (50), and Gehweiler et al. (51) all agreed that CT was especially valuable for detecting Jefferson fractures and in detecting laminar and posterior element fractures in general.

Congenital absence of the posterior arch of C1 and defects in fusion or segmentation may simulate fractures (50, 51) but are usually recognized on plain films obtained following various types of trauma to the head and neck. Otherwise these abnormalities would have gone unnoticed (52).

## HANGMAN'S FRACTURE

Judicial hanging is said to have been introduced into fifth centruy England by the Angles, Jutes, and Saxons (53, 54) and it was long presumed that

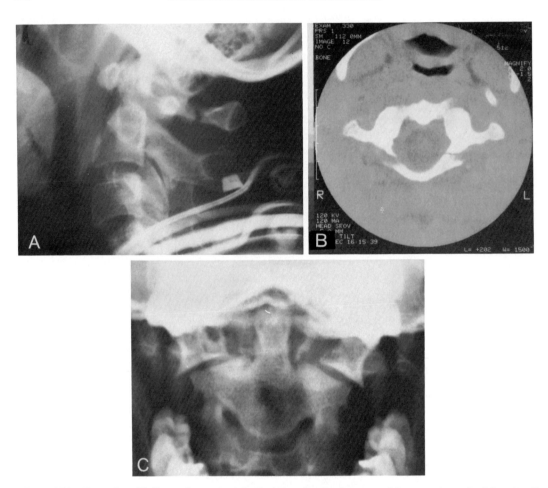

**Figure 4.20.**    Examples of Jefferson fractures. *A*, Lateral view showing fractures of the posterior arch of the atlas. *B* Similar case showing posterior arch fractures on CT. *C*, Classic open-mouth appearance showing spreading of the lateral masses of C1.

death occurred by strangulation. However, this appears only to occur with a "short drop" of only a few inches, whereas a "long drop" of close to 15 feet was reported by Paterson in 1890 to have produced near decapitation in one victim and complete decapitation in a second (53). Paterson described fractures through the pedicles of C2 following a drop of 6½ feet with fracture-dislocation, fracture of the transverse process of C2 on the left, and fractures of both transverse processes of C3. Rupture of the anterior and posterior longitudinal ligaments occurred, and the posterior antlantoaxial membrane and vertebral artery were torn. The spinal cord was ruptured at C2–3 and the C2 nerve roots and meninges were torn; however, the occipital bone, the atlas, the dens, the body of the axis, and the transverse ligament were intact. The fractured pedicles contin-

ued inferiorly into the body of C3. Fractures of this type are typical of hanging with the knot beneath the chin (submental knot), which produces a hyperextension of the neck, in contrast to the subaural knot, which produces a sharp lateral tilt and is more likely to produce a fracture through the body of the axis below the atlantoaxial joints. The hangman's fracture of the pedicles of C2 resulting from hyperextension injuries is therefore comparable to that resulting from a 6½ foot drop with a submental knot.

The hangman's fracture—which more correctly should be called the hanged man's fracture, since the executioner escapes unscathed—commonly occurs as a result of a motor vehicle accident in which an unrestrained motorist or one wearing only a lap belt jackknifes forward, flexing at the waist and striking his chin against the steering wheel with the neck extended or the face against the windshield (Fig. 4.21). Typically there are fractures through both pedicles of C2 where they have been avulsed from the body of the axis. Garber (48) is credited with characterizing the condition as traumatic spondylolisthesis. As with judicial hanging with a subaural knot, a hyperextension injury with a head tilted may result in the fracture extending into the body of the axis and into the temporal bone in the base of the skull. As with hyperextension injuries of the lower cervical spine, a disruption of the disc bond frequently occurs; however, the forward luxation of the body of C2 and the death-averting decompression of the upper cervical cord may actually spare the patient the devastating neurologic deficit seen with retrolisthesis. Trauma to the vertebral arteries at the time of injury has been reported to produce vertebrobasilar insufficiency with visual and brainstem signs.

## ATLANTOAXIAL DISLOCATIONS DUE TO LIGAMENT INJURIES

Since the odontoid process of C2 is bound to the anterior arch of C1, in order for the atlas to dislocate on the axis either the dens must break or be deficient or the ligaments that bind the anterior arch of C1 to the dens must be torn or be deficient from some other cause. The transverse ligament–odontoid system is therefore the main stabilizing bond of the atlantoaxial complex. While disrupting the transverse and alar ligaments can lead to lethal cord compression between the anteriorly displaced posterior arch of C1 and the upward projecting dens, a fracture through the base of the dens generally causes a less serious deformity without cord compression.

Traumatic atlantoaxial dislocation most commonly occurs with head injuries. Gehweiler et al., in reviewing the Duke series of 400 patients, found that in atlantoaxial dislocations due to trauma the dens fractured almost five times more frequently than atlantoaxial dislocations with tears of the transverse ligaments (18). They observed 11% of atlantoaxial dislocations with fracture of the dens and 2.5% without fracture. Those authors could not be certain of the incidence of nontraumatic dislocations. With our sizable population with infectious disease and others with rheumatoid arthritis, we also find more nontraumatic inflammatory disease–related displace-

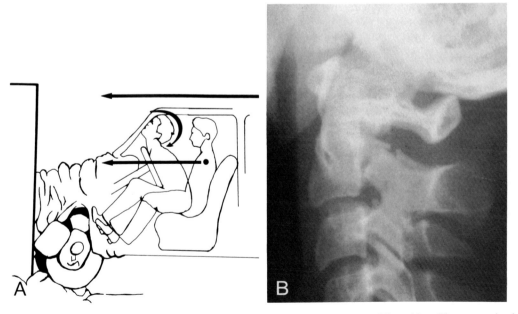

**Figure 4.21.** Hangman's fracture. *A*, Mechanism of "hangman" injury in an automobile accident. The unrestrained driver pitches forward, impaling the thorax on the steering wheel. If the face strikes the windshield before the vertex of the head does, the head is forced backward in hyperextension. This produces the cervical injury. (From Daffner RH: *Imaging of Vertebral Trauma.* Rockville, MD, Aspen Publishers, Inc, 1988.) *B*, Typical appearance of the traumatic spondyloschisis of C2, or hangman's fracture.

ments than traumatic displacements. These non-traumatic displacements may mimic those resulting from injury and are discussed further below.

## Rupture of the Transverse and Alar Ligaments

Steel (55) observed that the maximum normal translation of the odontoid posteriorly with respect to the atlas is 3 mm in adults, or 20% of the transverse diameter of the odontoid, and 4 mm in children, or 30% of the transverse diameter. The transverse ligament limits posterior movement of the dens. The alar ligaments limit rotation of the head and are a second line of defense in preventing posterior dislocation. The laxity of the alar ligaments is necessary to permit rotation, and this is taken up when the transverse ligament is deficient and the dens moves back a distance equal to its full transverse diameter. The safety zone or space between the back of the dens and the medulla on 100 normal air myelograms in adults and in 25 autopsied children was equal to or slightly greater than the diameter of the odontoid process. This constitutes the rule of thirds: one third cord, one third odontoid, and one third space. [Bailey proclaimed the rule of thirds as well having described it at a meeting at about the same time as Steel's abstract was presented (56).] Steel believed that the transverse ligament ordinarily ruptures laterally near its attachment to the anterior arch of the atlas rather than behind the dens.

In a biomechanical study of cadaver craniovertebral specimens, Fielding et al. (36) mounted C2 in epoxy and pulled C1 forward against the strength of the ligaments. These authors found the same 3-mm distance, or atlantodens interval (ADI), between the odontoid and anterior arch of C1 as Steel had reported. (The ADI is also called the predental space or middle atlantoaxial joint.) As the force increased, the transverse ligament ruptured abruptly, usually at its midportion (and not laterally as Steel had suggested), occasionally with an avulsion chip fracture. With the rupture of the transverse ligament, the ADI increased up to 5 mm. Continued force caused gradual disruption of the alar and other ligaments, increasing the ADI to 10 to 12 mm and leaving virtually no dead space. Since the force required to rupture the transverse ligament is roughly equal to that which may cause failure of the other ligaments, an individual with a deficient transverse ligament is in jeopardy of not being able to withstand a sec-

ond such injury. A minor injury or forced flexion with an ADI of 10 mm is therefore likely to be fatal. In postmortem cases studied by Steel in which an avulsed tip of the dens fatally traumatized the cord, the alar ligament was disrupted at the avulsed fragment while it was intact around the remainder of the odontoid process.

However, a deficient transverse ligament may not be visible on lateral roentgenograms, a sagittal "scout view" on CT, or sagittal MR imaging in the supine or neutral position and may only be evident on flexion-extension films. Because of the remarkable ability to study the cervical spine in orthogonal projections with MR imaging, we have also been able to study the neck in flexion and extension using this method. A sagittal section is performed with a thick sponge or pillow beneath the shoulders for the extension study, and another with sponges moved to a position beneath the occiput for the flexion examination. Needless to say, this should not be performed if there is imminent risk of cord compression by such maneuvers.

Penning suggested that the atlas be thought of as a ball bearing between the occiput and C2 (57). Motion at the atlanto-occipital joints is limited to up to 13° of flexion and 25° of extension, with no rotation and almost no lateral flexion possible (36, 58). The atlantoaxial joints permit about 10° of flexion-extension and 22–58° of rotation, with an average of 47°. Although the head can be turned up to 90°, most of this movement involves the lower cervical spine (58).

## Atlantoaxial Dynamics and Rotary Fixation

The joints between the atlas and the axis consist of two lateral atlantoaxial joints plus the atlantodental or middle atlantoaxial joint. Within normal ranges of rotation to either side, the dens maintains its close relationship to the anterior arch of the atlas. Thus in turning the head, the atlas pivots about the dens. For example, in turning the head to the right, the lateral mass of C1 on the left slides anteriorly and medially while the atlantoarticular mass of C1 on the ipsilateral right atlantoaxial joint rotates posteriorly and medially. This is readily appreciated if one considers the appearance in the axial plane, similar to that shown in Fielding and Hawkins Type I rotary fixation (see below).

Wortzman and Dewar (59) have pointed out that because of the oval or reniform shape of the contralateral left lateral mass, which swings forward with its long axis closer to the transverse plane, the left lateral mass will appear wider when seen on the AP open-mouth view. The space between this lateral mass and the odontoid process appears to get smaller. Sliding of the ipsilateral mass backward and downward may cause the joint to appear smaller on the open-mouth view with the head turned 15° to the left, while the upward and forward contralateral movement may make the joint appear wider (59). Previously Jacobson and Adler (60) had observed that turning the head 15–20° to one side is associated with a posteromedial offset of the ipsilateral lateral mass that normally exceeds the contralateral anteromedial offset.

The slope of the atlantoaxial joints does not permit pure lateral flexion. To accomplish tilting to one side there must be an accompanying rotation of C2 to the same side. For example, if the head is tilted to the right, there is rotation of C2 to the right, causing the spinous process to project to the left. If the lateral flexion occurs as a result of torticollis with muscle spasm, the head and atlas would tend to turn to the right with C2. In order to look straight ahead, the head is turned forward (i.e., to the left), and an open-mouth view will show the spinous process projecting to the left of the midline. On CT this may be quite subtle and confusing. The clue is an apparent tilting of the base of the skull despite the technician's best efforts to position the head straight. Clinically, a typical stance is recognizable whether the torticollis is due to injury or infection, with the head tilting and rotated like a cock robin with tilted head listening for a worm. It is thus necessary to understand the atlantoaxial dynamics to appreciate the CT and MR imaging appearance.

The rotary fixation of the atlantoaxial joint described by Wortzman and Dewar has been further defined by Fielding and Hawkins (61), who divided it into four categories (Fig. 4.22). Type I, the most common in these authors' experience, represents rotary fixation without anterior displacement of the atlas. The amount of rotational misalignment is within the normal range of the atlantoaxial dynamics described above. It is frequently seen in patients, especially children, with a torticollis following an injury. The atlanto-odontoid ligaments are intact. The dens acts as pivot. In Type II, the second most common in occurrence, there is deficiency in the transverse ligament with unilateral displacement of the lateral mass on one side. In the Type II anterior rota-

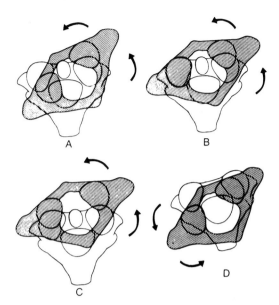

**Figure 4.22.** Atlantoaxial rotary fixation. *A*, Type I: rotary fixation without anterior displacement of the atlas. *B*, Type II: rotary fixation with anterior displacement of the atlas of 3 to 5 mm. One lateral mass of the atlas acts as a pivot. *C*, Type III: rotary fixation with anterior displacement of the atlas of more than 5 mm. *D*, Type IV: rotary fixation with posterior displacement of the atlas of the type seen in patients with fractured dens, os odontoideum, or rare cases of true absence of the dens. (From Fielding JW, Hawkins RJ: Atlanto-axial rotatory fixation. *J Bone Joint Surg* [*Am*] 59:37–44, 1977.)

tional misalignment, the ADI measures 3–5 mm in an adult. One lateral mass acts as a pivot while the other rotates anteromedially.

Type III was seen in less than one fifth of Fielding and Hawkins' cases. A fairly marked anterior rotational atlantoaxial subluxation of the two lateral and middle (atlantodental) articulations is present in this type, with forward displacement of the atlas greater than 5 mm indicating deficiency in the transverse and alar ligaments. In order for anterior atlantoaxial subluxation to occur all three joints must be involved. This is potentially the most dangerous of the four types. Type IV, the rarest form, represents a posterior rotational displacement seen in patients with fractures of the dens or in deficiencies of the odontoid (e.g., rheumatoid arthritis).

## ATLANTOAXIAL DISPLACEMENTS WITHOUT INJURY

The intact transverse ligament is normally stronger than the dens, which explains why fractures of the dens are more common than transverse and alar ligamentous disruptions. Nontraumatic atlantoaxial dislocations due to infection are "dead ringers" for those resulting from ligamentous injuries. They have been known for 160 years, since Sir Charles Bell reported an ulcer of the pharynx with a dislocation of the atlas (62). Similar cases were reported by Grisel (63) (the French still call the condition the "maladie de Grisel"), Desfosses (64), Coutts (65), Hess et al. (66), Sullivan (33), and Watson Jones (67), who published his two cases as "spontaneous hyperaemic dislocation of the atlas" and reviewed 14 others.

Sullivan's cases followed the flu or pharyngitis, and sore throat one to several weeks after the infection. He recognized that there was weakening of the lateral ligaments as well as the transverse ligament (33). Wilson found an average of 85.6% of such cases in patients under 13 years of age (68). Sullivan reviewed 56 cases and found that 76.8% of the patients were under 13 years of age, with an average age of 12.2 years (33). Watson Jones published a rare postmortem specimen of anterior atlantoaxial dislocation, shedding light on this condition. Virtually all of his cases and those of others have had infectious complaints of pharyngitis, tonsillitis, mastoiditis, middle ear disease, or tuberculous or pyogenic cervical adenitis (33,66,67). The most common associated condition was nasopharyngeal infection. The infections led to inflammation and decalcification of the insertion of the transverse and alar ligaments.

In addition to the infectious diseases incriminated in producing occipitoatlantoaxial dislocations, rheumatoid disease has been a frequently associated condition in our experience. Margulies et al. (69) reported the spontaneous dislocation of the dens in rheumatoid arthritis, as did Gleason and Urist (70).

Spitzer et al. (71) were the first to observe atlantoaxial dislocation in mongoloidism. Martel and Tishler studied 70 mongoloid subjects selected randomly; atlas dislocation was observed in 14 of 70 subjects of various ages (72). One also may see disc thinning and cervical Schmorl nodes in children with Down's syndrome. In 1965 Tishler and Martel had described 4 of 18 mongoloid individuals, mostly children, with dislocation of the atlas (72). Anterior atlantoaxial displacement has also been described in mucopolysaccaridosis type IV (73,74).

## FRACTURES OF THE ODONTOID PROCESS

To understand certain peculiarities about the odontoid process and anomalies associated with this region requires a brief word about the embryology of the craniocervical junction. The occipital bone forms from four sclerotomes, the most caudal of which develops into the proatlas or a separate bone between the occipital bone and atlas in reptiles and birds. In man the anterior arch of the atlas develops from the proatlas and the posterior arch from the first cervical sclerotome. The proatlas in man separates into an anterior arch of the atlas and the body of C1, which will become the dens. The axis forms from the second cervical sclerotome. The tip of the dens is formed by the ossiculum terminale, which is derived from the body of the proatlas and appears between ages 3 and 6 and fuses by age 12.

The posterior arch of the atlas forms from the first cervical sclerotome, usually fusing by age 3. Examples of nonfusion that may simulate fractures are discussed below. The body or anterior arch of C1 is separated from the neural arch by the neurocentral synchondrosis, which fuses at about age 7.

The primitive body of C1 will begin to fuse with that of C2 between ages 3 and 6, forming the odontoid process. This subdental synchondrosis, a remnant of the notochord, is situated at or above the level of the superior articular facets of C2, which distinguishes it from a fracture of the dens. When a fracture of the dens is suspected above the superior articular facets, a diagnosis of "synchondrotic slip" [Fielding et al.'s term (36)] should be considered. A persistent anterior arch of the proatlas may remain fused with the basion to form a so-called third or median occipital condyle—Lombardi's occipital vertebra (75). The anlage of the centrum of the proatlas that will form the tip of the dens appears at ages 2 to 5 and fuses with the dens between 10 and 13 years of age. When it remains as a separate ossicle, the ossiculum terminale (76), a defect will be seen in the tip of the odontoid in which the ossicle rests (77). Such an odontoid with a V-shaped defect is called a bicornuate dens and may be seen physiologically in young children.

### Os Odontoideum

The os odontoideum was first described by Giacomini in 1886 (78). It is currently believed to represent a nonfused hypertrophic remnant of the centrum of the proatlas and is associated with hypoplasia of the dens and absence of the distal ossification (58). The dens appears hypoplastic, with a dome-shaped superior surface, whereas the os odontoideum is round or oval in shape and usually lies close to the basion (dystopic) but is occasionally close to the dens (orthotopic). Its round inferior surface distinguishes it from an old ununited fracture (18). The association of a congenitally absent dens with a variety of neurologic syndromes has been noted by other authors as well (76). What at first inspection may appear to be a congenitally absent dens on closer inspection is seen to represent a dystopic os odontoideum. Braakman and Penning (20) noted the condition called "epiphysiolysis dentis" wherein a fractured dens may resorb with time, simulating a congenital absence of the dens. Like Gleason and Urist, we have also observed a number of patients with advanced rheumatoid arthritis with near total resorption of the dens, another cause for disappearance of the dens. The remnant may resemble an orthotopic os odontoideum.

## Types of Odontoid Fractures

A fracture through the base of the dens generally causes a less serious deformity without cord compression. With such a fracture, the odontoid remains bound to the anterior arch of the atlas and the ring of C1 and the dens will be carried forward, sparing the cord, which will not be compressed as it may be between a posteriorly displaced dens and an anteriorly displaced posterior arch of C1.

Anderson and D'Alonzo (79) studied fractures of the odontoid process and classified them into three types. Fracture of the upper part of the odontoid is called Type I. It is rare and probably represents an avulsion fracture by the alar ligaments of the proatlas or ossiculum terminale. It often appears as an oblique fracture through the odontoid tip. These should be treated conservatively.

Type II is the most common odontoid fracture, occurring in the base of the dens at or above the level of the superior facets of C2 (Fig. 4.23). The fragment may not appear displaced, but may angle or toggle in flexion and extension. This fracture may occur as a result of a flexion or extension injury. It is frequently unstable and leads to nonunion. Since it may not be associated with a pro-

found neurologic deficit, it may be picked up as an incidental finding. A Type II "fracture" in children may be actually related to a separation through the subdental synchondrosis, which is present up to age 3 and is usually closed by age 6. One explantion of the Type II fractures is the weakening of the dens at the site of the subdental synchondrosis.

Type III is a fracture at the base of the dens extending into the body of the axis (Fig. 4.24). This fracture passes through cancellous bone, is usually stable, and generally heals with union. Gehweiler et al. (18) referred to the Type II fracture as a "high" dens fracture and the Type III as a "low" dens fracture. In the lateral projection, the low dens fracture is seen to disrupt the Harris (axis) ring, whereas this ring is intact in the high dens fracture (79–81). This is a most useful sign since low dens fractures may not be visualized in the frontal projection. In children a fracture through the synchondrosis may be suspected if widening of the synchondrosis is present or there is forward tilting of the dens; slight posterior tilting of the dens may be seen normally.

The sometimes confusing differentiation between a persistent synchondrosis and a fracture has prompted Segall et al. (82) to suggest the use of the term "separate odontoid" to avoid the need of distinguishing a congenital os odontoideum from a posttraumatic lesion. However, the reader is reminded that fractures of the dens are usually below the level of the superior articular facets of C2, whereas the subdental synchondrosis is usually higher.

Although a fracture passing obliquely through the base of the axis may not be appreciated on plain films, an increased AP diameter of C2 on the lateral projection—Smoker and Dolan's "fat C2 sign" (83)—may alert the physician to the fracture, which will readily be confirmed on thin-section CT. The equivalent of the "fat C2"—a "fat articular mass"—is seen in an AP open-mouth view of a fractured lateral mass of C1 (Fig. 4.18B) and can be clarified by thin-section CT.

In addition to superimposition of normal structures such as the upper incisors simulating fractures of the dens, Mach bands are one of the most common causes of radiographic pseudofractures (Fig. 4.25). Ernst Mach (1838–1916), an Austrian physicist-philosopher-psychologist, discovered the phenomenon that bears his name. Mach bands are bright or dark "lines" representing a perceptual phenomenon that appears at the borders of

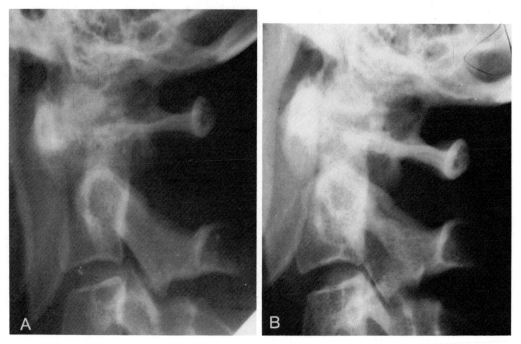

**Figure 4.23.**  Type II high dens fracture. *A*, High dens fracture before reduction in a 25-year-old woman injured in a motor vehicle accident. *B*, Reduction under fluoroscopy with the patient in a halo device.

structures of different optical or radiographic densities (84). They are also evident at the spaces between the corners of adjacent CT images on a clear film base.

## GUNSHOT WOUNDS

Another category of cervical trauma deserving brief comment is gunshot wounds of the cervical spine and spinal cord. Although they are no great diagnostic challenge, missile fragments can produce troublesome artifacts. Even those lodged within the spinal cord may be removed with some degree of recovery (85–87).

## CERVICAL TRAUMA WITH MINIMAL OBJECTIVE RADIOLOGIC FINDINGS

Following a neck injury objective evidence of a cause of neck pain with or without radiculitis may elude the neuroradiologist. Some of these more subtle and confusing conditions—such as nonlethal atlanto-occipital disruptions, fractures of vertebral pillars, and torticollis—have been described. Other such conditions include cerebellar tonsillar herniation and posttraumatic dissection of the vertebral artery. Whiplash injury (the cer-

vical acceleration-deceleration syndrome) has long been recognized as one such category. Some of these injuries have obvious CT abnormalities, as in Glenn's case of an ossified posterior longitudinal ligament producing cervical cord compression leading to quadriplegia after a "minor" whiplash injury (88). More subtle signs of whiplash may be detected by MR imaging, including posttraumatic synovitis of the apophyseal joints as well as the more obvious conditions already described in this chapter.

Patients with preexisting pathology such as multiple sclerosis, tumors, syringomyelia, and cervical spondylosis and chronic disc herniation with chronic nerve root or cord compression may experience an exacerbation of symptoms with acute cervical trauma (Fig. 4.5*B*). Chronic preexisting spondylotic ridging or disc herniation leaves little room for the spinal cord in the event of a hyperflexion injury. Epidural scarring from previous surgery may also become symptomatic following injury; a gadolinium-enhanced $T_1$-weighted MR image may confirm this diagnosis.

In other cases, confronted with equivocal and contradictory findings on a multitude of diagnostic studies in patients with unexplained disabling pain, a combined approach by the neuroradiolo-

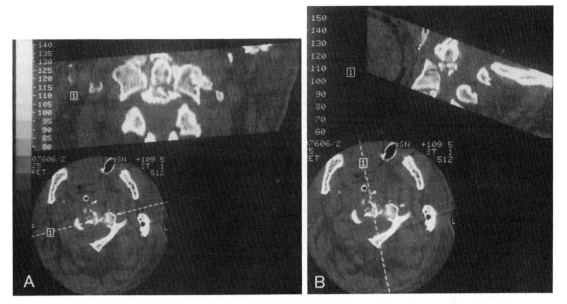

**Figure 4.24.** Type III fractures of the dens. Coronal (*A*) and sagittal (*B*) reformations show the fracture extends into body of the axis.

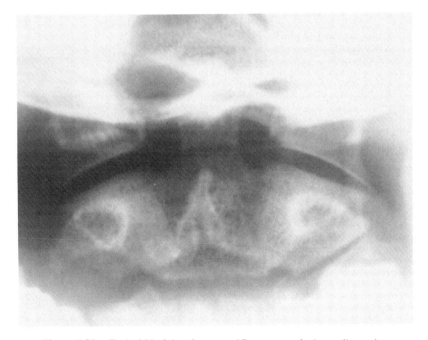

**Figure 4.25.** Typical Mach band seen on AP open-mouth view radiograph.

gist and algologist or pain management specialist may provide both diagnosis and therapeutic relief to the patient.

## SUMMARY

Radiologic imaging of conditions associated with painful trauma have been described. While CT and MR imaging have enhanced our diagnostic armamentarium, it must be recognized that each of the conditions in this chapter also may be diagnosed on plain films, tomography, and radionuclide studies. The choice of the safest and most cost-effective procedures should be coordinated between the referring physician and the neuroradiologist. The neuroradiologist with a full understanding of the organ system and skilled in the use of all neuroradiologic diagnostic modalities at his disposal offers the greatest likelihood of diagnosing the nature of painful cervical trauma. The referring physician should be wary of the diagnostician who concentrates on one modality, such as CT or MR imaging alone.

*Acknowledgments.* The author wishes to offer special thanks to Aspen Publishers for the use of Dr. R. H. Daffner's schematics and examples; to Churchill Livingstone for the use of Drs. Rogers and Lee's case; to the *British Journal of Surgery* for the use of Sir Geoffrey Jefferson's original schematics; and to the *Journal of Bone and Joint Surgery* for the use of Drs. Fielding and Hawkins' schematics of atlantoaxial rotatory fixation. I am also grateful to Dr. Kathy Maldjian for her considerable help in retrieving from our files so many of the cases evaluated for inclusion in the chapter.

## REFERENCES

1. Wales LR, Knopp RK, Morishima MS: Recommendations for evaluation of the acutely injured cervical spine: a clinical radiologic algorithm. *Ann Emerg Med* 9(8):422–428, 1980.
2. Rogers LF, Lee C: Cervical Spine Trauma. In Dalinka MK, Kaye JJ (eds): *Radiology in Emergency Medicine.* New York, Churchill Livingstone, Inc, 1984, pp 275–316.
3. Mirvis SE, Diaconis JN, Chirico PA, Reiner BI, Joslyn JN, Militello P: Protocol-driven radiologic evaluation of suspected cervical spine injury: efficacy study. *Radiology* 170:831–834, 1989.
4. Nichols CG, Young DH, Schiller WR: Evaluation of cervicothoracic junction injury. *Ann Emerg Med* 16:640–642, 1987.
5. Miller MD, Gehweiler JA, Martinez S, et al: Significant new observations on cervical spine trauma. *Am J Roentgenol* 130:659–663, 1978.
6. Evans DK: Dislocations at the cervicothoracic junction. *J Bone Joint Surg [Br]* 65:124–127, 1983.
7. Faerber EN, Wolpert SM, Scott RM, Belkin SC, Carter BL: Computed tomography of spinal fractures. *J Comput Assist Tomogr* 3(5):657–661, 1979.
8. Brant-Zawadski M, Miller EM, Federle MP: CT in the evaluation of spine trauma. *AJR* 136:369–375, 1981.
9. Handel SF, Lee Y-Y: Computed tomography of spinal fractures. *Radiol Clin North Am* 19:69–89, 1981.
10. Post MJ, Green BA, Quencer RM, Stokes NA, Callahan RA, Eismont FJ: The value of computed tomography in spinal trauma. *Spine* 7:417–431, 1982.
11. Keene JS, Goletz TH, Lilleas F, Alter AJ, Sackett JF: Diagnosis of vertebral fractures. A comparison of conventional radiography, conventional tomography and computed axial tomography. *J Bone Joint Surg [Am]* 65(4):586–594, 1982.
12. Post MJD, Green BA: The use of CT in spinal trauma. *Radiol Clin North Am* 21(2):327–375, 1983.
13. Boynton LW, Kalb R: Double lumen sign as demonstrated by computerized tomography in spine dislocations. *Spine* 8(8):910–912, 1983.
14. Shetty AK, Deeb ZL, Hryshko FG: Computed tomography of the spine. *J Comput Tomogr* 8(2):105–112, 1984.
15. Pech P, Kolgore DP, Pojunas KW, Haughton VM: Cervical spinal fractures: CT detection. *Radiology* 157(1):117–121, 1985.
16. Acheson MB, Livingston RR, Richardson ML, Stimac GK: High-resolution CT scanning in the evaluation of cervical spine fractures: comparison with plain film examinations. *AJR* 148:1179–1185, 1987.
17. Daffner RH: *Imaging of Vertebral Trauma.* Rockville, MD, Aspen Publishers, Inc, 1988.
18. Gehweiler JA Jr, Osborne RLL Jr, Becker RF: *The Radiology of Vertebral Trauma.* Philadelphia, WB Saunders, 1980.
19. Swischuk LE: Anterior displacement of C2 in children—physiologic and pathologic. (A helpful differentiating line). *Radiology* 122:759–763, 1977.
20. Braakman R, Penning L: *Injuries of the Cervical Spine.* London, Excerpta Medica, 1971.
21. Naidich JB, Naidich TP, Garfein C, et al: The widened interspinous distance: a useful sign of anterior cervical dislocation in the supine frontal projection. *Radiology* 123:113–116, 1977.
22. Roaf R: A study of the mechanics of spinal injuries. *J Bone Joint Surg [Br]* 42:810, 1960.
23. Penning L: Prevertebral hematoma in cervical spine injury: incidence and etiologic significance. *AJR* 136:553–561, 1981.
24. Templeton PA, Young JWR, Mirvis SE, et al: The value of retropharyngeal soft tissue measurements in trauma of the adult spine. *Skeletal Radiol* 16:98–104, 1987.
25. Whalen JP, Woodruff CL: The cervical prevertebral fat stripe: a new aid in evaluating the cervical prevertebral soft tissue space. *AJR* 109:445–451, 1970.
26. Williams CF, Bernstein TW, Jelenko C III: Essentiality of the lateral cervical spine radiograph. *Ann Emerg Med* 10:198–204, 1981.
27. Miller MD, Gehweiler JA, Martinez S, Charlton OP, Daffner RH: Significant new observations on cervical spine trauma. *Am J Roentgenol* 130:659–663, 1978.
28. Abel MS: Occult traumatic lesions of the cervical spine. *Crit Rev Clin Radiol Nucl Med* 7:469, 1975.
29. Vines FS: The significance of "occult" fractures of the cervical spine. *AJR* 107:493, 1969.
30. Alker GJ, Oh YS, Leslie EV, et al: Postmortem radiology of

head and neck injuries in fatal traffic accidents. *Radiology* 114:611–617, 1975.

31. Dally: Torticollis occipito-atlantoidien. Bull Gen Ther, LXXXIX: pp 354, 356, 388, 400, 1875.

32. Englander O: Non-traumatic occipito-atlanto-axial dislocation. A contribution to the radiology of the atlas. *Br J Radiol* 15(180):341–345, 1942.

33. Sullivan AW: Subluxation of the atlanto-axial joint: sequel to inflammatory processes of the neck. *J Pediatrics* 35:451–464, 1949.

34. Powers B, Miller MD, Kramer RS, Martinez S, Gehweiler JA: Traumatic anterior atlanto-occipital dislocation. *J Neurosurg* 4:12, 1979.

35. Lee C, Woodring JH, Goldstein SJ, et al: Evaluation of traumatic atlantooccipital dislocations. *AJNR* 8:19–26, 1987.

36. Fielding JW, Hensinger RN, Bjorkengren AG, Hershman EB: Cranioatlantoaxial injuries. In Taveras and Ferucci (eds). Philadelphia, JB Lippincott, 1989, vol 5, chpt 141.

37. Weir DC: Roentgenographic signs of cervical injury. *Clin Orthop* 109:9, 1975.

38. Zimmer AE and Shabtai K: The Basiepistropheal-odontoid line in the evaluation of the cranio-cervical junction, 1991. Submitted for publication.

39. Gammal TE, Brooks BS: Radiologic evaluation of the craniovertebral junction. In Taveras and Ferrucci (eds). Philadelphia, JB Lippincott, 1989, vol 5, chpt 79.

40. Eismont FJ, Bohlman HH: Posterior atlanto-occipital dislocation with fractures of the atlas and odontoid process. Report of a case with survival. *J Bone Joint Surg [Am]* 60:397, 1978.

41. Patzakis MJ, Knopf A, Elfering M, Hoffer M, Harvey JP: Posterior dislocation of the atlas on the axis. *J Bone Joint Surg [Am]* 56:1260–1262, 1974.

42. Haralson RH, Boyd HB: Posterior dislocation of the atlas on the axis without fracture. Report of a case. *J Bone Joint Surg [Am]* 51:561–566, 1969.

43. Sassard WR, Heinig CF, Pitts WR: Posterior atlanto-axial dislocation without fracture. Case report with successful conservative treatment. *J Bone Joint Surg [Am]* 56:625–628, 1974.

44. Jefferson G: Fracture of the atlas vertebra. *Br J Surg* 7:407–422, 1920.

45. Cooper, Sir Astley P: *A Treatise on Dislocations and on Fractures of the Joints.* London, Longman, Hurst, Rees, Orme and Brown, 1822, p 549.

46. Suss RA, Zimmerman RD, Leeds NE: Pseudospread of the atlas: false sign of Jefferson fracture in young children. *AJNR* 4:183–186, 1983.

47. Clark CR, Igram CM, El-Khoury GY, Ehara S: Radiographic evaluation of cervical spine injuries. *Spine* 13(7):742–747, 1988.

48. Keene GCR, Hone MR, Sage MR: Atlas fractures; Demonstration using computerized tomography. *J Bone Joint Surg [Am]* 60:1106–1107, 1978.

49. Kershner MS, Goodman GA, Perlmutter GS: Computed tomography in the diagnosis of an atlas fracture. *AJR* 128:688–689, 1977.

50. Stern E, Pontorero M, Bhansali D, Rocko J: Developmental anomalies of the atlas vertebra. *Perspec. Radiol* 4:42–49, 1991.

51. Gehweiler JA Jr, Daffner RH, Roberts L Jr: Malformations of the atlas vertebra simulating the Jefferson fracture. *AJR* 140:1083–1086, 1983.

52. Garber JN: Abnormalities of the atlas and axis vertebrae—congenital and traumatic. *J Bone Joint Surg [Am]* 46:1782–1791, 1964.

53. Duff C: *A New Handbook on Hanging.* London, A Melrose Ltd, 1954.

54. Schneider RC, Livingston KE, Cave AJE, Hamilton G: "Hangman's fracture" of the cervical spine. *J Neurosurg* 22:141–154, 1965.

55. Steel HH: Anatomical and mechanical considerations of the atlanto-axial articulations. *J Bone Joint Surg [Am]* 50:1481–1482, 1968.

56. Bailey RW: Paper read at the annual meeting of the American Orthopaedic Association, Boca Raton, FL, April 1968.

57. Penning L: *Functional Pathology of the Cervical Spine.* Baltimore, Williams & Wilkins Co, 1968.

58. Shapiro R, Youngsberg AS, Rothman SL: The differential diagnosis of traumatic lesions of the atlanto-axial segment. *Radiol Clin North Am* 11:505–526, 1973.

59. Wortzman G, Dewar FP: Rotary fixation of the atlanto-axial joint: rotational atlanto-axial subluxation. *Radiology* 90:479–487, 1986.

60. Jacobson G, Adler DC: Examination of the atlanto-axial joint following injury with particular emphasis on rotational subluxation. *AJR* 76(6):1081–1094, 1956.

61. Fielding JW, Hawkins RJ: Atlanto-axial rotatory fixation. *J Bone Joint Surg [Am]* 59:37–44, 1977.

62. Bell, Sir Charles: Case report of dislocation of the atlas in man with an ulcer of the pharynx. In: The Nervous System of the Human Body, Embracing the papers delivered to The Royal Society on the subject of nerves. 118:403, 1830.

63. Grisel P: Enucléation de l'atlas et torticolli nasopharyngien. *Presse Med* 38:50, 1930.

64. Desfosses R: Un eas de maladie de Grisel: torticollis nasopharyngien par subluxation de l'atlas. *Press Med* 38:1179, 1930.

65. Coutts MB: Atlanto-epistropheal subluxations. *Arch Surg* 29(2), 1934.

66. Hess JH, Bronstein IP, Abelson SM: Atlanto-axial dislocations unassociated with trauma and secondary to inflammatory foci in the neck. *Am J Dis Child* 49:1137–1147, 1935.

67. Watson Jones R: Spontaneous hyperaemic dislocation of the atlas. *Proc R Soc Med* 25:586–590, 1932.

68. Wilson MJ, Michele A, Jacobson E: Spontaneous dislocation of the atlanto-axial articulation including a case with quadriplegia. *J Bone Joint Dis* 22:698, 1940.

69. Margulies ME, Kata I, Rosenberg M: Spontaneous dislocation of the atlantoaxial joint in rheumatoid spondylitis. *Neurology* 5:290, 1955.

70. Gleason IO, Urist MR: Atlanto-axial dislocation with odontoid separation in rheumatoid disease. *Clin Orthop* 42:121–129, 1965.

71. Spitzer R, Rabinowitz JY, Wybar KC: Study of abnormalities of skull, teeth and lenses in mongolism. *Can Med Assoc* 84:567–572, 1961.

72. Martel W, Tishler JM: Observations on the spine in mongoloidism. *AJR* 97:630–638, 1966.

73. McKusick VA: *Heritable Disorders of Connective Tissue.* St. Louis, CV Mosby, 1972.

74. Burrows E, Leads N: Increased ADI in mucopolysaccharoidosis IV. In Heinz ER (assoc ed): *Neuroradiology (The Clinical Neurosciences,* RN Rosenberg, ed). New York, Churchill Livingstone, 1981, p 415.

75. Lombardi G: The occipital vertebra. *AJR* 86(2):260–269, 1961.

76. Rowland LP, Shapiro J, Jacobson HG: Neurological syndromes associated with congenital absence of the odontoid process. *Arch Neurol Psychiatry* 80:286–291, 1958.

77. Wollin DG: The os odontoideum. Separate odontoid pro-
    cess. *J Bone Joint Surg [Am]* 45:1459–1471, 1963.
78. Giacomini C: Sull' esistenza dell' "os odontoideum" nell'
    uomo. *G R Accad Med Torino* 49:24–28, 1886.
79. Anderson LD, D'Alonzo RT: Fractures of the odontoid
    process of the axis. *J Bone Joint Surg [Am]* 56:1663–1674,
    1974.
80. Harris JH Jr, Burke JT, Ray RD, et al: Low (type III) odon-
    toid fracture: a new radiographic sign. *Radiology* 153:353–
    356, 1984.
81. Harris JH Jr: *The radiology of Acute Cervical Spine Trauma.*
    Baltimore, Williams & Wilkins, 1978.
82. Segall HD, Ahmadi J, Zea C-S, Stanley P: Pathology of the
    craniovertebral junction. In Taveras and Ferrucci (eds).
    Philadelphia, JB Lippincott, 1989, vol 5, chpt 81.
83. Smoker WRK, Dolan KD: The "fat" C2: a sign of fracture.
    *AJNR* 8:33–38, 1987.

84. Daffner RH: Pseudofracture of the dens: Mach bands. *AJR*
    128:607–612, 1977.
85. Hubschmann OR, Krieger AJ, Lax F, Ruzicka PO, Zimmer
    AE: Syndrome of intramedullary gunshot wound with in-
    complete neurologic deficit: case report. *J Trauma*
    28(11):1600–1602, 1988.
86. Plumley TF, Kilcoyne RF, Mack LA: Computed tomogra-
    phy in evaluation of gunshot wounds of the spine. *J Comput
    Assist Tomogr* 3:362–372, 1979.
87. Mangiardi JR, Alleva M, Dynia R, Zubowski R: Transoral re-
    moval of missile fragments from the C1–C2 area: report of
    four cases. *Neurosurgery* 23(2):254–257, 1988.
88. Glenn WV Jr: State-of-the-art cervical magnetic resonance/
    computed tomography imaging. In Foreman SM, Croft
    AC (eds): *Whiplash Injuries—The Cervical Deceleration
    Syndrome.* Baltimore, Williams & Wilkins, 1988, pp 159–
    210.

# 5

# ELECTRODIAGNOSTIC STUDIES

*Arminius Cassvan and Avital Fast*

Whereas roentgenography, magnetic resonance imaging, and computed tomography studies evaluate structural changes and abnormalities in the soft tissues or bony structures of the cervical spine, electrodiagnostic studies evaluate the functional integrity of the neural elements. Frequently, the clinical complaints and radiographic findings do not correlate. Individuals suffering from significant amount of pain may have minimal radiographic changes. It has been shown that no statistically significant relationship may be found between degenerative changes in the cervical spine and level of pain (1). In a substantial number of asymptomatic individuals one may find disc narrowing, osteophytosis, and even protruded discs (2).

In patients with upper extremity pain, numbness, or sensory or muscular deficiencies, the electrodiagnostic studies may help localize the lesion as distal (peripheral or entrapment neuropathy) versus proximal (plexopathy, radiculopathy, myelopathy). The tests help in delineating the damaged structures (e.g., axon, myelin) and in predicting the prognosis. It should be stressed that these studies are performed as an extension of the clinical evaluation and therefore should not be performed by a technician.

The first sections of this chapter are devoted to electromyography (EMG) and nerve conduction studies (NCS). The second part will deal with somatosensory evoked potential studies (SEPs).

## NEEDLE ELECTROMYOGRAPHY

During the electromyographic examination, a needle electrode is inserted into various muscles of the neck and upper extremities; thus muscles innervated by the anterior and posterior rami are sampled. Following needle insertion, observations are made with the muscle at rest, during insertion/needle probing, and at minimal and maximal contraction.

Except for endplate and fasciculation potentials, normally innervated muscles are silent at rest. Moving the needle briskly while it is in the muscle elicits a very short burst of electrical activity, the insertional activity. These potentials are generated when the tip of the advancing electrode mechanically disrupts the muscle fibers' membrane. Normally, insertional activity is of short duration, lasting 300–400 msec, or the equivalent of the time the tip of needle moves in the muscle. A finding of "increased insertional activity" is nonspecific and thus of no real significance.

During minimal contraction the needle records action potentials generated from contracting motor units adjacent to the tip of the electrode. As the contraction becomes stronger the firing rate of the units recruited first increases and more motor units gradually join in, so that on maximal effort there is a full interference pattern.

Axonal damage results in loss of motor units. During more advanced stages there may not be enough motor units left in order to produce a complete interference pattern. In extreme cases, when most of the motor units are lost, no recruitment may be obtained. In these cases the oscilloscope displays a pattern typical of single motor units even when the muscle is maximally contracted.

The electromyographer must evaluate the amplitude, shape, and duration of the motor units. The great majority of the motor units are triphasic, but about 10–15% of them may be polyphasic (more than four phases). Increased polyphasicity may be seen in muscles undergoing subsequent reinnervation by the remaining viable motor units. This pattern may be observed frequently when evaluating an old injury.

Damage to the anterior horn cells or their axons leads to pathologic action potentials that may be picked up by the needle electrode while the muscles are at rest. These potentials are generated most frequently by discharging single muscle fibers and represent membrane instability. Originally denervation was considered the only reason for this spontaneous activation of single muscle fibers, but they have since been found in myopathies or metabolic disorders as well, so the term "denervation potentials" was abandoned. The recorded potentials appear as positive sharp waves or fibrillation potentials (Fig. 5.1). These potentials are initially noted about 1 week following injury in the paraspinal muscles and between 3–4 weeks following injury in the extremity muscles. If a patient displays pathologic potentials earlier than this following trauma, one may conclude that axonal damage causing membrane instability existed prior to the accident.

Complex repetitive discharges are also seen with the muscle at rest. These are complex waves resulting from spontaneous firing of muscle fibers with a frequency of up to 150/sec. They tend to be triggered by the movement of the needle electrode in the muscle. These potentials may indicate irritability and may be seen in radiculopathies.

A special type of spontaneous activity is represented by fasciculation potentials, the electrical expression of slow rate discharges of the entire or a part of a motor unit. They may take any shape and amplitude, being characterized only by their irregular, slow rhythm. They may be benign or malignant, the latter being associated with amyotrophic lateral sclerosis but also thyrotoxicosis and radiculopathies.

A diagnosis of radiculopathy may be established when the EMG abnormalities are found in a myotomal distribution. The presence of membrane instability changes in the paraspinal muscles also points toward a proximal lesion and helps in establishing the diagnosis. Cervical surgical procedures performed using the posterior approach damage the paraspinal muscles and may thus lead to abnormal electrophysiologic findings in these muscles. In these cases the findings may result from the surgical procedure and do not necessarily indicate the presence of a radiculopathy.

If the EMG changes are found to be limited to muscles innervated by one peripheral nerve, one can establish a diagnosis of polyneuropathy rather than radiculopathy.

## NERVE CONDUCTION STUDIES

## MOTOR CONDUCTION

Electrical stimulation of accessible peripheral nerves enables us to determine the latencies and conduction velocities of these nerves. A surface recording electrode is placed on a peripheral muscle, as a rule the muscle most distally innervated by a particular nerve (i.e., abductor pollicis brevis for the median nerve, abductor digiti minimi for the ulnar nerve, and extensor indicis proprius for the radial nerve). The respective nerve is then stimulated at least at two levels, a distal and a proximal one. Following stimulation, the electrical current travels along the nerve, reaches the motor point, and evokes a muscle contraction. The muscular response is registered by the recording electrode and displayed on the oscilloscope. The examiner then determines the amplitude, shape, and latency of the evoked response. When the peripheral nerve is stimulated at two levels the conduction velocity can then be obtained by dividing the distance between the stim-

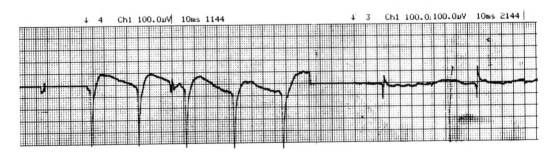

**Figure 5.1.**    Recorded potentials appear as positive sharp waves or fibrillation potentials.

ulated points by the latency difference obtained between the proximal and distal stimulation (Fig. 5.2). The conduction velocity is faster in proximal nerve segments because these have thicker myelin sheaths and because of the lower temperature distally (mainly a factor in conduction velocity in the lower limbs).

Proximal sites may be stimulated in conventional studies in order to assess conduction of proximal nerve segments or in the process of evaluating nerves such as the axillary or suprascapular. Attempts to perform needle stimulation of the cervical roots have been made and it has been claimed that this method may help in studying plexopathies (3).

In peripheral neuropathies of the demyelinating type (e.g., diabetic neuropathy) the conduction velocity may be significantly compromised. Peripheral neuropathies in which there are mainly axonal changes (e.g., alcoholic neuropathy) tend to affect the conduction velocity mildly. Commonly, axonal and myelin damage coexist.

### Late Responses—The "F" Wave

The "F" wave, so called because it was initially noted in the small muscles of the feet, is a late response seen during supramaximal stimulation of peripheral nerves. Following stimulation of a peripheral nerve the stimulus is conducted distally toward the muscle, thus eliciting the muscular response. At the same time the stimulus is also conducted antidromically toward the spinal cord. When the stimulus reaches the cord it triggers about 1–5% of the anterior horn cells. These in return send an impulse that travels distally to the muscle and constitutes the F wave. This wave is much smaller than the initial muscle response and varies in amplitude, shape, and latency. The determination of the fastest F response may help in the evaluation of proximal limb entrapments and/or radicular injury and in the assessment of segmental excitability (4–6). In many patients with radiculopathy, however, the F wave latency may remain within the normal range, so the usefulness of the F wave may be of limited value. In some cases a significant F wave latency difference between the ipsilateral and contralateral limbs may point toward a proximal lesion.

### SENSORY CONDUCTION

The sensory component of a mixed nerve or a pure sensory nerve can be recorded in a fashion

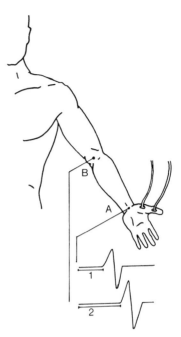

**Figure 5.2.** Peripheral nerve stimulated in at least two points to determine conduction velocity, which can be obtained by dividing the distance between the stimulated points by the latency difference obtained between the proximal and distal stimulation.

similar to that used for the motor component. The sensory electrodes record the evoked response from the sensory fibers (e.g., from the digital branches of the index or middle finger for the median nerve). Sensory conduction is frequently more sensitive and hence may be affected first in entrapment or peripheral neuropathies. The peripheral sensory nerves originate from cells located in the dorsal root ganglia. Any lesion at or distal to the dorsal root ganglia may affect the sensory evoked response and the sensory conduction. The presence of subjective sensory complaints or even an anesthetic finger with normal sensory evoked response and conduction velocity points toward a lesion located proximal to the dorsal root ganglia (e.g., herniated disc) (7, 8).

Sensory conduction may be of importance in establishing a differential diagnosis between brachial plexus injury and radiculopathy or spondylotic myelopathy. In brachial plexus lesions the injury is distal to the dorsal root ganglion. As a result the sensory potential may be significantly decreased in amplitude or absent altogether. In radiculopathies or myelopathies the lesion is located proximal to the ganglion and the sensory evoked response is as a rule normal.

In carpal tunnel syndrome, which may mimic radiculopathy or even coexist with a radiculopathy, prolonged sensory latencies may be the first observed abnormality.

## DIAGNOSIS OF SPECIFIC PATHOLOGIES

### RADICULOPATHY

Patients suffering from cervical radiculopathy are very frequently referred to the EMG laboratory. In practically all cases the peripheral conduction studies are normal, including the sensory conduction studies. Following extensive radicular damage, the F waves may be prolonged and thus point toward proximal pathology. EMG represents the most important part of the examination in establishing the presence of radiculopathy. The examiner is looking for EMG abnormalities in a radicular distribution. In selecting the muscles to be tested, the electromyographer will choose the ones innervated by different peripheral nerves that have a common root (e.g., brachioradialis, biceps, deltoid). One should keep in mind that there might be connections between adjacent motor rootlets with consequent overlap in motor innervation; thus EMG findings may occur at a higher or lower adjacent segment (9).

EMG abnormalities first appear in the paraspinal muscles as fibrillation potentials and/or positive sharp waves. These may appear 7–10 days following injury. One to 3 weeks later the same findings will be demonstrated in the proximal and then distal limb muscles. Denervation may take up to 6 weeks to occur in the most distal muscles of the extremities (10). If the EMG examination is done at a very early stage, the examiner must carefully look at the recruitment pattern. At this early phase denervation is still not expected to occur. However, the recruitment may be reduced and the firing rate increased while the recruitment interval is also modified accordingly. Although these findings are important and may be the only ones present at an early phase, they may frequently be overlooked by relatively less experienced or up-to-date electromyographers.

The importance of testing the paraspinal muscles cannot be overemphasized. Potentials expressing membrane instability ("denervation potentials") show up initially in the paraspinal muscles and, when present, indicate the presence of a proximal lesion affecting the posterior rami. In some cases with documented radiculopathy the EMG findings may be limited to these muscles.

One should, however, be careful in establishing a root level based solely on paraspinal muscle involvement since these muscles may be innervated by more than a single posterior primary ramus. Fibrillation potentials in these muscles are not synonymous with a herniated disc since they may be found in myelopathies, amyotrophic lateral sclerosis, diabetic radiculopathies, inflammatory and toxic myopathies, and metastatic infiltration of the posterior primary rami (11).

Many patients experience difficulties relaxing the paraspinal muscles during the EMG examination. We found that the prone position allows adequate relaxation of these muscles. We ask the patient to lean on his forehead and press down. The needle is then inserted adjacent to the spinous process all the way down toward the laminae. When studying C8 radiculopathies it is advisable to advance the needle using the EMG signal as a biofeedback to ascertain that the needle is in the muscle. This may help prevent the occurrence of pneumothorax.

Since peripheral nerve entrapments or polyneuropathies frequently occur in the presence of cervical radiculopathy, the electrodiagnostic studies and especially the sensory conduction study may help in establishing the correct diagnosis and guide the physician toward a sound therapeutic approach. Patients with peripheral entrapment neuropathy may have symptoms and findings proximal to the site of entrapment, as in radiculopathies—what is known as "double crush syndrome" (12). This combination may be more frequent than suspected on clinical grounds only and may help explain partial response to therapy directed toward one lesion only. A study of 100 patients with definite cervical root lesions was able to demonstrate that in 19% of cases there was a second lesion, such as a peripheral entrapment neuropathy or specifically carpal tunnel syndrome (8). The "combined lesion" may exist in cervical spondylotic myelopathy as well (13). The clinical picture may become even more complicated when myelopathy and radiculopathy occur simultaneously. Myeloradiculopathy secondary to spondylosis may develop acutely following trauma. Hyperextension injuries of the cervical spine or acute soft disc herniation may explain the combined pathology (14). Katirji et al. (15) correlated EMG findings in patients with definite cervical radiculopathy to metrizamide myelography/computed tomography findings. The radiologic studies were done within 3 months of the EMG studies. The authors found a 65% correlation between the involved segmental level as determined by their EMG studies and the radiologic findings. The correlation was higher (73.3%) for the C6 and C7 roots, which are the most commonly affected roots. This work emphasizes the usefulness of radiologic-electrodiagnostic correlations. In cases with multiple protruded discs or when there are extensive multilevel radiologic findings, the EMG abnormalities may determine the compromised neurologic level. This information may be important whenever surgical decompression is entertained.

Another study, performed on 24 patients with cervical disc prolapse confirmed radiologically, evaluated the value of different electrophysiologic tests (16). The authors found EMG abnormalities in 67% of the patients. Dermatomal SEPs revealed abnormalities on the affected side in 85% of the cases. Abnormal F wave responses were documented in 38% of the patients. In certain cases EMG abnormalities were demonstrated in the absence of sensory or motor deficits. Electrodiagnostic findings were present in the nonpainful side and at levels without disc prolapse.

Tackmann and Radu (17) found the F wave to be useless in their study, which included 20 patients. However, they found needle EMG abnormalities, in the form of fibrillation potentials and/or increased duration of motor unit action potentials and/or increased number of polyphasic potentials, in 19 subjects. The EMG results coincided with the affected root, as established clinically, in only 11 cases. Other investigators have shown that EMG findings correlate better with the clinical findings than radiographic studies (18).

We are not aware yet of similar studies correlating magnetic resonance imaging findings with electrodiagnostic abnormalities in patients with cervical radiculopathy.

## BRACHIAL PLEXOPATHY

Traumatic lesions involving the brachial plexus may occur separately or in conjunction with cervical injuries. Lesions involving the brachial plexus may clinically simulate cervical radiculopathy and confuse the less experienced clinician. The higher the lesion (i.e., in the trunk) the more difficult it will be to differentiate it from a root lesion. Involvement of the paraspinal muscles may be the only EMG finding that might help in establishing the level of injury. However, even cord injuries may clinically resemble root lesions and

pose a diagnostic challenge. Lateral cord lesions may mimic a C6 involvement, and injuries to the medial cord, from which the ulnar and the median nerves originate, may simulate a C7 or C8 root lesion (11, 19, 20).

If the evoked response obtained by sensory nerve stimulation is of normal amplitude, the lesion is, as a rule, located proximal to the dorsal root ganglion. Conversely, if the sensory nerve action potential displays a significantly reduced amplitude or is absent, the lesion must be at or distal to the dorsal root ganglion. Occasionally root lesions and brachial plexus injuries may coexist. In these cases the presence of paraspinal EMG abnormalities and compromised or missing sensory nerve action potentials may clarify the diagnosis. We should remember, however, that in many cases proper relaxation of the cervical paraspinal muscles is difficult to obtain, and there may be only a few fibrillations or positive sharp waves and at times no paraspinal abnormalities (11). In these cases it may be very difficult and at times impossible to differentiate between cervical radiculopathy and brachial plexus injury. SEP studies are of certain value in the evaluation of brachial plexopathies; the absence of SEPs may help document a complete tear of the brachial plexus (21). Moreover, in lesions involving the upper segments (e.g., the upper trunk) musculocutaneous and radial nerve SEPs may add useful information (22, 23). Since brachial plexopathies are only indirectly related to cervical trauma, no other related SEP studies are mentioned here.

## CERVICAL MYELOPATHY

Cervical myelopathy and cervical radiculopathy often coexist. Hyperextension injuries may cause acute myelopathy and radiculopathy in patients with preexisting cervical spondylosis (24). The clinical picture in patients with myelopathy should include hyperactive upper and lower extremity reflexes; however, in some cases with lower level stenosis hyperreflexia may be limited to the lower limbs. The presence of the Babinski reflex associated with impaired proprioception should direct the clinician toward the correct diagnosis (25). In these cases EMG studies may help in confirming the presence of concomitant radiculopathy and in ruling out motor neuron disease. In cases of cervical spinal stenosis, loss of anterior horn cells, as demonstrated by a decreased number of motor units and the presence of denervation, may be restricted to the stenosed cervical spinal level (26).

In the presence of diffuse denervation involving upper and lower extremity muscles extending much lower than the presumed stenosed cervical level, one should rule out amyotrophic lateral sclerosis, syringomyelia, spinal cord infarction due to vascular damage, and tumor affecting multiple roots.

## SOMATOSENSORY EVOKED POTENTIAL STUDIES

Painful cervical trauma does not as a rule result in electrophysiologic abnormalities. This type of finding is expected only if there is an associated neuropathic condition such as myelopathy or radiculopathy. The routine electroneuromyographic examination is the first to be performed in these cases, but if it is not contributory one resorts logically to somatosensory evoked potentials (SEPs). Evoked potential studies evolved in the last 15 years as useful diagnostic tools in central and peripheral nervous system dysfunction. SEPs are a series of small-amplitude electrical events recorded at the scalp or spinal level following stimulation of different nerves or dermatomes of the upper or lower limbs (27, 28).

The most useful procedure in the electrodiagnostic evaluation of a cervical radiculopathy or myelopathy remains the EMG examination of muscles in a root distribution. F wave evaluation has been shown to be of less benefit. However, these tests provide information exclusively about motor events in a radicular distribution, whereas the most frequently encountered clinical deficit relates to sensory modalities since pain, numbness, and tingling represent the most common complaints. In the lower limbs the H reflex allows an objective evaluation of the S1 segment, but there is no comparable routine sensory test for the upper limbs at any level. SEPs seem thus to be the procedure of choice in all of these cases. Indeed, they allow the evaluation of the afferent sensory impulses up through the roots to the spinal cord and further up to the cortex. In addition, in contrast with the lower limbs, where the lumbar potential is not consistently obtainable when using a noninvasive recording technique, the Erb point potential in the upper limbs (N9) is easy to obtain even after a few averaged sweeps and is extremely constant. It therefore seems that the evaluation of SEPs following stimulation of nerves of the upper extremities represents the ideal procedure in cases of clinically diagnosed cervical my-

elopathy or radiculopathy where electroneuromyographic examination is noncontributory.

The introduction of the concept of segmental stimulation by Eisen et al. (29) significantly changed the approach to somatosensory evoked response studies in radiculopathies. The authors advocated using sensory nerves, sensory branches of mixed nerves, or dermatomal patches in order to obtain specificity of stimulation at different root levels and avoid false-negative results due to the dilution of abnormal findings that can occur when stimulating a mixed nerve representing, as a rule, two or usually three roots. However, there is an opposite viewpoint. Although it is true that mixed nerves originate from two or more root levels and thus a monoradiculopathy may be masked by normal responses mediated through unaffected roots (30), it is also evident that mixed nerves are much larger in diameter than dermatomal twigs. Consequently mixed nerves are more sensitive to mechanical factors, and thus compression (31).

A search of the literature on SEP studies in cervical myelopathies or radiculopathies discloses a predilection for the use of mixed nerves by the vast majority of authors publishing in this domain, in definite contrast with similar studies in lumbosacral radiculopathies. In this latter area dermatomal stimulation has the upper hand, but with no striking difference in terms of number of studies as compared to those using sensory or mixed nerve stimulation. We are not aware of any possible explanation for these discrepancies.

When performing electrophysiologic studies in cervical versus lumbosacral radiculopathies, it is useful to keep in mind that, while in cervical radiculopathies careful differential diagnosis must be made to exclude brachial plexopathies, for which SEPs are equally important, in lumbosacral radiculopathies there is no real diagnostic "competitor" since lumbar plexopathies are of rare occurrence.

In order to be of definite clinical usefulness, an evoked potential must be consistently obtainable. By narrowing the filter bandpass or using digital filtering, or by using noncephalic monopolar recording versus cephalic bipolar recording (which is prone to phase cancellation), some authors (32–34) were able to obtain a few inconsistent, small-amplitude potentials. These potentials are usually not mentioned in the various published studies about the clinical yield of SEP testing in cervical entrapments of all sorts.

## MEASUREMENT TECHNIQUE

SEPs are recorded as a series of waves of varying amplitude and latency, depending on the location of the electrodes used. The waves are identified by their polarity—positive (P) or negative (N)—and latency (in milliseconds); for example, N9 is a negative wave with a latency of 9 msec. The essential waves, obtainable at nearly every trial when stimulating the major mixed nerves of the upper limbs, are N9 (the Erb point or brachial plexus potential), N13 (the cervical or cervicomedullary potential), and N19/20 (the cortical or thalamocortical potential). The N9 potential is of major importance as the "marker" or the reference point for latency measurements; this allows reliance on interwave rather than absolute values, which may be misleading since they depend on the patient's body size. The N9 potential represents "the time when the action-potential volley in the mixed peripheral nerve passes through some poorly defined point in the brachial plexus" (35). The electrode linkage recommended for the optimum visualization of this quite sizable potential is an electrode on the ipsilateral Erb point connected to an electrode on the contralateral Erb point. Another possible linkage for this potential is an electrode on the Erb point to a reference electrode on the forehead (Fz), a commonly used bipolar type of reference.

The N13 potential, labeled at times as P/N13, probably originates in more than one location but can grossly represent upper cervical and medullary structures (35). The best electrode linkage for this potential is an electrode on C2 or C7 (spinous processes of these two cervical vertebrae) to a reference electrode on the forehead.

The N19/20 potential also results from more than a neural generator; it can grossly represent activity generated at the thalamus, thalamocortical radiations, and cortex levels. It is followed by another wave, this time a positive wave at 22 or 25 msec, the P22/25. It is obviously of less use for cervical cord or root conditions, being of clinical usefulness for more rostrally located disorders such as cerebrovascular accidents and multiple sclerosis. The optimal electrode linkage in a cephalic, bipolar connexion is an electrode on C3 or C4, corresponding largely to the cortex representation of the left or right hand, respectively [a better position is 2 cm behind these points (C3' or C4')], to a reference electrode on the forehead.

Each laboratory should establish its own normal values and standard deviations by means of careful studies on a nonclinical population. At least 30 "normal" subjects, as equally distributed as possible in terms of sex and age, represents an appropriate sample.

## DIAGNOSIS OF PATHOLOGIC CONDITIONS—REVIEW OF THE LITERATURE

The first studies on SEPs in cervical entrapments dealt with cervical spondylosis and/or disc protrusion. The authors recorded from the cervical cord (evoked spinal electrogram) using an invasive method to reach the epidural space (36, 37). Abnormalities on the affected side translated into significantly reduced amplitude of the spinal potential with preserved normal latency.

Cervical spondylosis documented clinically and confirmed by radiologic investigation stimulated subsequent papers, this time on the noninvasive use of SEPs, mainly median nerve stimulation (38–41). Abnormal findings ranged from reduced-amplitude or absent P/N13 to prolonged N9 to P/N13 conduction time. Ganes (40) recorded peripheral, cervical, and cortical SEPs after median and ulnar nerve stimulation in 21 patients with cervical spondylosis and radiculopathy or myelopathy. There was a clinical-electrodiagnostic correlation in the sense that abnormalities were found only in cases with objective neurologic findings in patients with radiculopathies. However, there was no clear correlation for cases of myelopathy.

Stohr and Bluthardt (42) described a supraganglionic lesion pattern seen when recording SEPs with median or ulnar nerve stimulation in patients with cervical root lesions of an inflammatory, infiltrative, or traumatic nature. They noted a partial or total interruption of conduction from the Erb point to the cervical cord resulting in reduction or absence of N11 (a less consistently present wave) and N13.

In their paper on "segmental stimulation," published in 1983 (29), Eisen et al. studied patients with lumbosacral and cervical radiculopathy. They used sensory nerves for lower limbs stimulation while showing a preference for dermatomal patches for the upper limbs. Thirty-six patients with suspected or confirmed (by myelographic studies) root compression had electrophysiologic studies, including late responses and SEPs, and 78% revealed at least one abnormality.

Needle EMG displayed the higher diagnostic yield (75%), followed by SEPs (57%), and F waves (43%).

Two significant papers (43, 44) were published in 1986 by a group of Finnish authors. In the first paper, SEPs were recorded before and after surgical intervention for herniated cervical disc and radiculopathy or myelopathy (43). The median nerves were stimulated at the wrist using surface electrodes while recording from the Erb point, C7, and the inion, an unusual location for this type of test (C3 or C4 is more routinely used for the cortex location). The preoperative results were abnormal for all cases, as expected. The most significant improvement was registered 6–36 months after operation in 12 of 14 patients with radiculopathy and in 4 of 9 patients with myelopathy. However, a statistically significant difference in SEP values was proven only in radiculopathy, for two parameters such as amplitude of the N13 potential and relative amplitude difference of the same wave. It is therefore obvious that SEP abnormalities persist postoperatively in spite of clinical improvement in all patients.

The second paper from the same group compares surface noninvasive (skin) recording with epidural recordings at the level of C7 in cases with radiculopathy and radiculomyelopathy (44). The patients were divided into four subgroups according to the severity of the disease. A control subgroup was also used when comparing the skin and epidural SEPs. One of the differences between skin and epidural recording was that with the latter the N11 wave was seen consistently in addition to the consistently present N13, which was present in both types of recording. As expected, the skin recordings resulted in potentials of smaller amplitude than those of the epidural recordings. When comparing the two types of recordings in terms of mean latency and amplitude of the N13 wave, there was, in both cases, prolonged latency and decreased amplitude but more markedly so for the epidural recordings. A progressive decrease in the amplitude of N13 with the increase in severity of the disease was noted for epidural recordings, but the highest number of abnormalities (61%) was registered for the latency of N13.

Another contribution published by a group of researchers from the University of Hong Kong studied six Chinese patients suffering from cervical myelopathy due to ossification of the posterior longitudinal ligament documented radiologically (45). The cord compression was confirmed by myelography and SEP studies, which showed a good correlation with posterior column abnormalities. The SEPs appeared to be able to monitor the clinical course following treatment. Most of the paper is centered on pathogenic factors responsible for this particular pathologic entity.

Yiannikas et al. authored a paper on studies of 30 cases of cervical spondylosis (46). Their goal was to determine if SEP studies following median, ulnar, radial, and peroneal nerve stimulation may provide useful information in addition to that provided by needle EMG, NCS, and late responses. The patients were divided into three groups. The first group comprised 10 cases in which pain represented the major complaint but there were no neurologic signs. In this group all the procedures gave normal results. The second group comprised 10 cases presenting objective neurologic signs of root compression. The EMG studies were abnormal in nine of these cases, whereas SEP studies showed abnormalities only for five cases after radial nerve stimulation, the median and ulnar SEPs being normal. In the last group, comprised of 10 cases with a clinical picture of cervical myelopathy, seven had abnormal SEPs on median nerve stimulation and all had abnormal peroneal SEPs. The authors' conclusion is that EMG and SEP studies are of little value in patients with symptoms but no neurologic signs of root compression. In contrast, both tests are of definite value in patients with objective neurologic signs, with the EMG displaying more sensitivity. The reverse is true for cervical myelopathy, for which SEPs represented the most sensitive procedure.

Another conclusion in this study is that only radial nerve SEPs are diagnostically helpful in radiculopathies whereas, in addition to median nerve SEPs (contributory in 70% of cases), peroneal SEPs in the lower limb revealed the highest correlation in cervical myelopathy cases (46). On the basis of these findings it seems more useful to routinely perform lower limb SEPs before any other SEPs in cases of suspected cervical myelopathy. In addition, if lower limb SEPs are abnormal in a patient suspected of having root compression versus myelopathy, it is obvious that the latter condition is more likely the correct diagnosis. The specific abnormalities described by the authors were low-amplitude or absent P/N13 and even N19 waves in cases of radiculopathy and the same abnormalities plus prolonged EP/N13 conduction time in patients with myelopathy. For lower limb SEPs there was prolonged central conduction time and significant reduction in the scalp response amplitude in cases with myelopathic involvement.

Finding an electrophysiologic expression of pain represents a continuing concern for a good number of authors. A possible correlation with long-latency SEPs was obtained in one study, in which a 150–250-msec complex showed an increase in amplitude in parallel with an increase in pain intensity (47) and vice versa. However, there is a study in which short-latency SEPs seem to be involved as well (48). Indeed, delayed latency and increased amplitude of short-latency SEPs (less than 70 msec) were observed in the electrical distribution of painful dysesthesias in four patients with lesions in the proximal segments of the peripheral nervous system. One of the patients was diagnosed as suffering from painful spondylopathic cervical radiculopathy. The stimulated nerve in this case was the musculocutaneous. Unfortunately, the paper is specifically directed toward the painful character of the condition and does not really address the specific electrodiagnostic expression of pain. As is well known, numerous other papers are concerned with the diagnostic workup of neuropathic conditions in which pain represents the major element within the symptomatology.

As a rule, ulnar SEPs are used in the diagnosis of brachial plexopathies, including patients suspected of having thoracic outlet syndrome, since the ulnar SEP corresponds to the medial cord of the plexus (C8–T1 level). Ulnar SEPs have been found to be diagnostically sensitive also in cases of cervical myelopathy (49). The authors studied 57 patients with the clinicosurgical diagnosis of cervical myelopathy of the compressive type. Ulnar, median, and tibial nerve SEPs were compared and the ulnar SEPs proved to be the most useful, displaying a yield of 74%. The most common reported findings were reduced or absent cervical evoked responses and prolonged central conduction time. All cases with SEPs abnormalities were confirmed by median and tibial nerves stimulation. Median nerve somatosensory evoked studies were not helpful. Major cord involvement could be ruled out in patients with radicular symptoms by the presence of normal values for ulnar and tibial nerve SEPs.

One of the few studies on cervical radiculopathies in which the concept of segmental stimulation (29) was applied was published by Schmid et al. from Berne, Switzerland (50). They studied 28 cases and used wrist as well as finger stimulation in root distributions. Besides absolute latency, side-to-side difference was also taken into consideration. They analyzed side-to-side differences of N20/P25 amplitudes and of the N9–N13 interval conduction time. The results were disappointing: 68% of cases displayed false-negative findings on the symptomatic side and 36% of cases revealed false-positive findings on the asymptomatic side after nonsegmental nerve stimulation. When performing segmental stimulation 72% of the patients had false-negative findings on the symptomatic side while 23% displayed false-positive findings on the asymptomatic side. The authors' conclusion was that SEPs following mixed/sensory nerve and segmental stimulation do not reliably document clear-cut established unilateral radiculopathies with sensory and motor deficit. Therefore SEPs will not be helpful in the electrophysiologic workup of cervicobrachialgias of unknown etiology.

Another study with more positive results originated from Linz, Austria. It deals not only with evoked potentials but with the entire spectrum of electrophysiologic studies used in cervical disc prolapse confirmed radiologically (16). The SEP studies consisted of dermatomal stimulation and scalp recording from C4 to T2 (51). In 11 cases there were absent or distorted dermatomal SEPs (DSEPs). In eight cases of the 11 patients DSEP abnormalities displayed good correlation with the level of herniation, but three of these eight showed DSEP changes in adjacent segments as well. In another three of these eight cases the DSEP correctly lateralized the lesion but there was no correlation with the level of herniation. These six cases, with a less accurate diagnostic yield, included some radiologic findings with no clinical correlation. In the remaining two of these eight cases there were false-negative results on DSEP testing. The authors' conclusion is that EMG studies appeared to be less sensitive than DSEP studies in cervical root compression. Both EMG and DSEPs were considered as more useful, providing more information than clinical investigations and displaying existing abnormalities even in cases with no corresponding motor or sensory deficit.

A minimonograph on the electrodiagnostic examination of patients with radiculopathies was published by Wilbourn and Aminoff (11). Their criticisms concerning the value of SEPs in radiculopathies reside mainly in elements of dilution of results, such as "the long distance between the site of peripheral stimulation and the site at which the responses are generated" or the already-mentioned (30) masking of the focal conduction block in some fibers by the unaffected fibers from other roots. They also noted the extreme variations in the amplitudes of the evoked responses, both interside and intersubject, the lack of more precise localizing information when there are definite SEP abnormalities, and the fact that the presence of such abnormalities would not inform the diagnostician about the nature or age of a lesion in the sensory pathways. The authors are obviously partial to SEPs elicited by dermatomal rather than nerve trunk stimulation, stating that the latter are "diagnostically unhelpful," but do not give much credit to the former either, considering them "relatively insensitive." The only type of SEPs, as classified according to nerve selection, that the authors do not dismiss in spite of their "uncertain role" are the SEPs elicited by cutaneous nerve stimulation.

Electrophysiologic exploration of the motor tracts, first used in the fourth decade of this century (52), has made a significant impact in the development of noninvasive methods of investigating the central nervous system, especially with the introduction of magnetic stimulation (53). There is only one published contribution of which these authors are aware that deals with the use of motor potentials in cervical myelopathy by trauma or spondylosis (54). Thompson et al. studied six patients, three of them affected by cervical spinal cord trauma and the other three by cervical spondylosis and secondary myelopathy. The authors found that in five of the six cases there was an abnormal conduction in the central tracts, although the cortical SEPs in the same limb were normal in four of these patients. In the remaining case, in which there was normal central motor conduction, SEPs displayed abnormalities. Based on these results, the authors considered that the electrophysiologic examination of the motor pathways by cortical stimulation may be of considerable value in the diagnosis and treatment of patients with traumatic and compressive conditions of the spinal cord.

## CONCLUDING REMARKS

In the previous section, 18 studies were reviewed, 17 dealing with the use of somatosensory evoked responses and one on the use of motor potentials

in the electrodiagnosis of neuropathic disorders sometimes associated with painful cervical trauma. It must be kept in mind when dealing with the skepticism displayed by some authors quoted here that even more serious doubts were expressed regarding what we call today "routine EMG" up to 20–25 years after its introduction into clinical practice. The SEPs are relatively new tools and the motor potential studies very recent. Cortically stimulated motor responses are not yet approved for clinical use in this country; the only such study mentioned here originated in the United Kingdom, where the motor potentials were used first for clinical purposes (54). To give up the use of these advances in the area of noninvasive exploration of the peripheral and central sensorimotor pathways is obviously not an answer. Only 17 studies of the use of SEPs in the diagnosis of cervical conditions in less than 12 years is not enough to form a definite opinion about their value. Furthermore, the great majority of these studies point out the advantages of these procedures. For the same reasons, it is too early to decide about the usefulness of motor potentials in diagnosing cervical conditions. It is essential to continue using these tools with full knowledge of their realistically outlined limitations.

## REFERENCES

1. Gore DR, Sepic SB, Gardner GM, Murray MP: Neck pain: a long-term follow up of 205 patients. *Spine* 12:1–5, 1987.
2. Teresi LM, Lufkin RB, Reicher MA, et al: Asymptomatic degenerative disk disease and spondylosis of the cervical spine: MR imaging. *Radiology* 164:83–88, 1987.
3. Nerger AR, Busis NA, Logigian EL, Wierzbicka M, Shahani BT: Cervical root stimulation in the diagnosis of radiculopathy. *Neurology* 37:329–332, 1987.
4. Fisher MA, Shivde AJ, Teixera C, Grainer LS: The F response—a clinically useful physiological parameter for the evaluation of radicular injury. *Electromyogr Clin Neurophysiol* 19:65–75, 1979.
5. Fisher MA, Shahani BT, Young RR: Assessing segmental excitability after acute rostral lesions. 1. The F response. *Neurology* 28:1265–1271, 1978.
6. Eisen MA, Schomer D, Melmed C: The application of F-wave measurements in the differentiation of proximal and distal upper limb entrapments. *Neurology* 27:662–668, 1977.
7. Benecke R, Conrad B: The distal sensory nerve action potential as a diagnostic tool for the differentiation of lesions in dorsal roots and peripheral nerves. *J Neurol* 223:231–239, 1980.
8. Brandstater M, Fullerton M: Sensory nerve conduction studies in cervical root lesion. *Can J Neurol Sci* 10:152, 1983.
9. Marzo JM, Simmons EH, Kallen F: Intradural connections between adjacent cervical spinal roots. *Spine* 12:964–968, 1987.

10. Eisen A: Electrodiagnosis of radiculopathies. *Neurol Clin* 3:495–510, 1985.

11. Wilbourn AJ, Aminoff MJ: The electrophysiologic examination in patients with radiculopathies. (AAEE Minimonograph #32.) *Muscle Nerve* 11:1099–1114, 1988.

12. Upton ARM, Comas AJ: The double crush in nerve entrapment syndromes. *Lancet* 2:359–362, 1973.

13. Epstein NE, Epstein JA, Carras R: Coexisting cervical spondylotic myelopathy and bilateral carpal tunnel syndrome. *J Spinal Dis* 2:36–42, 1989.

14. Hoff JT, Wilson CB: The pathophysiology of cervical spondylotic radiculopathy and myelopathy. *Clin Neurosurg* 24:474–487, 1977.

15. Katirji MB, Rakesh A, Kantra TA: The human cervical myotomes: an anatomical correlation between electromyography and CT/myelography. *Muscle Nerve* 11:1070–1073, 1988.

16. Leblhuber F, Reisecker F, Boehm-Jurkovic H, Witzmann A, Deisenhammer E: Diagnostic value of different electrophysiologic tests in cervical disk prolapse. *Neurology* 38:1879–1881, 1988.

17. Tackmann W, Radu EW: Observations on the application of electrophysiological methods in the diagnosis of cervical root compressions. *Eur Neurol* 22:379–404, 1983.

18. Hong CZ, Lee S, Lum P: Cervical radiculopathy. Clinical, radiographic and EMG findings. *Orthop Rev* 15:433–439, 1986.

19. Marinacci AA: A correlation between the operative findings in cervical herniated disc with the electromyograms and opaque myelograms. *Electromyography* 6:5–20, 1966.

20. Wallace D: Disc compression of the eighth cervical nerve: pseudo ulnar palsy. *Surg Neurol* 18:295–299, 1982.

21. Aminoff MU, Olney RK, Parry GJ, Raskin NH: Relative utility of different electrophysiologic techniques in the evaluation of brachial plexopathies. *Neurology* 38:546–550, 1988.

22. Yiannikas C, Shahani BT, Young RR: The investigation of traumatic lesions of the brachial plexus by electromyography and short latency somatosensory potentials evoked by stimulation of multiple peripheral nerves. *J Neurol Neurosurg Psychiatry* 46:1014–1022, 1983.

23. Wilbourn AJ: Electrodiagnosis of plexopathies. *Neurol Clin* 3:511–529, 1985.

24. Wilberger JE, Chedid MK: Acute cervical spondylotic myelopathy. *Neurosurgery* 22:145–146, 1988.

25. Epstein NE, Epstein JA, Carras R: Cervical spondylosis, stenosis and myeloradiculopathy in patients over 65: diagnostic techniques and management. *Neurology Orthopaedics* 6:13–23, 1988.

26. Stark RJ, Kennard C, Swash M: Hand wasting in spondylotic high cord compression. An electromyographic study. *Ann Neurol* 9:58–62, 1981.

27. Chiappa KH, Choi S, Young RR: Short latency somatosensory evoked potentials following median nerve stimulation in patients with neurological lesions. In Desmedt JE (ed): *Progress in Clinical Neurophysiology.* Basel, Karger, 1980, pp 264–281.

28. Anziska B, Cracco RQ: Short latency somatosensory evoked potentials: studies in patients with focal neurological disease. *Electroencephalogr Clin Neurophysiol* 49:227–239, 1980.

29. Eisen A, Hoirch M, Moll A: Evaluation of radiculopathies by segmental stimulation and somatosensory evoked potentials. *Can J Neurol Sci* 10:178–182, 1983.

30. Katifi HA, Sedgwick EM: Somatosensory evoked potentials from posterior tibial nerve and lumbosacral dermatomes. *Electroencephalogr Clin Neurophysiol* 65:249–259, 1986.

31. Takano H, Tamaki T, Noguchi T, Nakakuwa K: Comparison of spinal cord potentials elicited by spinal cord and peripheral nerve stimulation. In Schramm J, Jones SJ (eds): *Spinal Cord Monitoring.* Berlin, Springer, 1985, pp 29–34.

32. Maccabee PJ, Pinkhasov EI, Cracco RQ: Short latency somatosensory evoked potentials to median nerve stimulation: effect of low frequency filter. *Electroencephalogr Clin Neurophysiol* 55:34–44, 1983.

33. Cracco RQ: Scalp-recorded potentials evoked by median nerve stimulation: subcortical potentials, traveling waves and somatomotor potentials. *Prog Clin Neurophysiol* 7:1–14, 1980.

34. Desmedt JE, Cheron G: Central somatosensory conduction in man: neuronal generators and interpeak latencies of the far-field components recorded from neck and right or left scalp and earlobes. *Electroencephalogr Clin Neurophysiol* 50:382–403, 1980.

35. Chiappa KH (ed): *Evoked Potentials in Clinical Medicine.* New York, Raven Press, 1983, pp 208–214.

36. Matsukado Y, Yoshida M, Goya T, Shimoji K: Classification of cervical spondylosis or disc protrusion by pre-operative evoked spinal electrogram. *J Neurosurg* 44:435–441, 1976.

37. Caccia MR, Ubiali E, Andreussi L: Spinal evoked responses recorded from the epidural space in normal and diseased humans. *J Neurol Neurosurg Psychiatry* 39:962–967, 1976.

38. Mastaglia FL, Black JL, Edis R, Collins DWK: The contribution of evoked potentials in the functional assessment of the somatosensory pathways. *Clin Exp Neurol* 15:279–298, 1978.

39. El-Negamy E, Sedgwick EM: Delayed cervical somatosensory potentials in cervical spondylosis. *J Neurol Neurosurg Psychiatry* 42:238–241, 1979.

40. Ganes T: Somatosensory conduction times and peripheral, cervical and cortical evoked potentials in patients with cervical spondylosis. *J Neurol Neurosurg Psychiatry* 43:683–689, 1980.

41. Siivola J, Sulg I, Heiskari M: Somatosensory evoked potentials in diagnostics of cervical spondylosis and herniated disc. *Electroencephalogr Clin Neurophysiol* 52:276–282, 1981.

42. Stohr M, Bluthardt M (eds): *Atlas der klinischen Elektromyographie und Neurographie.* Stuttgart, Kohlhammer, 1983.

43. Heiskari M, Siivola J, Heikkinen ER: Somatosensory evoked potentials in evaluation of decompressive surgery of cervical spondylosis and herniated disc. *Ann Clin Res* 18(suppl 47):107–113, 1986.

44. Heiskari M, Tolonen U, Nystrom SH: Comparison of somatosensory evoked responses from root and cord recorded by skin and epidural electrodes using stimulation of the median nerve in cervical radiculopathy and radiculomyelopathy. *Acta Neurochir (Wien)* 79(2–4):114–119, 1986.

45. Yu YL, Leong JC, Fang D, Woo E, Huang CY, Lau HK: Cervical myelopathy due to ossification of the posterior longitudinal ligament. A clinical, radiological and evoked potentials study in six Chinese patients. *Brain* 111:769–783, 1988.

46. Yiannikas C, Shahani BT, Young RR: Short-latency somatosensory evoked potentials from radial, median, ulnar and peroneal nerve stimulation in the assessment of cervical spondylosis. Comparison with conventional electromyography. *Arch Neurol* 43:1264–1271, 1986.

47. Chen ACN, Chapman CR, Harkins SW: Brain evoked potentials are functional correlates of induced pain in man. *Pain* 6:365–374, 1979.

48. Synek VM: Short latency somatosensory evoked potentials in patients with painful dysesthesias in peripheral nerve lesions. *Pain* 29:49–58, 1987.
49. Veilleux M, Daube JR: The value of ulnar somatosensory evoked potentials (SEPs) in cervical myelopathy. *Electroencephalogr Clin Neurophysiol* 68:415–423, 1987.
50. Schmid UD, Hess CW, Ludin HP: Somatosensory evoked potentials following nerve and segmental stimulation do not confirm cervical radiculopathy with sensory deficit. *J Neurol Neurosurg Psychiatry* 51:182–187, 1988.

51. Jorg J: *Die elektrosensible diagnostik in der Neurologie. Band 19: Schriftenreihe Neurologie.* Berlin, Springer-Verlag, 1977.
52. Adrian ED, Moruzzi G: Impulses in the pyramidal tract. *J Physiol (Lond)* 19:152–199, 1939.
53. Barker AT, Janlious R, Freeston II: Noninvasive magnetic stimulation of human motor cortex. *Lancet* 1:1106–1107, 1985.
54. Thompson PD, Dick JP, Anselman P, et al: Examination of motor function in lesions of the spinal cord by stimulation of the motor cortex. *Ann Neurol* 21:389–396, 1987.

# 6

# PSYCHOLOGICAL DYSFUNCTION IN CHRONIC CERVICAL PAIN

## An Introduction to Clinical Assessment

*Donald S. Ciccone and Roy C. Grzesiak*

Without always realizing it, the physician conducting a history and physical examination is simultaneously engaging in a relative weighting of both biologic and psychological factors. From the inception of multidisciplinary pain management, practitioners have urged concurrent evaluation of medical and psychological findings (1). Such a practice, of course, reflects the current belief that many, if not most, patients with chronic pain suffer from some form of psychological dysfunction. In our experience such dysfunction may significantly impair the ability of patients to reliably report on their signs and symptoms (2). Psychological influences, for example, may intervene to amplify or otherwise distort the perception of pain and, in so doing, compromise the patient's capacity for self-observation. In those cases in which pain is persistent or extends beyond the bounds of normal healing, the likelihood of psychological influence is greater and so may be the tendency for patients to engage in nonveridical reporting. As a result, patients may wittingly or unwittingly misstate their symptoms and display illness behavior in excess of that required by their physical injury. Under these circumstances, even a thorough examination may yield incomplete or misleading data that impede or preclude the task of differential diagnosis. Repeated examinations, even when conducted by the same physician, may

not yield the same physical findings. Even more troubling is the recent finding by Waddell (3) that treatment for chronic pain "is determined to a much greater extent than most physicians realize or would like to admit by the patient's distress and illness behavior" (p. 635). Obviously, illness behavior is not always a reflection of physical disease; it may instead be an expression of the patient's conscious or unconscious desire to communicate pain and suffering. Failure to recognize illness behavior may thus result in misdiagnosis and, in some unfortunate cases, iatrogenic disability.

It is important that physicians have some understanding and appreciation of the relationship between chronic pain on the one hand and psychological dysfunction on the other. The physician in the community hospital or in private practice does not always have the luxury of consultation with a psychologist or psychiatrist with expertise in chronic pain. The goal of this chapter, therefore, is to provide physicians with a brief introduction to the psychology of chronic cervical pain. Rather than maintain a stance of theoretical neutrality, we will rely exlusively on cognitive theory to explain the causes of psychological dysfunction (4). Specifically, we will argue that acute and chronic pain are fundamentally dissimilar and that many, if not most, of the symptoms associated with chronicity are the result of inaccurate or erroneous thinking by the patient. In the context of assessing psychological dysfunction, we will also explore the cognitive basis of both inappropriate illness behavior and emotional disorder. Finally, we will discuss individual differences in premorbid functioning that may predispose certain patients to a chronic as opposed to an acute course of illness.

## ACUTE VERSUS CHRONIC CERVICAL PAIN

Based on their review of the literature, Aryanpur and Ducker (5) estimated that, during any given month, approximately 10% of the population will develop neck pain, with or without radiation into the upper extremities. Similar in course to acute back pain, acute neck pain tends to resolve in approximately 1 month. Thus, about 70% of those who consult a doctor for neck pain of recent onset will follow a rapid, uncomplicated course. Most of the remaining patients will also respond favorably over time but a few, despite conservative or surgical care, will go on to become chronic. Of course, there may be unknown physical reasons for the failure of chronic patients to respond, but in many cases psychological dysfunction is a more plausible explanation. Along with Waddell (3), we believe that "acute pain, acute disability, and acute illness behavior are generally proportionate to the physical basis, and there may, indeed, be little objective evidence of any remaining nociceptive stimulus" (p. 636). Thus, the distinction we propose between chronic and acute pain is a qualitative and not a quantitative one since their etiologies are presumed to be different. Chronic pain is not merely associated with a more prolonged or protracted course but is "a completely different clinical syndrome from acute pain" (3).

The symptoms of chronic cervical pain may include any or all of the following: relatively intractable complaints of pain, a pattern of escalating disability and inactivity out of proportion to physical findings, excessive utilization of health care services, medication abuse, a preoccupation with somatic symptoms, and emotional distress (especially depressed mood). Few, if any, of these symptoms appear to have physical causes and thus further medical workup or intervention may be contraindicated.

The challenge for psychology has been to explain why certain patients develop chronic pain following the onset of acute injury while others do not. One of the earliest, and in our opinion one of the most convincing, explanations of chronic pain was put forward by Holmes and Wolff (6). Using an informal observational method to study the so-called backache syndrome, they attempted to correlate electromyographic activity in the lumbar spine with emotional responding in the experimental situation and with inferred characteristics of the patient's premorbid personality. They found "generalized and sustained hyperfunction of the skeletal musculature," reflecting chronic muscle tension and an abnormal pattern of muscle recruitment, among most of their patients with chronic back and neck pain. They attributed this pattern of muscle abnormality to their patients' strong desire to "win approval and support by 'doing for others', 'trying to please others', 'keeping the peace', and 'carrying heavy burdens of responsibility without complaint'" (p. 23). They observed that patients with chronic pain are in a "constant state of readiness" stemming from an apparent desire to anticipate and prepare for actions that may be instrumental in obtaining social approval. This tendency to always be "on guard and ready to take action" may place an extraordinary burden on skeletal muscles and thus threaten patients' ability to perform the very actions they believe they must if they are to "please others." A vicious cycle is established in which patients strive harder and harder to win approval by performing actions that aggravate and possibly prolong their abnormal muscle function. This pattern of inappropriate and excessive muscle use, which Holmes and Wolff found to be so prevalent, may thus: (a) directly cause chronic pain by slowly and insidiously inflicting microtrauma on skeletal muscles (7); and (b) explain the *psychological vulnerability* of certain patients to chronic pain following the onset of acute injury. This follows from the assumption that acute injury offers an opportunity to avoid burdensome and unwanted responsibility without incurring a loss of social support. This line of reasoning will be pursued further in a subsequent section on premorbid risk factors.

A more recent paper on the etiology of chronic neck and back pain by Sarno (8) lends added credibility to the notion of psychological vulnerability. Sarno found that: (a) stress-related ailments were prevalent in his sample; (b) the age distribution of patients was not consistent with a degenerative disease process; (c) patients in his sample were overly conscientious and thus exhibited the same "on guard" orientation originally observed by Holmes and Wolff; and (d) the onset or exacerbation of pain was often tied to recognized periods of increased stress. The role of traumatic injury in precipitating chronic pain, according to Sarno (8), is clearly "catalytic, not etiologic." Having established the psychological basis of chronic as opposed to acute pain, we are now prepared to address the issue of psychological assessment.

## CLINICAL ASSESSMENT OF PSYCHOLOGICAL DYSFUNCTION

A few caveats about psychological assessment may be in order at the outset of our discussion. First, patients who exhibit illness behavior in the absence of physical illness or injury are often assumed to be "malingering." The use of this term implies a conscious or deliberate attempt to deceive or manipulate the health care provider. According to a recent survey of orthopaedic and neurosurgeons, conscious deception or outright fraud committed by the patient is rare (9). The term "psychological dysfunction" is used instead of malingering, therefore, to acknowledge the unconscious nature of such illness behavior. This is not to suggest that economic and social rewards play no role in motivating patients but simply indicates that most are not aware that these contingencies exist. Second, the presence of psychological dysfunction in patients with chronic cervical pain does not preclude the possibility of concomitant pathophysiology. Patients may present with purely physical or purely psychological symptoms or, more often than not, a combination of both. Third, a psychological explanation for pain and disability should not be assumed simply because a physical lesion cannot be found.

In fact, there are three broad categories of information that may be used to support a "diagnosis" of psychological dysfunction. These can be defined as follows:

*Inappropriate illness behavior*—maladaptive coping responses characterized by physical disability that is disproportionate to the extent of injury and is accompanied by one or more of the following: excessive reliance on medical and nonmedical health service providers for relief of pain; improper use of narcotics, tranquilizers, or other addictive medications; body language (such as muscle guarding, bracing, facial grimacing, or rubbing) that effectively communicates pain and suffering in the presence of family members and health care providers; and persistent complaints of pain that extend beyond the bounds of normal healing, appear inconsistent with an anatomic distribution, and reflect an intensity that cannot be explained on the basis of objective pathophysiology.

*Emotional disorder*—periods of anxious, angry, depressed, or guilty mood severe enough to interfere with daily functioning and/or exacerbate the patient's experience of pain, possibly associated with: loss of interest in usual activities; social withdrawal; sleep and/or appetite disturbance; excessive worry or apprehension; avoidance behavior; palpitations; hyperventilation; sexual dysfunction; interpersonal and/or marital conflict; and irritability.

*Premorbid risk factors*—specific psychological, psychiatric, and/or biologic variables that may predispose patients to chronic pain-related disability, including: a history of hard-driving, work-oriented behavior associated with hyperactivity and/or excessive self-sacrifice; premorbid psychiatric disorder; premorbid substance abuse or dependency; prior history of chronic pain or other stress-related illness; and traumatic or otherwise stressful childhood experience.

Failure to recognize the foregoing symptoms and/or predictors of psychological dysfunction may undermine the effectiveness of otherwise appropriate medical intervention. For example, a patient with "chronic cervical sprain" may display exaggerated illness behavior in an unconscious effort to avoid work. Medical or physical therapy for the purpose of "pain relief" may have the unintended effect of legitimizing the patient's symptoms and reinforcing a tendency toward symptom magnification. The goal of this section is to sensitize the acute care physician to the role of psychological dysfunction in magnifying or otherwise distorting the physical symptoms that may be associated with cervical pain. Our plan is to specify a set of questions that can and should be answered by the physician during the course of clinical assessment. A set of representative questions corresponding to each of the above-mentioned categories will be presented along with a discussion of their diagnostic implication.

## INAPPROPRIATE ILLNESS BEHAVIOR

Until recently, there has been no way to reliably measure pain behavior or quantify the extent of inappropriate illness behavior exhibited by patients during physical examination. Specific "nonorganic" signs associated with such behavior have been widely recognized but never subjected to rigorous, empirical testing. Waddell, along with a number of his colleagues (10), has proposed a set of behavioral signs that may be associated with psychological dysfunction in patients with chronic low back pain. These so-called Waddell signs include: diffuse (nonanatomic) tenderness; improved straight leg raising when distracted; sensory less and/or motor weakness in a nonanatomic distribution; and excessive verbal complaints of pain or exaggerated facial grimacing during physical examination. Despite the subjective nature of this information, Waddell has reported adequate scoring reliability between independent physician examiners. Positive Waddell findings (i.e., three or more positive test results) were found to correlate with various measures of psychological dysfunction but were "separable from and independent of the standard physical findings of organic pathologic conditions" (p. 116). In particular, they found that objective nerve root irritation and compression as well as radiologic evidence of spinal pathology did not correlate with the presence or absence of illness behavior. Patients may be expected to exhibit both objective findings of spinal pathology and nonorganic signs of psychological dysfunction.

While the Waddell signs were developed for use with a low back pain population, they may be adapted for patients with chronic cervical pain as well. Rather than propose a formal scoring procedure analogous to the Waddell test, we propose that physicians simply consider each of the following questions during their initial medical examination:

1.  Are there persistent reports of pain extending beyond the bounds of normal healing?
2.  Is there a known physical cause of the patient's pain?
3.  Does the patient's report of pain appear proportionate to the suspected pathology?
4.  Is the distribution of pain, sensory loss, and/or motor weakness consistent with a dermatomal or myotomal distribution?
5.  Is the complaint of pain and/or tenderness specific and limited to a single skeletal or neuromuscular structure?

A more objective but less pragmatic approach to the assessment of pain behavior is the use of an observational scoring system (11). In a study of patients with chronic low back pain, Keefe and his associates were able to assess the frequency of guarding, bracing to avoid pain, grimacing, and rubbing or touching the site of pain (12). All of these behaviors were found to occur frequently during the course of physical examination and all were significantly more prevalent among patients receiving disability-related income.

Aside from an assessment of inappropriate pain behavior, it may also be useful to document the presence or absence of postural neglect. Of course, postural defects may be the result of ge-

netic factors or acquired structural abnormalities, but there may also be a relationship between posture and one's emotional state. Cailliet (13), for example, suggested that excessive stress may be associated with chronic flexion of the cervical and lumbar spine associated with "concurrent inhibition of the extensors." A failure to maintain proper cervical lordosis, for whatever reason, may result in a "forward head" with rounded shoulders. Such a posture may be etiologically related to abnormal muscle function and become a cause of chronic muscle tension, spasm, and/or pain (7, 14). Postural habits may thus predispose patients to chronic pain following traumatic injury or actually give rise to pain of insidious origin. Patients who routinely engage in prolonged sitting or forward bending at work (as in a clerical or data processing job) may be particularly at risk for developing a "postural syndrome."

The assessment of inappropriate illness behavior should also include a thorough analysis of "secondary gain." In virtually all cases of chronic musculoskeletal pain there are reward contingencies operating in the patient's environment tending to reinforce the maintenance of disability behavior. This is not to suggest that all patients are uniformly influenced by these contingencies but simply to make note of their existence. Moreover, most patients seem unaware that such contingencies are in any way related to their functional status. The most widely accepted explanation for the influence of external reward on illness behavior is the operant model proposed by Fordyce (15). In brief, this model holds that human behavior is under the control of its consequences. For example, if the consequences of disability behavior are positively reinforced (through financial gain, increased leisure time, or avoidance of unpleasant work activity) then such behavior is automatically strengthened and more likely to occur in the future. An important implication of this view is that unfavorable environmental conditions are directly responsible for controlling patient behavior. In our opinion, this model is not only incorrect from a scientific standpoint but potentially misleading to both patients and health care providers. It implies that patients do not bear responsibility for their own behavior and, in fact, are merely the victims of maladaptive reward contingencies. A more accurate (and therapeutically more appropriate) explanation of illness behavior is provided by cognitive theory (4). According to the cognitive model, inappropriate patient behavior is the result of irrational or inaccurate thinking. The cognitive premise is that we humans respond to our own internal construction of reality and that behavior is therefore inner-directed rather than externally controlled. Unfortunately, the inner direction we use to guide our behavior is sometimes based on faulty or illogical thinking. When this happens, our decision-making ability is compromised and we literally talk ourselves into self-defeating rather than self-enhancing behavior.

## The Cognitive Context of Illness Behavior

The distinction between operant and cognitive theory has practical implications for the process of assessment and for the manner in which we, as health care providers, view our patients. While the practicing physician need not be concerned with the details of cognitive assessment, it may be helpful to place the concept of "illness behavior" in a cognitive context. From this vantage point, unhealthy reward contingencies in the environment do not force or coerce patients into behaving inappropriately. In cognitive terms, it is the patient's responsibility to cope with such contingencies and avoid, insofar as possible, any behavior that is potentially injurious or self-defeating. Any failure to cope is attributed to faulty thinking, which can then be identified and corrected through cognitive restructuring therapy (16). For example patients may trigger inappropriate illness behavior by telling themselves:

"Pain is always a symptom of tissue damage."
"I must avoid all physical activity and give my body a chance to heal."
"My spine is very instable and likely to break if I push myself."

While these thinking "errors" are likely to be conscious, many others are held at an unconscious or tacit level of awareness. For example, many patients with physical restrictions are prone to irrational, self-condemning thoughts such as: "If I return to work and am unable to live up to my usual standards, I would think of myself as a total failure and lose all self-respect."

In our experience, negative self-rating is often an unconscious process that may nevertheless exert significant influence on patient behavior and result in unnecessary work avoidance. Other patients with similar thoughts may engage in excessive, hard-driving behavior (causing chronic muscle fatigue and strain) in a vain effort to prove their self-worth. In both cases, coping failure is probably the result of unconscious cognitive error, that is, equating self-worth with one's physical capacity and thereby inferring diminished self-worth as the result of physical incapacity or failure to perform at premorbid levels. If this cognitive view is correct than health care providers need not view patients with psychological dysfunction as victims of their environment but rather as active, albeit unwitting, participants in the process of symptom development.

## Eliciting Evidence of Psychological Dysfunction

Having established a psychological context for the assessment of patient behavior, it now seems appropriate to consider specific questions designed to elicit evidence of psychological dysfunction. The following questions are intended to extend the inquiry into patient behavior already in progress.

6. What behaviors does the patient perform to communicate pain and suffering to family members and health care providers? (E.g., How does the patient's spouse know when the patient is in pain?)
7. What specific behaviors are performed by the patient's spouse, friends, and/or family in response to the patient's pain behavior?

Increased attention and/or support from the patient's spouse or family is extremely common and is often contingent on an overt (publically observable) display of pain. This requires the patient to communicate pain through nonverbal and possibly exaggerated body language. The "secondary gain" at stake may be the symbolic significance associated with caregiving behavior (e.g., affection or approval) or it may be the caregiving behavior itself (e.g., a therapeutic massage or the application of a hot pack). In any event, the ability to manipulate one's social environment through nonverbal displays of pain is an attractive prospect to many patients, especially those in dire "need" of love or approval, and may, therefore, be a significant obstacle to physical rehabilitation.

8. What is the patient's current level of income and from what sources does the patient derive this money?

In the case of chronic back pain, Waddell (3) described the high incidence of disability among industrial workers as a "Western epidemic" associated primarily with socioeconomic factors. Based on his data, we would argue that many "disabled" workers do not suffer from a medical disorder but rather from a failure to cope adequately with physical, occupational, and/or interpersonal stress. Given the prevalence of pain-related disability in our society, we believe that even a cursory examination of patient behavior should include a complete account of all financial disincentives. The widespread availability of income protection insurance, under the auspices of workman's compensation statutes and the Social Security Administration, is clearly an environmental contingency with which many patients find it difficult to cope. Some patients seem to feel they are "entitled" to income protection and should not have to work if work-related activity increases their pain. Such patients may, consciously or unconsciously, convince themselves that disability insurance is not only their "right" but their only means of economic survival. In our experience, patients who avoid work unnecessarily usually do so without a conscious intent to defraud either their employer or their insurance company. More often than not they convince themselves of their disability status, and many actually become disabled as the result of adopting a dysfunctional (excessively inactive) life-style. A small number of patients who do not qualify for either income insurance or a government-sponsored subsidy may come to rely on their spouse or on loans from family and friends. We should remember that the longer the patient remains out of work and dependent on disability income, the more likely it is that he or she will remain disabled.

9.  Is the patient using, abusing, or dependent on an addictive drug (especially prescription narcotics or tranquilizers)?
10. Does the patient use alcohol as a means of controlling pain?

The use of narcotic analgesics, sedatives, hypnotics, and/or anxiolytic medications may be appropriate during the acute stages of neuromuscular injury or illness. Unfortunately, when the patient's pain extends beyond the bounds of normal healing, the use of such addictive medication may persist, often escalating into a pattern of abuse or dependency. The incidence of drug abuse in a chronic (nonmalignant) pain population has been estimated to be as high as 41%, with an additional 24% meeting the more stringent criteria associated with drug dependency (17). There are also data to suggest that patients who use narcotics or

sedatives tend to perceive themselves as more physically disabled and are more likely to have been operated on and/or hospitalized for their pain (18). Since patients routinely and consistently underreport their use of narcotics or other addictive substances, we suggest it may be more useful to focus on the type of medication the patient is using rather than on the amount reported. It should also be noted that long-term use of narcotics and/or sedatives may produce adverse side effects that include increased fatigue, irritability, and depression. Of course, these are also symptoms of the chronic pain syndrome the physician is attempting to treat. While there is some disagreement about the use of narcotics in this population (19), we think it is appropriate to consider detoxification an important goal of medical intervention. It is also essential to inquire about the patient's possible use or abuse of alcohol, especially when it is used as a method of controlling pain.

11. Who performs routine household chores such as food shopping, cooking, cleaning, and laundry?
12. How much of the patient's waking day is spent resting or reclining because of pain?

The rewards of pain-related disability clearly extend into the patient's home by providing a socially sanctioned excuse for avoiding virtually all household chores. It is important, therefore, to establish whether premorbid domestic responsibilities have been abdicated by the patient; if so, one should determine whether other members of the household (or friends) have taken over these duties. Disability status may also be associated with excessive inactivity and passive forms of recreation such as television viewing, frequent bed rest, and reading. The reason for this excessive inactivity, we believe, may again be traced to cognitive error of one kind or another. For example, despite the absence of objective findings, chronic pain patients seem to think about their pain in precisely the same way they think about an acute injury or illness (20). They implicitly believe there is a medical explanation for their pain as well as a medical cure and see themselves as mere "victims" of accidental injury or disease. Their pain is naturally construed as a signal of physical damage that can only be healed through bed rest and inactivity. Patients who have convinced themselves of their disability may also feel obligated to behave as if they were disabled by refraining from social activities, spending an inordinate amount of time in bed or resting, and, in general, performing behaviors they have come to expect of anyone suffering from an acute illness.

## EMOTIONAL DISORDER

When confronted with the prospect of chronic pain, restricted motion, and an altered life-style, patients often exhibit symptoms of inappropriate negative affect such as anxiety, anger, guilt, and/or depression. Any or all of these symptoms may effectively undermine the outcome of even the most appropriate medical treatment. Stress-induced autonomic arousal, for example, may eventually lead to sustained muscle tension, spasm, and pain, especially when it occurs in the context of a preexisting muscle injury (21). In this way, excessive stress may facilitate the development of a "pain-spasm-pain" cycle, directly exacerbating the patient's original injury and contributing to the establishment of a chronic pain syndrome. An equally important consequence of negative affect is its indirect influence on patient behavior. Patients may, for example, decide to engage in activities that necessitate excessive or inappropriate muscle use in a self-defeating attempt to avoid or minimize guilt. The assessment of negative affect is thus especially important in the context of chronic pain and should be addressed by the physician during the initial physical examination.

In our preceding discussion of pain behavior, we provided an introduction to cognitive theory in an effort to explain the psychological reasons for inappropriate illness behavior. Our goal in this section is to extend our discussion of cognitive theory to explain inappropriate affect as well. Before doing so, however, it may be useful to digress briefly for the purpose of explaining our use of the term "inappropriate." By referring to exaggerated illness behavior or guilt as inappropriate we do not necessarily wish to imply the presence of a psychological disorder or illness. We simply wish to indicate that such symptoms are self-defeating since they may directly as well as indirectly exacerbate the patient's pain. Thus, the term "inappropriate" does not reflect a diagnostic judgment so much as suggest a failure to cope adequately with an adverse set of medical or physical circumstances. We should note that there are "appropriate" emotional responses to pain that are thoroughly negative in their hedonic quality but do not directly or indirectly exacerbate pain or compromise the patient's response to medical intervention. Such appropriate emotional responses include concern, frustration, annoyance, and disappointment, regret, or grief following loss of physical function or inability to perform premorbid activities. Inappropriate emotions corresponding to these include anxiety, anger, hostility, and guilt or depression.

Along with exaggerated illness behavior, self-defeating affect may be the result of faulty or irrational thinking (4). When patients evaluate chronic pain as "unbearable," for example, they trigger a protective, autonomic response that is both unnecessary and disproportionate to the pain stimulus. While chronic pain may be highly aversive, it is by definition "bearable" since the patient has been bearing it for many months. The act of arbitrarily labeling pain as "awful" or as worse than it "should" be is called "awfulizing," and we believe it is frequently the cause of unnecessary pain-related stress. Just as patients talk themselves into self-defeating illness behavior, they also create needless emotional suffering by misinterpreting or otherwise thinking erroneously about their pain. We realize that physicians may not have the time or inclination to adequately assess all facets of the patient's adjustment status, but a few questions on this subject may provide valuable information bearing directly on the patient's medical condition. We have organized the following questions into three distinct categories of emotional "disorder" corresponding to anxiety, anger, and depression. Each category is prefaced with a set of questions designed to assess the patient's current emotional state. We should emphasize that these categories are not mutually exclusive and thus cannot be used for patient diagnosis or classification. We do not believe that patients can or should be defined in terms of their emotional responses to pain. Rather, our view is that emotional responding will depend on the particular constellation of rational and irrational beliefs that are "active" in the patient's mind at any given time. Patients may thus exhibit different emotional responses to the same stimulus on different occasions (depending on which beliefs happen to be "in use"). While some patients may be predominantly anxious, others may be both anxious and depressed.

### Anxiety

The first set of questions about emotional disturbance is designed to elicit information about the patient's current level of anxiety.

13. Does the patient report or exhibit signs of excessive worry, nervousness, or anxiety (e.g., rapid respiration or shortness of breath; chronic muscle tension, spasm, or tremor; excessive sweating or cold hands; palpitations; sleep disturbance)?

14. If the pain is of traumatic origin, does the patient dwell on or ruminate about the traumatic incident; experience flashbacks, sleep disturbance, or nightmares; and avoid situations (such as driving) that may reminiscent of the original trauma?

15. Does the patient report discrete periods of heightened anxiety or panic accompanied by such symptoms as shortness of breath, palpitations, feeling faint, or trembling and associated with an intense fear of dying, losing control, or going insane?

Anxiety is an emotional response to the anticipation of serious bodily injury or death. The ability to anticipate harm is a basic function of human cognition since it allows for the possibility of escape and/or increased physical readiness to cope with danger. From a cognitive standpoint, the perception of threat is sufficient to elicit increased physiological arousal, often referred to as an "emergency response," characterized by rapid and shallow breathing, increased blood pressure and heart rate, decreased gastric motility, and increased muscle tone. These short-term physiologic changes enable us to effectively engage in various self-protective behaviors, including "fight or flight" responses. Unfortunately, the cognitive mechanism responsible for triggering physiologic arousal is subject to human error and may needlessly elicit arousal (i.e., the physical symptoms associated with anxiety) even in the absence of any danger. We have already mentioned that many patients have a tendency to awfulize their pain, that is, to erroneously label it as threatening and thereby trigger an autonomic response that is both unnecessary and self-defeating. Such irrational thinking can occasionally be corrected through cognitive restructuring therapy and, in our opinion, this should be attempted when anxiety is a problem (16).

After sustaining a sudden cervical injury, patients may be at increased risk of developing a posttraumatic stress disorder involving frequent flashbacks of the traumatic incident; increased autonomic arousal associated with sleep disturbance, hypervigilance, and/or exaggerated startle response; and avoidance of situations or activities (such as driving) that may be reminiscent of the original trauma. The most salient symptom of this disorder is probably the occurrence of frequent and *intrusive* thoughts that cause the patient to reexperience or "relieve" the traumatic event.

The possibility of subtle closed-head injury should also be considered in all patients who present with a traumatically induced cervical sprain or "whiplash." The incidence of neuropsychological deficit in patients with chronic pain may be as high as 66% in the case of head and neck injury and 18% in the case of low back injury (22). It should be noted that subtle brainstem injuries secondary to cervical trauma will typically not be detected by either a mental status examination or computed tomographic scan or surface electroencephalographic recording. Nevertheless, patients may sustain subcortical damage following "hyperflexion-hyperextension" injury resulting in inattentiveness, distractability, losing one's train of thought, impairment in recent as well as short-term memory, and inability to maintain eye contact (22). Whenever head injury is involved, when the patient cannot recall an injury as a result of retrograde amnesia, and in virtually all cases of traumatic cervical injury, a screening examination by a qualified neuropsychologist may be appropriate.

Finally, we have found a relatively high incidence of panic disorder in patients with chronic pain and suggest that physicians be alert to this possibility. Panic disorder is a psychological dysfunction associated with discrete periods of intense anxious affect that the patient perceives as "uncontrollable." Although these attacks are discrete, transient events, the patient often becomes excessively apprehensive about the possibility that another one will occur. As a result, he scrupulously avoids any situation or circumstance that might trigger such an attack and in the process develops a tendency toward excessive avoidance behavior. The patient with panic disorder is often hypervigilant and acutely aware of normal internal (physiologic) events such as increased heart rate, shortness of breath, and fatigue during or following physical exertion. Such sensations are often construed as evidence that the patient's body is "out of control," that a heart attack is imminent, or that the patient is on the verge of "going crazy." The presence of persistent, uncontrollable pain in such a patient may thus be misconstrued as yet another signal of impending disaster. For this reason, patients with a predisposition to or actual history of panic may be at increased risk of either developing the disorder or relapsing following the onset of chronic pain.

## Anger

The next set of questions is designed to detect a problem with pain-related anger.

16. Does the patient report more frequent loss of temper and/or feelings of hostility following the onset of pain?
17. When pain increases or prevents the patient from engaging in a favorite activity or performing a routine chore, is there a tendency to feel angry and/or aggravated as opposed to frustrated?
18. Is the patient aware of any correlation between the onset of anger and an increase in pain symptoms (such as headache, muscle tension, or spasm)?

Patients who feel resentful about pain often see it as unfair, as if to suggest that nature were somehow obligated to be fair. The reason for their anger is their conviction that they "should" not be subjected to misfortune since they have done nothing to deserve it. Of course, this only makes sense if justice is in fact a universal imperative and nature is actually obligated to behave fairly. In reality, life is often unfair since people afflicted with pain and disability have often done nothing to warrant their bad luck. Anger thus stems from our failure to accept an unfortunate reality, namely that none of us are exempt from misfortune or, for that matter, from unfair treatment at the hands of others. While universal justice may be our preference, it is clearly not a necessity since the universe need not and often does not conform to our preferences. The tendency to confuse a personal preference with a law of nature is so common as to suggest that we humans may have a predisposition to think in this irrational manner. Nevertheless, for those individuals with neuromuscular injury or illness, this tendency is self-defeating since it may result in autonomic arousal that directly or indirectly exacerbates pain. Irrational "demands" are simply thinking habits and as such may be corrected, assuming the patient is motivated to correct them, through cognitive therapy.

## Depression

The last set of questions in this section is intended to identify patients who may have a problem with depression.

19. Does the patient exhibit symptoms of depression such as prolonged periods of depressed mood, loss of interest or pleasure in most or all activities, disturbance of sleep and/or appetite, psychomotor agitation or retardation, frequent fatigue or loss of energy, diminished ability to concentrate, recurrent thoughts of death or suicidal ideation, and feelings of hopelessness and/or worthlessness?
20. If the patient admits to suicidal ideation, has he formulated a plan and does he express serious suicidal intent?
21. When the patient fails to meet social or work-related obligations, does he tend to blame himself or feel guilty?
22. Does the patient frequently perform burdensome or otherwise unpleasant chores with the intent of helping others and/or winning social approval?

Many patients with chronic pain have a tendency toward depressed mood that complicates the course of their medical treatment but nevertheless falls short of meeting the criteria for either a major depression or any other psychiatric disorder as defined in the *Diagnostic and Statistical Manual of Mental Disorders*, revised third edition (DSM III-R). We will therefore use the term "depression" in this section to denote a specific emotional response to pain without necessarily implying the presence of psychiatric illness. Nevertheless, recent estimates appear to place the incidence of clinical depression in the chronic pain population as somewhere between 25% and 54% (23). The problem is so prevalent that Blumer and Heilbronn (24) have proposed defining chronic pain as merely a symptom of depressive illness. According to their model, patients with chronic pain do not become depressed because of their pain and disability but rather develop chronic pain because they are depressed. They propose a new diagnostic category called "dysthymic pain disorder," which they define as a psychological dysfunction stemming from the patient's immature and insatiable need for achievement and/or approval. While we view the Blumer and Heilbronn proposal as provocative and agree that many patients with chronic pain exhibit a premorbid tendency "toward excessive physical activity and over-achievement" (p. 198), we still believe that to equate chronic pain with depressive illness overstates the relationship. In our opinion, such a diagnosis does little to advance the cause of psychological assessment since it does not pin down the cognitive causes of either illness behavior or affective distress.

From a cognitive standpoint, depression usually stems from either self-blame (resulting in guilt) or self-pity, in which patients convince themselves that pain is so debilitating and long lasting as to preclude their ever living a "normal" or relatively happy life (25). Aside from negative self-rating (discussed below), the cognitive errors responsible for depression are primarily: (*a*) awfulizing the consequences of pain and associated physical limitations, as when patients view their circumstances as nothing short of catastrophic or devastating; and (*b*) "fortune telling" or negative forecasting, in which current pain and suffering are used to "prove" the existence of future pain and suffering. The result of these irrational thinking tendencies may be a profound sense of hopelessness resulting in any or all of the symptoms of depression (see Question 19). The extent to which patients are incapacitated by depression will depend entirely on the extent to which they actually believe their own irrational thinking. The frequency and severity of depressed mood may thus vary from mild and insignificant to extreme and even suicidal. As indicated in Question 20, patients who admit to suicidal ideation should be questioned carefully about their intent. There is obviously an ethical as well as a legal obligation to protect suicidal patients from themselves even if that entails involuntary commitment.

When pain and physical limitations force people to reduce or abandon their usual efforts to please others, the result is often an inappropriate sense of guilt. From our cognitive vantage point, guilt stems from an irrational tendency to blame or otherwise condemn oneself for having committed a wrongful act. Many of us tend to accept ourselves as worthwhile only so long as we fulfill certain obligations or meet certain conditions. When we violate one of these conditions and thereby fail to satisfy our own self-imposed standards of conduct, we irrationally rate ourselves as "bad" or, at least, as less worthy. Since humans are, by virtue of their biology, imperfect beings who are prone to mistakes, deficiencies, and physical limitations, such a philosophy is necessarily self-defeating and illogical. As a result of their conditional self-worth, many individuals feel compelled to perform tasks that are inherently unenjoyable but that effectively please others. Such tasks may be associated with excessive muscle use and result in chronic muscle fatigue and/or strain. In the presence of traumatic injury such inappropriate muscle use may contribute to muscle hyperactivity, spasm, and the persistence of pain. Nevertheless, many patients find it difficult to abandon these efforts since doing so would necessarily entail significant emotional pain in the form of guilt or self-blame. Many of our patients, for example, continue to perform heavy household chores or engage in strenuous work activities despite explicit medical advice to the contrary. Merely instructing such patients about appropriate physical restrictions is unlikely to deter them from persisting in their efforts to meet their perceived social "obligations." With appropriate psychological intervention, however, these patients may learn to cognitively dispute their irrational self-downing philosophy and begin placing their own health and well-being above the needs and interests of other people.

## Concluding Remarks

Before concluding our discussion of emotional disturbance we should note that many individuals who have not suffered neuromuscular injury or illness hold precisely the same irrational beliefs we have just attributed to patients with chronic pain. That is, they tend to equate their self-worth with their physical capacity, awfulize practical difficulties, however minor or major, and believe that present events may be used to predict the future. In some ways, therefore, the only difference between so-called normal individuals and those with chronic pain is that the latter have sustained a physical injury or illness while the former have not. Despite their cognitive similarity, however, patients and nonpatients may also differ on various cognitive dimensions such as the extent to which they feel obligated to perform burdensome or otherwise unpleasant chores in order to obtain social approval. The possibility that premorbid cognitive differences are implicated in the development of chronic pain will be addressed in the next section.

## PREMORBID RISK FACTORS

In susceptible individuals, acute cervical injury may trigger the onset of chronic pain and illness. At issue here is whether we can identify factors that render patients susceptible or vulnerable to such a chronic course. Aside from unaccounted for physical findings, what separates those who become chronic from those who do not may be their premorbid psychological history and their biologic vulnerability to stress-related medical disorder. We should stress at the outset that our ability to predict chronicity based on differences in premorbid functioning is limited at best. We will not attempt a comprehensive review of all known individual differences or risk factors since many, if not most, are of little value in predicting which patients ultimately become chronic. Nevertheless, there are a few risk factors that should be addressed in the interest of identifying possible psychological dysfunction. These include a hard-driving, work-oriented life-style characterized by excessive self-sacrifice and/or hyperactivity; premorbid history of depression or other psychiatric disorder; premorbid drug abuse or dependency; a preexisting chronic pain syndrome or other stress-related illness; early exposure to disability role models; and a history of sexual and/or physical abuse.

## Excessive Work-Oriented Behavior

23. Does the patient have a premorbid history of hard-driving, work-oriented behavior?

Many patients who go on to develop chronic pain following an acute injury or illness report a premorbid pattern of excessive self-sacrifice, hyperactivity, or overachievement (26–28). They often have a history of going to work at an early age, putting in frequent overtime hours, and holding more than one job at a time. They may have permitted or encouraged others to rely upon them excessively and, as a result, were routinely called upon and expected to perform special tasks or favors. These tasks were often burdensome in nature or at least not intrinsically rewarding for the patient. Following the onset of pain, this pattern of unrelenting self-sacrifice and overachievement typically comes to an abrupt halt with the patient becoming the recipient of special care instead of the provider (24). This role reversal is particularly striking and, in our experience, is quite prevalent among patients who develop chronic pain. The onset of physical injury or illness apparently offers these patients an opportunity to relieve themselves of their occupational and social obligations without any need for self-reproach and without any loss of social approval. From a cognitive perspective, they subscribe to an irrational philosophy in which self-worth is equated with work achievement and social acceptance is a prerequisite of self-acceptance. In effect, they believe they cannot afford to fail or disappoint others, so instead of saying to themselves "I want to do this" or "I'd like to do that" they erroneously think "I should do this" or "I have to do that." The performance of a routine task is thus elevated from a mere preference to an absolute necessity.

Patients with such a dire need for achievement or acceptance may often behave in accordance with a set of irrational, self-imposed demands such as:

"If someone is depending on me to accomplish something, I should not let them down."
"I should try to accomplish something every day."
"Once I make a commitment to do something, I must not break it."

Of course, such demands only apply so long as the patient is physically fit. So long as the patient continues to labor under such a philosophy, medical intervention is unlikely to succeed since it threatens a return to premorbid functioning. In the absence of cognitive change, patients may find it necessary to choose between remaining disabled and excessively inactive versus resuming an action-oriented life-style that is inherently unrewarding and, in addition, likely to exacerbate their neuromuscular injury or illness.

## History of Psychiatric Disorder

24. Does the patient have a history of depression or other psychiatric disorder?

In one recent study, the incidence of psychiatric disorder among patients with chronic pain was found to be approximately 50% (29). Of the 106 patients included in the study, 33% met the DSM III-R criteria for "Major Depression" and 15% were diagnosed as having "Hypochondriasis." This study also found the prevalence of depression and hypochondriasis to be more or less the same regardless of the presence or absence of organic pathology. Thus, psychiatric and organic pathology are not mutually exclusive but actually coexist frequently in a chronic pain population. Nevertheless, subjective estimates of pain intensity were found to correlate with severity of depressive illness, raising the possibility that psychiatric impairment may exacerbate, if not actually cause, the symptoms associated with chronic pain. Given the prevalence of depression and hypochondriasis in this population, it may be appropriate to screen patients for both of these "disorders." Criteria associated with depression have already been presented elsewhere in this chapter. A diagnosis of hypochondriasis is usually made when the patient is convinced of having a serious disease despite evidence to the contrary and despite frequent reassurances by a doctor. The patient is often anxious, is prone to "doctor shopping," and may feel that he is not receiving proper medical care. In referring to such hypochondriacal tendencies as a "disorder" we are simply using a convenient shorthand to convey what may actually be a constellation of irrational beliefs about disease.

Previous episodes of psychological dysfunction, especially depression, may render the patient vulnerable to inappropriate illness behavior following the onset of a painful traumatic injury. It is essential, therefore, to determine whether the patient has had psychiatric or psychological treatment in the past and, if not, whether anyone in his family has had such treatment. The occurrence of psychiatric or psychological disorder in a patient's family significantly increases his risk of developing either the same disorder or a related one. Regardless of how the disorder is transmitted, whether socially or genetically, the fact remains that psychological dysfunction is more likely when there is evidence of such dysfunction in the patient's family.

## Substance Abuse

25. Does the patient have a history of substance abuse or dependency?

Patients may be at increased risk of abusing prescription medication following the onset of pain if they have already abused such medication or other addictive drugs in the past. There is also reason to believe that premorbid drug abuse may be correlated with or even secondary to premorbid psychopathology (30). The correlation of depression with alcohol dependency, for example, has led to speculation that patients with limited coping resources may attempt to control their negative affect with psychoactive drugs. According to cognitive theory (31), patients who engage in addictive behavior exhibit a pattern of irrational thinking that resembles in certain respects the irrational thinking we have previously associated with inappropriate illness behavior. For example, patients with a substance abuse problem often make the following cognitive mistakes: (a) awfulizing negative emotion—a tendency to label negative mood states or feelings as "unbearable," resulting in an exceedingly poor tolerance for discomfort of any kind; (b) negative forecasting— a tendency to assume that past coping failures necessarily "prove" the patient to be incapable of change, resulting in feelings of helplessness and depression; and (c) self-blaming—a tendency to think less of oneself for behaving poorly or unsuc-

cessfully, resulting in depressed mood, an additional incentive to engage in substance abuse. Any or all of these thinking errors may effectively predispose patients to a chronic course following the onset of traumatic injury or illness. Specifically, such patients may awfulize their pain and inconvenience, predict a pattern of neverending pain, distress, and disability, and then damn themselves for being physically incapacitated, unproductive, and apparently unable to cope. In so doing, they may set the stage for depressive disorder, substance abuse, and other related symptoms of inappropriate illness behavior.

## History of Chronic Pain or Stress-Related Illness

26. Does the patient have a history of chronic pain or other stress-related medical illness?

A concurrent or premorbid diagnosis of fibromyalgia, myofascial pain, temporomandibular joint pain, migraine or muscle contraction headache, trigeminal neuralgia, postherpetic neuralgia, or any other chronic pain syndrome may be associated with the presence of psychological dysfunction. Even when such dysfunction is not etiologically significant, it may occur as a secondary phenomenon in response to pain. Prolonged exposure to pain, therefore, of whatever type and of whatever origin, is a risk factor that may signal the presence of inappropriate illness behavior and/or excessive autonomic arousal. We have already made the point that stress-related illness is more common among patients with chronic as opposed to acute pain (8). When it occurs premorbidly, such illness may reflect either a predisposition to stress or a biologic vulnerability to stress-induced injury. In a related vein, there is recent evidence to suggest that offspring of patients with fibromyalgia, a form of chronic musculoskeletal pain, may be at increased risk of contracting the disease (32). It is unclear whether such genetic influence is limited to cases of fibromyalgia or may extend to other forms of chronic pain as well. In any event, it may be useful to inquire about the presence of pain-related symptoms among members of the patient's family.

## History of Childhood Trauma or Stress

27. Was the patient exposed to chronic illness during childhood?

28. Did the patient sustain the loss of a loved one early in life?
29. Was the patient a victim of physical or sexual abuse?

Traumatic or otherwise stressful experiences in childhood appear to render some individuals more vulnerable to subsequent psychological dysfunction and may increase the risk of chronic pain following an acute injury or illness (33). Early and prolonged exposure to disability may also provide patients with an opportunity to acquire an extensive repertoire of illness behavior. Such patients may learn vicariously or through first-hand experience that overt displays of pain and suffering are routinely met with increased attention and avoidance of responsibility. Physical and/or sexual abuse or the loss of a parent or close relative at an early age (through death or divorce) renders the patient more vulnerable to emotional disorder as an adult and may set the stage for a failure to cope with subsequent injury (28).

## SUMMARY

Psychological dysfunction may either directly exacerbate or indirectly complicate the course of cervical pain and should be assessed during the initial physical examination. Our goal has been to sensitize the physician to selected signs and symptoms that may be associated with a chronic course of illness as opposed to an uncomplicated, acute injury. Toward that end, we have addressed three broad categories of information that may have a bearing on the presence or absence of psychological dysfunction: inappropriate illness behavior, emotional disorder, and premorbid risk factors. We further attempted to explain virtually all psychological symptoms in terms of their antecedent cognitive causes and, thus, adopted a frankly biased theoretical stance. We feel justified in doing so since: (a) most of the literature on chronic pain does not address the role of irrational cognition and is thus overly skewed in the opposite direction; and (b) evidence in favor of cognitive theory is compelling and, in our opinion, more persuasive than evidence for competing, noncognitive theories (4).

We have also argued that chronic pain is primarily the result of psychological dysfunction and not a symptom of physical disease. While many patients with chronic pain have demonstrable physical findings (34), often involving abnormal muscle function, these findings are rarely, if ever, sufficient to explain the persistence of pain sensation or the extent of pain-related disability. In fact, muscle hyperactivity, spasm, and other abnormalities may themselves be the result of inappropriate or hyperactive behavior (including postural neglect) as well as excessive autonomic arousal (6). Thus, the only physical findings in this population appear more consistent with a psychological than a biologic view of human illness. If we are ever to appreciate the clinical significance of chronic as opposed to acute cervical pain, we believe it will be necessary to abandon the search for a strictly biologic explanation.

By taking the time to evaluate the role of psychological dysfunction, the acute care physician may be in a position to effectively short-circuit the development of chronic disability. The questions raised in this chapter may help physicians to identify patients at risk of psychological involvement and thus in need of multidisciplinary treatment. Timely referral to a pain clinic, before a pattern of disability is established, can significantly enhance the prospects for restoration of function and return to gainful employment. Increased awareness of psychological issues in patients with chronic cervical pain will, we hope, encourage physicians to withdraw palliative medications and other pain-relieving modalities from those patients who present with behavioral or emotional symptoms of nonmedical origin. Continued medical treatment of these patients may encourage their pursuit of a medical solution to what often turns out to be a nonmedical problem.

*Acknowledgment.* The authors wish to extend their appreciation to Ralph E. Sweeney, Jr., M.D., Edward S. Rachlin, M.D., and Wen-Hsien Wu, M.D., for offering us the benefit of their considerable insight and expertise.

## REFERENCES

1. Sternbach RA: *Pain: A Psychophysiological Analysis.* New York, Academic Press, 1968.
2. Chapman CR, Bonica JJ: *Chronic Pain.* Kalamazoo, MI, Upjohn, 1985.
3. Waddell G: A new clinical model for the treatment of low-back pain. *Spine* 12:632–644, 1987.
4. Ciccone DS, Grzesiak RC: Cognitive dimensions of chronic pain. *Soc Sci Med* 19:1339–1345, 1984.
5. Aryanpur J, Ducker TB: Differential diagnosis and management of cervical spine pain. In Tollison CD (ed): *Handbook of Chronic Pain Management.* Baltimore, Williams & Wilkins, 1989, pp 320–334.
6. Holmes TH, Wolff HG: Life situations, emotions, and backache. *Psychosom Med* 14:18–33, 1952.
7. Middaugh SJ, Kee WG: Advances in electromyographic

monitoring and biofeedback in the treatment of chronic cervical and low back pain. In Eisenberg MG, Grzesiak RC (eds): *Advances in Clinical Rehabilitation.* New York, Springer, 1987, vol 1, pp 137–172.

8. Sarno JE: Etiology of neck and back pain: an autonomic myoneuralgia? *J Nerv Ment Dis* 169:55–59, 1981.

9. Leavitt F, Sweet JJ: Characteristics and frequency of malingering among patients with low back pain. *Pain* 25:357–364, 1986.

10. Waddell G, McCulloch JA, Kummel E, Venner RM: Nonorganic physical signs in low back pain. *Spine* 5:111–119, 1980.

11. Keefe FJ, Crisson JE: Assessment of behaviors. In Lynch NT, Vasudevan SV (eds): *Persistent Pain: Psychosocial Assessment and Intervention.* Boston, Kluwer, 1988, pp 61–73.

12. Keefe FJ, Wilkins RH, Cook WA: Direct observation of pain behavior in low back pain patients during physical examination. *Pain* 20:59–68, 1984.

13. Cailliet R: *Low Back Pain Syndrome.* Philadelphia, FA Davis, 1981.

14. Zohn DA: *Musculoskeletal Pain.* Boston, Little, Brown, 1988.

15. Fordyce WE: *Behavioral Methods in Chronic Pain and Illness.* St. Louis, CV Mosby, 1976.

16. Ciccone DS, Grzesiak RC: Cognitive therapy: an overview of theory and practice. In Lynch NT, Vasudevan SV (eds): *Persistent Pain: Psychosocial Assessment and Intervention.* Boston, Kluwer, 1988, pp 133–161.

17. Maruta T, Swanson DW, Finlayson RE: Drug abuse and dependency in patients with chronic pain. *Mayo Clin Proc* 54:241–244, 1979.

18. Turner JE, Calsyn DA, Fordyce WE, Ready LB: Drug utilization patterns in chronic pain patients. *Pain* 12:357–363, 1982.

19. France RD, Urban BJ, Keefe FJ: Long-term use of narcotic analgesics in chronic pain. *Soc Sci Med* 19:1379–1382, 1984.

20. Leventhal H, Meyer D, Nerenz D: The common sense representation of illness. In Rachman S (ed): *Medical Psychology.* London, Pergamon, 1980, vol 2.

21. Ciccone DS, Grzesiak RC: Chronic musculoskeletal pain: a cognitive approach to psychophysiologic assessment and intervention. In Eisenberg MG, Grzesiak RC (eds): *Advances in Clinical Rehabilitation.* New York, Springer, 1990, vol 3, pp 197–214.

22. Schwartz DP: Cognitive deficits. In Lynch NT, Vasudevan SV (eds): *Persistent Pain: Psychosocial Assessment and Intervention.* Boston, Kluwer, 1988, pp 23–41.

23. Getto CJ: Depression. In Lynch NT, Vasudevan SV (eds): *Persistent Pain: Psychosocial Assessment and Intervention.* Boston, Kluwer, 1988, pp 93–115.

24. Blumer D, Heilbronn M: Dysthymic pain disorder: the treatment of chronic pain as a variant of depression. In Tollison CD (ed): *Handbook of Chronic Pain Management.* Baltimore, Williams & Wilkins, 1989, pp 197–209.

25. Beck AT: *Depression.* Philadelphia, University of Pennsylvania Press, 1970.

26. Houdenhove BV, Stans L, Verstraeten D: Is there a link between 'pain-proneness' and 'action-proneness'? *Pain* 29:113–117, 1987.

27. Blumer D, Heilbronn M: The pain-prone disorder: a clinical and psychological profile. *Psychosomatics* 22:395–402, 1981.

28. Engel GL: Psychogenic pain and the pain-prone patient. *Am J Med* 26:899–918, 1959.

29. Benjamin S, Barnes D, Berger S, Clarke I, Jeacock J: The relationship of chronic pain, mental illness and organic disorders. *Pain* 32:185–195, 1988.

30. Mendels J: *Concepts of Depression.* New York, Wiley, 1970.

31. Greenwood V: RET and substance abuse. In Ellis A, Bernard ME (eds): *Clinical Applications of Rational-Emotive Therapy.* New York, Plenum Press, 1985, pp 209–235.

32. Pellegrino MJ, Waylonis GW, Sommer A: Familial occurrence of primary fibromyalgia. *Arch Phys Med Rehabil* 70:61–63, 1989.

33. Pennebaker JW: Traumatic experience and psychosomatic disease: explaining the effects of behavioral inhibition, obsession and confiding. *Can Psychol* 26:82–95, 1985.

34. Rosomoff HL, Fishbain DA, Goldberg M, Santana R, Rosomoff RS: Physical findings in patients with chronic intractable benign pain of the neck and/or back. *Pain* 37:279–287, 1989.

# 7

# ASSOCIATED CONDITIONS
# AND DIFFERENTIAL DIAGNOSIS

*John Aryanpur*

The patient with "pain in the neck" is commonly encountered in many different clinical situations. General practitioners, rheumatologists, orthopaedic and neurosurgeons, and rehabilitative medicine specialists all frequently treat and evaluate patients with complaints of acute or chronic cervical pain. The scope of this clinical problem is tremendous; a third of the population can recall a significant episode of severe neck pain within the past year (1) and it has been estimated that in any given month 10% of the population will experience an episode of pain in the neck (1). Epidemiologic studies reveal that one half to three quarters of all individuals report an episode of significant neck pain at some point in the past (2–4).

Pain in the neck is always debilitating, because unhindered neck mobility is a requisite for the majority of human occupational, recreational, and social activities. More than is realized, the neck is active in common daily activities—nodding, turning, lifting, and shaking hands. In a fundamental sense the neck acts as a mobile platform or fulcrum from which the highly refined sensory mechanisms of the head and face can be positioned to best interact with the world around us. Any disruption of normal neck function is therefore quickly appreciated as uncomfortable, and even painful. It is thus perhaps natural that the disparaging term "pain in the neck" has come to be so universally understood and employed in the description of unpleasant people or situations.

The human neck is a complex structure with multiple bony ligamentous, muscular, vascular,

and neural components. Trauma to or irritation of any of these components may produce the sensation of neck pain. In the course of investigating an apparent neck injury, coexistent pathologic processes such as degenerative osteoarthritis, joint and ligamentous laxity, inflammatory diseases of muscle, vascular insufficiency, and neural compression syndromes may also be discovered to be contributing significantly to the patients' neck pain. In addition, pathologic processes in other areas—such as the head, shoulder, diaphragm, or jaw—may cause pain that is referred to the neck and that is difficult to distinguish from primary cervical pathology. Finally, regardless of the severity or even the presence or absence of diagnosed underlying disease, all complaints of pain will be colored by numerous emotional and psychosocial factors particular to the individual patient. Thus the clinician investigating the complaint of neck pain requires a clear understanding of the potential structural and psychologic abnormalities underlying the pain complaint.

The relevant functional anatomy and biomechanics of the cervical spine have been reviewed in previous chapters, as have the various physical examination and diagnostic techniques that may be employed in the investigation of neck pain. In this chapter a framework for the evaluation of the patient with cervical pain is presented. This approach will allow the differentiation of cervical pain syndromes into several general categories, and suggest further investigations that should lead to a specific diagnosis. Subsequently, specific painful cervical conditions are reviewed individually.

## GENERAL CATEGORIES OF CERVICAL PAIN

Cervical spine pathology can involve muscle and ligamentous structrures, joints and bones, and nervous tissue. Often, one or more combinations of nerve, muscle, joint, or bone pathology will be present in an individual patient, complicating the diagnosis. In the vast majority of patients, however, specific pain presentations, coupled with characteristic history and physical findings, will allow the clinician to distinguish between primary injury to muscle, bone, and nervous tissue.

As in any clinical situation, several basic clinical questions must be answered in the evaluation of any patient with cervical pain before considering differential diagnostic possibilities. Information regarding the location, type, onset, and duration of the patient's symptoms is essential in directing the course of further investigation. Mechanical neck pain, dysphagia, and myelopathy of several months' duration, for example, might suggest a cervical spondylotic condition with anterior osteophytic compression of the esophagus. In contrast, posterior neck pain and cervical paraspinous muscle spasm in a individual recently involved in a motor vehicle accident would suggest an entirely different pathology, and would necessitate an entirely different approach to workup and initial treatment.

## ACUTE VERSUS CHRONIC PAIN

An obvious, but nonetheless important, distinction must be made between the "acute" and the "chronic" neck pain syndrome. The majority of patients seen by the general practitioner or emergency care physician will be of the "acute" nature. By far the vast majority of patients with the "acute" neck pain syndrome will ultimately prove to have suffered a cervical sprain, or whiplash, syndrome. Many such patients will report a specific traumatic event—such as a motor vehicle accident, lifting a heavy object, or turning the neck a certain way—from which they can date the onset of neck pain. In general, the duration of symptoms will have been 1 to 2 weeks or less, and the patient may even state that the pain has been slowly lessening. The pain itself is typically described as a posterior neck "tightness" or "spasm," often accompanied by headache, which severely restricts neck, shoulder, and upper extremity mobility. Not infrequently patients will complain of arm "weakness" or "numbness";

however on closer questioning and examination it will become obvious that the patient has confused disabilitating pain with neurologic impairment, and in fact no objective weakness or sensory disturbance is apparent. Physical examination often reveals cervical paraspinous muscle spasm only, and plain cervical radiographs are typically normal or at most exhibit straightening of the normal cervical lordotic curvature secondary to muscle spasm. Treatment of this condition with mild analgesics and muscle relaxants, avoidance of strenuous activity, short-term cervical bracing, and reassurance is nearly uniformly successful. Approximately 70% of patients who seek medical treatment for acute neck pain report improvement in or resolution of symptoms within 2 weeks of the initial visit (2).

These reassuring statistics however, do not, allay the need for comprehensive evaluation of every patient who presents with acute neck pain. Traumatic or spontaneous fractures/dislocations and disc herniations may be symptomatically indistinguishable from the more common cervical sprain syndromes. Furthermore, long-standing progressive cervical pathology, such as a slow-growing tumor, arthritic spinal degeneration, or occult infection, may present acutely in an otherwise well patient. Any unusual historical information or physical findings on initial evaluation should alert the clinician to the possibility of more serious underlying pathology, and prompt a more extensive initial workup. At a minimum, the patient with acute neck pain should undergo a general physical examination (with special attention to neck posture, mobility, and tenderness) as well as a neurologic examination. Since the consequences of missing serious cervical spine pathology are potentially devastating, a routine series of cervical spine radiographs should be obtained on all patients. More than 90% of unstable cervical spine lesions will be detected with a single cross-table lateral radiograph (5), and additional views will allow the appreciation of even more subtle pathology. In addition, even a normal cervical spine radiograph may prove useful as a baseline against which future films may be compared.

Although exceptions to any strict temporal criteria obviously exist, the patient with neck pain of greater than 2–3 weeks' duration may be considered to have the "chronic" neck pain syndrome. The heterogeneity of chronic pain-producing cervical pathologies makes it impossible to define a "characteristic" clinical presentation; however, salient features of the history and physical examination should suggest specific diagnostic possibilities. Association of the pain with trauma should prompt a search for occult articular or small process fractures, or chronic myofascial syndromes. The presence of coexistent chronic disease such as malignancy, rheumatoid arthritis, congenital abnormalities, or immunodeficiency states may shine light on the etiology of chronic neck pain. In cases in which thorough investigation reveals no obvious structural cause for neck pain, ongoing litigation or workman's compensation claims and other unrecognized secondary gains may be operative, creating the "amplified pain syndrome" (6). In general, patients with chronic neck pain syndromes will be referred to rheumatologic, orthopedic, or neurosurgical specialists for further evaluation and treatment. In addition to the investigations above, extensive evaluations utilizing magnetic resonance imaging, computed tomography, electrodiagnostic studies, and serologic investigations as described in previous chapters may be required before a final diagnosis is reached.

## PRIMARY PAIN PATTERN

A second critical distinction that must be made early in the evaluation of any patient with cervical spine pain regards the primary pattern or type of the pain complaint. A simplistic but not inaccurate categorization of cervical pain postulates three basic clinical pain patterns: the myotomal, sclerotomal, and dermatomal cervical pain syndromes. Classification of the patient's complaint in terms of these patterns can often simplify the differential diagnosis of neck pain.

The *myotomal pain pattern* is characterized by pain localized primarily to one muscle or muscle group. Movement of the neck in any direction exacerbates the pain, which is commonly described as an excruciating, sharp "spasm" or "stiffness." Often, the patient will also complain of occipital headache, probably due to constant contraction of the posterior neck musculature in an attempt to splint motion of the injured area. Physical examination reveals spasm of the injured muscle or muscle group with compensatory splinting of cervical motion. Palpation of the affected muscle characteristically reveals exquisite tenderness. Neurologic examination is normal and palpation of bony structures, although made difficult by muscle spasm, is painless.

The *sclerotomal pattern* of cervical pain may be similar to the myotomal pattern, but possesses certain important distinguishing characteristics related to the involvement of bone and joint structures. The pain itself is more typically described as "deep," "dull," or "aching" in quality. Neck motion aggravates the pain, and consequently splinting of the neck is commonly observed. Tension headache and jaw, shoulder, or scapular pain may also be observed as a result of sustained paracervical muscle spasm as well as referred pain patterns. Palpation may reveal focal muscle pain; invariably, however, this is accompanied by tenderness of underlying bony and joint structures. Pain that is reproduced by palpation of spinous processes in the posterior midline or by head compression or distraction maneuvers [Spurling's or "reverse Spurling's" tests (7)] is likely to be of bony or capsular origin. The neurologic examination is normal.

The *dermatomal pain pattern* is relatively uncommon, and signifies irritation or compression of neural tissue. For this reason prompt evaluation and treatment is required to forestall the development of permanent neurologic deficit. The patient may relate neck or shoulder pain as described above. In addition, however, the patient complains of arm, hand, or lower extremity symptoms such as pain, numbness, tingling, "clumsiness," stiff gait, or changes in bowel or bladder habits, all of which point to compromise of neurologic function. Radicular distribution of pain or sensory changes due to specific segmental or nerve root injury is common, and should be distinguished from patterns of referred pain from deeper structures. Physical examination will often reveal some element of cervical paraspinous muscle or bony tenderness, and mechanical pain may exist as discussed above. Neck motion may aggravate both the local and the radicular symptoms. Evidence of irritation of neural structures may be elicited by percussion (Tinel's sign) or by neck flexion or rotation (Lhermitte's sign). Neurologic examination may be normal, but often subtle changes in strength, sensation, or deep tendon reflexes may be detected by the careful examiner. For example, a decrease in fine or rapid alternating movements in the dominant hand may be the only sign of early motor involvement.

Obviously, these categorizations are not mutually exclusive, and may better be considered as gradations along a clinical spectrum. Many patients will present with combinations of the above patterns. For example, a patient with degenerative cervical osteoarthritis and neural foraminal stenosis causing cervical nerve root compression

**Table 7.1.**
**Categorization of Cervical Spine Pain**

| Duration of Symptoms | Pain Distribution | Example |
|---|---|---|
| Acute | Myotomal | Cervical sprain |
| | Sclerotomal | Fracture without neurologic deficit |
| | Dermatomal | Anterior spinal artery or central cord syndrome |
| Chronic | Myotomal | Chronic myofascial syndrome |
| | Sclerotomal | Bony tumor, osteoarthritis |
| | Dermatomal | Spinal cord tumor, primary neurologic disorder |

may well have symptoms and signs consistent with injury to muscular, bony, and neural structures. Diverse pathologies may contribute to the development of cervical muscle spasm and irritation, making this a nearly universal accompaniment of all complaints of neck pain. It is incumbent upon the clinician to determine as accurately as possible the position of each patient along this clinical gradation, and to reevaluate this assessment as frequently as the patients' changing clinical status may indicate. Table 7.1 outlines the basic differential diagnostic categorizations discussed above, and provides selected examples for each diagnostic category.

## ASSOCIATED CONDITIONS

An important and frequently overlooked cause of neck pain is referred pain from pathology in areas other than the neck itself. Temporomandibular joint syndromes, for example, may often present initially as lateral neck pain with decreased cervical mobility. Cardiac ischemic events classically involve left neck and jaw pain in addition to the more recognized substernal chest pain. Occipital neuritis is invariably associated with some degree of cervical paraspinous muscle spasm and pain, as are the tension and migraine headache variants.

In the trauma setting in particular, the clinician must be alert to the possibility of noncervical injury causing neck pain. The greater incidence of multisystem trauma related to high-speed vehicular accidents makes it increasingly likely that the trauma patient with neck pain will have suffered associated blunt abdominal or head injuries. A normal cervical spine radiographic series in a multitrauma patient with significant neck pain should at least prompt consideration of other possible etiologies for the pain, and may necessitate further diagnostic investigation. Traumatic diaphragmatic rupture, hemothorax, and upper mediastinal injures may cause shoulder and neck pain. Neck pain or stiffness in the obtunded patient with a basilar skull fracture or traumatic subarachnoid hemorrhage may be due solely to the head injury, or may indicate associated cervical injury undetected by the usual static plain radiographic views. Children, in particular, may complain of nonspecific neck pain with such injuries as a clavicular fracture or acromioclavicular separation. Children also have a significantly greater risk of radiographically nonapparent spinal injury because of their joint and ligamentous laxity and a relatively larger ratio of head to body weight (8). For this reason a high index of concern is warranted when dealing with any child with posttraumatic neck pain.

Although a full discussion of these associated conditions is beyond the scope of this chapter, the clinician treating patients with acute or chronic neck pain should be cognizant of these variations of cervical pain, and not hesitate to make referrals to appropriate specialists. Several more common noncervical pathologies that may cause neck pain are presented in the following pages.

## DIAGNOSTIC STUDIES

The evaluation of any complaint of neck pain must begin with plain films of the cervical spine. Frequently plain films will be sufficient to reveal pathologies such as osteoarthritis, osteoblastic or osteoclastic lesions, fractures, or dislocations. Oblique views allow visualization of the neural foramina and facets. When the question of cervical spinal stability arises, flexion and extension radiographs, always carefully supervised by an experienced physician, nay be diagnostic. Other views may be employed as needed, as discussed in previous chapters. With this initial radiographic information in hand, further radiographic, electrophysiologic, or laboratory studies may be rationally ordered.

Computed tomography (CT) remains the procedure of choice if detailed visualization of bony anatomy is required. Fractures, bony destructive processes, and osetophytic spurs are all easily evaluated with three-dimensional reconstructive techniques. Soft tissue and neural structures are in some circumstances adequately visualized with CT; however, in most cases the information obtained regarding soft tissue and spinal cord anatomy is insufficient. If soft tissue structures or neural tissues are the object of interest, routine myelography, intrathecally enhanced CT studies, and, more recently, magnetic resonance (MR) imaging studies are available. In most circumstances MR imaging offers the best anatomic information, and since it is totally noninvasive it has in recent years become the procedure of choice in evaluating the cervical spinal cord and soft tissues.

Radionucleotide scans, such as the gallium and leukocyte-tagged scans, are limited in anatomic resolution. They are, however, useful in the evaluation of possible spinal infections or neoplasms, particularly multiply myeloma. It should be remembered that these tests are fairly nonspecific and may remain abnormal for months after spinal injury or surgery.

Neurometric testing, including electromyographic (EMG) and nerve conduction velocity (NCV) techniques, are often useful in distinguishing the level and extent of injury to the nervous system. Following injury to a nerve or root, conduction velocities across the injured area will be abnormal. In contrast, evidence of denervation on EMG may take weeks to become apparent. Early in the disease course, therefore, NCV may be a more sensitive indicator of the level of disease.

Serologic investigations such as a complete blood count, sedimentation rate, protein electrophoresis, or rheumatoid screen may provide crucial information, and should be ordered early in the workup as dictated by the pertinent history and physical findings.

## SPECIFIC CERVICAL PAIN SYNDROMES

Based upon the history and physical examination, it should be possible to arrive at a tentative diagnosis in the vast majority of cases. Subsequent diagnostic studies will bolster or refute the initial clinical impression. Certain disorders that are common and should be familiar to every clinician are listed in Table 7.2 and are discussed below. This table is not all inclusive, but should serve to direct further investigation or referral to appro-

priate specialists. For a more comprehensive discussion of specific conditions in the differential diagnosis of cervical pain and corresponding treatment options the reader is referred to subsequent chapters of this text, or to one of the excellent review books on this subject (6, 9).

## CERVICAL TRAUMA

Mechanically the cervical spine may be considered a mobile platform that connects the head to the trunk. Sudden acceleration, deceleration, or rotation of the head or trunk will be transmitted through the cervical spine, resulting in the potential for serious cervical spine injury even with trauma that may superficially appear inconsequential. Based upon the mechanism of trauma, cervical spine injury may be divided into flexion, extension, rotation, or compression injuries. Each of these types is associated with a character-

**Table 7.2.**
**Pain Causing Disorders of the Cervical Spine**

Traumatic cervical pain syndromes
    Muscle sprain (whiplash)
    Fractures/dislocations
    Acute disc herniation ("soft disc")
    Spinal cord injury syndromes (anterior spinal artery
        and central cord syndromes, posttraumatic syrinx)
Degenerative osteoarthritis ("hard disc")
Tumors of the cervical spine
    Primary
    Metastatic
Tumors and chronic diseases of the cervical cord
    Intrinsic cord tumors
    Syrinx
    Intrinsic motor and sensory disorders
        Amyotrophic lateral sclerosis
        Spasmodic torticollis
        Multiple sclerosis
        Toxic/metabolic/vascular
Congenital spinal abnormalities
    Chiari malformations
    Klippel-Feil syndrome
    Os odontoideum
Rheumatoid arthritis and related conditions
    Polymyalgia rheumatica
    Ankylosing spondylitis
    Diffuse idiopathic skeletal hyperostosis
Infection
Referred pain syndromes
    Temporomandibular joint syndrome
    Occipital neuritis
    Reflex sympathetic dystrophy

**Table 7.3.**
**Fracture Patterns and Mechanisms**

| Mechanism of Injury | Fracture |
| --- | --- |
| Flexion | Anterior wedge |
| | Teardrop |
| | Anterior subluxation (unilateral or bilateral jumped facets) |
| | Clay shoveler's |
| Extension | Hangman's |
| | Posterior subluxation |
| | Articular process |
| Compression | Jefferson |
| | Wedge and burst |

istic set of fracture/dislocation patterns, as shown in Table 7.3.

In evaluating acute cervical spine trauma the historical facts alone are often sufficient to allow an educated guess as to the possible mechanism of trauma and resulting injuries to the patient. A history of a shattered windshield or bent steering wheel should indicate the possibility of cervical extension injury in the motor vehicle accident patient. Conversely, a diving accident or blow to the back of the head will most commonly result in a flexion injury. For these reasons, details of the traumatic event should be elicited carefully and accurately. In addition, in the current highly litigious climate a carefully recorded initial history and physical examination may prove very germane to later events.

Within each category of cervical spinal injury, the trauma itself may be divided into musculofascial, bony and ligamentous, and neurologic components. In general, the degree of injury will depend entirely upon the amount and direction of force transmitted to the cervical spine, and may not correlate with the severity of injury to other organ systems.

## Cervical Sprain (Whiplash)

By far the most frequent painful injury of the cervical spine is the cervical muscle sprain—more commonly referred to as a "whiplash" injury. Under normal conditions of movement and force the cervical muscles modulate many of the forces transmitted to the cervical spine via balanced contraction and relaxation. Sudden extremes of motion or force, however, may exceed the capacity of the cervical musculature to compensate, leading

to muscle sprain or rupture. Larger disruptive forces may cause bony and ligamentous damage in addition to the muscular injury. Classically the whiplash patient reports having been rear-ended in a motor vehicle accident; however, any sudden acceleration of the head relative to the body may cause this injury. The patient may walk away from the accident with no discomfort, only to notice the onset of neck pain several hours later. The pain associated with muscle sprain is usually described as an "aching" or "tightness" localized to the cervical paraspinous musculature. Exacerbation of the pain by neck motion is the rule. The pain usually reaches a maximum 2–3 days following the initial injury and then resolves slowly over 1–3 weeks. In the patient with a history of minor trauma, local neck pain with spasm and stiffness of cervical muscles, a normal neurologic examination, and normal plain films of the cervical spine the diagnosis of cervical sprain is usually appropriate. If any element in the history, physical examination, or radiographic studies is not consistent with the above then more serious cervical spine injury must be suspected, and further diagnostic workup is mandatory. As a corollary, traumatic neck pain that persists for more than 2–3 weeks following the injury should raise a red flag, and should be considered to be of bony or ligamentous origin until proven otherwise.

## Fractures/Dislocations

Trauma causing bony, articular, or ligamentous disruption is brought about by extreme abnormal movements or compressive forces in the neck. Although muscle and ligamentous structures provide some degree of protection from extremes of movement in flexion and extension, the cervical vertebrae are very vulnerable to axial compressive forces. These forces are commonly generated in diving and automobile accidents, accounting for the relatively high percentage of cervical spine injury in such instances. The actual injury from such forces is variable, and may cause ligamentous tear, bony fracture, or dislocation and malalignment depending upon the site of trauma and the force vectors involved. The pain associated with bony and ligamentous trauma is mechanical, sharp, and exacerbated by even the slightest cervical motion. In the absence of damage to neural structures radicular or dysesthetic pain should not be present. Significant paraspinous muscle spasm and tenderness is almost always present; however, the hallmark of bony or articular pathology is local bony tenderness on palpation. In general, plain cervical spine films will allow diagnosis of the majority of cases of traumatic cervical fracture or dislocation; however, in most cases further radiographic studies, including CT, are required to fully delineate the extent of the injury. Finally, in assessing spinal injury the presence or absence of spinal instability has important implications regarding further treatment plans and eventual patient outcome. Flexion or extension injuries of the cervical spine that disrupt both anterior and posterior elements are generally unstable and will require emergent reduction if displaced, followed usually by surgical stabilization.

Trauma may leave the patient neurologically intact and with plain radiographs that are normal. The majority of these patients will have muscle sprain injuries, and pain will resolve with the usual conservative therapies. In a small number of patients, however, disabling cervical pain will persist long after the apparent "muscle sprain." In these cases minor articular fracture or ligamentous or capsular rupture may be the source of pain. Abel, in a pre–CT era study, found radiographic evidence of small element articular fractures in many patients with chronic neck pain of previously undetermined etiology (10). With the advent of reconstructed and three-dimensional CT scanning progressively more subtle pathologies are being appreciated. In most such cases the patient can localize the discomfort accurately to the level of the lesion, and local injection of the damaged facets or ligaments with anesthetic agents may be both diagnostic and therapeutic.

The classification of cervical spine fractures/dislocations presented in Table 7.3 provides a framework for the discussion of specific fractures.

Cervical teardrop or anterior wedge fractures are associated with a *flexion-type injury*. These fractures are more common in the mid- to lower cervical spine, especially from C5 to T1, which is the transition area between the mobile cervical and the rigid thoracic spine. The vertebral body typically receives the brunt of the flexion force, and, depending upon the severity of the injury, either anterior wedging or compression of the entire vertebral body will result. In the later case, retropulsion of bone fragments into the spinal canal and compression of spinal cord or nerve roots is not uncommon. The mechanics of this type of injury make it likely that significant posterior element disruption will accompany the anterior fracture. Extreme flexion may cause distraction of posterior elements, with unilateral or bilateral facet dislocations, laminar or pedicle fractures, or rupture of interspinous and posterior longitudinal ligaments. These are obviously unstable injuries. A less severe type of flexion injury is the "clay shoveler's fracture" (Fig. 7.1 ). This is an avulsion fracture of the distal spinous process of C6, C7, or T1 caused by neck flexion in the setting of shoulder girdle muscle contraction, such as might occur during lifting a heavy object. Although

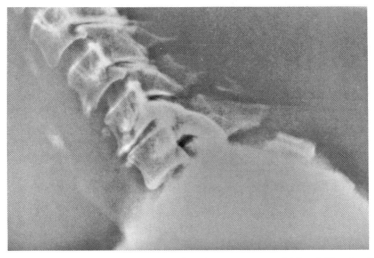

**Figure 7.1.**    Plain radiograph shows fractures through the spinous processes of C6 and C7: a clay shoveler's fracture.

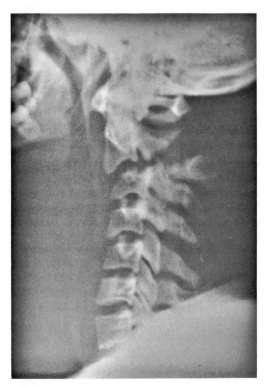

**Figure 7.2.** Plain radiograph shows fracture through the arch of C2 with subluxation: the hangman's fracture.

painful, these fractures are stable and not associated with neurologic deficits.

The prototypic *extension-type cervical injury* is a fracture through the neural arch of C2, the "hangman's fracture" (Fig. 7.2). In the classic fracture, with the knot of the hangman's rope secured under the chin, the weight of the free-falling body causes acute extension and distraction of the upper cervical spine. The result—bilateral fractures of the arch of C2 with dislocation—is uniformly fatal. Presently this type of injury is seen more commonly with less specifically focused trauma, such as that caused by collision with the windshield in motor vehicle accidents. The incidence of neurologic deficit with the modern-day hangman's fracture may be lower than that associated with flexion-type fractures, probably a reflection of the significantly higher early mortality of the hangman's fracture. Once again, fractures/dislocations of the posterior elements are frequent concomitants of this type of injury, and these are usually highly unstable fractures.

Direct axial compression of the cervical spine results in *compression fractures* such as the C1 compression fracture, or Jefferson fracture (Fig. 7.3). In this instance a blow to the head or a fall creates an axial compressive force that is directed inferiorly through the occipital condyles to the relatively fragile arch of C1. Bilateral or unilateral fracture of the C1 lateral mass and arch results. Fortunately, injury to neural tissue is rare with this mechanism of trauma, and disruption of posterior bony and articular elements is generally not encountered.

## Acute Disc Herniation

The application of severe flexion or axial compression forces to the cervical spine may rupture the disc annulus and cause prolapse of the nucleus pulposis into the spinal canal. In addition to the mechanical neck pain that results from a tear in the pain-sensitive external layers of the annulus, the prolapsed disc fragment may cause spinal cord or nerve root compression and resulting neurologic deficits. The patient with an acute cervical disc herniation, or "soft cervical disc," classically complains of neck pain and unilateral radicular neurologic symptoms after neck trauma. Unfortunately, if multiple bony injuries coexist, the disc herniation may be overshadowed on radiographic studies by bony abnormalities, and may be overlooked. Conversely, in the absence of bony injury, the clinician may not feel compelled to order the additional radiographic studies that allow detection of an acute disc herniation. In either case, the acutely herniated disc may be missed. A high index of suspicion for this particular pathology in

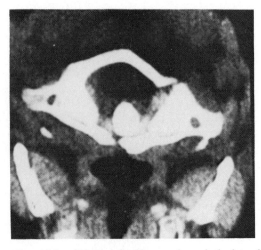

**Figure 7.3.** CT view of a fracture through the lateral mass and body of C1: the Jefferson fracture.

the patient with a history of neck trauma is indicated, and a careful review of MR or CT studies is usually sufficient to make the diagnosis.

## Spinal Cord Injury Syndromes

Finally, cervical spine trauma may cause injury to the nervous tissue itself. Although this most commonly occurs in the setting of cervical spine fractures, damage to neural structures may also occur independently of this, as in traumatic anterior spinal artery or central cord syndromes. Neck pain and the presence of neurologic deficit are presumptive evidence of traumatic cord/root injury. Severe dysesthetic radicular pain is frequent and may reflect either segmental spinal cord compression/ischemia or actual nerve root compression. With any severe spinal cord injury syndrome, an initial period of spinal shock may cause a flaccid plegia and areflexia that will mask the true extent of the deficits. Testing for sacral sensory sparing as well as the presence or absence of segmental spinal reflexes such as the bulbocavernosus or cremasteric are useful in determining whether the lesion is truly complete. In some cases, after the initial spinal shock has resolved some preservation of upper extremity sensory or motor function is noted. Proximal motor function may often be spared, but the fine motor control needed for adequate hand function is usually not recovered.

The *anterior spinal artery syndrome* is most frequently encountered in the setting of a flexion/compression-type injury with retropulsed bone fragments impinging on the anterior cord. Compression of the anterior spinal artery and ischemia in the distribution of that artery (anterior two thirds of the spinal cord, including gray matter and anterior and lateral funiculi) accounts for the classic picture of upper and lower extremity motor deficit, loss of pain and temperature sensation below the lesion, and preservation of position and gross tactile sensation. Recovery from this devastating lesion is unfortunately poor.

The *central spinal cord syndrome*, in contrast, is usually encountered in patients who have suffered hyperextension injuries of the cervical spine. Sudden neck extension in the elderly patient with cervical spondylotic degeneration is a common scenario. In this case, the cervical cord is driven by extension into anteriorly placed osteophytic bars or ridges. The result is cord contusion with disruption of penetrating radial arterial branches to the central gray region. Motor tracts descending in the lateral funiculus as well as ascending tracts

in the dorsal columns are typically spared, giving rise to the usual clinical picture of upper greater than lower extremity weakness and sensory deficit. Deficits may be fixed or may resolve over a period of hours to days, depending on the severity of injury.

A significant late sequela of spinal cord trauma is the development of *posttraumatic syringomyelia.* Damage to the central cord may lead to necrosis and, eventually, to frank cavitation of the central cord. The resulting syrinx may enlarge over months or years and cause slowly progressive segmental motor and sensory deficits. Dysesthetic radicular pain will slowly give way to a disassociated sensory loss and a lower motor neuron pattern of weakness as the lesion expands radially. The late progression of neurologic deficit in a spinal cord–injured patient should always suggest the possibility of a posttraumatic syrinx.

Whenever there is neurologic deficit in the presence of spinal trauma, adequate radiographic visualization of the spinal cord and thecal sac is essential for planning further treatment. Bony fragments, herniated discs, and epidural hematomas may all cause persistent cord compression and significant cord injury independent of that caused by the initial trauma itself. In all such cases intrathecally enhanced CT or MR scanning is therefore required.

## DEGENERATIVE OSTEOARTHRITIS

In normal individuals the cumulative trauma of daily wear and tear on mobile, weight-bearing joints such as the hips and knees causes progressive degenerative arthritic changes. This is all the more true for the cervical spine, which must support the 10–15-pound weight of the head through various maneuvers each day. Degenerative spondylosis, or osteoarthritis, of the cervical spine is common in all individuals over 50 years of age. Osteoarthritic changes of the vertebral column are usually associated with intervertebral disc degeneration and osteophyte formation (Fig. 7.4). Disc degeneration from acute or chronic repetitive trauma reduces the shock absorber effect of a well-hydrated intervertebral disc and causes abnormal stresses to be applied to the vertebral body, adjacent uncinate processes (joints of Luschka), and posterior facet areas. Over a period of time reactive osteophyte formation occurs along the abnormally stressed joint surfaces. Inflammation of joint linings and bony and cartilaginous exostoses may cause mechanical neck pain.

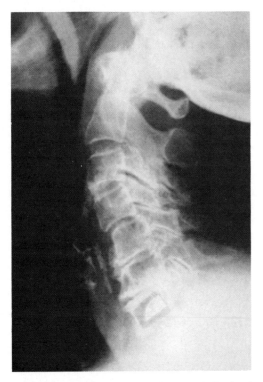

**Figure 7.4.** Plain radiograph of the cervical spine in this middle-age patient shows extensive osteoarthritic changes, loss of disc space height, and anterior and posterior lipping of vertebral bodies with osteophyte formation.

The lower, load-bearing areas of the cervical spine (C5–6 and C6–7) are the most common sites of degenerative cervical osteoarthritis.

Often, degenerative cervical spondylosis is totally asymptomatic. Mild to moderate degrees of disc degeneration or osteophyte formation are tolerated remarkably well by most individuals, and are common incidental findings on plain neck films. Occasionally, the patient with severe cervical osteoarthritis may experience neck pain triggered by activity, physical exertion, minor trauma, or even changes in weather. A rare patient may even suffer acute attacks with severe muscle spasm causing acute torticollis. This may be accompanied by a variety of symptoms—such as shoulder pain or stiffness or clicking sounds on neck motion—that should clue the examiner in to the sclerotomal, mechanical nature of the patients' pain. These painful episodes generally respond to symptomatic treatment and peak after a 2–3-day period. Total recovery is usual within 10–14 days.

If large enough or properly positioned, *osteophytic spurs* may cause compression of neural tissues, leading to the development of radicular

symptoms or myelopathy. Such lesions are commonly referred to as "hard discs," and are the most common cause of cervical radiculitis in the middle-age and elderly populations. Osteophytic spur formation off structures bordering the neural foramen, such as the uncinate process or facet joints, may cause foraminal stenosis and thereby compress or irritate exiting nerve roots. In addition to mechanical neck pain from joint disease, a prominent radicular or dermatomal component will also be present. Typically, patients with cervical root pain syndromes have neck and arm pain exacerbated by extension or turning of the head away from the painful side, both of which are maneuvers that stress the joint capsules and stretch the irritated root. Pain or numbness radiating over the shoulder or down the arm, weakness or sensory changes in the distribution of a particular nerve root, and appropriate reflex changes may all be encountered. The clinician should be familiar with the patterns of radicular pain in the cervical region. Cervical radiculitis may cause pain that radiates into the lower neck and shoulder (C4–5 roots) or down into the upper extremity (C6–T1 roots). These patterns are described in previous chapters. Unfortunately, differentiation between these patterns can sometimes be difficult in the clinical setting, and it is of more practical value to be able to recognize the possibility of nerve root irritation than to be able to specify exactly which root is involved. The predominantly radicular nature of these patients' symptoms and complaints is the key element of the history and physical examination.

Centrally placed hard discs off the posterior aspect of the vertebral body may impinge upon the anteroposterior diameter of the spinal canal. When combined with hypertrophied ligamentum flavum and articular capsule such impingement may be sufficient to cause cord compression and long tract signs and symptoms. This condition, termed "cervical spondylotic myelopathy" (11), represents the extreme of cervical degenerative osteoarthritis. The finding of neck pain, spastic gait, hyperactive lower extremity reflexes, and plain spine films demonstrating osteophytic spurring of the posterior aspect of cervical vertebral bodies should be sufficient to make a presumptive diagnosis. Further radiologic investigations that allow better delineation of cord and nerve root vis-à-vis bony anatomy are generally required.

Unfortunately, once osteoarthritic changes have reached the point of compression of neural tissue and radiculitis or myelopathy is present, remission of symptomatology is rare. Anti-inflammatory medications and mechanical stabilization by cervical bracing devices may prevent the progression of symptoms for a period of time; however, surgical intervention generally is the most expeditious way of effecting symptomatic relief, and has the added benefit of ensuring that further neural compression will not occur.

## TUMORS OF THE CERVICAL SPINE

Extramedullary neoplastic lesions of the cervical spine cause mechanical symptoms and localized pain due to bony destruction, and if large enough may compress neural tissue and lead to neurologic deficit. Tumors involving the cervical spine may be categorized into primary benign tumors, primary malignant tumors, and metastatic tumors. Malignant tumor metastases to bone are by far the most commonly encountered tumors of the cervical spine. A list of various tumor types is presented in Table 7.4.

The diversity of cervical spine tumors can be appreciated from Table 7.4; however, there are certain clinical characteristics common to patients with bony tumors of the neck. Pain resulting from the destruction of bony structures characteristically is described as "deep-seated" or "aching." The pain is initially mechanical in nature, and may be worse with motion. In addition, the pain is often worse at night. The patient may report falling asleep only to be awakened later by a deep, gnawing neck pain. Although the mechanism of such night pain is unclear, it may be caused by vascular engorgement and enlargement of the tumor during prolonged recumbency. Over time the pain typically increases in severity. If the tumor enlarges to impinge upon the spinal canal or neural foramina, or if bony destruction causes pathologic fractures, neurologic deficits may result. If the tumor irritates adjacent nerve roots a radiculopathy with motor and sensory deficits becomes apparent. As the tumor expands to fill a critical percentage of the cross-sectional diameter of the spinal canal a cervical myelopathy may appear. Occasionally a patient with a cervical spine tumor will present with the acute onset of neurologic symptoms without any significant history of pain; usually, however, the development of neurologic symptoms is clearly preceded by a period of mechanical neck pain.

A not infrequent scenario involves the patient with previously diagnosed malignancy who complains of axial neck or back pain. Every such patient—and in particular patients with tumors that frequently metastasize to the spine, such as breast, lung, prostate, and kidney tumors—must be promptly evaluated for spinal metastases. Cervical spine films with oblique views followed by CT scanning will reveal osteolytic or osteoblastic lesions, pathologic fractures, and abnormal soft tissue masses in the majority of cases. Definitive diagnosis requires tissue biopsy, either from the cervical lesion itself or, as is sometimes possible in metastatic lesions, from a more accessible tumor site.

**Table 7.4.**
**Tumors of the Cervical Spine**

Benign primary tumors
  Giant cell tumor
  Osteoblastoma
  Osteochondroma
  Eosinophilic granuloma
  Plasmocytoma
  Chondromyxoid fibroma
  Desmoid tumor
  Hemangioma
  Osteocartilaginous exostosis
  Rheumatoid pannus
Malignant primary tumors
  Chordoma
  Chondrosarcoma
  Osteosarcoma
  Ewing's sarcoma
  Aggressive solitary plasmocytoma
  Hemangiopericytoma
Metastatic
  Breast
  Prostate
  Renal
  Gastrointestinal
  Thyroid
  Lung
  Nasopharyngeal
Hematogenous metastatic process
  Multiple myeloma
  Lymphoma
  Hodgkin's disease

## TUMORS AND CHRONIC DISEASES OF THE CERVICAL CORD AND NERVOUS SYSTEM

### Intradural Spinal Tumors and Cavitary Lesions

Intradural or intramedullary lesions of the cervical cord may cause pain by a variety of mechanisms. Tumors of the spinal cord and theca may be classified into extradural extramedullary, in-

tradural extramedullary, and intradural intramedullary tumors. Extradural extramedullary tumors have been discussed above. Table 7.5 lists
intradural extra- and intramedullary spinal tumors.

*Extramedullary intradural lesions* such as menin-
giomas or neurofibromas characteristically erode
rather than destroy surrounding bone and often
do not cause the deep-seated bony pain associated
with primary bony tumors. The tumor may grow
to totally envelope a single nerve root with no apparent neurologic deficit on examination. As time
progresses, however, compression of the spinal
cord or nerve roots eventually becomes symptomatic. These tumors usually cause, at least initially,
predominately unilateral symptoms. Often the patient complains of unilateral radicular pain and
numbness only. Once again, as the mass grows
and the spinal cord is compressed signs and symptoms of myelopathy begin to predominate, and it
is usually at this point that the true nature of the
problem is appreciated.

*Intramedullary tumors* of the cervical spine are in
general slow-growing, infiltrative or expansile lesions. The most common intramedullary spinal tumors are spinal ependymomas and astrocytomas,
accounting together for 60–70% of all primary
spinal tumors (12). The spinal ependymoma is a
slow-growing tumor that originates from vestigial
ependymal cells lining the obliterated human central spinal canal. The tumor typically expands in a
superior inferior direction and radially, eventually compressing the spinal cord between it and
the confines of the spinal canal. Spinal astrocytomas are usually low-grade tumors that arise from
the neoplastic transformation of astrocytes. These
tumors are more infiltrative than ependymomas

**Table 7.5.**
**Intradural Intra- and Extramedullary Spinal Tumors**

Intradural intramedullary
  Astrocytoma
  Ependymoma
  Hemangioma
  Arteriovenous malformation
  Miscellaneous (lipoma, teratoma,
    ogligodendroglioma)
Intradural extramedullary
  Meningioma
  Neurofibroma
  Schwannoma
  Arteriovenous malformation
  Arachnoid cysts
  Metastatic tumors

and are consequently more difficult to treat surgically.

In general, pain is not the predominate presenting complaint of patients with such intramedullary spinal lesions. More commonly, these individuals will complain initially of subtle, seemingly
minor problems such as "tingling and numbness
in the hands," "difficulty opening bottles," or
"becoming more clumsy"—all reflecting the intrinsic cord pathology. Those patients who do
note pain often state that it is poorly localized and
dysesthetic or burning in quality. Pain is often
worse at night or in the early morning, for reasons
relating both to possible vascular engorgement
and increased nocturnal cerebrospinal fluid volume. The pain may also occasionally be exacerbated by activity, leading to the speculation that
increased blood supply to the tumor during exercise may aggravate ongoing compression. The
symptoms invariably progress, however, and
eventually gross motor or sensory disturbance is
apparent. Frequently obvious evidence of myelopathy such as extreme stiffness of gait, lower
extremity "jumping," or hyperreflexia are noted.
As the symptoms slowly progress medical attention is eventually sought. On examination the patient with an intramedullary spinal cord tumor
will have findings indicative of a centrally placed
spinal cord lesion. These may include the classic
suspended pain and temperature deficit, a disassociated sensory deficit, and long tract signs.

Besides the posttraumatic syrinx, which has
been discussed above, other *cavitary spinal lesions*
exist that may enter the differential diagnosis.
Many intrinsic spinal cord tumors, such as low-
grade spinal astrocytomas or ependymomas, will
demonstrate a cystic degeneration that may be
confused with a syrinx (Fig. 7.5). Congenital or
development syrinxes, such as those encountered
in patients with Chiari type I and II malformations
(discussed below), may also be encountered. In
such cases a careful history, supplemented by
newer imaging capabilities, may allow the correct
diagnosis to be reached.

Once the tentative diagnosis is made it may be
confirmed by radiologic studies. Myelography or
intrathecally enhanced CT are rapidly being supplanted by MR imaging as the study of choice in
the evaluation of suspected intrinsic cord lesions.

## Intrinsic Disorders of the Nervous System

Many primary neurologic disorders may cause
neck or arm pain that can be confused with the
more common cervical spine disorders discussed

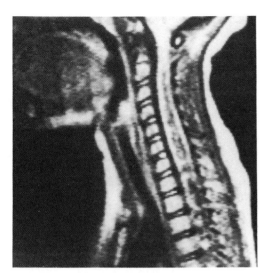

**Figure 7.5.** Mid-sagittal MR image through the cervical region demonstrates an extensive cystic, cavitary lesion of the spinal cord. This was a cystic spinal astrocytoma.

above. Multiple sclerosis, amyotrophic lateral sclerosis, poliomyelitis, and other infectious, toxic, metabolic, or vascular spinal cord insults may underlie a complaint of neck pain. In all these conditions, pain will go hand in hand with neurologic deficits, and the subacute onset of pain with neurologic deficit should suggest the possibility of intrinsic neurologic disease. In the acute setting in which cervical sprain, fracture, or dislocation must be ruled out, intrinsic neurologic disorders may be missed because of more obvious, but possibly irrelevant, spinal abnormalities.

*Multiple sclerosis* is a chronic demyelinating disorder of the central nervous system. Epidemiologic evidence suggests a possible infectious or autoimmune etiology. Poser et al., in a longitudinal study of patients eventually proven by autopsy to have multiple sclerosis, found that the onset of paresthesias was the first presenting symptom of the disease in a significant percentage (13). Painful paresthesias ranging from girdle-like pressure sensations to severe shooting dysesthesias have also been reported. In the later stages of the disease flexor spasms and other stresses on the spine may accelerate the development of osteoarthritic changes, leading to a superimposed cervical spondylosis. Rarely, however, do any of these patients need surgery.

*Amyotrophic lateral sclerosis* (ALS) is a progressive disease of unknown etiology involving descending motor tracts and anterior horn cells. Recent reports have suggested that exposure to certain plant toxins may play a role in the pathogenesis of at least one variant of amyotrophic lateral sclerosis (14). In this disease muscle fasciculations secondary to progressive denervation may lead to painful muscle cramps and spasms. Furthermore, since many of the middle-age individuals typically affected by ALS also have some degree of cervical spondylosis, in the early stages this disease may be difficult to distinguish from a cervical spondylotic myelopathy.

The *focal torsion dystonias*, of which spasmodic torticollis is the most common example, are a group of primary neurologic disorders of unknown etiology whose main symptom is painful continuous contraction or spasms of a muscle or muscle group. Spasmodic torticollis involves the cervical musculature, causing the patient to experience near-constant, often painful, unilateral or bilateral neck muscle contraction. Characteristically the head is rotated and flexed to one side. A jerking tremor may also exist. In the acute setting this disorder is commonly mistaken for cervical sprain or fracture/dislocation; however, as the condition persists the diagnosis becomes obvious. Accelerated cervical spondylotic changes are also quite common, and in late cases symptomatic nerve root compression may be present.

Numerous *neurotoxins* have been identified that can cause painful peripheral neuropathies as well as central nervous system injury. In our highly industrialized society the possibility of significant exposure to chemical toxins such as lead, mercury, and organophosphates must always be considered. A detailed inquiry into possible environmental exposures as well as appropriate screening serum tests are usually sufficient to make the diagnosis.

On rare occasions, *vascular insults* to the spinal cord may cause severe dysesthetic pain in a radicular or segmental distribution. This is most commonly encountered in the setting of abdominal aortic surgery, spinal trauma with vascular compromise, or occlusive vascular disease. Characteristically, in the early stages spinal cord ischemia causes a burning truncal pain that is poorly localized. Spinal infarction may occur within a matter of minutes to hours, guaranteeing a devastating neurologic deficit and poor ultimate prognosis.

## CONGENITAL SPINAL DISORDERS

Congenital disorders of ossification or neural tube formation may involve the cervical region. Unless they result in prominent deformities or functional deficits these disorders may remain un-detected at birth, and may become symptomatic only in the late teen or early adult years. The Chiari malformations, the Klippel-Feil syndrome, and os odontoideum are among the most fre-quently encountered of congenital disorders in-volving the cervical spine.

The *Chiari malformations* are a group of congen-ital malformations involving the midbrain, cere-bellum, and upper cervical spine. These malfor-mations are frequently associated with a host of other neural tube defects, including myelomenin-gocele, encephalocele, and hydromyelia. Al-though a full discussion of the various manifesta-tions of the Chiari syndromes is beyond the scope of this chapter, the cervical manifestations of this condition warrant further consideration. By far the most common type of Chiari malformation is the type I, or adult, Chiari malformation. In this condition the posterior fossa is characteristically small, with displacement of the cerebellar tonsils below the level of the foramen magnum. A failure of the primitive central spinal canal to close com-monly results in a cervical syrinx that communi-cates with the fourth ventricle via the obex (hy-dromyelia). Typically the patient with a Chiari type I malformation is an athletic young adult who notices an intermittent aching neck pain associ-ated with vague complaints of upper extremity numbness, tingling, or clumsiness. The neck pain may result from compression of the upper cervi-cal cord and roots by the herniated cerebellar tonsils, or may be caused by the progressively en-larging hydromyelia. The preponderance of der-matomal symptoms should lead the clinician to suspect involvement of the cervical spinal cord proper, and an MR imaging study or enhanced CT evaluation of this region is usually sufficient to make the diagnosis. The Chiari types II and III syndromes are considerably less common than the type I condition, and are invariably associated with a characteristic constellation of severe con-genital malformations that make the diagnosis ob-vious.

The syndrome of congenital blocked vertebrae, or *Klippel-Feil syndrome,* is a rare congenital con-dition that results in fusion or failure of articula-tion of one or more cervical spinal segments. The blocked or fused vertebrae themselves are not painful; however, the immobility caused by a blocked cervical segment invariably results in su-pranormal stresses on the articulations above and below the fusion site. The superior articulation in particular often suffers accelerated degenerative

changes with osteophyte formation. This can lead to a radiculitis and/or myelopathy. Plain cervical radiographs will reveal the blocked vertebrae as well as any associated osteoarthritic changes.

*Os odontoideum* is a failure of fusion of the dens to the body of C2. Controversy exists as to whether this condition is truly congenital or is a consequence of unrecognized trauma in the neo-natal and childhood years. In any case, the failure of fusion of the dens to the body of C2 results in spinal instability at the C1–2 junction (Fig. 7.6). This instability is typically apparent during neck flexion, and may reduce spontaneously in exten-sion. In mild cases the degree of C1–2 subluxa-tion may be less than 2–3 mm and may be clinically inapparent. In more severe cases the subluxation may be much more significant and any minor neck trauma resulting in sudden flexion may cause pro-found neurologic deficits.

## RHEUMATOID ARTHRITIS AND ASSOCIATED CONDITIONS

The connective tissue disorders are a heteroge-neous group of chronic inflammatory diseases of bone and joints. Rheumatoid arthritis, ankylosing spondylitis, and polymyalgia rheumatica are among the connective tissue disorders that com-monly affect the cervical spine. These disorders may cause cervical spine pain by one of several mechanisms. Inflammation of articular surfaces and mechanical neck pain is common early in the disease course. Subsequent joint inflammation may lead to exuberant pannus formation and neu-ral compression or to abnormal bone deposition and fusion, or may cause progressive articular and ligamentous laxity and spinal instability.

*Rheumatoid arthritis* is a chronic inflammatory arthropathy of presumed autoimmune or infec-tious etiology. The prevalence of this disorder in the United States is roughly 1–3% of the popula-tion. Although rare juvenile forms exist, cervical spine involvement is more frequently encoun-tered in the elderly patient with rheumatoid ar-thritis. The progressive joint inflammatory and destructive changes that bring about the charac-teristic distal extremity deformities may also affect the vertebral column. The cervical spine is com-monly involved, especially in the C1–2 area. Chronic inflammation of articular surfaces at the occiput–C1 and C1–2 junctions may lead to exu-berant pannus formation, bony destruction, and ligamentous laxity. In more advanced cases, at-lanto-occipital subluxation, basilar invagination,

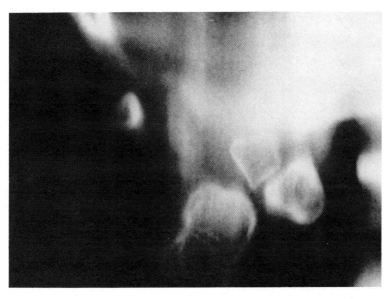

**Figure 7.6.** Tomogram through the C1–2 area reveals a smooth rounded ossicle separated from the body of the axis that travels as a unit with the atlas during flexion. This is an os odontoideum.

and atlantoaxial subluxation are not uncommon. As in any primary bony or articular disorder of the cervical spine, mechanical neck pain is the initial presenting symptom. Morning pain and stiffness and stiffness after inactivity are the hallmarks of this condition. Progressive ligamentous laxity and mechanical pain may lead to compensatory cervical muscle contraction, and occipital headache and muscle spasms may ensue. Extremes of bony and ligamentous instability may allow cord compression, lower cranial nerve palsies, myelopathy, and facial numbness. In the presence of this instability trivial trauma may cause acute, devastating neurologic deficit. In advanced cases the diagnosis of rheumatoid arthritis is often made by physical examination alone; however, early in the disease course serum tests such as the erythrocyte sedimentation rate and rheumatoid factor screens may help to confirm the clinical impression. Radiologic evidence of rheumatoid arthritis may be obtained on plain spine films; but these films may be unimpressive early in the disease.

*Polymyalgia rheumatica* is a syndrome of pain and stiffness of the neck, shoulder, and lumbar/pelvic regions. In its early stages it may be mistaken for rheumatoid arthritis. Most common among the elderly, it may manifest as acute or subacute mechanical neck and shoulder pain. Again, morning stiffness and increase in symptoms with inactivity are common. The physical examination is often normal or may reveal only focal muscle or articular tenderness to palpation. As with the other connective tissue disorders, serologic abnormalities (particularly an elevated erythrocyte sedimentation rate) are characteristic.

*Ankylosing spondylitis* is an inflammatory joint disorder with a striking predilection for the cartilaginous joints of the axial skeleton. The main pathologic features involve abnormal bone metabolism with deposition of bony syndesmophytes and spontaneous fusion of ligamentous and facet structures. Although commonly associated with the lumbosacral spine, ankylosing spondylitis may also involve the neck (Fig. 7.7). Initially the patient may complain of pain and stiffness in the neck and shoulders. Morning stiffness is often present and tends to improve with exercise during the day. There may be a mild associated peripheral arthritis. Progressive restriction of cervical mobility develops as spinal fusion advances. The abnormally fused spine acts as a long lever arm during trauma, and fractures through the fused area are quite common. In the absence of trauma, compression of neural structures is rare. Diagnosis may be made on the basis of plain spine films. The well-described association of ankylosing spondylitis with the HLA-B27 histocompatibility antigen type makes this type of testing useful as well.

Although not strictly an inflammatory connective tissue disorder, *diffuse idiopathic skeletal hyperostosis* (DISH) is included in this discussion since it

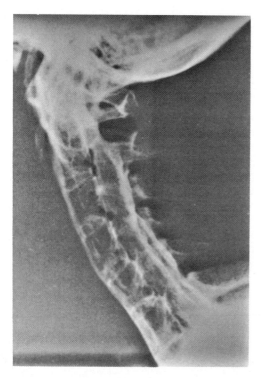

**Figure 7.7.**  Plain radiographs reveal the extensive cervical spinal fusion and bony syndesmophytes characteristic of ankylosing spondylitis.

is often confused with ankylosing spondylitis. In contrast to the pan-fusion characteristic of ankylosing spondylitis, DISH primarily involves the anterior vertebral body. DISH is a hyperostotic disorder that affects the anterior longitudinal ligament of the spine (15). Ossification of this ligament results in syndesmophytes and abnormal spinal fusion, with sequelae similar to those encountered in patients with ankylosing spondylitis.

## INFECTIONS

Infections of the cervical spine are rare, but the consequences of missing this diagnosis are potentially devastating. Presently in this country vertebral column infections most commonly occur in the setting of spinal surgery or after major spinal trauma. The introduction of skin organisms such as staphylococci or streptococci into a cervical surgical wound may seed devitalized bone or muscle and eventually progress to osteomyelitis or a disc space infection. Fractures of the cervical spine, particularly in patients with brittle bone such as the elderly or those with ankylosing spon-

dylitis, may lacerate the esophagus and cause a prevertebral abscess that eventually involves bony structures.

Primary vertebral infections are rare in this country except in specific host populations. In young patients streptococcal infections of the nasopharyngeal and tonsillar area may if untreated spread into the retropharayngeal space and cause vertebral or disc space infections. Among individuals with sickle cell disease or splenic dysfunction staphylococcal osteomyelitis may be encountered. In the older or immunosuppressed patient reactivation of tuberculosis may result in bony seeding and Pott's disease. Finally, patients with malignancy or who are otherwise immunosuppressed may develop more esoteric bacterial or fungal infections of the spine.

Initially cervical spinal infections may be relatively asymptomatic. As the infection progresses and an immunologic reaction is mounted, fever, sweats, and other constitutional symptoms may develop. Mechanical neck pain and paraspinous muscle spasm, often with radiation to the shoulders and back of the head, is a common early symptom. Patients may demonstrate severe restriction of neck motion as a result of pain. These complaints are often present for weeks or months, and may be mistakenly attributed to the normal postsurgical or posttraumatic healing process before the correct diagnosis is eventually made. If the infection tracks into the prevertebral space, dysphagia, dysphasia, and hoarseness may occur. Myelopathy is a late and ominous sign, suggestive of epidural compression and possible epidural abscess.

Unfortunately, bony changes usually take 3–6 weeks to become apparent on plain radiographs, and are often nonspecific. For this reason many infections are not diagnosed until relatively late stages, by which time medical and surgical treatment may be rendered more difficult. Whereas neoplastic processes of the spine characteristically originate in bone and spare the disc space, infection usually begins in the disc space and subsequently spreads to adjacent bone. Radionucleotide bone scanning using gallium, technetium, or labeled white cells is often useful in locating the area of inflammation; however, the relative nonspecificity of these tests makes them difficult to interpret in the patient who has recently undergone surgery or suffered trauma. Obviously, laboratory findings of an elevated white blood cell count or erythrocyte sedimentation rate will point to possible infectious processes as well. In most cases, however, the ultimate microbiologic diagnosis may require aspiration or open biopsy and drainage of the infected area. Recent protocols have advocated an aggressive initial approach including biopsy, drainage and curettage, and concomitant bony fusion. The infectious organism may thereby be identified and appropriate antimicrobial coverage instituted.

## REFERRED PAIN SYNDROMES

The problem of pain referred to the cervical region has been alluded to earlier in this chapter. Many noncervical pathologies may directly or indirectly bring about cervical pain. The syndromes more commonly encountered by the general practitioner include the temporomandibular joint (TMJ) syndrome, occipital neuritis, and the reflex autonomic dystrophies.

*Inflammation or irritation of the TMJ* may develop idiopathically or may be the result of chronic stresses to the joint resulting from an imbalance in masticatory motor function. Characteristically the patient describes severe pain in the region of the angle of the jaw and retroauricular area. This pain may radiate down the neck and posteriorly into the occipital region, and on occasion neck pain may the only symptom. Although the neck pain may appear to originate from cervical elements, once the correct diagnosis is entertained it is generally possible to demonstrate exacerbation of symptoms by minor jaw motion or palpation.

*Occipital neuritis* is an inflammatory condition of the greater occipital nerve, a branch off the C2 root. Pain in the occipital area with concomitant posterior cervical muscle spasm is characteristic. Usually exquisite point tenderness is present over the greater occipital nerve itself. Miscellaneous cervical pathologies may cause occipital neuritis, possibly via cervical spinal muscle contraction and compression of the greater occipital nerve as it passes through the occipital aponeurosis. Conversely, primary injury to the nerve itself, as in trauma or peripheral neuropathy, may cause severe occipital pain and lead to compensatory cervical paraspinous muscle splinting. Local anesthetic blocks of the affected nerve may be both diagnostic and therapeutic.

*Reflex sympathetic dystrophy* is a term applied to a syndrome of posttraumatic pain, hyperalgesia, hyperesthesia, and autonomic changes in an injured extremity. The syndrome may follow major or apparently minor trauma to an extremity, and may be seen with upper extremity/neck injuries such as an avulsion injury of the brachial plexus. Characteristically, the patient develops pain at the site of the injury that persists and eventually acquires a burning or shooting, dysesthetic quality. With time, the pain appears to spread to involve the whole extremity, and secondary changes such as hyperesthesia and hyperpathia develop. Emotional state and psychological stresses may exacerbate symptoms. Vasomotor changes in the affected extremity are common, and may range from hyperhidrosis and vasodilatation to cyanosis and trophic changes of muscle and joints. While numerous theories of etiology have been proposed, the pathophysiologic events underlying this syndrome are not understood. Clinical evidence suggests that early diagnosis and appropriate treatment of this condition may prevent the development of some of the more debilitating autonomic sequelae.

**REFERENCES**

1. Lawrence J: Disc degeneration, its frequency and relationship to symptoms. *Ann Rheum Dis* 28:121, 1969.
2. British Association of Physical Medicine: Pain in the neck and arm. *Br Med J* 1:253, 1966.
3. Hult L: Cervical, dorsal and lumbar spinal syndromes. *Acta Orthop Scand [Suppl]* 17:1, 1954.
4. Hult L: The Munkford Investigation. *Acta Orthop Scand [Suppl]* 16:1, 1954.
5. McSwain N, Martinez J, Timberlake G: *Cervical Spine Trauma. Evaluation and Acute Management.* New York, Thieme Publishers, 1989, p 47.
6. The Cervical Spine Research Society: *The Cervical Spine.* London, J.B. Lippincott Co, 1983.
7. Spurling RG, Scoville WB: Lateral rupture of cervical intervertebral discs. *Surg Gynecol Obstet* 78:350, 1944.
8. Pang D, Wilberger JE Jr: Spinal cord injury without radiographic abnormality in children. *J Neurosurg* 57:114, 1982.
9. Bland J: *Disorders of the Cervical Spine.* Philadelphia, WB Saunders, 1987.
10. Abel M: *Occult Traumatic Lesions of the Cervical Vertebrae.* St. Louis, Warren H. Green, 1971.
11. Wilkinson M: *Cervical Spondylosis: Its Early Diagnosis and Treatment.* Philadelphia, WB Saunders, 1971.
12. Wilkins R, Rengachary SP: *Neurosurgery.* New York, McGraw-Hill, 1985.
13. Poser C, Presthus J, Horstal O: Clinical characteristics of autopsy proven multiple sclerosis. *Neurology* 16:791, 1966.
14. Spencer P, Nunn P, Hugan J, et al: Guam amyotrophic lateral sclerosis-parkinsonism-dementia linked to a plant excitant neurotoxin. *Science* 237:517, 1987.
15. Resnick D, Niwayama G: Radiographic and pathological features of spinal involvement in diffuse idiopathic skeletal hyperostosis (DISH). *Radiology* 119:559, 1976.

## SECTION II

# THERAPEUTIC TECHNIQUES

# 8

# SELECTED PHYSICAL MEDICINE MODALITIES

*Rajka J. Soric*

Before attempting to treat a patient suffering from a painful cervical trauma, the specifics of the underlying pathology should be established. Differentiation between a soft tissue injury and bony or articular damage is imperative, because the clinician may precipitate a neurologic disaster by prescribing an inappropriate treatment modality.

Classification of clinical injuries is based on different criteria. Injuries are differentiated according to the severity as mild, moderate, severe, and most severe on the basis of the duration of the "symptom-free period." An intelligently obtained history and a thorough physical examination in most instances suffices in differentiating a simple soft tissue injury from a trauma that has produced a neurologic deficit.

The quality of the pain described by the patient is always subjective but may help in establishing the correct diagnosis. Details about the onset of the pain, its localization, and possible radiation must always be known to the examiner, as well as aggravating and ameliorating factors. Careful inquiry about a patient's bowel and bladder habits and sexual function is necessary because a patient often will not volunteer such information. Various radiologic and electrophysiologic tests represent reliable diagnostic tools that offer further help in establishing the exact diagnosis.

Once the type and extent of the underlying pathology is established, treatment goals can be defined. In most instances, after the control of severe pain has been achieved, restoration of function becomes the major area of interest.

Bland differentiated four parameters that contribute to pain perception: nociception, pain sensation, suffering, and pain behavior (1). While nociception and pain sensation characterize primarily the acute phases of an illness, the suffering and pain behavior are characteristics of chronic painful disorders. In conditions of acute and severe pain following a cervical trauma, various physical modalities are used in an attempt to decrease or alter nociception. If done successfully, this reduces the incidence of secondary complications, and therefore shortens the overall morbidity.

As is true for any other therapy, physical agents and various manual techniques have their limitations. Early recognition of such limitations is important, because this will allow the clinician to alter the treatment early in the course of the illness, minimizing the chance for developing pain behavior that is so closely related to chronic pain syndrome. Unfortunately, physical therapy tends to be abused and habit-forming in patients with cervical pain. The effectiveness of the prescribed modality is best evaluated by regular clinical assessments of patients. While doing so, one should keep in mind the power of the placebo effect as well as the limited value of the patient's subjective symptoms.

The following physical modalities are discussed with respect to their use in patients suffering from acute cervical trauma:

Cervical orthoses
Heat
Cold
Exercise
Electrotherapy
Laser therapy

113

Mobilization techniques and biofeedback and relaxation techniques are discussed elsewhere in this text.

## CERVICAL ORTHOSES

As with any injury that results in pain, splinting is a frequent and effective method of treatment for the cervical spine. It is done in an attempt to reduce the mobility of the cervical spine, minimize the pain and associated muscle spasm, diminish the weight-bearing force through the cervical spinal segments, and protect the neural structures (1, 2). The use of spinal orthoses for painful neck trauma in a neurologically intact patient should be considered as a temporary measure only.

There are three basic types of cervical orthoses currently in use. The choice of orthosis should depend primarily upon the condition of the patient. In reality, however, choices are usually made on the basis of a clinician's personal preference.

**Soft Collars.** The most frequently used soft collars are the cervical ruffs and foam collars. Both are cheap and easily obtainable. Patients find them comfortable, and the compliance rate is therefore excellent. While these orthoses do not provide stability for the neck nor do they help unload the spine to any degree, they serve as a reminder to the patient to limit neck and head motions. This is achieved through sensory feedback and results in pain reduction. The additional advantages of psychological satisfaction and localized heat contribute to the therapeutic effect of soft collars. In most cases, soft cervical collars are used only for a few days after the injury.

**Semirigid Collars.** The Philadelphia collar is probably the most popular semirigid cervical orthosis. It is tolerated by patients almost as well as the soft collar, and yet it adds an additional benefit of motion control of the midcervical segment (1). It does not, however, reduce the weight-bearing stress through the cervical spine. Semirigid orthoses are usually made of plastazote and polyethylene. They come prefabricated, but minor individual adjustments are possible.

**Rigid Orthoses.** The four-poster, SOMI (sterno-occipital–mandibular immobilization), and halo orthoses are examples of rigid cervical supports. Use of rigid orthoses in patients with soft tissue injuries is very limited. By and large, they are bulky and heavy and require head as well as thoracic and/or lumbar extensions that ensure optimal spinal stabilization. Depending upon the direction of the movement that one wishes to re-strict and the level of the segment that needs to be immobilized, the choice of a rigid orthosis will vary.

Efforts to provide immobilization for the spine date back to Hippocrates (1). For years an injury to the cervical spine automatically implied a lengthy immobilization. This rationale has been changing over the past years, as it was established that some of the hypothetical advantages of the cervical orthoses do not exist. In fact, a detrimental effect of prolonged and constant use of the cervical support has been well identified (1). As also noted by Thomas (3), Mealy et al. have shown in their double-blind study a reduction of pain and improved mobility of the cervical spine in patients who were not treated with cervical orthoses after an injury, but instead began early mobilization exercises (4). Other authors suggested, on the basis of animal studies, that faster revascularization and recovery result from early mobilization of the injured muscle (5).

If a cervical orthosis is prescribed, it is imperative that the patient be advised regarding its proper use. The cervical spine should always be maintained in slight flexion. This allows separation of the posterior facet joints and helps to maintain the patency of the intervertebral foramina. Prolonged use of the collar is never indicated and may, in fact, precipitate additional problems. The patient should remove the brace periodically and perform range of movement and isometric exercises. This will help prevent contracture formation and ensure a good alignment. It may also prevent the development of psychological dependence.

## HEAT

Heat is probably the most frequently used modality for the treatment of acute cervical pain. Its therapeutic benefit is based upon its local as well as distant effects.

The most potent local effect of heat is vasodilatation. Following the injury, swollen muscle bundles or tonically contracted muscles may cause localized ischemia, resulting in the slow removal of cell metabolites. These stimulate the release of various "pain substances" that lead to increased vascular permeability, localized edema, and, at a later stage, tissue fibrosis (5). Heat applied locally to such an area will promote vasodilatation and hence stimulate the rapid removal of tissue irritants by enhancing the cellular metabolic rate.

This will ultimately result in a quicker resolution of the inflammatory reaction, as well as a decrease in the pain. The counterirritant effect of heat provides additional analgesic properties via the "gate mechanism" in the substantia gelatinosa (6). Within a few minutes of heat application, the painful muscle spasm begins to diminish. This is thought to be due to excitation of the exteroceptors of the skin and a subsequent effect on the spindle mechanism (7).

Locally applied heat is a valuable adjunct for other types of treatments. For example, it alters the viscosity of the synovial fluid and distensibility of the collagen fibers, thus making stretching exercises more effective (8).

The physiologic response to locally applied heat will depend upon the obtained tissue temperature, the duration of the hyperthermia, and the size of the treatment area (1). According to Hoff's law, chemical reactions increase by two to three times for each temperature increase of 10°C (1). This has an important clinical implication in situations of total body heating. The blood pressure may drop, the respiratory rate rises, and the fluid losses may increase. This may in extreme cases lead to dehydration and a dangerous rise in the core temperature.

There are two major groups of heat modalities. Superficial agents can raise the temperature of the skin and subcutaneous tissues only, while deep heating modalities reach the deep-seated joints and muscular layers. The physiologic effects, however, remain the same.

Of the superficial agents, the most frequently used one is the *hydrocollator pack*. Cotton housing containing a silicone gel can easily conform to the shape of the neck and will emit heat for approximately 20 minutes. The temperature of the hydrocollator pack when ready for use reaches 65°C. This temperature would inevitably cause a burn if the pack was applied directly to the skin. At least two layers of protective toweling is mandatory to prevent any thermal damage (1). The heat in the hydrocollator pack is transmitted by conduction and does not penetrate below the skin layer (9).

Electric *heating pads* that a patient can use at home are a good alternative to hydrocollator packs. Their disadvantage, however, is that they do not cool spontaneously, thus putting the patient at the risk of developing burns (10).

*Shortwave diathermy* converts 17.12-MHz wavelength radio waves into heat. Its depth of penetration depends upon the tissue composition and the choice of applicator. The magnitude of penetration or conductivity is a function of the thickness of the subcutaneous fat layer and the water content of the tissue (1). At best, shortwave diathermy will heat the superficial muscle layer only (11). Since the presence of metal in the electromagnetic field may cause excessive selective heating, pacemakers and various surgical implants are considered contraindications for this modality (11). Another disadvantage of shortwave diathermy is the inability to accurately control the amount of delivered energy.

Of all the heating modalities, *ultrasound* is the one most frequently used for patients suffering from acute cervical pain. Sonic energy with a frequency of 0.8–1.0 MHz is converted to heat. Most of the therapeutic effects are due to selective heating of the interfaces between tissues of different acoustic impedance and coefficients of absorption (11, 12). The greatest advantage of ultrasound over all of the other heating modalities is its superior depth of penetration and accurate dosimetry (expressed as watts per square centimeter). One should always keep in mind, however, that ultrasound can easily produce tissue damage. Because it is most often delivered to the area that does not contain thermal receptors, tissue cavitation and local burns are not uncommon. This problem can be successfully prevented by the proper application method. Ultrasound has the additional disadvantage of a restricted treatment field. Because of the small size of the sound head in the transducer, only a limited surface area can be treated at a time. The need for the active involvement of a therapist makes it an expensive modality as well (7). For a long time it was thought that the presence of metallic implants was a contraindication for the use of ultrasound. It has been proven, however, that metal and bone are equally dense to ultrasound and such precautions are no longer necessary (13). The presence of plastics, such as methylmethacrylate and high-density polypropylene, is still considered a contraindiction for its use.

*Phonophoresis* is a variant of ultrasound treatment. A biologically active substance mixed with a coupling medium is forced through the skin during the ultrasound application. A limited number of animal studies and clinical trials have been done with this modality to date, and it is too early to pass judgment about its effectiveness (9).

Generalized or *total body heating* offers another treatment option for a patient with a painful neck. The sedating effect and general relaxation are considered to be the most significant end results of such therapies (1, 11).

## COLD

Cryotherapy is continually gaining popularity as an effective treatment modality. Its analgesic effect and depth of penetration are superior to those of heat. Furthermore, cryotherapy is inexpensive and easy to apply. Fat acts as an insulator, not allowing the muscle layer to warm up immediately after the ice pack is removed. This ensures a longer cooling effect and longer lasting analgesia.

Cold decreases the inflammatory response by diminishing the metabolic rate. This in turn reduces the blood supply to the cooled area (14). Vasoconstriction further contributes to the reduced blood flow. Muscle spasm decreases as a result of the decreased sensitivity of the muscle spindle (7). The neuronal excitability diminishes as well, resulting in a reduced conduction velocity (15, 16). The counterirritant effect of cold contributes to its direct analgesic effect achieved through the gate mechanism (6).

Muscle spasm and pain are the two most troublesome symptoms in patients suffering from an acute cervical strain. Because both are successfully controlled by ice, patients should be encouraged to use this modality more often. This is particularly true during the initial 24–48 hr after the injury, since ice lessens the extent of tissue hypoxia and limits the edema (17).

A plastic bag filled with ice or ice water wrapped in a towel and applied to the affected area is the most common form of cold application. The duration of the treatment averages 15–20 min and may be repeated several times a day. Commercially available frozen gels are reusable and better conform to the shape of the neck. If applied directly to the skin, they can cause frostbite. To prevent this, a gel pack should be wrapped in a protective towel and then applied to the skin surface.

Vapocoolant sprays are another frequently utilized method of cold application. Usually ethyl chloride or fluoromethane sprays are used. By virtue of quick evaporation, they produce a significant, albeit superficial, cooling effect and transient analgesia. The spray is used most commonly in combination with stretching—the "spray and stretch" technique (18). It is important to position the neck so that the muscle being treated can be maximally stretched as soon as the analgesic effect of the evaporated spray takes hold. In an attempt

to reduce the incidence of muscle soreness, warming of the skin following the completion of therapy may be very helpful.

## EXERCISE

Even though the importance of exercise in the management of acute cervical pain is well established, the types of exercises and the timing of their introduction after the injury still remain rather controversial issues. Exercise programs aimed at restoration and improvement of an individual's functional level are still not prescribed frequently enough for patients with an acute cervical trauma. Such an approach may be justified in the early phases after the injury, but should not be condoned later on. Because of the pain in the neck, patients have a tendency to decrease their overall level of function, which eventually leads to significant deconditioning. Flexibility diminishes while ligamentous and capsular structures shorten (19). Ultimately, this results in a biomechanical dysfunction that may promote the development of secondary complications.

Immediately after the injury, it is often necessary to rest the cervical region because any type of exercise will simply be too painful. Gentle manual stretching should be started as soon as the acute pain subsides. With a gradually diminishing intensity of pain, other goal-specific exercises must be introduced. Range-of-movement exercises for the neck should be started as early as possible and should be combined with mobilization exercises of the shoulders for optimal results. The earliest restriction of movement following an injury is usually that of extension of the cervical spine. If intervention does not occur early on, movement in all directions will eventually diminish; after an extended period of time contractures will develop.

A significant amount of confusion exists when describing *range-of-movement and stretching* exercises. Both are performed in an attempt to elongate the shortened tissue. Conventionally, however, it is assumed that stretching exercises are performed by another person or a mechanical force, whereas the range-of-movement exercises can be, and most of the time are, performed by the patient (20). In order to be therapeutic, the stretching must be slow and prolonged, allowing the muscle fiber to relax and elongate. If preceded by the application of a vapocoolant spray, these exercises are referred to as the "spray and stretch" technique (18).

Of all the strengthening exercises, the *isometric* type is generally preferred in the treatment of acute painful conditions. An individual's hand acts as an external force that prevents the movement of the neck, thus limiting the pain. These exercises are done in an attempt to maintain the normal agonist-antagonist capability. Therefore they are absolutely essential in patients who wear a collar (1). Performing the exercises two to three times a day, six to 10 times in each direction, is the usually prescribed routine. Caution should be exercised in patients who have diastolic hypertension, because isometric exercises may aggravate the problem.

*Isotonic* exercises, so often prescribed for other body parts, are not widely utilized in the treatment of an acute cervical trauma. The same holds true for the *isokinetic* type, in which exercises are done against a machine that assures a constant speed and resistance throughout the range of movement (21). Lewitt and Simons have suggested "post-isometric relaxation" as the best exercise technique for acute myofascial pain (22). The muscles are first placed in a stretched position, which is followed by isometric contraction and then relaxation. A gentle stretch completes the cycle. With this technique, they claim 94% immediate, albeit transient, pain relief (22).

A frequent problem encountered in patients following a cervical trauma is abnormal posture. This is the basis for the mechanical pain that may develop if postural deficiencies are not corrected. The most common postural abnormality of the cervical spine is characterized by forward projection of the head and protraction of the shoulders. This seems to be a position of comfort after an acute injury. In addition to muscle tightness, this posture causes compression of the apophyseal joints and an excessive lordotic curve (1). It may contribute to impingement of the suboccipital nerves, resulting in a headache. Recognition of the possible long-term complications of an altered posture is very important, since tonic contraction of the trapezii, which inevitably is a part of the clinical picture, and altered physiologic cervical lordosis may give rise to chronic pain. Postural reeducation utilizing visual feedback, and stretching and strengthening exercises for the neck and upper back, when done regularly, will result in a clinical improvement.

Cervical spine alignment during the night is another issue that must be addressed by the clinician treating a patient with acute cervical pain. Habits of sleeping on a thick pillow must be discouraged, and the patient should be instructed to use ruffs and later special cervical pillows that help maintain anatomic alignment.

## ELECTROTHERAPY

Electrical stimulation used for therapeutic purposes can closely approximate physiologic changes at the site of a cell membrane. The ultimate effectiveness of such electrical stimulation depends upon the intensity, duration, and waveform of the stimulus.

Faradic, or alternating, current may be used for stimulation of the peripheral nerves, altering the transmission of the painful stimuli and contributing to pain modulation. It can also be used for stimulation of the motor nerves, simulating a normal muscle contraction. This enhances the metabolic rate and vascular supply and helps eliminate the waste products. The end result of such treatment is control of pain and muscle spasm.

The physiologic effects of galvanic, or direct, current depend upon the active electrode. The effects of direct current at the negative pole include softening of the tissues, increase in nerve irritability, and vasodilatation. At the positive pole, the effects of galvanic current include diminished nerve irritability, vasoconstriction, and local analgesia (23).

Since its introduction in 1967, transcutaneous electrical nerve stimulation (TENS) has become over the years the most popular electrical device with analgesic properties. The exact mechanism of analgesia produced by TENS still remains unexplained (20). On the basis of Melzack and Wall's gate theory, it is thought that TENS provides a nonnoxious afferent stimulus that travels via the thick, myelinated A fibers, activating the interneurons of the substantia gelatinosa that in turn presynaptically inhibit the transmission of nociceptive stimuli to various suprasegmental levels (20). Unfortunately, this theory fails to explain phenomena such as prolonged analgesia after the termination of treatment.

The central biasing mechanism provides an explanation for the TENS-induced analgesia in conditions characterized by an altered or absent afferent input. TENS supplements this sensory deficit and allows the pain-modulating function of the reticular formation to operate (22, 24, 25). The effect of TENS on the release and concentration of endorphins and enkephalins in the peripheral circulation as well as the cerebrospinal fluid has been extensively studied and is believed to play a major role in the mechanism of analgesia produced by this modality (26–28).

TENS units produce stimuli with currents between 0 and 100 mA, pulse rates between 1 and 200 Hz, and pulse widths from 10 to a few hundred milliseconds. Variations of these parameters most likely have a bearing on the mechanism of action by which analgesia is achieved (29).

The superior analgesic effect is achieved by a stimulation setting characterized by a high rate, long width, and high amplitude. This "conventional TENS" or "HI-TENS" unit most likely produces analgesia by raising the cerebrospinal fluid level of endorphins, as well as altering the transmission of the painful stimuli via the gate mechanism (20). The low-frequency stimulation with "acupuncture TENS" utilizes larger pulse widths and lower frequencies. The analgesic effect is reversible by the intravenous administration of naloxone, and therefore is considered to be due to the enhanced release of $\beta$ endorphins only (29, 30).

As in other painful conditions, the efficacy of TENS for the control of acute cervical pain is limited by nerve adaptation (31). By changing the stimulation parameters or electrode placements, this problem may be rectified (20). The placement of the electrodes is chosen by trial and error. The most frequent sites include acupuncture points, the distribution of spinal roots, peripheral nerves, trigger points, or simply painful areas. In treating patients with acute cervical pain, caution must be exercised that the electrodes are not placed over the carotid sinus or epiglottis (20).

## LASER THERAPY

Light amplification by the stimulated emission of radiation (laser) is gaining popularity in the treatment of various acute and chronic conditions. High-power or "hot" lasers have been extensively used in surgical specialties for quite some time. Their therapeutic effect is based upon the transformation of the absorbed light energy into heat that produces tissue damage. The "cold" laser, in contrast, does not cause any tissue damage.

The exact mechanism of action of this modality is still not known. Stimulated collagen production, altered DNA synthesis, and accelerated wound healing have been proposed on the basis of experiments done in rodents. Similar results have not been confirmed in humans (10, 32). Additional explanations for the mechanisms of action include relief of arterial spasm, excitation of the

mitochondrial membranes, and enhanced levels of serotonin (20).

Some authors consider low-power laser therapy a painless and safe form of acupuncture and recommend its use in chronic myofascial pain syndrome (33, 34). Very little research has been done regarding the use of the laser in acute cervical trauma. Consequently, strong evidence to support its efficacy is lacking. However, if the effects of the laser on healing prove to be superior, one can argue that for this reason it should be used more regularly. The "grid technique" of application would probably be the most appropriate (33). If the laser is used for its analgesic properties, the "point stimulation technique" would be preferred (35).

### REFERENCES

1. Bland JH: *Disorders of the Cervical Spine. Diagnosis and Management.* Philadelphia, WB Saunders, 1987, pp 236–278.
2. Harris JD: Spinal orthoses for pain and instability. In Bedford JD (ed): *Cervical Orthoses in Orthotics etcetera.* Baltimore, Williams & Wilkins, 1981, pp 100–122.
3. Thomas HG: Cervical spondylosis. *Med Clin North Am* 34:6213–6222, 1989.
4. Mealy K, Brennan H, Fenelon GCC: Early mobilization of acute whiplash injuries. *Br Med J* 292:656–657, 1986.
5. Sheon RP, Moskowitz RW, Goldberg VD: *Soft Tissue Rheumatic Pain—Recognition, Management, Prevention,* ed 2. Philadelphia, Lea & Febiger, 1987, pp 16–26.
6. Melzack R, Wall PD: Pain mechanisms: a new theory. *Science* 150:971–979, 1965.
7. Phull PS: Management of cervical pain. In DeLisa JA (ed): *Rehabilitation Medicine—Principles and Practice.* Philadelphia, JB Lippincott, 1988, pp 749–764.
8. Lehmann JF, Brunner GD, Stow RW: Pain threshold measurements after therapeutic application of ultrasound, microwaves and infrared. *Arch Phys Med Rehabil* 39:560–565, 1958.
9. Lehmann JF, Stonebridge JB, DeLateur BJ, Warren CG, Halar E: Temperature distributions in the human thigh, produced by infrared hot pack and microwave applications. *Arch Phys Med Rehabil* 47:291–299, 1966.
10. Basford JR: Physical agents and biofeedback. In DeLisa JA (ed): *Rehabilitation Medicine—Principles and Practice.* Philadelphia, JB Lippincott, 1988, pp 257–275.
11. Lehmann JF, DeLateur BJ: Therapeutic heat. In Lehmann JF (ed): *Therapeutic Heat and Cold,* ed 3. Baltimore, Williams & Wilkins, 1982, pp 404–562.
12. Horvath SM, Hollander JL: Intra-articular temperature as a measure of joint reaction. *J Clin Invest* 28:469–473, 1949.
13. Lehmann JF, Lane CE, Bell JW, Brunner GD: Influence of surgical metal implants on the distribution of the intensity in the ultrasonic field. *Arch Phys Med Rehabil* 39:756–760, 1958.
14. Perkins JF, Li M-C, Hoffman F, et al: Sudden vasoconstriction in denervated or sympathectomized paws exposed to cold. *Am J Physiol* 155:165–178, 1948.
15. Lippold OCJ, Nicholls JG, Redfearn JWT: A study of the afferent discharge produced by cooling a mammalian muscle spindle. *J Physiol (Lond)* 153:218–231, 1960.
16. Coppin EG, Livingstone SA, Kuehn LA: Effects on hand-

grip strength due to arm immersion in a 10 C water bath. *Aviat Space Environ Med* 49:1322–1326, 1978.

17. Schanbel HJ: The local use of ice after orthopedic procedures. *Am J Surg* 72:711–714, 1946.

18. Travell JG, Simons DG: Background and principles. In *Myofascial Pain and Dysfunction. The Trigger Point Manual.* Baltimore, Williams & Wilkins, 1984, pp 5–44.

19. Sheon RP, Moskowitz RW, Goldberg VD: *Soft Tissue Rheumatic Pain—Recognition, Management, Prevention,* ed 2. Philadelphia, Lea & Febiger, 1987, pp 301–314.

20. Soric R, Devlin M: Role of physical medicine. In Tollison CD (ed): *Handbook of Chronic Pain Management.* Baltimore, Williams & Wilkins, 1988, pp 147–162.

21. DeLateur BJ: Exercise for strength and endurance. In Basmajian, JV (ed): *Therapeutic Exercise,* ed 3. Baltimore, Williams & Wilkins, 1978, pp 227–233.

22. Lewitt K, Simons DG: Myofascial pain: relief by postisometric relaxation. *Arch Phys Med Rehabil* 65:452–456, 1984.

23. Sawyer M, Zbieranek C: The treatment of soft tissue after spinal injury. *Clin Sports Med* 5(2):388–405, 1986.

24. Bowsher D: Role of the reticular formation in responses to noxious stimulation. *Pain* 2:361–378, 1976.

25. Mayer DJ, Price DD: Central nervous system mechanisms of analgesia. *Pain* 2:379–404, 1976.

26. Stratton SA: Role of endorphins in pain modulation. *J Orthop Sports Phys Ther* 3:200–205, 1982.

27. Sjoelund BM, Eriksson MB: The influence of naloxone on analgesia produced by peripheral conditioning stimulation. *Brain Res* 173:295–301, 1979.

28. Sjoelund BM, Eriksson MB: Endorphins and analgesia produced by peripheral conditioning stimulation. *Adv Pain Res Ther* 3:587–592, 1979.

29. Barr JO, Nielsen DN, Soderberg G: Transcutaneous electrical nerve stimulation characteristics for altering pain perception. *Phys Ther* 66(10):1515–1521, 1986.

30. Huges GS, Lichstein PR, Whitlock D, et al: Response of plasma beta-endorphins to transcutaneous electrical nerve stimulation in healthy subjects. *Phys Ther* 64(7):1062–1066, 1984.

31. Gersh MR, Wolf SL: Applications of transcutaneous electrical nerve stimulation in the management of patients with pain. *Phys Ther* 65(3):314–322, 1985.

32. Basford JR, Hallman HO, Sheffield CG, MacKey GL: Comparison of cold quartz ultraviolet, low-energy laser and occlusion in wound healing in a swine model. *Arch Phys Med Rehabil* 67:151–154, 1986.

33. Waylonis GW, Wilke S, O'Toole D, Waylonis DA, Waylonis DB: Chronic myofascial pain: management by low-output helium-neon laser therapy. *Arch Phys Med Rehabil* 69:1017–1020, 1988.

34. Stillwell GK: *Therapeutic Electricity and Ultraviolet Radiation,* ed 3. Baltimore, Williams & Wilkins, 1983.

35. Goldman JA, Chiapella J, Casey H, et al: Laser therapy of rheumatoid arthritis. *Lasers Surg Med* 1:93–101, 1980.

# 9

# MANIPULATION AND MOBILIZATION

*Preston B. Fitzgerald*

Although spinal mobilization was demonstrated as long as 2000 years ago in ancient Chinese pictures and writings (1), the field of spinal manipulation and mobilization is not without controversy. Not until recently has scientific literature exhibited any interest in the effects of its treatment or in its scientific rationale. Because of the placebo effect of the "hands-on" type of treatment, many physicians have thought that results have occurred coincidental to the normal healing response to the pathology or because of some other unexplained phenomenon. Since the latter 1800s, spinal manipulation has been used in various clinical settings by osteopaths, bone setters of Europe and Canada, and chiropractors in the United States. Recently, physiatrists and physical therapists have started to utilize this method of clinical treatment.

Manipulation and mobilization differ in several aspects. Mobilization means "taking the joint to its limit of passive range of motion" (2). Mobilization requires a lesser skill level than does manipulative processing. It requires less training and can generally be handled by the physician in an office. Cassidy et al. have provided an understanding of the concept of manipulation by stating that it is "a process of physiological movement which goes beyond the passive range of motion in the paraphysiological zone" (2). Manipulative treatment requires extensive study, numerous years of hands-on experience, and an understanding of the joint capsule, its line of drive, the articulation and the physiologic zone, and the relationship of the articular capsules (3). Contraindications to both are always evident and are based on the un-

derlying pathophysiology that inhibits manipulation or mobilization.

This author does not agree with some of the past treatises on manipulation and the controversy surrounding the technique. Precluding the effects of spinal mobilization, there is new evidence of considerable interest in the field of spinal manipulative treatment that comes from Viedman and his fellow researchers at the Institute of Occupational Health, Helsinki, Finland. It shows that rest, or the lack of mobilization of the joints, not only delays healing but can also cause degenerative osteoarthritic changes that can be measurable within 1 week (4). This chapter is restricted to discussion of a limited treatment modality that may offer some benefit in restoring functional integrity to a traumatized cervical spine in a controlled clinical environment.

Clinical experience has indicated that spinal mobilization in cervical trauma is best used when the objective is to increase mobility and decrease the patient's pain response. Conditions that would warrant spinal mobilization are hyperflexion/hyperextension injury to the cervical spine from either anterior or posterior impact, which does not generally involve the pathophysiology that a lateral hyperflexion/hyperextension injury would involve (5). The obvious distinction is in the capsular region and the relationship of the zygapophysis, with manipulation being provided on the geometric orientation of the vertebral segment's articulation. This manipulation mechanism is defined in this chapter, and history, physical examination, and appropriate radiologic considerations are used to determine who would

120

be a proper candidate for spinal manipulation in cases of cervical trauma.

## CLINICAL EVALUATION

The attending physician should consider the history and physical examination of utmost importance in the patient's clinical evaluation. Based on all the variables that can occur in the myriad of trauma to the cervical spine, the clinical evaluation will provide the attending physician an opportunity for observation and a plan for a rational treatment protocol. If used properly, it can eliminate hours of confusion. Areas that should be covered during the clinical evaluation are the patient's history (including chief complaints, traumatic history, past history, and family history), general behavior, mood, general appearance, general complaints, and a complete physical examination.

## HISTORY

The history should be performed by the attending physician on the patient's initial visit. It is the basis for both the patient's care and the tentative working diagnosis for deciding whether to administer manipulation or mobilization. Questions that should be addressed are: What was the patient's condition before the injury? What amount of pain and suffering is directly attributable to the present injury? Recording the patient's history is an accurate measurement by which information is extracted from the patient in his or her own words. This history will establish the basis for accurate diagnosis and clinical impression, which is utilized in formulating a plan for manipulation and mobilization after cervical trauma.

The history is divided into four areas: chief complaints, traumatic history, past history, and family history (6).

### Chief Complaints

During the examination, the patient's complaints must address, in his or her own terms, the reasons for which he or she sought care in the office.

### Traumatic History

Each patient should be questioned regarding the type of injury, the impact, and the involvement of other objects in and around the area of trauma. Specific questions should be asked; for example,

were eyeglasses knocked off in the injury? These objective findings are valuable in understanding the degree of impact and also the causal factor of impact. Traumatic history must include whether the patient was wearing seat belts or a shoulder harness, any supportive safety gear to absorb blunt trauma to the head, or any other device that would interfere with a more significant trauma.

### Past History

This portion of the history would include information regarding any previous injuries to the neck, particularly to the neuromusculoskeletal system in the neck area. Each significant injury must be documented, and a review of medical files would be appropriate. The documentation should include the date of injury, the type of treatment that was administered, the point of medical improvement, and the rate of improvement at the time of discharge. Past history should also include surgeries, medications, hospitalizations, and any other complications. Knowledge of the patient's use of medication is of great benefit in spinal manipulative treatment because it allows the physician to be aware of a particular type of medication that might warrant caution in manipulative processing. For example, pain medication can alter the patient's physiologic muscle tension and alter and increase ranges of motion. Therefore, the physician must be aware of the types of medications being taken and their pharmacologic effects for the patient's safety. Also, particular pathologies, such as rheumatoid arthritis, significant ankylosis, or irritation or injury to the ligamentous structures, should warn of contraindications for manipulative treatment. It is very important to evaluate contraindications for manipulation or mobilization in the past history.

### Family History

A complete family history should include all medical and orthopaedic disorders. Once again, the family history could provide a foundation for ruling out manipulative treatment by identifying medical contraindications as noted above.

## GENERAL BEHAVIOR

Certain questions regarding general behavior should be answered, such as: Is the patient's demeanor straightforward? Does he lose his concentration? Does she express behavior that is inappropriate in nature? Straightforward answers to questions given should be documented verbatim in the patient's chart.

## MOOD

Does this person experience any anxiety reaction, phobias, aggression, or hostility that should be recorded? Some patients, particularly those with head injuries or posttraumatic concussion syndrome, will exhibit inappropriate behavior and will not be able to clinically assess the time, date, or place. Under rare conditions such as this, the examiner should consider immediate referral for neurologic or neuropsychological evaluation.

Questioning individuals close to the patient will be invaluable in helping to determine if there has been a change in memory or sensory orientation. Once again, this type of information is of utmost importance and may provide information that contraindicates manipulation and mobilization. For example, a symptom of cognitive confusion could be related to significant carotid artery disease—a direct contraindication to manipulation and mobilization. A comprehensive diagnostic evaluation is required before any treatment.

## GENERAL APPEARANCE

Many examiners often ignore the general appearance of the patient. This is unfortunate because they could observe many alterations. The listing of the patient's head, the varying degree of asymmetry of the muscle masses under trauma, areas of edema and hemorrhage, and any alteration of the patient's movement to a guarded stance are all of utmost importance.

The patient's general appearance can give much information to the examiner. The physician must take time to observe any type of symptom or postural structural change that could give any information as to the degree of physical alteration. The examiner should carefully observe the general appearance of the patient as part of the initial examination.

## GENERAL COMPLAINTS

The general question that the examiner now needs to answer is, does the clinical picture or history of trauma correlate with the symptomatic picture? It is very significant to observe whether there exists such a correlation, given that cervical injuries frequently result from automobile accidents and given the litigious nature of our society.

## PHYSICAL EXAMINATION

A physical examination can vary in its degree of thoroughness. In considering the patient for manipulative treatment, the physician should use the vital signs and general appearance of the patient as criteria for the basic essential assessment. The vital signs, consisting of the patient's temperature, pulse rate, blood pressure, height, and weight, should be routinely determined. An indication of idiopathic hypertension or an extreme fever would warrant elimination of a patient as a candidate for manipulative processing, given the generally accepted contraindications of manipulation and mobilization (7).

### Palpation Examination

**General Principles.** Palpation is an examination by the observer to evaluate structural integrity, neuromuscular integrity, and normal muscle tone of the spine in its presenting profile.

A thorough evaluation of the anatomic and physiologic structures of the cervical spine is extremely important. From a spinal manipulative standpoint, the three-dimensional understanding elicited by the examiner is of great benefit (8). This three-dimensional understanding is comprised of the examination of muscle symmetry, the underlying osseous structures, and the neurovascular placement. From this comprehensive evaluation, the examiner is then able to mentally form a realistic model for the patient being considered for manipulation or mobilization. Considering the orientation of the zygapophysis, the muscle tone and density, and the neurologic status, the examiner can prepare for an appropriate manipulation of the patient.

The purpose of adequate palpation is to compare symmetrical skeletal structures, bilateral muscle groups, and ranges of motion. Myotendinotic changes are detected by a deep pressure and massaging type of palpation. This is called *goding*, or symmetrical-type palpation.

The examination should begin with the superficial tissues and progress into the more moderate and deeper muscle groups of the cervical spine. The examination should be performed exactly at the site where the pain is perceived by the patient. As the examiner continues, he or she should note the duration or intensity of the pain. The end result is that the examiner is able to provide a three-dimensional comprehensive view of the cervical spine for evaluation (9).

Before relying on palpation to determine the criteria for mobilization, we must also reflect that each and every tissue change does not necessarily mean that there is an abnormal irritant or an abnormal muscle group involved. One must perform a comprehensive palpation examination, and then correlate it with both radiographic and physical exam findings to determine a differential diagnosis.

**Cervical Spine Palpation Examination.** The examination of the cervical spine should consist of palpation of four cervical areas: anterior cervical musculature, posterior cervical musculature, interspinous spaces, and related areas. The palpation examination should start with the outside continuity of the skin structure, working to the intermediate and deep muscle groups of the cervical spine. It should be started in a focus of the upper neck along the greater occipital area, working out into the posterior and anterior muscle groups from cephalad to caudad. Particular notice should be taken of areas of differences in sensation to the patient, differences of light touch, areas of swelling, and variations in surface temperature (10).

*Anterior Cervical Musculature.* The anterior cervical musculature is the area most commonly injured in the acceleration phase of cervical trauma (11). Palpation of the anterior cervical region could give indications of variance in muscle size from swelling or muscle atrophy. It should include both the movement of the neck in the swallowing phase as felt on palpation by the examiner and more superficial movement felt in response to digital palpation of the intermediate and deep musculature. This examination will check for muscle density change in taut and tender fibers of the muscle groups (11).

*Posterior Cervical Musculature.* This examination should start from the superficial areas and move more posteriorly and into the deep and intermediate musculature. Following observation and digital palpation, extension and flexion of the neck should be felt by the examiner with the hands on the neck muscles, with the patient's forehead resting forward and the examiner's hand supporting the weight of the head (2). The decelerative-phase injuries are most commonly noted in the posterior cervical muscle groups. On examination

the musculature may be found to be torn, swollen, or injured. The degree of damage is somewhat lessened in the posterior cervical area as a result of the anatomic structure and the physiologic strength of the ligamentum nucha.

*Interspinous Spaces.* The interspinous spaces should be examined for altered movement to rule out stretching or injury to the interspinous ligaments. Once again, the examination is performed with the patient's head resting in the examiner's right or left arm. The head should be moved with a rocking motion as the examiner locates each vertebral segment, feeling for the separation or lack thereof of the interspinous space.

*Related Areas.* After the examination has been performed, the spinous processes should be palpated to note any area of particular tenderness or abnormal movement. If there is any abnormal movement, one must suspect fracture and conduct appropriate testing and evaluation at that point.

## RANGES OF MOTION

A number of opinions exist as to the value of a range-of-motion examination in the cervical spine. Many examiners believe that there are hard concurrent data to substantiate standard ranges of motion. However, ranges of motion will vary with the individual, age, and muscle density. Many congenital factors also contribute to the problem of physical exam observation of range of motion (13). Range of motion must be evaluated very carefully prior to mobilization or manipulation because clinical evidence of a hypermobile spine would be a contraindication to manipulative treatment. A hypomobile spine with no evidence of any contraindications to manipulation is a prime candidate for mobilization to increase mobility if the physical exam warrants it.

In determining ranges of motion, one must consider the following criteria: osseous problems, rotation present in a restrictive movement, whether there is pain on isometric contracture, and whether there is evidence of any surrounding paravertebral musculature involvement. Such factors are known to restrict the range of motion of the cervical spine.

Range of motion can assist in differentiating the pain that arises from a joint from that which arises from a muscle. Isometric contracture will cause pain in a facet joint even if the joint does not move.

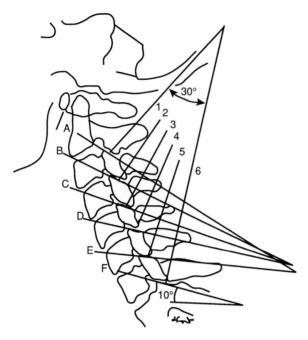

**Figure 9.1.** Coupled action of lateral flexion and axial rotation is due to the oblique orientation of the facet joints. (Adapted from Kapandji IA: The vertebral column as a whole. In: *The Physiology of the Joints. Vol 3: The Trunk and the Vertebral Column.* New York, Churchhill Livingstone, 1974, p 201.)

Figure 9.1 illustrates a fairly typical facet orientation for consideration of line of drive for spinal manipulation. This diagram also illustrates the lateral flexion and axial rotation that can occur in the movement of the cervical spine during its consideration for mobilization or manipulation (14).

### Increased Range of Movement

In an important new study Cassidy et al. (15) documented increased ranges of movement in the cervical spine following a single adjustment (16). The study involved 51 patients with unilateral neck pain, some acute and some chronic, 40 (80%) of whom had "substantial limitation of activity" due to pain. The subjects were given a single rotational cervical adjustment on the side of pain. Pre- and post- ranges of movement were measured by a cervical goniometer, a measuring device worn on the head that is standard equipment for range-of-movement measurements in health sciences. There was a marked increase in range of movement in various planes—on the same and opposite sides as the injury—in rotation, flexion and extension, and ipsilateral and contralateral bending. The most noticeable improvement was in rotation (16). The investigators also reported a significant decrease in pain. Using refined methods of statistical analysis, they have been able to show a most important connection: the decrease

in pain is positively linked to the increased range of movement (16).

In a related study, LaFrance and Cassidy (17) have also found significant increases in rotational range of motion in the cervical spine following a single adjustment using asymptomatic subjects. Treatment consisted of a single rotary cervical adjustment with contact on C2. Pre- and post-ranges of movement were again objectively measured by goniometer (16).

### HEAD AND NECK INJURIES

Mobilization of the tender areas in the posterior musculature and osseous structures should be defined during the physical examination. Management of patients with head and neck injuries consists of both evaluation of the injuries to rule out any ligamentous instability and treatment of any muscle tears of the fibers. The symptoms can start to occur in the sternocleidomastoid and within 24 hr the patients start to experience significant muscle swelling.

The brachial neuralgias are usually the result of soft tissue injuries, most commonly a contracture of the scalenes group. They do not exactly revolve around injury to the brachial plexus but are more of an entrapment syndrome. Patients who have been involved in rear-end collisions have similar injuries and, as has been shown by Wickstrom and

Larocca (18), can start having pain in the shoulders, numbness in the hands and arms, and paresthesias.

## RADIOGRAPHIC EVALUATION

The chiropractic profession recognizes that diagnostic radiographic examinations, while offering inestimable benefits to the knowledge that is made avaiable, have risks and possible detriments that must be weighed against those benefits. The academic/scientific community in chiropractics stands on record that there should always be clinical evidence of need for diagnostic radiographic examinations before they are performed. Use of radiography as a routine procedure or on the basis of a patient's self-referral is not good practice and is not condoned (19).

When performing a radiographic examination, a minimum of three views in an accelerative/decelerative-type injury or trauma to the neck will enable the examiner to observe the facets and the spinal integrity (Table 9.1). They will also reveal contraindications to manipulative treatment or any pathologies that may be evident that would predispose the patient to further aggravation following such treatment.

In head and neck injuries for which the physical examination reveals structural alteration, the three basic views should consist of an anteroposterior cervical, open-mouth cervical, and lateral cervical (20). If no widening of the intervertebral disc space or bone damage is suspected, an additional flexion/extension lateral view should be obtained (21). If radiculopathy is evident, right and left anterior oblique views are indicated in addi-

**Table 9.1.**
**Radiologic Features in Whiplash Injuries[a]**

Alignment abnormalities
   Alordosis
   Arcual kyphosis
   Segmental flexion/extension
   Anterolisthesis
   Apophyseal joint space widening
   Widening interspinous spacing (fanning)
Soft tissue abnormalities
   Increased prevertebral space
   Acute loss of disc height
   Displaced prevertebral fat stripe
   Vacuum cleft sign (extension) (25)

[a]Adapted from Yochum TR, Lindsay JR: Radiological features in whiplash injuries. In: *Essentials of Skeletal Radiology.* Baltimore, Williams & Wilkins, 1987, p 442.

tion to the above-mentioned views (22, 23). Certainly the right and left anterior oblique views should be reviewed to rule out any foraminal encroachment or any osteophytic formation before any type of manipulative treatment is employed, both for the patient's safety and for examiner reliability in determining the course of treatment. One of the cardinal rules in radiology is, when in doubt, always take multiple cervical views to determine safety of manipulative treatment and to enable appropriate consideration of underlying pathologies or the suspicion of fractures.

If the anteroposterior, open-mouth, lateral, and lower cervical views reveal no osseous pathology, but one suspects anterior or posterior cervical muscle spasm rigidity, a Davis series (seven views of the cervical spine) with both flexion and extension should be obtained, in addition to right and left anterior oblique views. A pillar view is also important where one cannot radiographically isolate or reveal the absolute angle of the cervical area or where low-grade fracture is suspected. Certainly, this would be left to the discretion and professional experience of the examiner.

Consideration of a computed tomography scan would be indicated after a minimum of 6 weeks of manipulation therapy to further understand underlying soft tissue pathology. Magnetic resonance imaging is also acceptable for this purpose. The clinician must utilize professional judgment.

## CERVICAL BIOMECHANICAL CONSIDERATIONS

Manipulations should be employed in those patients who have a component of aberrant flexion, extension, right and left lateral flexion, or rotation lordosis. The manipulation is directed to the angle of the zygapophysis to free up the restriction of movement as well as to restore appropriate cervical biomechanical relationships. Delaying movement in the cervical spine can cause fibrous adhesions in and around the bony structure and lesions in the surrounding muscle groups, resulting in restrictions of movement and pain on movement (3). Hohl believes that there can be delayed degenerative changes in 60% of the patients who have experienced a rapid accelerative/decelerative impact injury (24).

In a normal physiologic state in the cervical spine, a lordosis is the rule rather than the exception. Consideration based on clinical experience has indicated that in a kyphotic curvature, or lack of some lordosis, the individual can appear to have degenerative joint disease. The hyperlordotic neck is certainly a poor candidate for manipulative processing, because any hyperlordosis or kyphosis is a contraindication for manipulative processing unless arcual kyphosis is induced by contracture of the longus colli musculature.

## PATHOPHYSIOLOGY OF ACCELERATION/ DECELERATION IMPACT INJURIES

It is interesting to note that head positioning during trauma is of great importance in considering the degree of damage to the neck that must be evaluated. This is particularly true in the type of accelerative/decelerative impact that occurs as a result of the increased speed of vehicles and increased vehicle usage on the highway.

The specific nonpathologic injury produced by a − Gx accelerative force transmitted indirectly to the head via the spinal column consists of tissue damage at the zone of maximum stretch at the atlanto-occipital area, as defined by Unterharnscheidt (25) in his study on Rhesus monkeys. He noted very few injuries or lesions of the axons or myelin sheaths. According to this study, the first thing that occurs is that a substantial amount of kinetic energy is built up during the acceleration phase when the monkey is in the flexed position and the head is rotating forward. In this motion, called the "concertina effect," the head is held in a position with the chin low toward the thorax and the cervical spine more in a flexed position. After impact, the neck makes a hyperflexion movement backward during the deceleration phase. This phenomenon must also occur in human pathology. Following such trauma the patient would have injury to the joints or to the soft tissue structures of the spinal cord and would not be a candidate for mobilization or manipulation; this patient would best be held immobile.

## NEUROBIOLOGIC MECHANISMS IN MANIPULATIVE THERAPY OF ALTERED JOINT FUNCTION

In the spinal column, the mobile segments of the bony structure of the cervical spine consist of apophyseal joints and discs. Many manipulators consider the manipulative processes as being directed at the mechanism of the disc. There is another school of thought that supports the idea that manipulation would act much the same way in segments where there are no discs, particularly in the extremity skeletal joints. For example, a

jammed elbow can be corrected by traction manipulation. Traction manipulation would be administered to decrease the pain response and decrease the pressure in the synovial capsule. Based on clinical experience, manipulative treatment is considered to be of benefit in skeletal joints as well. Therefore, spinal manipulative treatment seems to be of primary benefit in the treatment of altered joint function.

Understanding altered joint function has many benefits. As research becomes more sophisticated and as interest in pursuing the effects of manipulative treatment for altered joint function becomes greater, more scientific treatises will appear on this subject.

It is very likely that the manipulative neurophysiologic mechanisms play as important a role in the manual therapeutic treatment as does the mechanical correction of the segmental dysfunction. Figures 9.2 and 9.3 attempt to present this model schematically (26).

Spinal manipulative treatment in and of itself is a diagnostic profile for the treatment of altered joint function. If the patient starts to make an improvement within the first month, the diagnosis of altered joint function is certainly appropriate. In other words, the early stages of manipulative processing are much like any diagnostic test. The patient's response to treatment, based on the manipulative processing and comparative examinations, is clinically evaluated to determine the healing response. If altered joint function is a scenario, which Figure 9.3 clearly illustrates by normal orientation of the facet angles in the cervical area, then the patient should make some improvement with manipulation.

## DIFFERENTIAL DIAGNOSIS AND DEFINITION OF RADICULAR AND SPONDYLOGENIC PAIN (NONRADICULAR PAIN SYNDROMES)

In the acute cervical trauma with a radicular-type syndrome, there is poor clinical differential diagnostic impression. One often finds a very confused picture when testing for the radicular pain syndrome. Particular attention must be paid to motor and sensory disturbances. These can be exhibited by areas of decreased pain perception, hypesthesias, and paresthesias, but they add very little to understanding the clinical picture (27). Radicular pain would not warrant electromyographic studies to determine if the pain is truly a radiculopathy until enough time has passed that edema

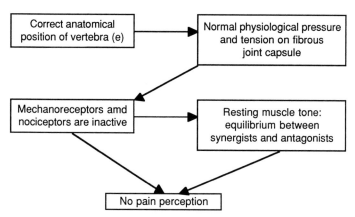

**Figure 9.2.** Model for receptor activity when vertebrae are in the correct position. (Adapted from Dvorak J, Dvorak V: *Manual Medicine Diagnostics.* Stuttgart, Georg Thieme Verlag, 1984, pp 49–50.)

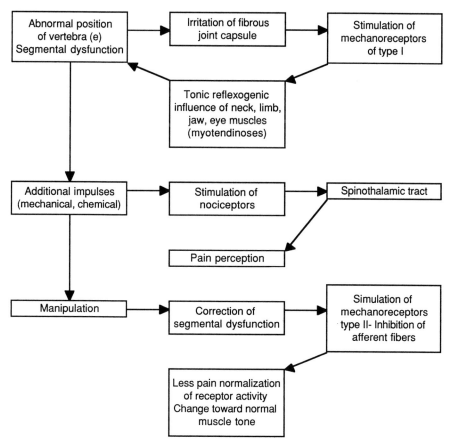

**Figure 9.3.** Model for receptor activity when vertebrae are in abnormal position (segmental dysfunction). (Adapted from Dvorak J, Dvorak V: *Manual Medicine Diagnostics.* Stuttgart, Georg Thieme Verlag, 1984, pp 49–50.)

can subside. Gross motor alteration is detectable, but more subtle neurologic deficits, such as scleratogenous referred pain, that can mimic true radicular pain are more difficult to detect. Many times the cervical spine will have referred pain that occurs upon various mechanical/chemical stimuli of different spinal and paraspinal cervical structures. This is the reason some of the important experimental neurologic work by Korr (28), Simmons (29), and Wyke (30, 31) has attempted to categorize the soft tissue changes that occur in functional disturbances at the parietal joints. These changes are often described as inflammatory soft tissue rheumatism.

A variety of approaches are taken in different healing professions. The chiropractic theory of subluxation directs the treatment toward relieving the nerve impingement. The neurosurgeon tends to focus on decompressing the discal area for alleviation of pain. The result is further confusion and a decrease in the diagnostic profile in treatment.

## TRAUMATIC ARTHRITIS

Direct trauma to the joint causes soft tissue changes to the synovial membrane, which becomes congested, edematous, and hemorrhagic. At the same time an outpouring of the synovial fluid continues. The latter may contain serum and fiber, which give a deep amber color to the fluid. If the tissues are torn, extravasation into the joint cavity varies from a minute amount, detected either microscopically or chemically, to frank hemorrhage. Synovial fluid interferes with the clotting mechanism of the blood so that the mixture to a large extent remains liquid. Once the synovial fluid is released outside the synovial capsule, synovial inflammation occurs. If resorption of synovial inflammation is complete, over a period of time, the joint could return to normal activity (32).

Various other factors militate against the restoration of normal joint physiology and anatomy. If blood clots are present and deposited in the depths of the synovial fluid, they organize into adhesions (33). This is the major factor in the propensity for traumatic arthritis. It is at this time that irregularities of the surface of the joints would become more pronounced and further radiographic consideration would be in order. Turek (33) hypothesized that early implementation of mobility and supportive physiologic therapeutics, such as traction and stretching of the involved joint, can diminish the enhancement of

synovial inflammation and may decrease the irregularity of the articulation affected.

## TREATMENT

Many times the cervical spine will have referred pain that occurs as a result of various mechanical/chemical stimuli of different spinal and paraspinal cervical structures. The time frame in which spinal mobilization can be effective to prevent symptoms is generally three to five sessions.

Physical therapy, such as ultrasound and high-voltage positive-electrode galvanic stimulation, is required for the reduction of edema and muscle contraction when periarthritis has occurred as the result of trauma. Mobilization along the angle of articulation to the point of passive range of motion, within 1–2 weeks after trauma, may assist in the prevention of periarthritis and lesions. The motion can assist in the reduction of muscle atrophy.

## ORTHOPAEDIC TESTING

Orthopaedic tests have been developed to reproduce the patient's symptoms in order to better understand the clinical picture. For understanding altered joint function, these tests are designed either to increase pressure in the zygapophysis or to stretch the paravertebral muscle groups. Four orthopaedic tests often used for determining altered joint function are the Fitzgerald compression test, Jackson's compression test, cervical distraction, and shoulder depression.

## FITZGERALD COMPRESSION TEST (FIG. 9.4)

The examiner stands at the lateral aspect of either side of the patient. With the patient's head extended backward, the examiner compresses, with a direct pressure, at the posterior aspect of the skull. The test should compress the neck and stimulate the articular facets that would be related to disc disease, pain-sensitive structures, or nerve root irritation. A significant increase in any combination of neck, shoulder, or anterior cervical tenderness in the described position would be a positive test finding.

## JACKSON'S COMPRESSION TEST (FIG. 9.5)

In Jackson's compression test, the patient is instructed to rotate the head to either the right or

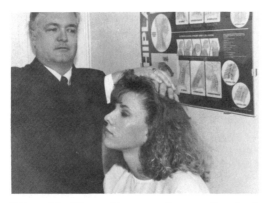

**Figure 9.4.** Fitzgerald compression test. Test developed after years of clinical practice by P. B. Fitzgerald. Review of literature did not reveal any orthopaedic test that tested for altered joint function and produced positive reproduction of pain in test results.

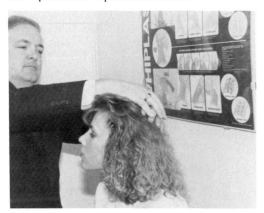

**Figure 9.5.** Jackson's compression test. (From Mazion JM: *Illustrated Manual of Orthopedic Signs/Tests/Maneuvers for Office Procedure.* Orlando, FL, Daniels Publishing Co, 1980, p 295.)

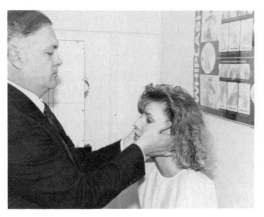

**Figure 9.6.** Cervical distraction. (From Mazion JM: *Illustrated Manual of Orthopedic Signs/Tests/Maneuvers for Office Procedure.* Orlando, FL, Daniels Publishing Co, 1980, p 259.)

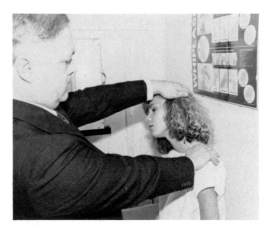

**Figure 9.7.** Shoulder depression. (From Mazion JM: *Illustrated Manual of Orthopedic Signs/Tests/Maneuvers for Office Procedure.* Orlando, FL, Daniels Publishing Co, 1980, p 355.)

the left, and the examiner, with the patient's head at maximum rotation, places pressure at the base of the head downward. The pressure causes compression of the intervertebral disc space. Reproduction of pain is a positive finding (34).

## CERVICAL DISTRACTION (FIG. 9.6)

Cervical distraction consists of a continuous vertical pressure with the examiner supporting the mandible and the occiput. A positive finding of increased pain indicates a muscle injury (35).

## SHOULDER DEPRESSION (FIG. 9.7)

Shoulder depression is tested by placing one hand on the base of the muscle groups surrounding the cervical spine and placing pressure opposite the head, with the patient in a seated position. The combination of movements either elicits pain in the muscles or indicates adhesions around the dural sheaths of the nerve root (36).

## MANAGEMENT OF A PATIENT

Two issues must be considered before initiating manipulation and mobilization: the safety of the treatment and the risk of a delayed diagnosis that would require medical treatment (37). Neither alleged danger has ever been substantiated as significant and, in a chapter devoted to safety, the New Zealand Commission concludes that spinal manipulative treatment is "remarkably safe" (37).

The one significant risk arising from chiropractic treatment is vertebral artery syndrome (VAS) following cervical adjustment, which may lead to stroke. The incidence and mechanisms of VAS are reported better in chiropractic literature (38–40) than elsewhere (37). The risk is extremely remote, however—about 0.0002% or two to three cases per million treatments—figures with which medical specialists agree (41, 42). This compares with a 1–2% risk of paralysis from neurosurgery on the cervical spine (15,000 cases per million) (43), which is often performed for similar degenerative conditions (37).

Chinese researchers have found some correlation between visual disturbances and the effect of spinal manipulation. It is hypothesized that there is change in the neurovascular component of the spinal cord that causes neuronal alteration of the optic chiasm (44).

All the physiologic therapeutic modalities are used to prepare the patient to undergo spinal mobilization or manipulation. Successful management of these cases requires careful evaluation in which the framework is laid for rational therapy of any condition that the presenting pathology might require (45). Before a treatment program for an accelerative/decelerative injury can be initiated, it must be determined that there is no hemorrhage from the carotid artery or any abnormal neurologic deficit arising from the traumatic insult. The degree and intensity of the impact should be evaluated and correlated with the physical and objective examination to determine the degree of manipulative treatment that needs to be implemented. After laying the framework and making an evaluation as to the type of trauma sustained by a patient, the physician should implement a clinical course of treatment consisting of gentle spinal mobilization to help decrease resistance to movement and restore functional integrity.

Of great importance in the management of these injuries is preparatory manipulative treatment to prepare the soft tissues and surrounding structures in order to provide a decreased resistance to movement. Spinal mobilization should be administered based on the clinician's past experience, in a gentle fashion, within the first week of treatment but not initially. The patient should be able to be taken through gentle ranges of motion to determine any restrictions of movement.

There are certain time frames that are beneficial in implementing therapeutic modalities. Certainly, within the first 72 hr ice should be administered to the area of affliction to vasoconstrict the tissue and to provide a decreased pain sensation to the surrounding external subcutaneous tissue (46). The second phase, in addition to ice, would include the implementation of high-voltage galvanic stimulation at a location where the patient's skin does not appear contracted. Such physiologic therapeutics should be applied to the point at which the patient is most comfortable, but not until the surrounding tissue begins contracture. This therapy should be administered for a minimum of 30 min preparatory to manipulative or mobilization treatment, depending on the condition of the patient. After 72 hr ultrasound would be an excellent choice of preparatory therapy for manipulation or mobilization (46). Following the above form of treatment, some type of imbibition, either disc distraction or mechanical traction, is very beneficial and preparatory and provides joint-controlled mobility.

It has been this author's experience that a 4–12-week treatment course can help restore joint movement in a controlled fashion in an accelerative/decelerative injury or in any patient for whom there are clear findings in favor of spinal mobilization. In a more complicated case the manipulative processing can be utilized for up to 120 days to help restore joint integrity. The patient should be evaluated at least once every 10 visits regarding the need for continued clinical treatment. If there is no response (increasing mobility or decreasing myospasms), then manipulative treatment probably will not be of benefit. However, there are always exceptions to this rule.

A treatment course should consist initially of one mobilization every day for a period of about 2 weeks after trauma. The frequency of manipulation is then reduced to three times per week with at least 1 day between treatments for a period of 4–6 weeks. After this initial period of time and after another evaluation has been performed, manipulative treatment should be reduced to probably once per week for a 1-month cycle, or performed on an as-needed basis to prevent recurring symptoms. If a cervical injury patient is not making clinical progress at this time, a secondary diagnostic profile, such as a magnetic resonance imaging or computed tomography scan, could be utilized to determine if further problems of the neck, such as ligamentous derangement, exist or to visualize soft tissue patterns that cannot be seen on normal radiographic examination.

Manipulative treatment should be a very slow process in the initial stages and should be utilized more aggressively as the patient can tolerate it. It must be remembered that all manipulative treatment requires interaction with the patient, close visual monitoring, and extensive physical exam preparation to establish a baseline against which to compare the healing response.

## MANIPULATIVE TECHNIQUES

It is impossible to list all variations of manipulative techniques, but some of the specific manipulations for head and neck injuries are outlined here. Generally, in cervical trauma or head injuries the type of manipulative technique that is administered would be a specific short-levered, high-velocity thrust (47). Normally the contact is made with the small portion of the hand, but the thumb can also be the force that delivers a thrust. The

spinal segment above or below the location of thrust should be stabilized by the clinician's hand to limit its passive range of motion. The high-velocity thrust is delivered with the contact hand to the short lever area of the vertebra (i.e., transverse process, spinous process, or mamillary process) in the direction in which the correction should be made (48).

Figures 9.8 through 9.15 demonstrate some of the basic principles of spinal manipulative treatment to the cervical and occipital regions.

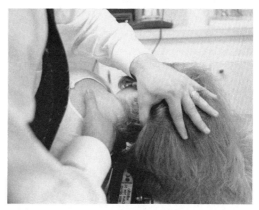

**Figure 9.10.** Body manipulation of C3–5 with thenar eminence stabilization of the segments above. The manipulator, using the thenar eminence portion of the hand, moves the segmental bony region, thrusting posterior to anterior with line of drive determined by facet orientation.

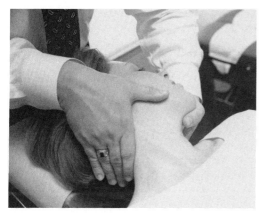

**Figure 9.8.** Body manipulation of C3–5 with occiput stabilization. The movement is a quick lateral thrust of the hand, posterior to anterior, with line of drive determined by facet orientation.

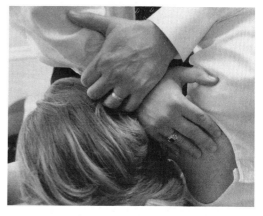

**Figure 9.11.** Atlas-axis manipulation along a line of drive consistent with stabilization of C3–4 using manipulation drop for absorption of the recoil. This manipulation is done at a 45° angle with the lateral aspect of the knife edge of the hand moving quickly through the area. It is a lateral thrust with line of drive determined by facet orientation. The patient should not experience any discomfort during this manipulation.

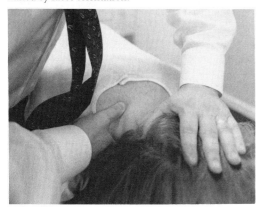

**Figure 9.9.** Thumb manipulation of C6–7 while stabilizing segments above and below. This manipulation is administered with a rapid thrust of the thumb against the C6–7 posterior lateral area, with line of drive determined by facet orientation.

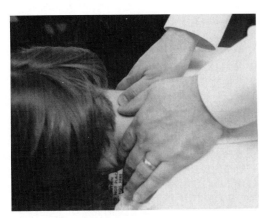

**Figure 9.12.** Bilateral manipulation of C5–6 using the thumbs in alignment with the angle of the zygapophysis. This movement is a quick, rapid thrust of the hand forward, posterior to anterior, with line of drive determined by facet orientation.

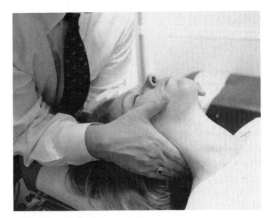

**Figure 9.15.** Disc distraction mobilization of C3–5. While cupping the occiput with the thenar eminence, an intermittent traction movement is performed until engagement of isometric contracture is achieved.

## CONTRAINDICATIONS TO MANIPULATION

The techniques that have been described in this chapter require years of training and hands-on experience and should not be implemented callously or without a great degree of caution. The field of spinal mobilization and manipulation requires as much training as does surgery. In the hands of a skilled clinician, manipulation is generally a very safe procedure.

The following is a list of contraindications for manipulation of cervical spine injuries: unstable fractures, severe osteoporosis, multiple myeloma, osteomyelitis, primary bone tumors, metastatic bone tumors, Paget's disease, any progressive neurologic deficit, spinal cord tumors, central intervertebral disc herniations, hypermobile joints, rheumatoid arthritis, Reiter's syndrome, anticoagulant therapy, congenital bleeding disorders, and acquired bleeding disorders. Even in the presence of these underlying pathologic processes, soft tissue mobilization may still be possible.

Finally, the most important contraindications to manipulative treatment are inadequate physical and spinal examination, and secondarily, poor training that does not consist of a minimum of 2 years of academic training and 1 year of internship after basic postgraduate training.

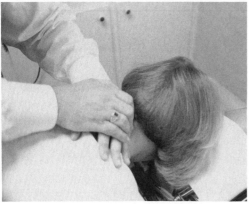

**Figure 9.13.** Manipulation of C5–6 with knife edge of hand. The angle of the hand is aligned with the angle of the zygapophysis spinous process it contacts. The thrust is posterior to anterior, with the line of drive determined by facet orientation.

### REFERENCES

1. Xing Chen Boa: Notes from lecture given at Railway Hospital, Bejing, China, July, 1987.
2. Cassidy JD, Kirklady-Willis WH, McGregor M: Spinal manipulation for the treatment of chronic low back and leg pain: an observational study. In Bueger AA, Greenman PE (eds): *Empirical Approaches to the Validation of Spinal Manipulation.* Springfield, IL, Charles C Thomas, 1985.

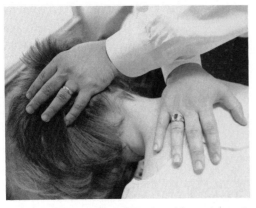

**Figure 9.14.** Occiput mobilization with traction to the lower cervical vertebrae. This is a stretching movement.

3. Viedman T: Experimental models of osteoarthritis: the role of immobilization. *Clin Biomechanics* 2:223–229, 1987 (and the various papers by Viedman there referenced).

4. Schafer RC (ed): *Basic Chiropractic Procedural Manual*, ed 4. Arlington, VA, American Chiropractic Association, 1984.

5. Katayama K: Histopathological study of the whiplash injury. *J Jpn Orthop Assoc* 4:439–453, 1970.

6. Bates B: *A Guide to Physical Examination*, ed 2. Philadelphia, PA, JB Lippincott, 1979; 17:297–298.

7. Arnold LE: *Chiropractic Procedural Examination.* Seminole, FL, Seminole Printing, 1979, pp 7–65.

8. Schafer RC: *Chiropractic Management of Sports and Recreational Injuries.* Baltimore, Williams & Wilkins, 1986, pp 209–218, 219–228.

9. Dvorak J, Dvorak V: *Manual Medicine Diagnostics.* Stuttgart, Georg Thieme Verlag, 1984, pp 49–50.

10. Gates D: *Correlative Spinal Anatomy.* Lakemont, GA, CHB Printing & Binding, 1977, pp 100–122.

11. Kapandji IA: *The Physiology of the Joints*, ed 2. New York, Longman, Inc, 1974, pp 216–227.

12. Kapandji IA: *The Physiology of the Joints*, ed 2. New York, Longman, Inc, 1974, pp 230–242.

13. Kapandji IA: *The Physiology of the Joints*, ed 2. New York, Longman, Inc, 1974, pp 246–247.

14. Foreman SM, Croft AC: Biomechanics: kinematics of the lower cervical spine (C3–C7). In *Whiplash Injuries—the Cervical Accelerative/Decelerative Syndrome.* Baltimore, Williams & Wilkins, 1988, p 27.

15. Cassidy JD, Quon J, LaFrance L: Effect of manipulation on pain and range of motion in the cervical spine. (in press)

16. Smith-Chapman D: Increased range of movement. *The Chiropractic Report* 3(3):4 (No. 15), 1989.

17. LaFrance L, Cassidy JD: The effects of manipulation on the range of motion of the cervical spine. (in press)

18. Wickstrom J, Larocca H: Trauma: head and neck injuries from acceleration/deceleration forces. In Ruge D, Wiltse LL (eds): *Spinal Disorders: Diagnosis and Treatment.* Philadelphia, Lea & Febiger, 1977, p 350.

19. Cunningham JW, Johnston WW: *Occupational Medicine and Legal Sourcebook*, 1985, p 12.

20. Yochum TR, Lindsay JR: *Essentials of Skeletal Radiology.* Baltimore, Williams & Wilkins, 1987, pp 13–17.

21. Yochum TR, Lindsay JR: *Essentials of Skeletal Radiology.* Baltimore, Williams & Wilkins, 1987, p 21.

22. Turek SL: *Orthopaedics Principles and Their Application*, ed 4. Philadelphia, JB Lippincott, 1984, vol 1, p 452.

23. Turek SL: *Orthopaedics Principles and Their Application*, ed 4. Philadelphia, JB Lippincott, 1984, vol 2, p 19.

24. Hohl M: Soft tissue injuries of the neck. *Clin Orthop Rel Res* 109:42–49, 1975.

25. Unterharnscheidt F: Pathological and neuropathological findings in rhesus monkeys subject to −Gx and ±Gx indirect impact acceleration. In Sances A, Thomas DJ, Ewing CL, Larson SJ, Unterharnschedit F (eds): *Mechanisms of Head and Spine Trauma.* Goshen, NY, Aloray, 1986.

26. Dvorak J, Dvorak V: *Manual Medicine Diagnostics.* Stuttgart, Georg Thieme Verlag, 1984, pp 47–48.

27. Korr IM: Proprioceptors and the discussion of mechanisms of manipulative therapy. In Korr IM (ed): *Neurobiologic Mechanisms in Manipulative Therapy.* New York, Plenum, 1978.

28. Korr IM: Proprioceptors and somatic dysfunction. *J Am Osteopath Assoc* 74:638, 1975.

29. Simmons DG: Muscle pain syndromes. *Am Phys Med* 54:289, 1975; 55:15, 1976.

30. Wyke BD: The neurological basis of thoracic spinal pain. *Rheum Phys Med* 10:356, 1967.

31. Wyke BD: Neurology of the cervical spinal joints. *Physiotherapy* 65:72, 1979.

32. Turek SL: *Orthopaedics Principles and Their Application*, ed 4. Philadelphia, JB Lippincott, 1984, vol 1, pp 451–452.

33. Turek SL: *Orthopaedics Principles and Their Application*, ed 4, Philadelphia, JB Lippincott, 1984, vol 1, p 451.

34. Mazion JM: *Illustrated Manual of Orthopedic Signs/Tests/Maneuvers for Office Procedure.* Orlando, FL, Daniels Publishing Co, 1980, p 295.

35. Mazion JM: *Illustrated Manual of Orthopedic Signs/Tests/Maneuvers for Office Procedure.* Orlando, FL, Daniels Publishing Co, 1980, p 259.

36. Mazion JM: *Illustrated Manual of Orthopedic Signs/Tests/Maneuvers for Office Procedure.* Orlando, FL, Daniels Publishing Co, 1980, p 355.

37. Smith-Chapman D: The chiropractic profession. In *Chiropractic: a Referenced Source of Modern Concepts: New Evidence.* Palmerton, PA, Practice Makers Products, Inc, 1988, pp 29, 30.

38. Kleynhans A: Complications of and contraindications to spinal manipulative therapy. In Haldeman S (ed): *Modern Developments in the Principles and Practice of Chiropractic.* New York, Appleton-Century-Crofts, 1980, pp 359–384.

39. Terrett A: Vascular accidents from cervical spinal manipulation: report on 107 cases. *J Aust Chiropractors' Assoc* 17(1):15–24, 1987.

40. Terrett A: Vascular accidents from cervical spinal manipulation: the mechanisms. *J Aust Chiropractors' Assoc* 17(4):131–144, 1987.

41. Gutman G: Injuries to the vertebral artery caused by manual therapy. *Manuelle Medizin* 21:2–14, 1983. (Abstract only in English)

42. Dvorak J, Orelli P: How dangerous is manipulation to the cervical spine? *Manual Medicine* 2:1–4, 1985.

43. *Rocha v Harris*, 39 CCLT 279, 283 (1987). [A Canadian case, expert testimony of Dr. Lawrence Clein, neurosurgeon.]

44. Yichi Yang: Notes from lecture given at the Hospital of Traumatology, Bejing, China, July, 1987.

45. Turek SL: *Orthopaedics Principles and Their Application*, ed 4. Philadelphia, JB Lippincott, 1984, vol 1, pp 451–452.

46. Schafer RC: *Chiropractic Management of Sports and Recreational Injuries.* Baltimore, Williams & Wilkins, 1986, pp 161–186.

47. Langley JC: Spinal manipulation and the reduction of pain. In Tollison CD (ed): *Handbook of Chronic Pain Management.* Baltimore, Williams & Wilkins, 1989, p 170.

48. Langley JC: Spinal manipulation and the reduction of pain. In Tollision CD (ed): *Handbook of Chronic Pain Management.* Baltimore, Williams & Wilkins, 1989, pp 111–119.

## 10

# NERVE BLOCKS
# AND INVASIVE THERAPIES

*Winston C. V. Parris*

The cervical segment of the vertebral column is exposed to a variety of traumatic injuries and mechanical lesions that may develop into chronic pain syndromes. These injuries may be direct or indirect, major or minor, superficial or deep, either musculoskeletal alone or involving the central nervous system. The natural lordosis of the cervical spine, along with its relative increased range of motion and the mechanical effect of supporting the head, produce degenerative changes that may ultimately result in progressive musculoskeletal pathology (1). These pathologic changes may contribute to chronic cervical back pain with a variety of organic and behavioral sequelae. Nerve block therapy is a major component of the invasive modalities used to treat chronic cervical pain syndromes.

In addition to their therapeutic use, nerve blocks may be used, in selected circumstances, for diagnostic, prophylactic, and prognostic purposes (2). The placebo effect of nerve blocks, as in any medical therapy, is not to be underestimated in susceptible patients. Performance of nerve blocks should be associated with certain prerequisites to ensure patient safety and to minimize the risk of associated complications. These prerequisites include: (*a*) adequate (preblock) evaluation of the patient; (*b*) baseline determination of vital signs (pulse, blood pressure, respiration, and general observation of the sensorium); (*c*) understanding of the pathogenesis of the disease process associated with the pain; (*d*) knowledge of the pharmacology of the drugs used to perform the nerve block; (*e*) technical competence in the performance of the nerve block; (*f*) ready availability of

resuscitative equipment and drugs; (*g*) certification in advanced cardiac life support (ACLS); and (*h*) facilities for patient observation after nerve block administration.

Many experts insist that the placement of an intravenous line is mandatory prior to the performance of a major nerve block. This recommendation, although medicolegally prudent, is controversial. The protagonists argue that the correction of hypotension and the institution of resuscitation are facilitated by the presence of an intravenous line, and this is correct. However, the added cost of intravenous lines with fluids, the discomfort associated with venous access, the risk of local infection with phlebitis, and the possibility of vasovagal syncope (3) in susceptible patients are relative contraindications to the insertion of intravenous lines. Moreover, the administration of intravenous lines in patients with distinct behavioral components of chronic cervical back pain reinforces dependency on the "medical model" of pain management and adversely interferes with the dynamics of pain rehabilitation (4). All these reasons make the acquisition of venous access controversial at best and possibly unnecessary in some cases. It is important to stress, however, that there are selected patients (e.g., moderately obese patients, cachectic and dehydrated patients, patients with inaccessible veins secondary to previous chemotherapy, patients with unstable respiratory or cardiovascular diseases) who require the elective insertion of intravenous lines prior to the performance of any invasive nerve block. The ultimate decision lies with the physician performing the nerve block and his judgment of what are considered acceptable standards of practice for a particular patient in a given location.

The following nerve blocks may be used for the management of chronic cervical back pain:

1. Cervical epidural steroid injection
2. Suprascapular nerve block
3. Stellate ganglion block
4. Cervical trigger point injection
5. Occipital nerve block
6. Epidural blood patch
7. Cervical plexus block
8. Accessory nerve block

Other miscellaneous invasive therapies that may be used for the management of selective chronic cervical back pain include:

1. Neurolytic blocks
2. Selected cryotherapy
3. Acupuncture
4. Dorsal column stimulation
5. Deep brain stimulation
6. Surgical procedures

It is important to stress that nerve blocks and other invasive therapies are best administered in concert with the multidisciplinary evaluation and management of the chronic pain patient. Further, the normal progression from simple, noninvasive modalities to complex and invasive ones should be observed unless a particular procedure is specifically indicated. All the above-mentioned nerve blocks and invasive therapies are discussed in this chapter along with their indications, potential complications, and clinical relevance.

## CERVICAL EPIDURAL STEROID INJECTION

Lumbar epidural steroid injections (5) have been used since the turn of the century for the treatment of low back pain. However, the use of epidural steroid injections in the cervical region (6) has only gained popularity in the past 10 years. This modality has been used for treating patients with a variety of chronic cervical pain syndromes, including cervical radiculopathy. The good news is that many patients who would have undergone cervical laminectomies can now be treated successfully with cervical epidural steroid injections.

The technique for cervical epidural steroid injection is basically the same as for the lumbar region except for important anatomic considerations. While the axes of the lumbar spinous processes are roughly parallel to the axis of the lumbar spine, the cervical spinous processes (with the exception of C7) form an angle of approximately 45° with the axis of the cervical spine. The C7 spinous process is almost perpendicular to the axis of the cervical spine. The presence of a slight cervical lordosis and the fact that the C7–T1 interspace is the largest (7) make access to the cervical epidural space relatively easy. Further, the cervical cord is narrowest in the C7 region and the epidural space is correspondingly widest at that level. The negative pressure in the cervical epidural space is most pronounced at the C7–T1 interspace because of its proximity to the thoracic cavity. All these anatomic features make the C7–T1 interspace, and to a lesser extent the C6–7 interspace, the ideal points of access to the cervical epidural space.

It is mandatory to ensure strict aseptic precautions during the performance of this nerve block since compromise of sterility may result in serious complications, including meningitis, myelitis, and encephalitis (8); all of these complications are potentially fatal. The block is ideally performed with the patient in the sitting position and with the neck flexed forward so that the chin rests on the manubrium of the sternum. An assistant may be used to make sure that the thoracic spine is kept as erect as possible and to avoid hyperflexion of the neck. This assistant can also be used to support the patient, especially if vasovagal syncope should occur. The prone position is also used for the performance of cervical epidural steroid injection, with the upper chest supported by one or two pillows depending on the size of the patient. These pillows facilitate flexion of the neck. This position is desirable in patients who are prone to developing syncopal episodes, but precludes the use of the hanging drop technique for identification of the epidural space. The lateral position is seldom used since it is associated with a high incidence of inadvertent dural puncture.

The needle is inserted in the midline close to the superior aspect of the C7 spinous process and advanced meticulously in 1-mm increments until the ligamentum flavum is reached. The epidural space is identified by the loss of resistance technique with air or normal saline or by the hanging drop technique (9). Both techniques are associated with false-positive identification. It is the author's impression that the loss of resistance technique with air is the safer and more reliable technique. The loss of resistance technique with normal saline has the potential disadvantage of masking inadvertent dural puncture, and this makes it more complication-prone than the loss of resistance technique with air. Since the cervical epidural steroid injection is a "single shot" procedure not requiring epidural catheter insertion, a 22-gauge needle is used for the injection. A resistance-free syringe or "pulsator" syringe is used to demonstrate loss of resistance in identifying the epidural space.

Radiograpic studies (10) have shown that it takes approximately 10–12 ml of contrast medium to spread cephalad to C2 and caudad to T4 if injected at the C7–T1 interspace in the epidural space. A mixture of local anesthetic and depot steroid preparations are used and a variety of different dosage schedules have been recommended (11). Lidocaine 1.0%, mepivacaine 2.0%, and bupivacaine 0.25% have been used with good results. The purpose of this local anesthetic concentration is to avoid major motor nerve blockade and achieve maximal sympathetic with adequate sensory blockade, thus providing almost immediate pain relief. Seven to 8 ml of 0.25% bupivacaine achieves the goal easily. Two to 3 ml of 4% methylprednisolone (Depomedrol, 80–120 mg) is frequently used, although triamcinolone acetate (Aristocort, 50 mg) has been used as the steroid injectate. Special care should be exercised to ensure that the dura is not inadvertently punctured, because the introduction of methylprednisolone into the intrathecal space may produce severe neurologic complications (12).

The frequency of administration of cervical epidural steroid injection is controversial (13), with recommendations ranging from one injection every other day to a single injection. Since the depot steroids are slowly released in the body following injection, their effects are not immediate. For example, it takes approximately 6–10 days before the full therapeutic effects of epidural methylprednisolone are manifested. This slow release has the beneficial effect of minimizing the systemic toxic effects of the steroid injection (14). There is actually no well-established scientific rationale for the injection of steroids into the epidural space. It appears that this practice became firmly established long before controlled studies on the efficacy and mechanism of action of steroids were performed (15). In a retrospective study done by Rosen et al. (16), 40 patients with chronic low back pain secondary to herniated lumbar discs and spinal stenosis were reviewed. All patients received one to five injections of epidural steroid (methylprednisolone) by the same anesthesiologist. Follow-up at 8 months posttreatment showed that 10 patients (25%) were asymptomatic, 13 patients (32%) obtained varying degrees of pain relief, and 17 patients (43%)

received no pain relief. Further, the study showed that 12% of patients eventually had to undergo surgery and that half were dissatisfied with epidural steroid injections as a form of treatment.

The mechanism of action of epidural depot steroid in relieving pain is believed to be the anti-inflammatory effect of the steroids (17). The net effect is the probable decrease in neural and perineural inflammation together with the inhibition of periradicular adhesions and fibrosis. The evidence for these effects is inferential at best. The local anesthetics injected into the cervical epidural space provide some immediate relief that may last for several hours. As the local anesthetic effect wears off, however, many patients may complain of increased pain. Fortunately, this hyperalgesic state is short lived (2–3 days) and is usually followed by increasing periods of sustained pain relief in some patients. In our practice, we perform a single cervical epidural steroid injection with a mixture of 7 ml of 0.25% bupivacaine and 3 ml of 4% methylprednisolone and reevaluate the patient at the end of 3–4 weeks. If there is no subjective pain relief, another therapeutic option is explored. If there is some measurable pain relief but unacceptable residual pain, the procedure may be repeated at that time. No more than two cervical epidural steroid injections are performed during a 6-month period. This conservative approach minimizes the development of steroid-induced side effects or complications.

Dilke et al. (18) have demonstrated that epidural steroids are far superior to placebo in patients with lumbar nerve root compression syndromes. This study showed that patients with acute or early chronic pain syndromes get more benefit than patients with long-standing chronic pain. Consequently, it appears that early intervention with cervical epidural steroid injection is indicated in patients with painful cervical injuries or subacute cervical degenerative disease processes. Dirksen et al. (19) suggested that cervical epidural steroid injections may be effective in treating reflex sympathetic dystrophy. The postulated mechanism of action of this modality is the correction of the dysregulation of the spinal input-output sensorimotor reflex via a corticosteroid-mediated supraspinal and possibly perispinal effect (20). If this postulate is substantiated clinically (and initial case reports seem to support that hypothesis), then the rationale for using cervical epidural steroids to treat patients with painful (trauma-induced) cervical syndromes that have progressed to reflex sympathetic dystrophy may be justified.

This mechanism is different from the anti-inflammatory effect previously ascribed to steroids.

The injection of corticosteroids in the cervical epidural space is associated with a variety of complications (Table 10.1), some of which are serious while others are not. Most of the complications are preventable if adequate pre–nerve block patient evaluation is undertaken and if proper attention is paid to nerve block technique. Notwithstanding, complications will occur and it is important to recognize them early, treat them effectively, and constantly reassure the patient and family. Further, prior to the actual performance of the nerve block, informed consent should be obtained while outlining to the patient and family all the potential risks and complications of the procedure. In a recent review of complications of cervical epidural steroid injections (21), it was shown that inadvertent dural puncture was the most serious complication of this procedure. The incidence of this complication in skilled hands is approximately 0.5% (22). The major clinical implication of this complication is the development of severe postural headache. Treatment consists of strict bed rest, increased oral and intravenous fluid administration, the use of oral and intramuscular narcotics, and continued neurologic observation. If these conservative measures fail after 24–48 hr, then a cervical epidural blood patch with approximately 7 ml of autologous blood is performed. Success rates of epidural blood patch range from 92% to 99% (23). For this reason the epidural blood patch technique is preferred over saline epidural injection to treat post–dural puncture headache.

Vasovagal syncope was more common than inadvertent dural puncture in Waldman's study (21), but was more self-limiting and less incapacitating. This complication is usually associated with a high patient anxiety, which may be reduced by patient education and relaxation strategies. In our institution, a videotape on pain management issues is shown to all new chronic pain patients, and nerve blocks and their administration are included as one of the topics highlighted and discussed. In many cases this presentation serves to allay the patients' fears and anxiety. Patients who are still anxious and apprehensive after this exposure, and patients who have a history of vasovagal phenomena, receive their cervical epidural steroid injection in the prone position after intravenous access is secured. When vasovagal syncope occurs, it is treated with the patient in the Trendelenburg position, using intravenous fluids and incremental doses of an appropriate vasopressor (e.g., ephedrine 5–10 mg intravenously).

Superficial infection at the site of the injection may occur in a few patients, especially those who are immunocompromised. Thus, strict aseptic precautions should be maintained during the performance of this procedure. Following unrecognized inadvertent dural puncture, serious effects may result if the local anesthetic–methylprednisolone mixture is injected into the subarachnoid space. First, a total spinal block may occur with respiratory arrest and circulatory collapse. It should be stressed that this serious complication is almost always fully reversible and totally correctable if recognized early and managed properly. Anesthesiologists, by nature of their training and experience, are best suited to manage these complications. Endotracheal intubation with ventilatory support may be required for several hours, and appropriate circulatory support may also be necessary. Second, the methylprednisolone could produce severe neurologic complica-

**Table 10.1.**
**Complications of Cervical Epidural Steroid Injections**

Early complications
  Intravascular injection (seizures, peripheral vascular collapse, cardiac arrest)
  Vasovagal syncope
  Inadvertent dural puncture
    Total spinal block
    Post–dural puncture headache
  Inadvertent puncture of cervical spinal cord
  Severe hypotension secondary to "high" epidural block
  Bradycardia secondary to "high" epidural block
  Transient neurologic deficits
Late complications
  Epidural hematoma
  Anterior spinal artery thrombosis
  Epidural abscess
  Superficial infection at injection site
  Nausea and vomiting
  Increased pain and stiffness of neck
  Abdominal distention
Complications due to steroids
  Steroid psychosis
  Suppression of adrenocortical axis
  Idiosyncratic reaction
  Pseudotumor cerebri
  Allergic or anaphylactic reactions
  Osteoporosis
  Vertebral compression fracture

tions that may develop several days or weeks after the nerve block. The presence of polyethylene glycol (24) and possibly myristyl-γ-picolinium chloride in methylprednisolone may produce neurotoxic effects that may result in irreversible nerve damage (e.g., chronic arachnoiditis). These complications require early consultation and treatment by a neurologist.

There are certain vascular phenomena that may occur secondarily to cervical epidural steroid injections (see Table 10.1), including anterior spinal artery thrombosis, epidural hematoma, and intramuscular injection. Epidural hematoma should be managed by neurosurgical consultation, and the drastic sequelae can be adequately treated if early surgical intervention is implemented. Inadvertent intravenous or intra-arterial injection may produce a variety of neurologic and cardiovascular complications ranging from dizziness to cardiac arrest. The onset of tinnitus is a very reliable indicator of impending seizures. These seizures are best treated with increments of intravenous sodium thiopental 25 mg or diazepam 2.5 mg. Anterior spinal artery syndrome is usually diagnosed after it is too late to do anything effective about it. However, neurologic and radiologic consultations are useful in excluding other potentially correctable lesions or in limiting the existing lesion. The utilization of a variety of specialists in managing the complications emphasizes the need for a multidisciplinary approach to pain management, not only for initial evaluation of patients, but also for consultation on management problems as they occur.

Other rare complications of cervical epidural steroid injections include direct trauma to the cervical spinal cord, inadvertent "high" epidural block, epidural abscess, transient central nervous system deficits, nausea and vomiting, dyspnea, severe hypotension, bradycardia, increased pain and stiffness of the neck, facial flushing, transient subjective upper extremity weakness, and abdominal weakness. Steroid psychosis, idiosyncratic reactions, and suppression of the adrenocortical axis may be due to the systemic effects of the steroids per se and are usually not dose related. Osteoporosis and vertebral collapse with neurologic sequelae (25) may also occur with large doses of methylprednisolone.

## SUPRASCAPULAR NERVE BLOCK

Many patients with chronic cervical pain secondary to trauma or arthropathy may develop resid-

ual shoulder pain in addition to the original cervical pain or after resolution of that pain. This shoulder pain may be more intense than the original cervical pain; it may be localized to the shoulder area or may radiate to the proximal aspect of the affected upper extremity. This syndrome may be treated successfully with a series of suprascapular nerve blocks. The suprascapular nerve block is performed by injection of 10 ml of 0.25% bupivacaine one fingerwidth superior to the midpoint of the spine of the scapula. Paresthesias are sought as the needle enters the suprascapular fossa, and the resulting sharp pain is experienced over the acromial aspect of the shoulder. One milliliter of 4% methylprednisolone may be added to the local anesthetic (if an inflammatory component is present), and the mixture is injected after the elicitation of paresthesias.

Potential complications of suprascapular injections include: (a) intravascular injection, (b) pneumothorax, and (c) muscle atrophy (26) with associated cosmetic changes of the periscapular area. Intravascular injections may be avoided by meticulous observation of the technique of aspirating after injecting 2-ml increments of the local anesthetic–steroid mixture. If blood is observed, the injection is stopped and a new location is sought, again using paresthesia to the acromion of the shoulder as the endpoint. Pneumothorax can be avoided by flexing the upper extremity on the side of the nerve block at the elbow and placing the hand on the opposite shoulder. This action initiates the elevation and rotation of the scapula from the posterior chest wall and increases the distance from the skin to the chest wall, thus reducing the possibility of pneumothorax (27). Injection of bupivacaine and other local anesthetics may cause localized muscle atrophy, which may result in worrisome cosmetic changes to the periscapular area. While no specific treatment is available or necessary, reassurance of the patient is required since the atrophied muscle usually regenerates in 6 weeks. The suprascapular nerve block facilitates the implementation of progressive physical therapy as part of the rehabilitation protocol of the chronic cervical back pain patient.

## STELLATE GANGLION BLOCK

Thermographic evaluation and clinical experience have demonstrated that some patients with chronic cervical back pain secondary to trauma may develop pain radiating from the posterior neck area to the shoulder area and distally down the corresponding upper extremity. Most of the time this pain radiation pattern is unilateral, but it can infrequently be bilateral. The factors contributing to this development are not clear. Nevertheless, the characteristic hyperpathic pain and the corresponding hypothermic pattern on thermography suggest that the pain may be sympathetically mediated (28). Working on this assumption, patients who demonstrate these symptoms and in whom upper extremity pain is unrelieved by cervical epidural steroid injections may receive a series of stellate ganglion blocks on the same side as the upper extremity pain. It must be emphasized that this approach is utilized in collaboration with the comprehensive management (29) of chronic pain patients with in-depth psychological analysis. In other words, not all patients with upper extremity pain would receive nerve blocks since issues of pain behavior, secondary pain, workers' compensation, Social Security disability, and litigation would have to be evaluated along with the clinical and laboratory evidence (including thermography) of pain.

Like all invasive nerve blocks, strict aseptic precautions are taken during the administration of stellate ganglion blocks. An anterior paratracheal technique (30) is used with the needle directed in a perpendicular direction toward the anterior tubercle of the transverse process of the sixth cervical vertebra (Chassaignac's tubercle). This location is sought by identifying the cricoid cartilage, which is at the same anatomic level as Chassaignac's tubercle. Although the stellate ganglion is in fact located at the level of the seventh cervical vertebra, the block is performed at the level of the sixth cervical vertebra so as to minimize the chances of a pneumothorax since the dome of the parietal pleural membranes lies in close proximity to the stellate ganglion (especially on the right side). Ten milliliters of 0.25% bupivacaine is used in our institution to perform stellate ganglion blocks, and this relatively large volume is used so as to extend caudad to the stellate ganglion along the prevertebral fascia. Thus, this nerve block may be more accurately described as a cervicothoracic sympathetic block rather than a stellate ganglion block, although the latter name is more commonly used. After initial contact with the transverse process, the needle is withdrawn approximately 2 mm and an aspiration test performed to determine if a blood vessel has been punctured. The vertebral artery is the most susceptible vessel, and 1 ml of local anesthetic injected in this vessel could produce dramatic grand mal–type convulsions.

Therefore if any blood is observed in the syringe on aspiration, the needle should be immediately and completely withdrawn and repositioned. It is important to identify the carotid artery prior to performing the block and to retract it laterally.

Signs of a successful stellate ganglion block include ptosis, enophthalmos, and miosis: this is called Horner's syndrome. Other clinical features include anhydrosis, conjuctival hyperemia, unilateral engorgement of the nasal mucosa, hoarseness, and flushing of the skin over the face, neck, upper chest, and upper extremity on the side of the block. Complications of stellate ganglion block (31) include injection into the vertebral artery with immediate convulsions, intradural injection with respiratory and cardiovascular arrest, hematoma of the neck, neuralgia of the chest wall and upper arm, phrenic nerve block, pneumothorax (rare), and osteitis of the transverse process. Bilateral stellate ganglion blocks are never recommended since inadvertent bilateral recurrent laryngeal nerve block may produce loss of laryngeal reflex with airway compromise. No statistics are available to determine the efficacy of stellate ganglion blocks in patients with upper extremity pain radiating from cervical back pain. However, this approach appears logical after thermographic documentation of the sympathetic dysfunction.

## CERVICAL TRIGGER POINT INJECTION

In sports and automobile injuries, cervical pain may occur following sudden cervical hyperextension or "whiplash." The dull aching pain in the back of the head or neck or both is usually musculoskeletal in origin and due to soft tissue injury of ligamentous tissue and muscle. The trapezius (upper segment) is the most commonly involved muscle, although other posterior extensor muscles (splenius capitis, mastoid attachment of sternocleidomastoid, levator scapulae, and scalenus posterior) may be the site of injury (32). These traumatized muscles usually heal over a 1–3-month period, but in some patients chronic pain develops and persists for several years. Physical examination of the occipital region of the head and the posterior neck may reveal tender areas or myofascial trigger points (33) that may be hyperirritable and painful when compressed.

The classical features of a trigger point include (a) positive "jump" sign, (b) skinfold hyperesthesia, (c) increased hyperemia, and (d) palpable nodule. Because this region of the body is partially covered by hair, these features may not always be elicitable. Nevertheless, trigger point injections may be very effective in controlling the pain in these locations. The mechanism of action of trigger point injections, or more fundamentally the pathogenesis of trigger points, is not clear. Travell and Simons (34) have speculated on the pathogenesis of trigger points, but their precise mechanism of producing pain is far from understood. Fine et al. (35) recently demonstrated that the analgesic effects of trigger point injections may be reversed by naloxone. This observation implies that the endogenous opioid system is involved. Lewit (36) also demonstrated that "needling" of trigger areas without local anesthetic injection may produce analgesia. These findings all suggest that the pain relief is not solely due to a local anesthetic effect.

Trigger point injections are performed after appropriate skin cleansing with antiseptic solution (alcohol or Betadine). Two to 3 ml of 0.25% bupivacaine is injected into the trigger area, and 0.5–1.0 ml of 4% methylprednisolone may be added to the local anesthetic in cases in which an inflammatory component is suspected. Pain relief is usually immediate and may persist for a period much longer than the expected duration of the local anesthetic. This procedure may be performed at several sites and is relatively complication free if the clinician adheres to the principle of frequent aspirations (to avoid intravascular injections). Superficial infection, muscle atrophy, and intravascular injections are infrequent complications of trigger point injections.

## OCCIPITAL NERVE BLOCK

In chronic cervical back injuries, residual pain may persist in the more cephalad aspect of the posterior extensor muscles or in the occipital area of the scalp. A greater occipital nerve block may be performed to relieve the associated chronic pain. After skin cleansing with an antiseptic agent, the branches of both the greater and lesser occipital nerves may be blocked by infiltration along the middle third of a line (superior nuchal line) from the mastoid process to the greater occipital protuberance. Five milliliters of 0.25% bupivacaine or equivalent local anesthetic (with or without steroid) is used for this nerve block. An area of analgesia from the occiput to the vertex may result. This nerve block is not associated with major complications other than intravascular injections, which can be avoided by intermittent aspirations while injecting.

## EPIDURAL BLOOD PATCH

Dural puncture, deliberate or inadvertent, may be associated with severe incapacitating headache. Occasionally, the worst pain is not in the head but in the cephalic region of the cervical spine. This pain is usually aggravated by ambulation and relieved by recumbency. If conservative measures fail to relieve the headache, an epidural blood patch (37) may be used to treat the afflicted patient. This procedure is ideally conducted as a two-person technique.

After one assistant has inserted an epidural needle close to the site of dural puncture, the other assistant withdraws about 12 ml of autologous blood from the patient's forearm for injection into the epidural space. Both procedures are conducted using strict aseptic precautions. The blood is injected into the epidural space at a steady rate and pain relief is usually experienced shortly afterward. The mechanism of action of the epidural blood patch is not clear. Several theories (38) have been proposed, including the sealant effect, the mechanical splinting effect of the blood in the epidural space, and a biochemical effect resulting from the injected blood.

## CERVICAL PLEXUS BLOCK

The cervical plexus is formed by connecting branches of the anterior primary rami of the upper four cervical nerves. The plexus consists of a superficial component that innervates the skin over the occipital area of the neck and from the chin to the clavicle. A deep portion of the cervical plexus distributes branches to the cervical vertebral muscles and strap muscles of the neck. The diaphragm is innervated by the fourth cervical nerve (phrenic nerve) and is therefore subjected to paresis if bilateral deep cervical plexus block is performed. Although not commonly utilized, deep cervical plexus block can be used to decrease muscular spasm in the cervical prevertebral muscles and the strap muscles of the neck. These muscles are usually traumatized during neck injuries and may be the site of inflammatory changes secondary to degenerative cervical arthropathy.

Deep cervical plexus block may be performed by using a "single needle" technique at the C4 level with the needle pointed in a medial and slightly caudal direction until contact with the gutter between the anterior and posterior transverse processes is reached. The C4 level is the point at which a horizontal line from the lower border of the mandible (with the head in a neutral position) intersects the vertical line from the mastoid process to Chassaignac's tubercle. Eight milliliters of 1.0% lidocaine or 0.25% bupivacaine is used for the deep cervical plexus block and digital pressure is maintained distally in the interscalene groove with the patient in a horizontal or moderate Trendelenburg position. Complications of this nerve block include intra-arterial (vertebral artery) injection, epidural or subdural injection, phrenic nerve block, and cervical sympathetic chain block.

## ACCESSORY NERVE BLOCK

Accessory nerve block is infrequently performed in everyday pain management. It may be utilized in patients with myofascial pain syndrome that is confined to the trapezius muscle. The accessory nerve is the 11th cranial nerve, and it emerges from the posterior border of the sternocleidomastoid muscle to traverse the posterior triangle of the neck and to enter the trapezius muscle at the junction of the middle and inferior third of its anterior border. The nerve is blocked by introducing a needle at the junction of the superior and middle thirds of the lateral border of the sternocleidomastoid muscle and injecting 10 ml of 0.25% bupivacaine in that area. Accuracy of the block is facilitated by a nerve stimulating device. There are a few complications associated with this procedure and its main indication is for painful spasms of the neck muscles.

## MISCELLANOUS INVASIVE THERAPIES

As a general rule, *neurolytic blocks* are usually reserved for patients with terminal cancer pain. In selected patients who are desperate with severe intractable pain, neurolytic blocks of appropriate peripheral nerves may be performed as a last resort. The nerves selected for these neurolytic blocks should be peripheral in location and consistent in distribution. The suprascapular and occipital nerves are ideally suited for chemical neurolysis in patients with intractable, nonresponsive, cervical muscle pain. Informed consent should be obtained from the patient and the family. As with local anesthetic blocks, strict aseptic precautions must be taken, and radiologic (fluoroscopic) confirmation of correct needle placement is obtained for accuracy and medicolegal considerations. The neurolytic agent used in our institution is 6% phenol in 10% glycerine. However, absolute alcohol may be used, although its administration is associated with intense postblock burning resulting

from alcohol neuritis. *Thermal neurolysis or cryotherapy* of these nerves may be used in certain patient groups using the same principles.

*Acupuncture* (39, 40) should also be considered as an invasive therapy since it involves the introduction of multiple fine needles into the skin through specific points. The needles may be left in place, twirled for varying intervals, or electrically stimulated (electroacupuncture). This technique is indigenous to Chinese medicine and is frequently misused or abused in Western medical practice. However, in skilled hands and with appropriate subjects it can be used for chronic cervical back pain. Although the mechanism of action of acupuncture is not well understood, it is believed to be a form of hyperstimulation analgesia (41). The current increase in the prevalence of AIDS mandates that, where reusable needles are employed, practitioners of acupuncture impose strict techniques for resterilization of needles. This serves not only to avoid spread of the HIV virus from patient to patient but also to prevent contamination of medical and nursing personnel.

Ever since the publication of the gate control theory by Melzack and Wall (42) in 1965, a variety of nerve stimulation techniques have evolved for treating chronic intractable pain. This development coincided with the disillusionment with contemporary neurosurgical techniques (cordotomy, rhizotomy, neurectomy, tractotomy) available for treating chronic pain at that time. Research and clinical experience gained from using transcutaneous electrical stimulation in stimulating peripheral nerves led to the practice of electrical stimulation of the spinal cord. The technique used to stimulate the spinal cord may be implemented via laminectomy or with percutaneously inserted epidural electrodes. The electrode implantation is usually temporary and the site of implantation variable depending on the etiology of the pain syndrome. Proper patient selection for these techniques is crucial if satisfactory results are to be optimized. Patients with major psychological or psychiatric problems (43) should be excluded from treatment with this modality.

*Dorsal column stimulation* has gained some popularity as an alternative modality for treating difficult chronic pain patients, but in general its long-term efficacy is still undetermined (44). Dorsal column stimulation is associated with a variety of complications that include intermittent or irregular stimulation (secondary to electrical leakage), radicular dysesthesia, and infection. The application of dorsal column stimulation for chronic cervical back pain is limited because inadvertent stimulation of C4 (phrenic nerve) may result in undesirable side effects (45). Most of the clinical experience gained in the use of this technique has been from the management of lower thoracic and lumbar pain syndromes. The general consensus for the most effective use of dorsal column stimulation is to restrict its use to patients with localized pain and in whom there is no major psychological, behavioral, or psychiatric dysfunction. Further, the device should have multipolar electrodes and should be placed percutaneously in the epidural space above the dermatomal pain segments (46). Successful placement is usually assured if stimulation of the region produces paresthesia in the painful segments without radicular irritation.

*Deep brain stimulation* is a modality of pain management reserved for patients with intractable, unremitting pain who have relatively normal psychological profiles and for whom none of the conventional modalities of pain management has provided satisfactory pain relief. Thus, patient selection is probably more crucial than in dorsal column stimulation in order to optimize efficacy. The technique of deep brain stimulation is not new. It was first reported by Heath (47) in 1954, and since then several reports have addressed its possible clinical usefulness for treatment of intractable chronic pain patients (48–50). Its invasiveness and potential for major complications have restricted widespread application, however, and the advent of other techniques for treating chronic pain patients has further restricted its use. Research in specific target areas of the brain for stimulation is currently being conducted (51) in several centers around the world, and it is possible that more information may provide a better understanding of the specific application of this modality.

Some patients with chronic cervical back pain associated with brachial plexus avulsion have benefited from periaqueductal-periventricular stimulation of the brain (52), which is based on the hypothesis that the stimulation utilizes the endogenous opioid mechanism. More specifically, some of these patients have been reported to obtain significant pain relief from the stimulation of the thalamic sensory relay nuclei (the ventralis posteromedialis) and the internal capsule. As neurologic stereotactic techniques improve, procedures such as deep brain stimulation may become more routine and more effective for selected chronic pain management. At the present time there are unacceptable complications (53) associated with the procedure, including electrode mal-

function, meningitis, encephalitis, hemiparesis, motor dysfunction, abnormal eye movements, intracerebral hemorrhage, and intraventricular hemorrhage. The future may be bright for this modality of pain management if current research trends continue.

There are a variety of conventional *surgical procedures* that have been used to treat chronic cervical pain syndromes. The most common of these procedures include cervical laminectomy and cervical cordotomy (54). As surgical techniques have been reevaluated and the relationships between postoperative pain relief and laminectomy have been reexamined, it has become obvious that criteria for all back surgery (including cervical laminectomy) must be redefined. The newer diagnostic techniques such as magnetic resonance imaging, the metrizamide-enhanced computed tomography scan, and bone scanning have provided sharper definitions of the vertebral column in relation to the contiguous structures. These techniques may contribute to decreasing unnecessary surgery and speed up the process when surgery is indicated. However, caution is still required and the multidisciplinary evaluation of the patient is still a good way, if not the best way, to manage the chronic cervical pain patient.

## CONCLUSION

Several nerve block techniques have been described that may be useful in managing the chronic cervical pain patient. Since the typical patient with traumatic cervical pain is young and is expected to have a long, productive life, the need for irreversible invasive techniques is very restricted. The intense flurry of research activity in pain management both in the United States and abroad may revolutionize the currently available techniques for pain management. With the discovery of newer pharmacologic agents, older techniques may be rejuvenated and principles of pain management enhanced. The future does indeed look bright for progress to be made in the management of chronic pain in general and chronic cervical pain in particular.

## REFERENCES

1. Abenhaim L, Siussa S, Rossignol M: Risk of recurrence of occupational back pain over a three-year follow-up. *Br J Ind Med* 45:829–833, 1988.
2. Parris WCV: Nerve block therapy. In Brena SF, Chapman SL (eds): *Chronic Pain: Management Principles. Clinics in Anesthesiology.* Philadelphia, WB Saunders, 1985, pp 93–109.
3. Graham DT: Prediction of fainting in blood donors. *Circulation* 23:901–906, 1961.
4. Sanders SH: Component analysis of a behavioral treatment

program for chronic low back pain. *Behav Ther* 14:697s–705, 1983.

5. Kepes ER, Duncalf D: Treatment of back ache with spinal injections of local anesthetics, spinal and systemic steroids. A review. *Pain* 22:23–47, 1985.

6. Warfield CA, Biber MP, Crews DA, Gwarakanath GK: Epidural steroid injections as a treatment for cervical radiculitis. *Clin J Pain* 4:201–204, 1988.

7. Rowlingson JC, Kirschenbaum LP: Epidural analgesic techniques in the management of cervical pain. *Anesth Analg* 65:938–942, 1986.

8. Bromage PR: Complications and contraindications. In: *Epidural Analgesia*. Philadelphia, WB Saunders, 1978, pp 13–15, 469–471.

9. Purkis IE: Cervical epidural steroids. *Pain Clinic* 1:3–7, 1986.

10. Jackson R: *The Cervical Syndrome*, ed 2. Springfield, IL, Charles C Thomas, 1958.

11. Cousins MJ, Bromage PR: Epidural neural blockade. In Cousins MJ, Bridenbaugh PO (eds): *Neural Blockade*. Philadelphia, JB Lippincott, 1988, pp 253–360.

12. Dawkins CJM: An analysis of the complications of extradural and cordal block. *Anaesthesia* 24:554–563, 1969.

13. Winnie AP, Hartman JJ, Meyers HL Jr, Ramamurthy S, Barangan V: Pain clinic: intradural and extradural corticosteroids for sciatica. *Anesth Analg* 51:990, 1972.

14. Knight CL, Burnell JC: Systemic side effects of extradural steroids. *Anaesthesia* 30(5):593–594, 1980.

15. Cuckler JM, Bernini P, Wiesel S, Booth R, Rothman R, Pickens G: The use of epidural steroids in the treatment of lumbar radicular pain. *J Bone Joint Surg [Am]* 67:63, 1985.

16. Rosen CD, Kahanovitz N, Bernstein R, Viola K: A retrospective analysis of the efficacy of epidural steroid injections. *Clin Orthop* 228:270–272, 1988.

17. Sekel R: Epidural depo-medrol revisited. *Med J Aust* 4:688–693, 1984.

18. Dilke TEW, Burry HC, Graham MER: Extradural corticosteroid injection in the management of lumbar root compression. *Br Med J* 2:635–637, 1973.

19. Dirksen R, Rutgers MJ, Coolen JM: Cervical epidural steroids can reflect sympathetic dystrophy. *Anesthesiology* 66:71–73, 1987.

20. Duncan GE, Stumpf WE: Target neurons for (3)H-corticosterone in the rat spinal cord. *Brain Res* 307:321–326, 1984.

21. Waldman SD: Complications of epidural cervical nerve blocks with steroids: a prospective study of 790 consecutive blocks. *Reg Anaesth* 14:149–151, 1989.

22. Cronen MC, Waldman SD: Cervical epidural steroid nerve block in the palliation of pain secondary to intractable muscle contraction headache (abstract). *Headache* 28:314–315, 1988.

23. Waldman SD, Feldstein GS, Allen ML: Cervical epidural blood patch for treatment for cervical dural puncture headache. *Anesthesiol Rev* 14:23–25, 1987.

24. Nelson DA, Vates TS, Thomas RB: Complications from intrathecal steroid therapy in patients with multiple sclerosis. *Acta Neurol Scand* 49:176–188, 1973.

25. Usubiaga JE: Neurologic complications following epidural anesthesia. *Int Anesthesiol Clin* 13:2, 1975.

26. Parris WCV, Dettbarn WD: Muscle atrophy following bupivacaine trigger point injection. *Anesthesiol Rev* 16(3):50–53, 1988.

27. Parris WCV: Suprascapular nerve block: a safer technique. *Anesthesiology* 72:580–581, 1990.

28. Pochaczevsky R: Liquid crystal thermography of the spine and extremities. *J Neurosurg* 56:386–395, 1982.

29. Brena SF, Chapman SL: Chronic pain: a logarithm for management. *Postgrad Med* 72:111–117, 1982.

30. Moore DC: In: *Regional Block*. Springfield, IL, Charles C Thomas, 1967.

31. Bonica JJ: *The Management of Pain*. Philadelphia, Lea & Febiger, 1953.

32. Travell J, Rinzler SH: The myofascial genesis of pain. *Postgrad Med* 11:425–434, 1952.

33. Weinberger LM: Traumatic fibromyositis: a critical review of an enigmatic concept. *West J Med* 127:99–103, 1977.

34. Travell JG, Simons DG: *Myofascial Pain and Dysfunction. The Trigger Point Manual*. Baltimore, William & Wilkins, 1984.

35. Fine PG, Milno R, Hare BD: The effects of myofascial trigger point injections are naloxone reversible. *Pain* 32:15–20, 1988.

36. Lewit K: The needle effect in relief of myofascial pain. *Pain* 6:83–90, 1979.

37. Crawford JS: Experiences with epidural blood patch. *Anaesthesia* 35:513–521, 1980.

38. Szeinfeld M, Ihmeidan IH, Moser MM, Machado R, Klose KJ, Serafini AN: Epidural blood patch: evaluation of the volume and spread of blood injected into the epidural space. *Anesthesiology* 64:820–822, 1986.

39. Melzack R, Stillwell DM, Fox EJ: Trigger points and acupuncture for pain. Correlations and implications. *Pain* 3:3–23, 1977.

40. Nathan PW: Acupuncture analgesia. *Trends in Neurosciences* July, pp 21–23, 1978.

41. Soper WY, Melzack R: Stimulation produced analgesia: evidence for somatotopic organization in the mid-brain. *Brain Res* 251:301–311, 1982.

42. Melzack R, Wall PD: Pain mechanism: a new theory. *Science* 150:971–979, 1965.

43. Long DM, Erickson D, Campbell J, North R: Electrical stimulation of the spinal cord and peripheral nerves for pain control—ten years experience. *Appl Neurophysiol* 44:207–217, 1981.

44. Pineda A: Dorsal column stimulation and its prospects. *Surg Neurol* 4:157–163, 1975.

45. Krainick JU, Thorden U, Strassburg HM, Wenzel D: The effects of electrical spinal cord stimulation on spastic movement disorders. *Adv Neurosurg* 4:257–260, 1977.

46. Krainick J, Thorden U, Riechert T: Pain reduction in amputees by long-term spinal cord stimulation. *J Neurosurg* 52:346–350, 1980.

47. Heath RG: *Studies in Schizophrenia*. Cambridge, MA, Harvard University Press, 1954.

48. Pool JL, Clark WD, Hudson P, Lombardo M: *Hypothalamic-Hypophyseal Interrelationships*. Springfield, IL, Charles C Thomas, 1956.

49. Gol A: Relief of pain by electrical stimulation of the septal area. *J Neurosurg Sci* 5:115–120, 1967.

50. Ervin FR, Brown CE, Mark VH: Striatal influence on facial pain. *Confinia Neurologia* 27:75–86, 1966.

51. Gerhart KD, Yezierski RP, Fang VR, et al: Inhibition of primate spinothalamic tract neurons by stimulation in ventral posterior lateral (VPL) thalamic nucleus: possible mechanisms. *J Neurophysiol* 49:406–423, 1983.

52. Plotkin R: Results in 60 cases of deep brain stimulation for chronic intractable pain. *Appl Neurophysiol* 45:173–178, 1982.

53. Hosobuchi Y: Subcortical electrical stimulation for control of intractable pain in humans. *J Neurosurg* 64:543–553, 1986.

54. Rosomoff HL, Carroll F, Brown J, Sheptac P: Cordotomy: technique. *J Neurosurg* 23:639–644, 1965.

# 11

# BIOFEEDBACK AND RELAXATION THERAPIES

*Barry A. Reich*

## BIOFEEDBACK THERAPIES

> A sensation of feeling always becomes conscious when the sensorium commune is attentive to it.
>
> Johannes Muller (1)

In the mid-sixties a new era in the field of physiologic control was born—"biofeedback." According to Birk (2) the term "feedback" was coined by the mathematician Norbert Weiner and concisely defined by him as "a method of controlling the system by reinserting into it the results of its past performance." Biofeedback is a process in which the "system" is biologic and where the feedback is mediated by a man-made detection device. The signal is amplified and displayed on instruments rather than being present as an inborn feedback loop inherent in the organism.

Biofeedback is presently accepted as a fundamental learning system in which an individual learns to make certain responses upon receiving immediate information (feedback) regarding his own physiologic processes. By making a correct response or successively approximating the correct response over a series of trials (treatments), the individual is moved closer to his goal (physiologic control). By analogy, an individual using biofeedback equipment is like a dart thrower aiming at a target and able to see immediately if he has over or underthrown the target, versus the dart thrower who is blindfolded and given no visual or auditory information about his throw. Assuming an equal initial competency level, it becomes easy to reason that the thrower with feedback about each attempt at the target will probably be more successful. We may therefore assume that being able to discriminate a physiologic occurrence can enhance or maximize one's ability to learn control over that occurrence. However, for control to be obtained the physiologic event must be available to "conscious control." Second, the control must be discriminable so that the individual is ultimately able to reproduce and emit the established control without being constantly monitored by a biofeedback device during his usual daily activities.

Biofeedback offers the individual the ability to discriminate information that is normally at a level unavailable to the senses. Biofeedback becomes a "window" to view our own physiology and thus, supplied with this information, effect and influence voluntary control over the physiology. By becoming aware of the previously undetectable physiologic fluctuations the patient being taught biofeedback training can establish a regulatory repertoire to permit harmony of mind and body. It is this recital of learned experience that is used to restore the individual's optimal homeostatic function. It is interesting to note that after many individuals have learned the biofeedback process necessary to establish physiologic regulation, continued conscious application of the process may become unnecessary to maintain the regulation (3–6). It is as if what was once a conscious act becomes over time a reflexive homeostatic equilibrium activity.

According to Furedy and Riley (7) we may consider narrowing the term "biofeedback" to be applicable in behavioral medicine "only if it is the contingent signal ('feedback') from a biological function that has led to the increase in control of

144

that function." Biofeedback, like any learning situation, appears to be regulated by individual differences such as motivation, difficulty of task, amount of time spent on learning the skill, massed versus spaced practice, and optimizing the learning environment. Marinacci and Horande (8) stated that "repeated trials and patience on the part of both examiner and patient are essential in obtaining the best result."

Biofeedback is a process that addresses a combination of physiologic and psychological concepts. Not only does it give the individual the accessibility to learn applied physiologic control, but it also offers the individual the suggestion and perception of control over bodily function. It has been demonstrated by Bandura (9) and Holroyd (10), among others, that when individuals have an expectation or belief that they can control or influence a course of events (the cause of their pain), they will demonstrate increased persistence and effort. This persistence increases the chances of successful biofeedback learning and intervention. The concept of belief in an internal locus of control, "self-efficacy," and enhanced outcome expectation allows the patient to view himself less as a victim of discomfort but more as the captain of his fate. In essence, being able to reduce one's negative expectations about pain and discomfort allows for a reduction in sympathetic and parasympathetic nervous system arousal. Flor et al. (11) studied the reduction of pain as reported by rheumatology patients receiving a number of different treatments. Those patients who were in the biofeedback treatment condition reported a perceived ability to "control the pain" and thus the authors gave a major weighting to the contribution of the psychological factors at work within the biofeedback training paradigm.

There are two types of reaction to pain, the physical and the psychological. Each can be a primary effect or a contributing effect in terms of expression and continuation of a patient's reported pain. Obviously direct injury to soft tissue or to nerves causes involuntary recruitment of surrounding processes. As a patient experiences pain and discomfort an associated involuntary pain-tension-pain cycle usually evolves. This cycle may cause pain in addition to that caused by the original trauma. For example, increased muscle tonicity becomes evident not only in the region of trauma but, for many patients, in the surrounding musculature as well. The resultant excessive sympathetic nervous system activity contributes to overall generalized muscle tension. In addition, generalized muscular tension is usually positively correlated with psychological stress. The patient's prior experience with pain and present state of psychological well-being can often be observed as symptom correlates. Thus to successfully intervene in the pain process experienced by a patient, a procedure that can address the two areas would be most efficacious. Biofeedback lends itself to this use. Nouwen and Solinger (12) have proffered that patients may change attitudes toward pain as a result of biofeedback training. Providing the patient does not gain secondarily from continued pain or the expression thereof, the reduction in autonomic nervous system arousal mediated by direct and indirect control is perceived as a psychological calming and is also experienced in conjunction with a reduction in associated muscle tension activity.

## BIOFEEDBACK THERAPY FOR CERVICAL PAIN

Biofeedback becomes a treatment of choice when cervical pain can be ascribed to the following conditions: psychological stress disorder (e.g., idiopathic/psychogenic torticollis), skeletal muscle dysfunction (e.g., cervical sprain), tissue ischemia, or a combination of these etiologies (e.g., cervical myofascial syndrome) (13, 14). Additionally, since neurogenic pain usually involves skeletal muscle dysfunction secondarily, such an etiology also lends itself to intervention via biofeedback methodology. Biofeedback can also be successfully utilized as an intervention modality when specific muscle training is believed to be beneficial, as well as when stress management or reduction of overall tension level is sought. Additionally, electromyographic (EMG) biofeedback has been demonstrated to result in a decrease of plasma adrenocorticotropic hormone and to enhance production of $\beta$-endorphins (15).

Since the word "trauma" pertains to a physical/psychic insult or injury, biofeedback and relaxation therapy become applicable as posttraumatic treatments when we view the patient's symptomatology within the following framework. After a patient has received a physical trauma to the head, neck, shoulder, or thoracic region it is not unusual for muscle and/or neurogenic-type pain to persist with a constellation of symptoms and distress that is relatively consistent in description by patients. Cervical spine injuries have been noted to account for the most frequent of all spine traumas (16). Extreme or sudden unexpected cervical flexion-elongation, hyperextension, rotation, compression, and/or axial loading occurring alone or in tandem can produce severe discomfort. Localized tenderness of the neck, stiffness, stabbing or sharp pain upon rotation, extension, and flexion, dull ache at rest, and warm throbbing-type pain have all been identified with frequency by the posttraumatic patient.

The cervical trauma may produce sensations that are experienced in regions away from the neck (e.g., cephalic, otologic, ocular, radicular, cerviobrachialgic). The symptoms, while generally limited to those described above, have the capacity to run the gamut from minor to incapacitating depending upon the extent of the precipitating insult and the degree to which the patient's own internal mechanisms express the pain perception. Saper (17) noted that even minor cervical trauma "can bring about the development of a set of characteristic symptoms, with striking consistency from patient to patient, but varying greatly in intensity and extent to which they cause disability." It is unusual when physical trauma to the neck does not result in some pain, which is often persistent in spite of an occasional absence of demonstrable physiologic pathology. In addition, the posttrauma period can often be associated with psychological symptoms. These may include personality changes, emotional lability, irritability, increased fatigue, hyper/hyposomnia, and depression.

Following a cervical trauma the symptoms expressed are usually due to (a) abnormality of muscle(s) tonus (including, but not limited to, spasm, irritability, and recruitment); (b) injury to the cervical plexus: the great auricular nerve, the anterior cervical cutaneous nerve, the lesser occipital nerve, and the supraclavicular nerve; (c) associated tissue ischemia; and (d) psychological stress reaction. de Vries (18), Bonica (personal communication, 1988), Mense and Stahnke (19), Travell and Simons (20), Lance (21), and Jackson (22) have all pointed out the importance of including the concepts of ischemia and vasoconstriction as contributing to musculoskeletal pain. In this case the contracting muscle(s) may act in a manner to compress the intramuscular blood vessels, shunting the blood flow. At the same time the contracted muscle increases the rate of metabolism, putting additional demands upon the oxygenated blood supply. The intramuscular blood flow being restricted by muscle contraction is unable to respond to the circulatory demand and pain increases. The greater the metabolism of the muscle

tissue (e.g., tonus level) the more the pain increases. The accumulation of algogenic chemicals released in situ (e.g., bradykinin, histamine, potassium, prostaglandin, and lactic acid) is generally at a rate proportional to the experienced pain (23–25).

## BIOFEEDBACK TRAINING PROCESS

With the biofeedback process the emphasis is placed upon the patient inasmuch as biofeedback depends upon the concept of self-regulation. The practitioner or clinician becomes the tutor, the catalyst, the lubricant that assists the patient toward rehabilitation and a state of physiologic, and occasionally psychological, equilibrium. The patient himself becomes the active or primary component in the rehabilitation process. Biofeedback becomes a part of the patient's armamentarium that can be used without fear of addiction, tolerance, or withdrawal. It is never temporarily out of stock at the pharmacy. Once trained, wherever the patient goes he takes his biofeedback knowledge with him; it cannot be forgotten at home. However, the patient must be trained via a method that will maximize the biofeedback learning to generalize outside the training venue.

A person generally does not first learn to drive a car on a crowded interstate expressway. Initially the novice driver is proctored on a quiet side street or a deserted parking lot. The driver then moves on to busier streets and avenues as his confidence builds. Finally, as his experience and skill permit, the driver becomes eager to tackle the interstates, bound only by his fuel tank and the horizon. Likewise, in biofeedback training the patient is best guided via a system of successive approximations. This stepwise learning has as its goal specific learned physiologic control. Goals for each session become more demanding to complete. A graduated set of tasks and performance criteria should be arranged to ensure continuous progress and retention of skills. Situations are varied during the training to maximize the learning and the generalization of the learned skills. For example, in EMG biofeedback training body positions must be varied to maximize the applicability of the learned control to the actual daily activities undertaken by the patient. Simply teaching the patient to relax a specific muscle while in an optimal nondemanding environment and in a static position has little practicality or relevance to the person's actual daily environment with its specific demands. Within the training paradigm the clinician should become less involved over time so that the patient can perceive the success obtained as reinforcing a sense of personal efficacy.

During the training process it is important to assess the physiologic baseline that the patient presents upon starting each session. The EMG levels at the start of each session become valuable indicators of sustained learning and ultimate success, for it is the sustained and maintained physiologic control between training sessions that indicates application of the learned behaviors to the patient's everyday activity schedule without disruptive tonus dysfunction.

While Peck and Kraft (25) found that continual practice was necessary to maintain pain reduction via EMG training, recent comprehensive and longitudinal studies have shown otherwise (3, 6, 26). It is desirable that the skills and physiologic state obtained via the specific biofeedback training protocol become a natural, automatic, reflexive component of the patient's physiologic repertoire. Although it is necessary for a patient to practice at home during the beginning of physiologic skills acquisition, many pain patients have demonstrated that the learned control often becomes part of the natural homeostasis of the individual without continued practice. Successful patients indicated pain reduction 5 years after being discharged from active treatment, with only 14% of these patients indicating the continued daily practice of biofeedback learning (3, 26). Basmajian (27) has also related the ability of subjects to display conscious motor unit control in the absence of continued visual or auditory feedback and without the necessity of daily practice.

Hudzinsky and Levenson (28) found that the variables of sex, number of sessions attended, age at time of treatment/program participation, and "locus of control" significantly affected outcome measures of success. Others have found that the ability of the individual to become a consummate learner of muscle control via EMG biofeedback protocols does not seem influenced by age, race, sex, socioeconomic status, education level, IQ, or manual skill (26, 27). In a 5-year longitudinal study on over 1000 pain patients Reich (26) found that the specific variables providing the best prediction of success with biofeedback training were (a) how long the underlying physical pathology had been present without successful intervention prior to initiating biofeedback, and (b) the number of biofeedback training sessions attended by the patient. Other researchers have also noted that the number of training sessions given/at-

tended is correlated with the pain relief obtained and maintained by the patient (8, 29). Basmajian (5) indicated that a high presenting level of nervousness in the patient may negatively affect a successful outcome.

Earlier it was mentioned that tension can manifest itself as additional physiologic dysfunction. Ferraccioli et al. (15) indicated that fibromyalgia patients who presented with depression and/or overt psychosomatic background were less likely to report a reduction of pain obtained via EMG biofeedback than similarly diagnosed pain patients without any noted psychological disturbance. This result held steady under conditions of "true" versus contrived EMG readings. The patients who were not depressed and who learned control in the "true" biofeedback condition revealed the most significant improvement. However, Stilson et al. (30) indicated that no differences were noted in the success rate of EMG training for normal subjects versus psychiatric subjects in the learning of conscious muscle tonus control.

After the practitioner has evaluated the patient and determined that biofeedback training is appropriate in the rehabilitation process, a treatment strategy should be planned. The treatment strategy should contain detailed protocols outlining the specific methods and goals for the individual patient. Knowledge of the patient's occupation and daily activity profile must be incorporated into the treatment protocol. It is this knowledge that permits the skilled clinician to develop a training procedure that will allow for biofeedback control of muscle activities involved in the patient's daily regimen to be approximated and learned in an efficacious manner.

With the advent of newer sophisticated computerized biofeedback equipment, detailed records indicating success within and between sessions can be easily kept and analyzed. Adjustments to threshold levels and degrees of difficulty can be modified to maximize the successful physiologic skills acquisition of the patient. It must be understood that the acute or chronic pain patient generally has a lowered threshold of frustration. Since biofeedback is a learning procedure that requires the active participation of the patient it is necessary to make the initial training tasks easy. The clinician must be sensitive to the individual's ability to learn so as not to increase the patient's frustration and thus ensure failure. "Self-efficacy" as described by Bandura (9) plays a most important role in the biofeedback process and appears to permit a system of internal reward that allows for enhanced and more rapid acquisition of learned physiologic control. The learning situation must allow the patient to feel that some control in the perception of pain can be obtained. As change in the targeted physiologic response becomes effected by the patient, the internal cognitive components become more significant in the continuance, precision, and generalizability of the response (7).

## ELECTROMYOGRAPHIC BIOFEEDBACK

Modern EMG usage may be traced back to the 1940s, at which time the procedure was recognized as a tool for research and rehabilitation within the field of physical medicine. Marinacci (31) and Hefferline (32) reported that subjects were capable of utilizing feedback displays of motor unit activity to produce changes in a predetermined direction. Harrison and Mortensen (33) measured isolated activity of motor units in the tibialis muscle with surface electrode EMG and noted that individuals were able to maintain such activity on command. Thus EMG was utilized as a feedback modality allowing the subjects upon volition to increase the frequency and amplitude of motor units. Since the early 1960s independent research by Basmajian et al. (34, 35), Booker et al. (36), Brudny et al. (37), Stoyva and Budzynsky (38), Johnson and Garton (39), Miller (40), Herman (41), and Surwit and Keefe (42) has demonstrated the efficaciousness of application of EMG biofeedback for neuromuscular rehabilitation. However, for biofeedback to yield the desired results the patient must be able to balance motivation with passivity, for the more a patient "tries" to produce a desired neuromuscular response the more he may prevent himself from obtaining the goal by generating excessive sympathetic muscle tension in his attempts. "Straining or pushing" a response often creates additional muscle activation or acts in a manner that does not allow for complementary muscle groups to compensate for a dystonic condition. It is the process of "allowing" or "cognitively willing and believing" in the desired motor function that more often yields the intended activation or relaxation of the targeted muscle. Breznitz (43) intimated that without hope there is no life. In biofeedback training, without belief there is little possibility of change. Davidson and Schwartz (44) stated that if both psychological and physiologic relaxation are present the resulting relaxation achieved will be more pronounced.

Rather than try to ferret out the individual contributions of the physiology-psychology dichotomy, we must view the process as inherently "contaminated" and accept that biofeedback therapy combines both in a complementary fashion.

Early research paradigms generally were concentrated around the concept that training in one muscle group (typically the frontalis) would generalize within the individual and be experienced as a lowered level of stimulation throughout the entire physiology (38). As the field became more advanced in studying the physiologic response it was shown that such generalization does not seem to be the case. A lowering of the tonus in the frontalis muscle does not appear to be correlated with a lowering of the individual's overall level of physiologic activation (45–49). Shedivy and Kleinman (50) demonstrated that various nuchal muscles and the frontalis muscle would vary independently of each other, although a trend was noted. The researchers found that the sternocleidomastoid and semispinalis/splenius muscles were not significantly influenced by increasing or decreasing the tonus in the frontalis. Fridlund et al. (47) found no generalization from training in the frontalis muscle to the nuchal muscles or muscles in the forearm or leg regions. Shedivy and Kleinman specifically picked the nuchal muscles because of their role in torticollis and muscle contraction headache. Learned control is usually experienced only in the specific muscle(s) successfully trained (50, 51). Yet this control may be plentiful, as Kato and Tanji (52) demonstrated with the ability of subjects to learn the isolated control of greater than 286 motor units, producing volitional contraction without the incorporation of any neighboring units.

Information reported by Ladd et al. (53) indicates that single motor unit inhibition relies upon a learned response that may generalize across muscles, but voluntary contraction responses are specific to the skeletal muscle involved. Training involuntary contraction in a muscle does not lessen the time or trials required for training associated muscles or those located in areas orthogonal to the training. Thus successful use of biofeedback therapy can be a laborious undertaking if paretic and spastic conditions exist along with involvement of extensive synergistic and oppositional muscle groups. However, since Budzinsky and Stoyva (54) stated that EMG biofeedback could hasten and enhance the learning of muscle relaxation, the relevance of this technique has become recognized in the field of tonic rehabilitation. Qualls and Sheehan (55), in an extensive review of the literature, stated that "from the evidence reviewed so far, it is clear that the efficacy of EMG biofeedback as a technique for reducing levels of tension in the target muscle is well documented."

## Background Knowledge for the Practitioner

A good working knowledge of muscle anatomy, physiology, and kinesthesiology is a must for the successful biofeedback practitioner. For example, recent research (56–58) has indicated that muscle temperature may affect the readings obtained via EMG biofeedback. In addition, it has been pointed out by Hellebrandt et al. (59) that there is a "reflex positioning" of the head as the upper limbs are being used, and Basmajian (60) pointed out that the neck is constantly affected by any muscle action or stress in the upper limb. Because pain can often create a guarded posture, the resultant poor posture creates EMG readings that must be interpreted by the clinician. An elevated reading may indicate postural difficulties and may not indicate the existence of a spasm condition. Often positioning the patient in a corrected alignment is all that is necessary to observe normal testing EMG levels in the specific muscle being measured. Middaugh and Kee (61) have demonstrated that for patients with low back pain an "elevated EMG during quiet standing most often represents inappropriate muscle use rather than muscle spasm." In such cases biofeedback may be utilized to assist the patient in learning appropriate postural dynamics, assisting in the overall physical rehabilitation of the patient. It is of note that Reich (62) did not find elevated EMG tonus in the nuchal regions of cervical pain patients to be due to simple postural positioning; rather, he found that it was generally attributable to objective muscle hyperactivity following use.

In addition, an awareness of associated physiologic concepts is complementary to the EMG biofeedback clinician's background. These concepts include those proffered by Travell and Rinzler (63) indicating that referred pain patterns and trigger points can arise from deep muscle and ligaments within the body. For example, bilateral frontal headache and postural dizziness are often sequelae of injury to the clavicular division of the sternocleidomastoid. McNab (64) as well as Travell and Simons (20) have postulated that ulnar distribution parethesia may be a direct result of

spasm in the scalene muscles. Graff-Radford et al. (65) demonstrated chronic headache as a referred pain originating in the upper trapezius, sterocleidomastoid, splenii, and suboccipital muscles. Occipital headaches are a common symptom following cervical trauma and may include the vertex and temporal regions. The knowledge of referred pain patterns assists the biofeedback clinician to identify muscles of importance.

It must be clearly understood that an individual muscle rarely acts in an independent manner but generally reflects functional group activity. As discussed by Middaugh and Kee (61), it is one's knowledge of the complex motor patterns involving multiple muscle groups that permits the practitioner to approach and to successfully administer EMG biofeedback training.

## Reliability of EMG Readings

The literature to date offers many contradictory studies indicating the presence of abnormal EMG readings appearing with consistency in patients who present with musculoskeletal pain. Jette et al. (66) did not measure any abnormal spontaneous resting myoelectric activity in the upper trapezius muscles of subjects who stated they were experiencing severe neck pain. Research by Bush et al. (67) indicated that musculoskeletal pain patients who also presented abnormal EMG levels were the exception rather than the rule. Yet, Nouwen (68) indicated evidence of EMG levels in the muscles of pain subjects. Pozniak-Patewicz (69) found that 96% of "cephalic pain" subjects consistently demonstrated significant elevation of electrical activity in neck muscles during a pain episode. In addition, this study found that the amplitude of elevation varied by sex: Female subjects displayed action potentials that were three times higher than those for males ($p = .001$). The author found no association for age and electrical activity. Hudzinski and Lawrence (70) not only found elevated EMG tonus levels for pain patients but also found significant age correlations. Their research included observed tonus levels in the masseter, sternocleidomastoid, and second cervical muscle regions. To further complicate the picture, Peck and Kraft (25) found that EMG tonus reduction may be learned via biofeedback training and yet not be correlated with any reduction in reported pain.

Recent research at our facility at the Nassau Pain and Stress Center as well as independent investigations by Ahern et al. (71), Miller (72),

Cohen et al. (73), and Middaugh and Kee (61) indicate that it is inappropriate to use baseline, static EMG readings as a sole index of muscle pathology for musculoskeletal pain patients. Based upon research on over 1000 cervical and low back pain patients, Reich (62) found that a significant difference could be observed in most pain patients versus the "normal" population when readings taken before and after functional activity were compared. A significant nonvoluntary sustained elevation of muscle tonus levels can be observed in pain patients following even minimal activity and/or movement. This delayed return to resting potentials is usually not observed in the "normal" no-pain group. This difference was often observed even when the static baseline EMG levels indicated no difference. Ahern et al. (71) found that static posture absolute EMG levels were nondiscriminant. The researchers noted significant differences when observing dynamic movement EMG levels. These readings clearly discriminated between chronic low back pain patients and nonpatient controls.

In a 1989 study by Arena et al. (74) EMG levels were measured employing a number of different postural positions. A consistent and reliable pattern of surface paraspinal EMG levels was noted by the researchers. The readings proved to be diagnostically discriminant for five different types of low back pain patients versus a control group. Results by Middaugh and Garwood (75) demonstrated that while only 65% of cervical pain patients revealed elevated EMG tonus levels during quiet sitting baseline measurements, approximately 90% of cervical pain patients revealed abnormal EMG levels when tested following repeated movement activity. Reich (62) found that only 20% of cervical myofascial pain patients demonstrated a significant elevation of surface EMG activity in nuchal region muscles at resting baseline, whereas only 4% of a control nonpain population evidenced the same elevation. However, when this same observation was made after a test maneuver consisting of 15 minutes of isometric exercise of the cervical spine, 97.2% of the pain population presented with significant elevation and irritability. Sustained abnormal elevation was observed in only 5.5% of the nonpain population following the same exercise routine. These observations were noted for the trapezius and sternocleidomastoid muscle groups as measured by surface electrode EMG. Such findings clearly indicate the necessity for including functional activity as part of the biofeedback protocol.

It is interesting to note that Simons (13) has identified the upper trapezius and sternocleidomastoid muscles as being frequently responsible for a referred pain pattern in patients presenting with myofascial pain syndromes. Bentgtsson et al. (76) noted that the trapezius muscle is often involved in patients complaining of muscle pain related to primary fibromyalgia. In addition, Bischoff and Traue (77) have demonstrated that myogenic headache can result from tonic abnormalities consisting of phasic dysfunction, such as muscular hyperirritability to certain stimuli and a delay in the recovery periods following muscular exertion of the neck muscles. These headaches were often correlated with limited ability to turn the head. Haynes et al. (78) found that for subjects indicating muscle contraction headache, cervical EMG and frontalis EMG readings were not significantly different at rest. However, when presented with a stressor during a headache, a significantly greater number of subjects evidenced elevated cervical readings but not frontalis readings.

Thus the measurement of EMG activity during initial baseline for musculoskeletal pain patients should not consist solely of individual static readings but must involve a number of criteria to assess appropriateness of biofeedback as a training intervention.

## Developing EMG Biofeedback Protocols

It is generally accepted that individuals who have experienced cervical trauma exhibit EMG levels that are either elevated, asymmetric, and/or hyperirritable, when compared to individuals who have not experienced such trauma (11, 61, 62, 69, 79). It is the learned voluntary control over these abnormal EMG patterns that is the basic tenet of EMG biofeedback rehabilitation training. Most EMG biofeedback protocols are concerned first with inhibiting or reducing any hypertonicity and then address movement and activities that facilitate volitional recruitment.

Cervical trauma often results in discomfort experienced in the neck, shoulder, arms, and suboccipital region of the head and occasionally over the vertex and temporal regions (80). Resulting muscle trauma will generally not only manifest itself with symptomatology in the nuchal region but also with cephalalgia. Headache associated with the cervical syndrome is one of the most common presenting patient complaints (81). In a recent study of headache patients being treated for posttraumatic headache, 43.6% reported receiving a "whiplash-neck injury" (82).

As reported by Winston (83), cervical trauma can also manifest itself as a "migrainous" type headache. Historically the syndrome of "migraine cervicale" (84) was thought to be due to trauma that acted in a manner to hyperflex the cervical spine. It has recently been proposed that other types of cervical injuries can also produce "migraine"-like symptoms (83). Cervical-induced headache may therefore have both vascular and muscular components. Biofeedback is a treatment that has been of demonstrated success for both muscle contraction and vascular headache (3, 6, 85).

In 1973 Brudny et al. (86) applied EMG to specific training regimens for nine patients suffering from spasmodic torticollis. He concluded "that external sensory information, reflecting closely the functional state of affected muscles, could apparently augment or substitute for a defect in the servo-mechanism of patterned volitional movements and aid in reestablishing the integrity of sensory motor interaction." Brudny (87) offered the hypothesis that the proven success of EMG biofeedback in the restoration of muscle function may be due to the combination of visual and auditory information. He stated that the specific form of the EMG information pattern is instructed by the therapist, and that the muscle potential–brain connection may represent the most direct inphase biofeedback loop possible between the muscles, the brain, and the environment. He believed this to be the key to the facilitation of learning. Therefore, Brudny proposed that the phrase "physiological information processing" may be a better definition for the conceptual construct of how biofeedback is assimilated.

Basmajian (5) stated that the exact neural pathways permitting improved performance via biofeedback training remain unknown. He suggested two possibilities: the first, that biofeedback allows the development of new neural pathways, he discounted in favor of a second, more likely explanation, that "old persisting cerebral and spinal pathways" are "mobilized" via the biofeedback training modality. At whatever level the higher learning function takes place it is the direct, learned control of resting and active muscle state that is the desired outcome (5). Basmajian further stated that EMG biofeedback appears to be "particularly suitable" for treatment of torticollis, which appears to receive much support from the work conducted by Cleeland (88, 89).

In 1969 Jacobs and Felton (90) examined patients who had recently experienced neck injuries that had resulted in painful muscle spasm. The authors found that the injured patients could learn to reduce tonus levels more quickly by using biofeedback instrumentation than by simply "feel" or by depending on the body's own existing internal sensors. When compared to the reduction of tonus levels in the nuchal muscle achieved by uninjured subjects, the injured patients demonstrated a comparable amount of relaxation, although there was significant difference in the rate of learning. Leplow (91) studied the utility of EMG biofeedback versus "nonfeedback instructed self control" on reducing tonus levels in the hypertrophied sternocleidomastoid in patients suffering from idiopathic torticollis spasmodicus. Results indicated that the EMG biofeedback condition was significantly superior to the instructed self-control condition, leading to reduced EMG tonus levels.

Prior to utilizing EMG biofeedback protocols in the rehabilitation of the cervical pain patient, the clinician should fully map the region of symptomatic complaint, including the areas relating to known dermatome radiation patterns. All possible pathophysiologic etiologies contributing to the perception of pain should be identified so as to establish an individualized treatment course for reestablishing voluntary control. Determining the usefulness of EMG biofeedback for the cervical pain patient should not be done on the basis of the subjective complaint of "muscle spasm" or "pain" alone.

In a recent study Suurkula and Haag (92) measured surface EMG activity in female factory workers with shoulder and neck pain/disorders that resulted from trauma induced by repetitive daily assembly work. The EMG measurements were used in an effort to quantify any differences in those subjects presenting with neck pain/disorders versus those without pain. All pain subjects presented with symptomatology characteristic of "occupational cervicobrachial disorder" as described by Maeda (93). EMG readings taken of the descending portion of the trapezius and the infraspinatus muscle consistently revealed significant differences between subjects who reported pain versus those who reported no discomfort. Greater differences were observed in the infraspinatus muscle regions versus the trapezius regions for those patients reporting neck pain. Since from a biomechanical point of view it may be expected that the trapezius muscle would be of greater importance, the authors hypothesized that this finding indicated a referred pain phenomenon in the genesis of nuchal pain. They postulated that local ischemia from repetitive muscle movements may be a precipitating factor in work-related neck disorders. Photoplethysmographic and thermal biofeedback protocols can be used for pain resulting from ischemia and are discussed later in the chapter.

Specific muscles of interest in cervical trauma/pain syndrome include, but are not limited to, the trapezius, sternocleidomastoid, splenius capitis, semispinalis capitis, rectus capitis, capitis obliquus, longus colli, longissimus cervicis, levator scapulae, sternohyoid, longus coli, scalene, and minor rhomboid. While activity of some of the aforementioned muscle groups is not measurable by surface electrode EMG, it should be understood that the deep as well as the surface muscles may contribute to a cervical dysfunctional/pain syndrome. Unfortunately the deep structures do not lend themselves to simplistic surface electrode biofeedback procedures. The reader is directed to Basmajian's *Muscles Alive* (94) for a detailed description of the role each muscle takes in providing support and movement of the neck.

Motor examination of the deltoids, biceps, and triceps, wrist extension and flexion, hand grasp, and finger abduction and adduction can all reveal specific cervical spine problems. It is important that these activities be observed and if necessary rehabilitated with biofeedback protocols.

When initiating biofeedback, resting levels of the muscle and the contralateral muscle should be noted in sitting, supine, prone, and lateral positions. It is important not only to address the specific tonus levels of the musculature but to assess the bilateral (a)symmetry present as well. Especially important is dynamic, active muscle testing with the assessment of the ability of the muscle(s) to cocontract in functionally appropriate groups, act synergistically in complex motor patterns, and to return to resting state after activity (e.g., flexion, extension, and rotation of associated joint(s), as applicable). Triano and Schultz (95) have clearly demonstrated the importance of assessing the flexion-relaxation response in musculoskeletal pain patients. Generally, any significant elevation in resting tonus level, hypoactivity, asymmetry, abnormal pattern of concurrent recruitment of synergists, temporal delay in return to baseline level after activation, or hyperirritability (spontaneous discharge) indicates the presence of operational conditions amenable to EMG biofeedback intervention.

## Case Examples

**Case 1.** An unmarried 27-year-old female patient was referred by her orthopaedic surgeon. The patient presented with a 5-year history of unremitting torticollis (to the left) subsequent to physical trauma (whiplash injury) received in a motor vehicle accident. When the episode first occurred the patient had radiographs taken at a hospital emergency room and was told that they were nonremarkable. The patient was notified that she had received a "soft tissue whiplash injury." Intervention via bed rest, nonsteroidal anti-inflammatory drugs, muscle relaxants, benzodiazapines, physical therapy (consisting of ultrasound, iontophoresis, cervical traction, and massage), trigger point injections, and transcutaneous electrical nerve stimulation were unsuccessful. Since her condition proved refractory, a magnetic resonance (MR) image and a computed tomography (CT) scan were performed. Initial CT results were thought to indicate that a cervical fusion had occurred spontaneously at C5–6 as a result of the chronicity and angle of cervical spine misalignment. However, follow-up with MR imaging indicated that the condition was caused by a severe disc herniation (Fig. 11.1).

The patient's complaints were constant daily pain, described as "sharp and intense," in the nuchal, shoulder, and thoracic regions. Her range of motion was severely limited in flexion, extension, and rotation. The patient's normal station involved keeping her head rotated to the right in a fixed position of 35° (Fig. 11.2). The patient was disabled. Additionally, she was clinically depressed secondary to her unremitting pain and postural deformity. There was no prior relevant medical or psychological history.

Initial surface EMG readings confirmed static resting elevation of tonus levels and asymmetry over the regions of the splenus capitis, semispinalis capitis, sternocleidomastoid, longissimus cervicus, longus colli, trapezius, levator scapulae, and supraspinatus muscles. After minimal isometric exercise the sternocleidomastoid and upper trapezius muscles revealed an inability to return to resting tonus levels. Continuous involuntary sustained activity was observed to be in excess of 100 times expected levels. During this time the patient also indicated subjective complaints of se-

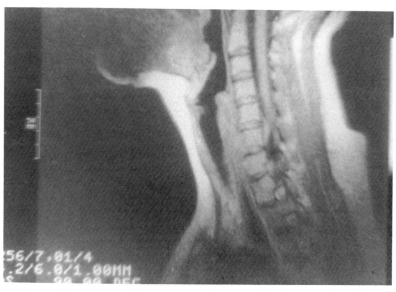

**Figure 11.1.** MR image of cervical spine of patient in case 1. Note elongated mass of C5–6 disc material impinging on the thecal sac.

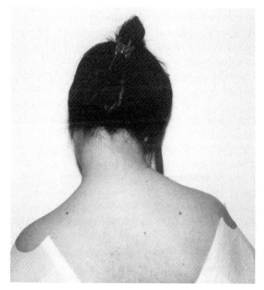

**Figure 11.2.** Photograph of patient's posture prior to biofeedback intervention.

vere pain, which prevented additional isometric testing.

The patient was introduced to a biofeedback protocol consisting of individual unilateral muscle training with the patient directed in techniques to reduce the involuntary elevated tonus levels. Figure 11.3 presents a graphic representation of

such training for the right sternocleidomastoid muscle. The patient was instructed to lower the visual display feedback by decreasing right sternocleidomastoid activity. The patient was then instructed to move her head as close to midline position as possible and then repeat the whole process. Thus a successive approximation "shaping" technique as outlined by Cleeland (89) was utilized. After the patient was able to demonstrate three successive days of sustained and maintained readings within the "normal reference range" for the specific muscle, treatment was directed toward the next abnormal muscle. Upon completion of instruction in reducing tonus levels of each individual unilateral muscle to normal reference range readings, training proceeded to the use of multichannel hookups that displayed appropriate synergistic and oppositional muscle dynamics under various postural attitudes. At the same time training was taking place the patient was titrated from all medications (Valium, Flexeril, and Motrin). Training was carried out over a 20-month period. Each training session consisted of 35 trials of 1.5 min each separated by a 10-sec intertrial timeout. The patient received training two times per week.

As can be noted in Figure 11.4, the patient presents today with normal posture symmetry and has full unrestricted range of motion. Pain is virtually absent and occurs only after an extended

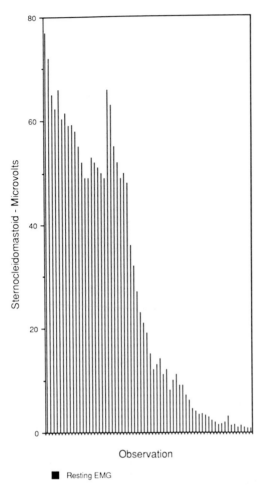

**Figure 11.3.** Graphic representation of patient's presenting EMG tonus level for the right sternocleidomastoid muscle across training sessions.

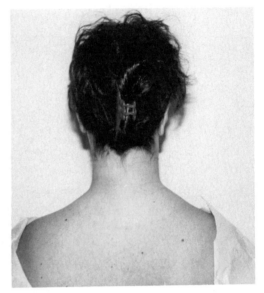

**Figure 11.4.** Photograph of patient's posture upon discharge from biofeedback treatment program.

day's activity that involves extensive use of her upper extremities. The patient is no longer using any medications. In this specific case the need for surgery was avoided with restoration of function and comfort level.

**Case 2.** A 38-year-old female with a 36-month history of neck pain was referred by her neurologist. The patient was employed as a computer operator and was required to work at a computer console for approximately 50% of the work day, and to work at her desk using the telephone for the remaining 50%. The patient had a 12-year history of nerve deafness in her right ear that has been progressive. The patient believed that her neck problem was due to the daily trauma of her work environment. Her work day was 11 hours long. The patient denied any history of nervous or

mental problems and indicated no family history of neurologic disease. Prior to coming to our center the patient underwent a CT scan of the cervical spine from the occiput to C4 that was negative. The patient had been seen by her family physician, chiropractors, orthopaedists, neurologists, a physiatrist, a pyschiatrist, an accupressurist, physical therapists, and a nutritionist prior to her referral for treatment via biofeedback. Her condition had remained refractory to all previous interventions, including medications (e.g., diazepam, cyclobenzaprine, methocarbamol, amitriptyline, Artane, Symmetrel, Clonopin, diflunisal), massage, manipulation, cervical traction, use of Philadephia and soft collars, exercises (isometric and range of motion), and ultrasound. Her orthopaedist had suggested that she undergo a muscle neurectomy but she wished to avoid that procedure.

The patient was on disability leave from her job when she presented at our center. Her head was turned severely to the right, and the left sternocleidomastoid was in spasm and warm to the touch. No discreet masses could be palpated. Passively there was full range of motion of the head. Under her own power the patient evidenced restricted range of motion in terms of rotation, extension, and flexion. She indicated severe sharp pain in her nuchal, shoulder, and occiput regions. EMG examination to obtain baseline readings via surface electrodes indicated significant elevation of tonus levels overlying the sternocleidomastoi-deus (bilateral, but higher on the left), semispi-nalis capitis, longus capitis, levator scapulae, tra-pezius, and supraspinatus muscles. Readings were taken of the sternocleidomastoideus, and read-ings on the left side were over 50 times normal ref-erence range whereas those on the right side were only eight times normal. After the most minimal activity the patient complained of severe pain and felt she "lost control of the head as if in the movie 'The Exorcist.'" EMG readings obtained at this point were elevated over 120 times the normal reference range. After activity it would take the patient 15–30 min of quiet relaxation in a chair in a reclined, head-supported position for any re-duction in tonus levels to be observed.

Training initially consisted of teaching the pa-tient to assume a postural position that would per-mit some lowering of the persistently elevated tonus and hypertrophic state observed in the ster-nocleidomastoid and upper trapezius muscles. As soon as any lowering in tonus was observed, a pe-riod of irritability and high-frequency tremor would follow. Via a system of graduated subtasks followed with resting sessions, continuous sus-tained muscle control was learned. Activation of muscles was increased for longer periods, with the patient reducing her fears of dysfunction along the way. Hypesthesia at the C6–7 level dimin-ished. The patient returned to her prior job able to fulfill all activities 8 months after treatment had commenced.

**Case 3.** A 47-year-old male experienced severe pain in his neck and arms following a lifting acci-dent at his place of work. Conservative measures consisting of bed rest, nonsteroidal anti-inflam-matory drugs, physical therapy, and chiropractic yielded no reduction of symptomatology. Pain continued to increase and was experienced as ra-diating into the fingers of his left hand, with sig-nificant numbness of the left index finger. Pain in his neck was experienced with flexion, extension, and rotation to the left. On examination the left triceps reflex was noted to be absent. Biceps re-flexes were observed as 2+. Algesia and astasia were noted over the left C7 dermatome with 3/4 weakness of the triceps and wrist extensors on the left and 4/5 weakness of the biceps on the left. A myelo-CT scan provided evidence of a lesion at the C6–7 level on the left side.

The patient underwent a hemilaminectomy of C6 and C7 on the left side. The disc was noted to have extended (fragments) from underneath the C6 root and had intruded into the foramen under the C7 nerve root. The patient had been placed upon steroids postoperatively.

After surgery the patient continued to experi-ence pain and sensory disturbance along the C7 and, to a slight degree, C6 dermatome on the left side. The patient indicated pain primarily in the left cervicothoracic junction, with point tender-ness noted. The left triceps reflex remained ab-sent, and the left biceps reflex continued to be de-pressed as compared to the right. A postoperative CT scan was said to reveal no evidence of reher-niation of the disc. The patient was referred for biofeedback by his neurosurgeon with a diagnosis of "postsurgery myofascial syndrome."

The patient presented for biofeedback com-plaining of "severe disabling daily neck pain." Sta-tion and gait were guarded concerning the cervi-cal spine. Static baseline surface electrode EMG testing of the upper trapezius, splenius capitis (bi-lateral), and sternocleidomastoid (bilateral) yielded patterns consistent with a mild guarding. Minimal cervical isometric activity elicited an ex-pression of discomfort from the patient and a sig-nificant pattern of elevation, asymmetry, and ir-ritability in the same muscles. A program of multichannel EMG training was adopted permit-ting the patient to view activity in reciprocal mus-cles while being directed with postural positioning of his head. The patient was instructed to use the multichannel display to assist him in the voluntary inhibition of the spastic muscles in the shortened range and to keep the muscles silent while the head was passively supported in a supine position. Initially the patient had great difficulty allowing the neck musculature to relax and not recruit ex-cessive tonus activity in the surrounding regions. However, with the help of the visually displayed EMG patterns the patient was able to gain voli-tional control of independent muscle activity that was accompanied by a subjective pain reduction. A total of 46 treatments consisting of three 15-min sessions was required prior to mastery of muscle self-regulation. The patient subsequently returned to his prior occupation as an architec-tural designer and is able to draft at his table for a standard work day without experiencing discom-fort.

## PHOTOPLETHYSMOGRAPHIC AND THERMAL BIOFEEDBACK

It is generally accepted that peripheral skin tem-perature is directly related to vasodilation/con-striction. In addition, the reflected pulse height (blood volume pulse) measurement obtained via photoplethysmography (PPG) is assumed to be a correlate of vasospastic activity present. PPG biofeedback indicates the relative volume of blood flowing through the arteries in the area of pain. Also included in the PPG measurement is the interbeat interval (IBI), which measures the time (generally reflected in seconds) between heartbeats. By attending to a tone or visual signal the patient can learn to dilate blood vessels in the area or tissues associated with the pain etiology. These measurements may be used to assist the patient who is experiencing musculoskeletal pain (due to ischemia) to learn greater physiologic control.

Muscle spasm may be the product of decreased circulation to the muscle fibers with resultant ischemia and buildup of waste products (23). Bancroft and Milken (96) indicated that muscle ischemia directly followed muscle contraction and resulted in hyperemia during the relaxed state. However, the literature is extremely sparse in the area of applying PPG feedback to the rehabilitation of musculoskeletal pain and resultant ischemia. Most of the literature concerning this type of biofeedback has been limited to studies investigating migrainous headache and Raynaud's disease/phenomenon. Since the application is similar, it is worth giving a brief summary of this use.

Adler and Adler (97), Andrasik and Holroyd (98), Blanchard et al. (6), and Reich (3) have all indicated the long-term success of biofeedback interventions for muscle contraction, vascular, and mixed-type headache. Biofeedback for these conditions basically consists of thermal, EMG, and PPG biofeedback. For contraction headache patients, training usually consists of EMG biofeedback of frontalis and/or upper trapezius muscles. The goal for the patient is a successful lowering of any elevated tonus levels noted along with sustained control. For migraine and mixed-type headache patients, training usually consists of thermal and PPG protocols to assist the patient in vasocontrol. In some cases vasodilation is the goal and for others vasoconstriction becomes important. Approximately 75–88% of muscle contraction headache patients and approximately 78–94% of migraine/vascular headache patients report long-term (60-month) sustained improvement. Most of the headache patients report very infrequent and nonsystematic use of the biofeedback techniques originally learned. This seems to be in agreement with the statement proffered earlier that the learned behavior seems to be incorporated into a reflexive homeostatic condition.

Migraine headache has principally been considered a "vascular" headache, although the recent zeitgeist has incorporated a neurogenic (biogenic amine) component, decreased platelet serotonin. It is now popularly believed that a perturbation of the neurotransmitter 5-hydroxytryptamine plays a functional role in the etiology and expression of this debilitating type of cephalalgia (99). Since serotonin has been shown to play a major role in pain moderation, depression, and myofascial disorders, it appears that a commonality may be noted. It has been postulated by a number of clinicians (83, 84, 100, 101) that migraine-type headaches appear to be precipitated by cervical trauma, thus giving rise to the term "cervical migraine" (84).

Raynaud's disease is considered to be a primary functional disorder of the cardiovascular system presenting with intermittent bilateral vasospasms of the extremities (hands and feet). A. G. Raynaud (102) proposed that the most logical cause of the disease was overreactivity of the sympathetic nervous system. Raynaud's phenomenon is a syndrome that appears secondary to a number of vascular and musculoskeletal diseases (e.g., lupus erythematosus, carpal tunnel syndrome, systemic sclerosis). Pariser et al. (103) investigated the ischemia associated with Raynaud's phenomenon in a population of patients presenting with migraine and muscle contraction headaches. The results indicated 18.3% of the migraine patients and 13.4% of the muscle contraction headache patients also had Raynaud's phenomenon. These results compare with a 7% prevalence of Raynaud's phenomenon in the general population. It is obvious that a vasospastic component is associated with both types of headache, which can often result from cervical trauma.

It is interesting to note that both migraine headache sufferers and those afflicted with Raynaud's disease/phenomenon appear to be predominantly female. Females are three times more likely than males to experience migraine headache (105) and five times more likely to experience Raynaud's disease/phenomenon. Similarly it should be noted that cervical pain syndromes appear to be predominantly experienced/reported by females (80, 104; Reich, unpublished data, 1989). In only one study (105) was the prevalence rate of cervical disorder (cervicogenic headache) the same for male and female sufferers. In addition, female cervical pain patients appear to demonstrate lower recovery rates than males (106). In utilizing PPG and thermal biofeedback for these conditions the clinician attempts to establish a voluntary mediated control of the peripheral vasculature to increase the blood volume, thereby augmenting the peripheral blood flow.

Ischemic pain associated with musculoskeletal dysfunction must be considered when addressing the pain patient. The mechanism of either primary or secondary circulatory involvement in the cervical pain syndrome has also been mentioned (56, 92, 107, 108). In a current research project under development at our pain center, abnormal PPG readings indicating circulatory involvement have been noted in 75% of females presenting with cervical pain. Of males presenting with cervical pain, 58% were observed to have significant vasoconstriction in the nuchal regions identified by the patient as painful (Table 11.1). With the awareness of these findings an investigation was undertaken to assess the contribution that PPG training might offer in the reduction of perceived pain for the cervical trauma patient. A single-blind protocol was developed in which the patient was not aware if he or she was receiving actual or contrived feedback information. Analyses indicated significant reduction in intensity of pain only for the subjects in the true biofeedback group who actually learned appropriate vasodilation. All patients in the contrived feedback group (those given erroneous data) and in the true biofeedback group who were not able to learn vascular control did not have any significant decrease in reported pain. Table 11.2 presents the data for this study. Interestingly, female patients tended to

display more vascular involvement than the male subjects in the study. Females appeared to demonstrate an additional, although nonsignificant, trend: greater pain was experienced during the first 2 days preceding menses and continued into the first 2 days following menses. Rouleau and Denver (109) utilized thermal biofeedback to assist patients experiencing fibrositis in reducing pain by means of learned control over vascular flow. Results appeared encouraging but no longitudinal follow-up was offered.

Additional research is needed to establish reliable findings concerning the role of ischemia in musculoskeletal disorders and the amenability of the ischemia to control via PPG feedback techniques.

## ELECTROENCEPHALOGRAPHIC BIOFEEDBACK

It has been noted that individuals who are experiencing a calm and relaxed (nonsleep) state emit alpha brainwaves in the frequency of 8–13 Hz as recorded by surface electrode at the occipital-parietal site. Alpha patterns are also correlated with a "relief from attention and concentration" (110). Hypnosis and relaxation training were often used as pain control interventions and were noted to be associated with increased slow brainwave activity. Thus it was initially believed that the utility of electroencephalographic (EEG) biofeedback was to assist the patient in learning to achieve a state of deep mental calm. The concept rested on the premise that a calm patient would evidence a lowered perception of pain.

In 1975 Melzack and Perry (111) compared the effects of EEG biofeedback, hypnosis, and a combination of the two on refractory chronic pain of physical origin. All treatments were reported to reduce the pain symptoms significantly. However, the combined treatment offered the best pain reduction (36%), followed by the hypnosis alone (22%), and finally the EEG biofeedback (10%). These results are in contrast to those obtained by Reich (3), which demonstrated superior pain reduction via EMG and thermal/PPG biofeedback for headache patients versus treatment with hypnosis alone or hypnosis in combination with the biofeedback. Perhaps the methodologic differences in the two studies (e.g., type of pain, method and type of biofeedback) reflect the divergence of the obtained results.

Unfortunately alpha biofeedback seems to be very susceptible to artifactual movement and oc-

**Table 11.1.**
**Number of Patients with Cervical Pain Demonstrating Vasospasm**

|        | Total | Vasoconstriction |
|--------|-------|------------------|
| Male   | 31    | 18 (58%)         |
| Female | 40    | 30 (75%)         |

$\chi^2 = 2.29$ (nonsignificant).

**Table 11.2.**
**Number of Cervical Pain Patients with Vasoconstriction Reporting a Reduction of Pain by Treatment**

|        | True Biofeedback | Contrived Biofeedback |
|--------|------------------|------------------------|
| Male   | 5/9    (56%)     | 1/9    (11%)           |
| Female | 10/15 (67%)      | 2/15 (13%)             |

ular occurrences. These phenomena limit the interpretive value of EEG biofeedback in pain control. Some individuals have concluded that EEG patterning is so coarse and vague that they compare its reliability to a person listening to events on the other side of the globe by placing an inverted cup on the ground beneath his feet. Perhaps what holds the most promise for the future in the field of EEG biofeedback is the investigation of discrete event-related potentials, as recently investigated by Spiegel et al. (112) and Miltner et al. (113).

Voluntarily induced changes in event-related potentials, in addition to voluntarily induced slow brain potentials, have shown efficacy in changing pain-related behavior (114–116). Many researchers have demonstrated that observed EEG event-related potentials are correlated with subjective pain reports (117–120). Event-related potentials appear to be correlated with the various intensities of noxious stimuli. By using biofeedback to mediate changes in amplitude and changes of polarity of somatosensory electrical brain activity, subjects have noted modification of the pain perception. In a recent study Miltner et al. (113) investigated the ability of 10 healthy adult males to learn biofeedback of event-related potentials as a method of controlling the perception of experimentally induced pain caused by intracutaneous electrical stimulation. Results not only confirmed the ability of the subjects to utilize the biofeedback to learn control of the event-related potentials but were also correlated with a significant reduction in subjective pain reports. Post hoc analysis indicated that the subjects effected biofeedback control via individually chosen "cognitive strategies" consisting of concentration, relaxation, and positive shared experiences. The experimental protocol was constructed to control and assess for the intervening variable of habituation to the noxious stimulus. The results obtained were interpreted by the authors as demonstrating the role that "complex psychological aspects, i.e., attentional aspects, cognition, processing of stimulus information and response preparation" have in pain control in addition to the neurophysiologic aspects of stimulus processing. Additional research is needed in this field and is discussed later in this chapter as the concepts apply to the techniques of analgesic hypnosis. Research studies utilizing these concepts as applied to pain resulting from cervical trauma are absent from the literature.

## RELAXATION THERAPIES

Through the involvement of the imagination and by reference to previous experiences we become able to place what we sense sometimes within ourselves and sometimes outside us.

Johannes Muller (1)

There are two ways to react to stress: you can either be laid back—or laid out.

Robert Orben (121)

Relaxation has been called the "aspirin of behavioral medicine" (122) because of its almost global applicability to the variety of pain disorders. However, in my experience the initial offering of relaxation to the pain patients appears to them as a most bitter pill to swallow. Probably the most difficult advice to be followed by a patient in pain, when instructed by a doctor, is to relax. Most frequently the retort is, "How can I relax when I'm experiencing so much pain?" or "That's easy for you to say but impossible to accomplish." Patients are usually resentful and are annoyed by such advice. Yet if the clinician can explain the relationship of relaxation to the sensation of pain and offer direction and procedures that can be followed to accomplish such goals, pain moderation can be achieved for many patients. When properly taught, relaxation is a skill that can be extremely useful in reducing the frequency, intensity, and duration of pain episodes.

As early as 1872 it was pointed out by Mitchell (123) that pain had a direct influence upon "both body and mind." Simons (13) states that "psychological stress is frequently expressed as increased muscle tension which mechanically overloads the muscles." Schwartz (124) related that the basis for relaxation is that it can allow for a calming caused by "disregulation." He states that disregulation is basically the deleterious effect of biologic and psychological stressors upon the individual's state of homeostasis. Blumenthal (125) proffered that relaxation therapies have been proven successful "as determined by a variety of outcome criteria in physiological, behavioral, and subjective response domains including changes in physiological responsivety, overt symptomatology, and self-report." Jessup et al. (126) found that for some pain patients relaxation training compared favorably with biofeedback in the reduction of discomfort. Basmajian (5) found that the combination of relaxation utilized in concert with biofeedback is of benefit because pain patients experience a significant amount of emotional stress that contributes to the continuation of any psychophysiologic pathology.

Lichstein (127), Marzuk (128), Borgeat et al. (129), Silver and Blanchard (130), and Beiman et al. (131) have stated that biofeedback is not superior to the relaxation techniques. Lacroix et al. (132) examined the effects of EMG biofeedback, relaxation training, a combination of the two, and no treatment (a control group) on the frequency of muscle contraction headache in patients with cervical and low back pain. All three treatment groups showed significant pain relief versus the control group. The relaxation training group appeared to maintain the lessened headache symptomatology the best when observed 6 months later. Smith (30) found that for headache patients a combination of biofeedback and relaxation training achieved results superior to either given alone. In contrast, Reich (3) found consistently greater reduction in pain for patients treated via biofeedback as compared to three kinds of relaxation procedures (hypnosis, progressive relaxation training, and autogenic training). Biofeedback training alone achieved the greatest reduction in frequency, intensity, and duration of self-reported pain events. A subpopulation of patients was given a combined treatment of relaxation training and biofeedback. This group did not fare as well as the biofeedback alone group in reduction of pain episodes. The combined biofeedback/relaxation training and relaxation training alone groups showed significant reduction in pain as compared to a no treatment control group. These findings remained stable 36 months after discharge from treatment.

In a study involving headache patients, Sorbi and Tellegen (133) compared the treatment modalities of relaxation training and "stress-coping training." A significant reduction in headache activity was found for both of the groups but important differences were noted in the perceptions and beliefs of the two sets of subjects. Patients in the relaxation group stated a greater awareness of stress and awareness of medication use, while the patients in the "stress-coping training" group perceived a learned "control" over stress. In an assessment 8 months later the different perceptions were no longer noted. Other researchers (134–136) found that different types of relaxation training generally resulted in pain reduction and self-reported improvement. Some researchers (137, 138) argue that all of the relaxation techniques are basically the same and differ only in name, not effect.

Relaxation as a therapeutic regimen to gain control over physiologic functions is far from new. The early teachings of Kebhalistic mysticism, Christianity, Taoism, Shintoism, Zen, and Yoga have utilized various exercises and techniques for thousands of years to provide individuals with a basis for consciousness altering and to help achieve a psychological/physiologic peace and sense of integrity/harmony.

## PROGRESSIVE MUSCLE RELAXATION/ AUTOGENIC AND SIMILAR THERAPIES

In 1938, working at Harvard University, Edmund Jacobsen (139) ushered into the field of psychology the concept that muscle relaxation therapy—progressive muscle relaxation—could be utilized as a basis for reducing and even eliminating anxiety in addition to reducing disease. Via his process of progressive muscle relaxation patients were instructed to successively tense and relax various muscle groupings to achieve a state of comfort. It was upon this basis that the theoretical development of a balance between the musculoskeletal system and the psychological state of an individual was brought to the attention of a burgeoning field, later termed "behavioral medicine" (2). Jacobsen was among the first investigators to note that electrical activity could be recorded from muscle that appeared to be at rest. In addition, he recorded the effect that the imagination had upon electrical activity of the resting muscle. He noted that when he directed a resting patient to imagine a muscle in use, electrical activity could be measured from the muscle even though there was no appearance of visual movement (140). At approximately the same time Schultz and Luthe (141) were developing the concept of "autogenic training." Central to both methods is the concept of deep muscle relaxation. Also active in this area of research was Burrow (142) with his theory of "cotention," which demonstrated the ability of individuals to lessen physiologic distress via a cognitive pathway. The contribution of Wolpe (143) was his approach of "systematic desensitization," which enabled an individual to control the physiologic correlates associated with an anxiety state.

The basis for success with these techniques is the principle of teaching subjects to become aware of subtle internal cues and to use cognitions about these cues to bring about a desired change

in their psychophysiologic state. By means of relaxation the patient can establish contact with his
body sensations and with this awareness develop
skills to accept or alter these sensations. Building
upon this central core concept of relaxation, Lazarus (144) introduced a "visual imagery" approach to assist individuals to achieve a deep state
of relaxation. In addition the concept of meditation and/or transcendental meditation has been
successfully demonstrated to permit individuals
to obtain a calming of physiologic functioning
(145, 146) and should be included in the field of
relaxation therapies. Relaxation may consist of
any of the aforementioned theories or be as simple as deep (diaphragmatic) breathing utilized by
the patient as a pain coping mechanism.

Interaction between the individual's cognitive
state and perception of pain is well accepted. In
any multidisciplinary pain program presently employed at any major hospital or private clinic,
treating the psychological component of pain is
considered of equal importance to physiologic rehabilitation. In many cases the mind sets the lead
for the body to follow. Bradley et al. (147) applied
biofeedback in combination with cognitive behavioral therapy as a pain reduction technique for
subjects suffering from rheumatoid arthritis. The
results of his study clearly indicated that self-re-
ports of pain intensity and depression significantly decreased for subjects receiving the treatment versus those who received only standard
medical treatment. However, while a significant
difference was observed between the two groups
for pain behavior, disease, and anxiety at posttreatment assessment, the differences were not
maintained at time of follow-up assessment 1 year
later. It was postulated that the "coping strategies" learned and applied by the patients permitted the initial posttreatment results to be observed. Thus attitude and relaxation appear to
play a significant role in the rehabilitation of pain
patients. Reich (unpublished data, 1989) and
Middaugh and Garwood (75) have independently
demonstrated that reactivity in the upper trapezius and splenius capitis muscles is very sensitive
to the emotional state of the patient. Bischoff and
Traue (77) reported that "even in situations of
purely psychological stress the phasic muscle activity in the neck region can reach 10% to 20% of
the maximum contraction."

It is generally accepted that anxiety and/or
emotional tension may act in a manner to specifically exacerbate and increase both musculoskeletal and ischemic cervical pain. The concept pre-

sented earlier of the pain-tension-pain cycle must
not be forgotten when addressing the patient. Patients frequently manifest traits of anxiety, frustration, and depression secondary to any injury
that causes distress or a perceived loss of function.
Usually, the more disabling the injury the more do
psychological variables come into play. Sternbach
(148), Weisenberg (149), and Fordyce (150) related that most pain is automatically associated
with a state of anxiety and ultimately depression.
This psychological dysfunction adds to the pain
spiral and may perpetuate pain beyond recovery
rates normally expected for pain solely due to
physical trauma.

Hockersmith (151) demonstrated that chronic
pain patients acted in a behavioral manner that
sustained back pain and low back muscle tension
even after the original physiologic trauma was resolved. Dunn and Blazar (80) stated that a positive
Tinel's sign may be present over innervated
nerves for years after the original injury. For the
cervical pain patient this reaction is of even
greater importance because of the specific reactivity of the nuchal muscles as demonstrated in the
studies of Reich (unpublished data, 1989) and
Middaugh and Garwood (75). Any stressful environmental condition, or even the perception of
one, stands a good chance of increasing musculoskeletal tonus. Simply being aware of the muscle
tension usually experienced in one's neck when
driving home in a rainstorm after a full day's work
demonstrates such nuchal reactivity. Given any
underlying preexistent pathophysiology, pain
may be increased manyfold.

Conversely, with relaxation the body generally
responds with lowered muscle tonus, more regulated respiration, increased oxygenation of the
blood, dilation of the peripheral vasculature, shift
in blood flow from the skeletal muscles to the di-
gestive organs, increased gastrointestinal motility,
reductions in lactic acid, catecholamines, and
adrenaline, and more regulated EEG patterns.
Relaxation training offers the patient increased
control over awareness, perceptions, and physiology of pain. As Turk et al. (152) suggested relaxation may reduce pain via five specific pathways:
(a) by reducing the patient's muscular tonus and
the pain associated with same; (b) by occupying the
patient's attention—directing it away from the
pain; (c) by reducing anxiety, which reduces any
associated tension; (d) by providing the patient
with a specific activity he can perform to control
the pain perception; and (e) by assisting the patient to obtain rest and needed sleep. Blumenthal

clinician should become less involved over time so that the patient can perceive the success obtained as reinforcing a sense of personal efficacy.

During the training process it is important to assess the physiologic baseline that the patient presents upon starting each session. The EMG levels at the start of each session become valuable indicators of sustained learning and ultimate success, for it is the sustained and maintained physiologic control between training sessions that indicates application of the learned behaviors to the patient's everyday activity schedule without disruptive tonus dysfunction.

While Peck and Kraft (25) found that continual practice was necessary to maintain pain reduction via EMG training, recent comprehensive and longitudinal studies have shown otherwise (3, 6, 26). It is desirable that the skills and physiologic state obtained via the specific biofeedback training protocol become a natural, automatic, reflexive component of the patient's physiologic repertoire. Although it is necessary for a patient to practice at home during the beginning of physiologic skills acquisition, many pain patients have demonstrated that the learned control often becomes part of the natural homeostasis of the individual without continued practice. Successful patients indicated pain reduction 5 years after being discharged from active treatment, with only 14% of these patients indicating the continued daily practice of biofeedback learning (3, 26). Basmajian (27) has also related the ability of subjects to display conscious motor unit control in the absence of continued visual or auditory feedback and without the necessity of daily practice.

Hudzinsky and Levenson (28) found that the variables of sex, number of sessions attended, age at time of treatment/program participation, and "locus of control" significantly affected outcome measures of success. Others have found that the ability of the individual to become a consummate learner of muscle control via EMG biofeedback protocols does not seem influenced by age, race, sex, socioeconomic status, education level, IQ, or manual skill (26, 27). In a 5-year longitudinal study on over 1000 pain patients Reich (26) found that the specific variables providing the best prediction of success with biofeedback training were (a) how long the underlying physical pathology had been present without successful intervention prior to initiating biofeedback, and (b) the number of biofeedback training sessions attended by the patient. Other researchers have also noted that the number of training sessions given/attended is correlated with the pain relief obtained and maintained by the patient (8, 29). Basmajian (5) indicated that a high presenting level of nervousness in the patient may negatively affect a successful outcome.

Earlier it was mentioned that tension can manifest itself as additional physiologic dysfunction. Ferraccioli et al. (15) indicated that fibromyalgia patients who presented with depression and/or overt psychosomatic background were less likely to report a reduction of pain obtained via EMG biofeedback than similarly diagnosed pain patients without any noted psychological disturbance. This result held steady under conditions of "true" versus contrived EMG readings. The patients who were not depressed and who learned control in the "true" biofeedback condition revealed the most significant improvement. However, Stilson et al. (30) indicated that no differences were noted in the success rate of EMG training for normal subjects versus psychiatric subjects in the learning of conscious muscle tonus control.

After the practitioner has evaluated the patient and determined that biofeedback training is appropriate in the rehabilitation process, a treatment strategy should be planned. The treatment strategy should contain detailed protocols outlining the specific methods and goals for the individual patient. Knowledge of the patient's occupation and daily activity profile must be incorporated into the treatment protocol. It is this knowledge that permits the skilled clinician to develop a training procedure that will allow for biofeedback control of muscle activities involved in the patient's daily regimen to be approximated and learned in an efficacious manner.

With the advent of newer sophisticated computerized biofeedback equipment, detailed records indicating success within and between sessions can be easily kept and analyzed. Adjustments to threshold levels and degrees of difficulty can be modified to maximize the successful physiologic skills acquisition of the patient. It must be understood that the acute or chronic pain patient generally has a lowered threshold of frustration. Since biofeedback is a learning procedure that requires the active participation of the patient it is necessary to make the initial training tasks easy. The clinician must be sensitive to the individual's ability to learn so as not to increase the patient's frustration and thus ensure failure. "Self-efficacy" as described by Bandura (9) plays a most important role in the biofeedback process and appears to permit a system of internal reward that allows for enhanced and more rapid acquisition of learned physiologic control. The learning situation must allow the patient to feel that some control in the perception of pain can be obtained. As change in the targeted physiologic response becomes effected by the patient, the internal cognitive components become more significant in the continuance, precision, and generalizability of the response (7).

## ELECTROMYOGRAPHIC BIOFEEDBACK

Modern EMG usage may be traced back to the 1940s, at which time the procedure was recognized as a tool for research and rehabilitation within the field of physical medicine. Marinacci (31) and Hefferline (32) reported that subjects were capable of utilizing feedback displays of motor unit activity to produce changes in a predetermined direction. Harrison and Mortensen (33) measured isolated activity of motor units in the tibialis muscle with surface electrode EMG and noted that individuals were able to maintain such activity on command. Thus EMG was utilized as a feedback modality allowing the subjects upon volition to increase the frequency and amplitude of motor units. Since the early 1960s independent research by Basmajian et al. (34, 35), Booker et al. (36), Brudny et al. (37), Stoyva and Budzynsky (38), Johnson and Garton (39), Miller (40), Herman (41), and Surwit and Keefe (42) has demonstrated the efficaciousness of application of EMG biofeedback for neuromuscular rehabilitation. However, for biofeedback to yield the desired results the patient must be able to balance motivation with passivity, for the more a patient "tries" to produce a desired neuromuscular response the more he may prevent himself from obtaining the goal by generating excessive sympathetic muscle tension in his attempts. "Straining or pushing" a response often creates additional muscle activation or acts in a manner that does not allow for complementary muscle groups to compensate for a dystonic condition. It is the process of "allowing" or "cognitively willing and believing" in the desired motor function that more often yields the intended activation or relaxation of the targeted muscle. Breznitz (43) intimated that without hope there is no life. In biofeedback training, without belief there is little possibility of change. Davidson and Schwartz (44) stated that if both psychological and physiologic relaxation are present the resulting relaxation achieved will be more pronounced.

Rather than try to ferret out the individual contributions of the physiology-psychology dichotomy, we must view the process as inherently "contaminated" and accept that biofeedback therapy combines both in a complementary fashion.

Early research paradigms generally were concentrated around the concept that training in one muscle group (typically the frontalis) would generalize within the individual and be experienced as a lowered level of stimulation throughout the entire physiology (38). As the field became more advanced in studying the physiologic response it was shown that such generalization does not seem to be the case. A lowering of the tonus in the frontalis muscle does not appear to be correlated with a lowering of the individual's overall level of physiologic activation (45–49). Shedivy and Kleinman (50) demonstrated that various nuchal muscles and the frontalis muscle would vary independently of each other, although a trend was noted. The researchers found that the sternocleidomastoid and semispinalis/splenius muscles were not significantly influenced by increasing or decreasing the tonus in the frontalis. Fridlund et al. (47) found no generalization from training in the frontalis muscle to the nuchal muscles or muscles in the forearm or leg regions. Shedivy and Kleinman specifically picked the nuchal muscles because of their role in torticollis and muscle contraction headache. Learned control is usually experienced only in the specific muscle(s) successfully trained (50, 51). Yet this control may be plentiful, as Kato and Tanji (52) demonstrated with the ability of subjects to learn the isolated control of greater than 286 motor units, producing volitional contraction without the incorporation of any neighboring units.

Information reported by Ladd et al. (53) indicates that single motor unit inhibition relies upon a learned response that may generalize across muscles, but voluntary contraction responses are specific to the skeletal muscle involved. Training involuntary contraction in a muscle does not lessen the time or trials required for training associated muscles or those located in areas orthogonal to the training. Thus successful use of biofeedback therapy can be a laborious undertaking if paretic and spastic conditions exist along with involvement of extensive synergistic and oppositional muscle groups. However, since Budzinsky and Stoyva (54) stated that EMG biofeedback could hasten and enhance the learning of muscle relaxation, the relevance of this technique has become recognized in the field of tonic rehabilita-

(125) stated that "relaxation therapy may be viewed as a general approach designed to restore the individual to a stable homeostasis through a process of self-regulation."

## HYPNOSIS

Some individuals may think it appropriate to include the concept of hypnosis within the relaxation modalities. Since the 1950s, when the British Medical Association (1955) and the American Medical Association (1958) endorsed hypnosis as a viable medical technique, a great deal of attention has been given to the use of this form of therapy in affording pain moderation. According to *Newsday* (May 9, 1989) it is estimated that currently over 20,000 doctors are utilizing hypnosis as a therapeutic modality in the United States.

Franz Anton Mesmer (1734–1815) is credited as being the father of medical hypnosis. As developed and refined by Bernheim (153), Janet (154), Charcot (155), Breuer and Freud (156), Hilgard (157), Tart (158), and Barber (159, 160), hypnosis is basically a state of altered consciousness that allows for extension or heightening of suggestibility within the individual. It was used for its analgesic properties as early as the 19th century by the British surgeon James Espdaile in several thousand operations to provide anesthesia. At that time chemical anesthesia was not developed as a standard procedure and was not in common use.

Hypnosis has been utilized in the field of behavioral medicine to permit a patient to become deeply relaxed so as to produce analgesia with a variety of pain perceptions or to develop the patient's insight and understanding concerning his symptoms and behaviors. The individual's threshold for pain can be raised as result of the hypnotic procedure. Wall (161) stated that hypnosis can be utilized to "provide an extraordinarily effective blockade" between afferent inputs and the effector mechanisms, thereby providing the patients with anesthesia. Melzack and Perry (111) also noted that hypnosis is effective in altering the perception of painful stimuli. However, the primary factor affecting the degree of pain reduction to be expected is the hypnotic susceptibility of the subject. Hilgard and Hilgard (120) demonstrated that the more hypnotically responsive a subject, the more likely a reduction in the perceived pain. After giving a test of hypnotic responsiveness, the Hilgards divided their subjects into three groups indicating different levels of hypnotic susceptibility—high, medium, and low. All patients were exposed to a painful stimulus (ischemic pain induced by cold water) and treated with a hypnotic analgesic technique. Pain was reduced by one third or greater in 67% of the high group, whereas only 13% of the low group indicated pain reduction of one third or more. It is important to note that the low susceptibility group still experienced some success, with 44% indicating a reduction in perceived pain of 10% or more. Similar results were obtained by McGlashan et al. (162) in a study utilizing experimentally induced ischemic pain. Not only were significant differences observed in subjects defined by susceptibility, but significant differences were also observed for highly susceptible subjects who were given hypnosis or a placebo. Erickson (163) has concluded that the basic tenet of hypnosis is that a state of intensified attention and heightened receptiveness to a set of ideas permits an alteration in the perception of and overt behavior in response to specific events.

It may be stated that hypnosis basically consists of two parts, an induction followed by suggestions. It has been proposed that the induction is simply a relaxation procedure and all pain reduction observed may be explained by the relaxed state obtained by the patient undergoing the induction procedure. However, Hilgard and Hilgard (120) have demonstrated that the induction alone devoid of specific analgesic suggestions does not appear to reduce pain "any more than it reduces other sensory functions." Furthermore, in the same study they indicated that it was the specific procedural arrangement of analgesia suggestions following the induction that resulted in the observed pain reduction.

Spiegel et al. (112) examined the effects of hypnosis on event-related potential amplitudes of somatosensory perceptual distortion. This specific sensory modality was chosen because of its applicability to the field of pain control (120, 164). Subjects who were found to be highly susceptible to hypnosis, by standardized screening devices, displayed significant task-related changes in the amplitudes of their somatosensory event-related responses. Results indicated that the amplitude of the $P_{100}$ and $P_{300}$ event-related potentials were increased during "hypnotic attention" and reduced significantly during "hypnotic obstruction." These results were not found for the low susceptibility group. It was suggested that hypnotic analgesia was mediated via an alteration in the perception or processing of the stimulus as being painful rather than the subject's discriminating the detection of the stimulus as being present or not present. That hypnosis is capable of altering the amplitude of event-related potentials, thereby producing a change in subjective pain intensity, suggests that this technique, as with biofeedback, appears beneficial in the self-regulation of pain and could assist in the rehabilitation of symptoms resulting from cervical trauma.

Recently Houle et al. (165) examined the efficacy of hypnosis versus relaxation induced suggestions for analgesia to create a perceived reduction of noxious stimulation. Experimental pain was induced via cold pressor and noxious tooth pulp stimulation. The two stimuli were chosen because of their qualitative differences based upon the types of nerves activated and the mode of stimulus activation. Cold pressor stimulation is thought to activate a number of nociceptive and nonnociceptive fibers and is experienced as a progressive cold leading to severe pain. In contrast, electrical tooth pulp stimulation acts primarily upon small fibers, producing a brief, variable sensation. Twenty-eight subjects rated the strength and the unpleasantness of both noxious stimuli before and after receiving the specific pain reduction treatment. A significant reduction of reported unpleasantness and strength of stimulus was reported for both treatments when used for tooth pulp stimulation. However, a significant reduction of unpleasantness but not strength of noxious stimulus was reported for cold pressor pain. The authors noted that the subject's susceptibility to hypnosis was not a significant factor. Importantly, the research appears to indicate that these pain reduction treatments produced analgesia dependent upon the nature of the noxious stimulus.

In an experiment conducted by Carasso et al. (166), 26 cervical headache patients were treated with medical hypnosis, relaxation training, and group therapy. Results indicated that when specific suggestions and exercises were included for the back and neck muscles, 95.66% of the patients reported significant improvement in the pain condition. Fifty-two percent reported complete relief and only one patient reported no change. Longitudinal follow-up revealed a stable rate of remission 10 months after discharge from treatment. It is interesting to note that all subjects participating in this study had previously been treated with more traditional treatments and yet symptoms had proved refractory prior to intervention via hypnosis.

## SUMMARY

Since the early 1900s investigators have sought techniques to gain voluntary control over physiologic events that have appeared to be mediated involuntarily. Bair (167) reported in a 1901 edition of *Psychological Review* that he had developed a rudimentary device attached to a kymograph to assist persons to learn voluntary control over ear movements. Bair undertook the study as a means to assess "the nature of the will." This chapter has presented some of the most important and recent findings concerning the field of biofeedback and relaxation therapies as they relate to "voluntary" control over the painful sequelae of cervical trauma. The various types of biofeedback and relaxation therapies have demonstrated some effectiveness in the treatment of muscular, vascular, and neurogenic pain disorders. Treatment has been utilized not only in the reduction of pain but also to assist the patient to obtain greater control over diminished physiologic function. While it is evident that these various approaches share some common elements, there is a notable lack in the literature of their application to the management of cervical related pain. Although headache and low back pain studies are preponderant in the biofeedback and relaxation therapy literature, few researchers have extended what appear to be useful and cost-effective treatment modalities to cervical pain rehabilitation. The Foundation for Research in Head Pain and Related Disorders (168) acknowledges the role of biofeedback and suggests its use as a first-round treatment for migraine and muscle contraction headache. While some of these headaches may be related to and/or caused by cervical trauma, rehabilitation (via biofeedback) of any underlying cervical pathology has been for the most part neglected.

EMG, EEG, thermal, and PPG biofeedback and the relaxation therapies offer the clinician a noninvasive, self-regulatory mechanism for moderation of pain. A great diversity of methodology and resultant findings have been reported by many researchers in the field. While conflicting claims exist for the treatments outlined above, improvement has very often been observed and maintained for many years after discontinuing the intervention and maintained even in the absence of continued medication. There are no deleterious side effects associated with the treatments. According to Lake (169) "there is accumulating evidence that biofeedback is a cost-effective treatment that has been shown to lead to a substantial reduction in medical and hospital expenses for some people." However, at this juncture the evidence demands continued research to provide the clinician with a better understanding, thereby yielding greater utility and effect. There is little doubt that the techniques of biofeedback and the relaxation therapies will continue to offer clinical efficacy as pain moderators. The important concept inherent in such intervention is that the techniques described place the responsibility for treatment on the patient. Self-efficacy and a sense of internal locus of control become established within the patient. It is hoped that, as the techniques become improved and refined via convergent and discriminant validation studies, the cervical trauma patient will benefit from greater reduction of pain and enhanced rehabilitation.

## REFERENCES

1. Muller J: *Handbuch der Physiologie des Menschen*. Coblenz, Verlag von J. Holscher, 1837.
2. Birk L: *Biofeedback: Behavioral Medicine*. New York, Grune & Stratton, 1973.
3. Reich RA: Non-invasive treatment of vascular and contraction headache: a comparative longitudinal clinical study. *Headache* 29(1):34–41, 1989.
4. Reich BA: Biofeedback treatment of 684 chronic pain patients: a clinical assessment. Presented at the Vth World Congress on Pain of the International Association for the Study of Pain, Hamburg, Germany, August 1987.
5. Basmajian JV: Research foundations of EMG biofeedback in rehabilitation. *Biofeedback Self Regul* 13:275–298, 1988.
6. Blanchard EB, Applebaum E, Guarnieri P, Morrill B, Detinger MP: Five year prospective follow-up on the treatment of chronic headache with biofeedback and/or relaxation. *Headache* 27:580–583, 1987.
7. Furedy JJ, Riley DM: Classical and operant conditioning in biofeedback. In White L, Tursky B (eds): *Clinical Biofeedback: Efficacy and Mechanisms*. New York, The Guiford Press, 1982.
8. Marinacci AA, Horande M: Electromyography in neuromuscular re-education. *Bull LA Med Soc* 25(2):57–71, 1960.
9. Bandura A: Self-efficacy: toward a unifying theory of behavioral change. *Psychol Rev* 84:191–215, 1960.
10. Holroyd KA: Stress, coping, and the treatment of stress related illness. In McNamara JR (ed): *Behavioral Approaches in Medicine: Applications and Analysis*. New York, Plenum, 1979.
11. Flor H, Haag G, Turk DC, Koehler H: Efficacy of EMG biofeedback, pseudotherapy, and conventional medical treatment for chronic rheumatic back pain. *Pain* 17:21–31, 1983.
12. Nouwen A, Solinger JW: The effectiveness of EMG biofeedback training in low back pain. *Biofeedback Self Regul* 4:103–111, 1979.
13. Simons DG: Myofascial pain syndromes of the head, neck and low back. In Dubner R, Gebhart GF, Bonds MR (eds):

*Proceedings of the Vth World Congress on Pain*. Amsterdam, Elsevier, 1988.
14. Evaskus DS, Laskin DM: A biochemical measure of stress in patients with myofascial dysfunction syndrome. *J Dent Res* 51:1464–1466, 1972.
15. Ferraccioli G, Ghirelli L, Scita F, et al: EMG-biofeedback training in fibromyalgia syndrome. *J Rheumatol* 14(4):820–825, 1987.
16. Green BA, Callahan RA, Klose KJ, et al: Acute spinal cord injury: current concepts. *Clin Orthop* 154:125–135, 1981.
17. Saper JR: *Help for Headaches: A Guide to Understanding Their Causes and Finding the Best Method of Treatment*. New York, Warner Books, 1987.
18. de Vries HA: Quantitative electromyographic investigations of the spasm theory of muscle pain. *Am J Phys Med* 45:119–134, 1966.
19. Mense S, Stahnke M: Responses in the muscle afferent fibers of slow conduction velocity to contractions and ischemia in the cat. *J Physiol (Lond)* 342:383–397, 1983.
20. Travell J, Simons DG: *Myofascial Pain and Dysfunction: The Trigger Point Manual*. Baltimore, William & Wilkins, 1983.
21. Lance JW: *Mechanism and Management of Headache*, ed 3. London, Butterworths, 1978.
22. Jackson R: *The Cervical Syndrome*, ed 4. Springfield, IL, Charles C Thomas, 1978.
23. Mense S: Slowly conducting afferent fibers from deep tissues: neurobiological properties and central nervous actions. *Prog Sens Physiol* 6:139–219, 1986.
24. Dorpat TL, Holmes TH: Mechanisms of skeletal muscle pain and fatigue. *Arch Neurol Psychiatry* 74:628–640, 1955.
25. Peck CL, Kraft GH: Electromyograph biofeedback for pain related to muscle tension. *Arch Surg* 112:889–895, 1977.
26. Reich BA: Biofeedback in pain syndromes. Presented at the 3rd International Conference on Neurogenic and Musculoskeletal Pain, New York, November 1988.
27. Basmajian JV: Man's posture. *Arch Phys Med Rehabil* 46:26–36, 1965.
28. Hudzinski LG, Levenson H: Biofeedback behavioral treatment of headache with locus of control pain analysis: a 20-month retrospective study. *Headache* 25:380–386, 1985.
29. Smith WB: Biofeedback and relaxation training: the effect on headache and associated symptoms. *Headache* 27(9):511–514, 1987.
30. Stilson DW, Matus I, Ball G: Relaxation and subjective estimates of muscle tension: implications for a central efferent theory of muscle control. In Shapiro D, Stoyva J, Kamiya J, Barber TX, Miller N, Schwartz GE (eds): *Biofeedback and Behavioral Medicine*. Chicago, Aldine, 1979/80.
31. Marinacci AA: *Clinical Electromyography: A Brief Review of the Electrophysiology of the Motor Unit and Its Application to the Diagnosis of Lower Neuron Diseases, Perpheral Neuropathy and the Myopathies*. Los Angeles, San Lucas Press, 1955.
32. Hefferline RF: The role of proprioception in the control of behavior. *Trans NY Acad Sci* 20:739–764, 1958.
33. Harrison VF, Mortensen OA: Measurement of motor units in the tibialis anterior by EMG [abstract]. *Anat Rec* 136:207, 1960.
34. Basmajian JV: Control and training of individual motor units. *Science* 20:662–664, 1963.
35. Basmajian JV, Kulka CG, Marayan MG, Takebe K: Biofeedback treatment of foot drop after stroke compared with standard rehabilitation technique: effects on volun-

tary control and strength. *Arch Phys Med Rehabil* 56:231–236, 1975.

36. Booker HE, Rubow RT, Coleman PJ: Simplified feedback in neuromuscular retraining: an automated approach using electromyographic signals. *Arch Phys Med Rehabil* 50:631–625, 1969.

37. Brudny J, Grynbaum BB, Korein J: Spasmodic torticollis: Treatment by feedback display of the EMG. *Arch Pys Med Rehabil* 55:403–408, 1974.

38. Stoyva J, Budzynski TH: Cultivated low arousal: an antistress response? In DiCara LV (ed): *Recent Advances in Limbic and Autonomic Nervous System Research.* New York, Plenum, 1974.

39. Johnson HE, Garton WH: Muscle re-education in hemiplegia by use of electromyographic device. *Arch Phys Med Rehabil* 54:320–322, 1973.

40. Miller NE: Biofeedback evaluation of a new technic. *N Engl J Med* 290:684–685, 1974.

41. Herman R: *Neuromotor Control Systems: A Study of Physiological and Theoretical Concepts Leading to Therapeutic Application.* (Final report, 23P-551 15/3-03.) Philadelphia, Temple University School of Medicine, December 1977.

42. Surwit RS, Keefe FJ: Electromyographic biofeedback: behavioral treatment of neuromuscular disorders. *J Behav Med* 1:13–24, 1978.

43. Breznitz, H: Hope: researcher finds hope eases stress, effects outcome. *Am Psychol Assoc Monitor* 4:18, 1984.

44. Davidson RJ, Schwartz GE: The psychobiology of relaxation and relaxed states: multi-process theory. In Mostofsky DI (ed): *Behavior Control and Modification of Physiological Activity.* Englewood Cliffs, NJ, Prentice-Hall, 1976.

45. Carlson JB, Basilio CA, Heukulani JD: Transfer of EMG training: another look at the general relaxation issue. *Psychophysiology* 20:530–536, 1983.

46. Whatmore GB, Whatmore NJ, Fisher LD: Is frontalis activity a reliable indicator of the activity in other skeletal muscles? *Biofeedback Self Regul* 6:305–314, 1981.

47. Fridlund A, Fowler S, Pritchard D: Striate muscle tensional patterning in frontalis EMG biofeedback. *Psychophysiology* 17:47–55, 1980.

48. Davis P: Electromyographic feedback: generalization and the relative effects of feedback, instructions, and adaptation. *Psychophysiology* 17:604–612, 1980.

49. Alexander AB: An experimental test of assumptions relating to the use of electromyographic biofeedback as a general relaxation technique. *Psychophysiology* 12:656–662, 1975.

50. Shedivy DI, Kleinman KM: Lack of correlation between frontalis EMG and either neck EMG or verbal ratings of tension. *Psychophysiology* 14:182–186, 1977.

51. Cotton DHG, Lawson JS: A factor analytic investigation of muscle tension: implications for EMG training. Paper presented at the 3rd Annual Meeting of the Society for Behavioral Medicine, Chicago, Illinois, March 1982.

52. Kato M, Tanji J: Volitionally controlled single motor units in human finger muscles. *Brain Res* 40:435–437, 1972.

53. Ladd H, Johnsson B, Lindegren U: The learning process for fine neuromuscular control in skeletal muscles of man. *Electromyog Clin Neurophysiol* 12:213–223, 1972.

54. Budzynski TH, Stoyva JM: An instrument for producing deep muscle relaxation by means of analog information feedback. *J Appl Behav Anal* 2:213–237, 1969.

55. Qualls PJ, Sheehan PW: Electromyograph biofeedback as a relaxation technique: a critical appraisal and reassessment. *Psychol Bull* 91:21–42, 1981.

56. Merletti R, Sabbahi MA, DeLuca CJ: Median frequency of the myoelectric signal: effects of muscle ischemia and cooling. *Eur J Appl Physiol* 52:258–265, 1984.

57. Hagberg M: Muscular endurance and surface electromyogram in isometric and dynamic exercise. *J Appl Physiol* 51(1):1–7, 1981.

58. Pertrofsky JS, Lind AR: The influence of temperature on the amplitude and frequency components of EMG during brief and sustained isometric contractions. *Eur J Appl Physiol* 44:189–200, 1980.

59. Hellebrandt FA, Hout SJ, Partridge MJ, Walter CE: Tonic neck reflexes in exercise of stress in man. *Am J Phys Med* 41:45–55, 1962.

60. Basmajian JV: Methods of training the conscious control of motor units. *Arch Phys Med Rehabil* 48:12–19, 1967.

61. Middaugh SJ, Kee WG: Advances in electromyographic monitoring and biofeedback in the treatment of chronic cervical and low back pain. In Eisenberg MG, Grzesiak RC (eds): *Advances in Clinical Rehabilitation.* New York, Springer, 1987, vol 1, pp 137–172.

62. Reich BA: Biofeedback for pain. In *Proceedings of the International Symposia on Neurogenic and Myofascial Pain.* New York, Franklin Hospital Medical Center, 1986.

63. Travel J, Rinzler SH: The myofascial genesis of pain. *Postgrad Med J* 11:425–434, 1952.

64. MacNab I: The "whiplash syndrome". *Orthop Clin North Am* 2:389–403, 1971.

65. Graff-Radford SB, Reeves JL, Jaeger B: Management of chronic head and neck pain: the effectiveness of altering factors perpetuating myofascial pain. *Headache* 27:186–190, 1987.

66. Jette DU, Falkel JE, Trombly C: Effect of intermittent, supine cervical traction on the myoelectric activity of the upper trapezius muscle in subjects with neck pain. *Phys Ther* 65(8):1173–1176, 1985.

67. Bush C, Ditto B, Feuerstein M: A controlled evaluation of paraspinal EMG biofeedback in the treatment of chronic low back pain. *Health Psychol* 4:307–321, 1985.

68. Nouwen A: EMG biofeedback used to reduce standing levels of paraspinal muscle tension in chronic low back pain. *Pain* 17:353–360, 1983.

69. Pozniak-Patewicz E: "Cephalic" spasm of head and neck muscles. *Headache* 15:261–266, 1976.

70. Hudzinski LG, Lawrence GS: Significance of EMG surface electrode placement models and headache findings. *Headache* 28:30–35, 1988.

71. Ahern DK, Follick MJ, Council JR, Laser-Wolston N, Litchman H: Comparison of lumbar paravertebral EMG patterns in chronic low back pain patients and non-patient controls. *Pain* 34:153–160, 1988.

72. Miller DJ: Comparisons of electromyographic activity in lumbar paraspinal muscles of subjects with and without chronic low back pain. *Phys Ther* 65:1347–1354, 1985.

73. Cohen MJ, Naliboff BD, Schandler SL, McArthur C: Comparisons of electromyographic response patterns during posture and stress tasks in chronic low back pain patients and controls. *J Psychosom Res* 30:131–141, 1986.

74. Arena JG, Sherman RA, Bruno GM, Young TR: Electromyographic recordings of 5 types of low back pain subjects and non-pain controls in different positions. *Pain* 37(1):57–65, 1989.

75. Middaugh SJ, Garwood MK: A new approach to the key muscle hypothesis in EMG biofeedback. Presented at the 20th annual meeting of the Association for Applied Psy-

chophysiology and Biofeedback, San Diego, California, March 17–22, 1989.

76. Bengtsson A, Henriksson KG, Larsson J: Muscle biopsy in primary fibromyalgia. *Scand J Rheumatol* 15:1–6, 1986.

77. Bischoff C, Traue HC: Myogenic headache. In Holroyd KA, Scholte B, Zenz H (eds): *Perspectives in Research on Headache*. Lewiston, NY, CJ Hogrefe, Inc, 1983.

78. Haynes SN, Gannon LR, Cuevas J, Heiser P, Hamilton J, Katranides M: The psychophysiological assessment of muscle-contraction headache subjects during headache and nonheadache conditions. *Psychophysiology* 20:393–399, 1983.

79. Krusen EM: Cervical pain syndromes. *Arch Phys Med Rehabil* 49:376–382, 1968.

80. Dunn EJ, Blazar S: Soft-tissue injuries of the lower cervical spine. *Instr Course Lect* 36:499–512, 1987.

81. Edmeads J: Headaches and head pains associated with diseases of the cervical spine. *Med Clin North Am* 62:533–544, 1978.

82. Barnat MR: Post traumatic headaches I: demographics, injuries, headache and health status. *Headache* 26:271–277, 1986.

83. Winston KR: Whiplash and its relationship to migraine. *Headache* 27(8):452–457, 1987.

84. Bartschi-Rochaix W: *Migraine Cervicale: Das Encephale Syndrom Nach Halswirbeltrauma*. Berne, Verlag Hans Huber, 1949.

85. Diamond S, Montrose D: The value of biofeedback in the treatment of chronic headache: a four year retrospective study. *Headache* 24:5–18, 1984.

86. Brudny J, Grynbaum BB, Korein J: New therapic modality for treatment of spasmodic torticollis. *Arch Phys Med Rehabil* 54:575, 1973.

87. Brudny J: Biofeedback in chronic neurological cases: therapeutic electromyography. In White L, Tursky B (eds): *Clinical Biofeedback: Efficacy and Mechanisms*. New York, The Guiford Press, 1982.

88. Cleeland CS: Biofeedback and other behavioral techniques in the treatment of disorders of voluntary movement. In Basmajian JV (ed): *Biofeedback: Principles and Practice for Clinicians*, ed 3. Baltimore, William & Wilkins, 1989.

89. Cleeland CS: Behavior techniques in the modification of spasmodic torticollis. *Neurology* 23:1241–1247, 1973.

90. Jacobs A, Felton GS: Visual feedback of myoelectric output to facilitate muscle relaxation in normal persons and patients with neck injuries. *Arch Phys Med Rehabil* 50:34–39, 1969.

91. Leplow B: Some mechanisms underlying biofeedback training in patients with idiopathic torticollis spasmodicus [abstract]. *Biofeedback Self Regul* 13:76, 1988.

92. Suurkula J, Haag GM: Relations between shoulder/neck disorders and EMG zero crossing shifts in female assembly workers using test contraction method. *Ergonomics* 30(11):1553–1564, 1987.

93. Maeda K: Occupational cervicobrachial disorder and its causative factors. *J Hum Ergol* 6:193–202, 1977.

94. Basmajian JV: *Muscles Alive*. Baltimore, Williams & Wilkins, 1967.

95. Triano JJ, Schultz AB: Correlation of objective measures of trunk motion and muscle function with low-back disability ratings. *Spine* 12:561–565, 1987.

96. Bancroft H, Milkin J: The blood flow through muscle during sustained contraction. *J Physiol (Lond)* 97:17, 1939.

97. Adler CS, Adler SM: Biofeedback psychotherapy for the treatment of headaches: a 5 year follow-up. *Headache* 16:189–191, 1975.

98. Andrasik F, Holroyd KA: Specific and nonspecific effects in the biofeedback treatment of tension headache: 3 year follow-up. *J Consul Clin Psychol* 51:634–636, 1983.

99. Anthony M, Lance LW: The role of serotonin in migraine. In Pearce J (ed): *Modern Topics in Migraine*. London, Heinemann, 1975.

100. Simons DJ, Wolff HG: Studies on headache: mechanisms off chronic posttraumatic headache. *Psychosom Med* 8:227–242, 1946.

101. Vijayan N: A new post-traumatic headache syndrome: clinical and theraputic observations. *Headache* 17:19–22, 1977.

102. Raynaud AG: *De l'Asphyxie Locale et de la Gangrene Synchequie des Extremites*. Paris, Rignoux. 1862.

103. Pariser KM, Bana DS, Molloy PJ, Messinger HB, Graham JR: Raynaud's phenomena in patients with classic migraine and tension headaches [abstract]. *Headache* 26:324, 1986.

104. Sexton RO, Maddock RC: When headache pain strikes. *Med Hypnoanalysis* 4(1):31–42, 1983.

105. Pfaffenrath V, Dandekar R, Pollmann W: Cervicogenic headache—the clinical picture, radiological findings and hypotheses on its pathophysiology. *Headache* 27(9):495–499, 1987.

106. Hohl M, Hopp E: Soft tissue injuries of the neck: factors influencing prognosis. *Orthop Trans* 2:29, 1978.

107. Hagberg M: Local shoulder muscle strain—symptoms and disorders. *J Hum Ergol* 11:99–108, 1982.

108. Bjelle A, Hagberg M, Michaelsson G: Occupational and individual factors in acute shoulder-neck disorders among industrial workers. *Br J Ind Med* 38:356–363, 1981.

109. Rouleau J, Denver DR: Electromyography (EMG) and temperature biofeedback of the "Pure Fibositis Syndrome." In *Proceedings of the Biofeedback Society of America 11th Annual Meeting*. New York, The Biofeedback Society of America, 1980, pp 142–145.

110. Brown B: *New Mind, New Body—Biofeedback: New Directions for the Mind*. New York, Harper & Row, 1974.

111. Melzack R, Perry C: Self-regulation of pain: the use of alpha-biofeedback and hypnotic training for the control of chronic pain. *Exp Neurol* 46:452–469, 1975.

112. Spiegel D, Bierre P, Rootenberg J: Hypnotic alteration of somatosensory perception. *Am J Psychiatry* 46:749–754, 1989.

113. Miltner W, Larbig W, Braun C: Biofeedback of somatosensory event-related potentials: can individual pain sensations be modified by biofeedback-induced self-control of event-related potentials? *Pain* 35:205–213, 1988.

114. Miltner W, Larbig W, Braun C: Biofeedback of visual evoked potentials. *Int J Neurosci* 29:291–303, 1986.

115. Dowman R, Rosenfeld JP: Operant conditioning of somatosensory evoked potentials (SEP) amplitude in rats. I. Specific changes in SEP amplitude and a naloxone-reversable somatotrophically specific change in facial nociception. *Brain Res* 333:201–212, 1985.

116. Finley WW: Biofeedback of very early potentials from the brain stem. In Elber T, Rochstroh B, Lutzenberger W, Birbaumer N (eds): *Self Regulation of the Brain and Behavior*. Heidelberg, Springer, 1984.

117. Bromm B: Pain-related components in the cerebral potential. Experimental and multivariate statistical approaches. In Bromm B (ed): *Pain Measurement in Man: Neurophysiological Correlates of Pain*. Amsterdam, Elsevier, 1984.

118. Chapman CR, Jacobsen RC: Assessment of analgesic states: can evoked potentials play a role? In Bromm B (ed): *Pain Measurement in Man: Neurophysiological Correlates in Pain.* Amsterdam, Elsevier, 1984.

119. Buchsbaum MS, Davis GC: Application of somatosensory event related potentials to experimental pain and the pharmacology of analgesia. In Lehmann D, Callaway E (eds): *Human Evoked Potentials: Applications and Problems.* New York, Plenum, 1979.

120. Hilgard ER, Hilgard JR: *Hypnosis in the Relief of Pain.* Los Angeles, William Kaufman, Inc, 1975.

121. Orben R: Urgent message. Salt and pepper. *The Wall Street Journal,* May 11, 1989.

122. Russo DC, Bird PO, Masek PJ: Assessment issues in behavioral medicine. *Behavioral Assessment* 2:1–18, 1980.

123. Mitchell SW: *Injuries of Nerves and Their Consequences.* Philadelphia, JB Lippincott, 1872.

124. Schwartz GE: Psychosomatic disorders and biofeedback: a psychobiological model of disregulation. In Maser JD, Seligman MEP (eds): *Psychopathology: Experimental Models.* San Francisco, WH Freeman, 1977.

125. Blumenthal JA: Relaxation therapy, biofeedback, and behavioral medicine. *Psychotherapy* 22(3):516–530, 1985.

126. Jessup BA, Neufeld RWJ, Merskey H: Biofeedback therapy for headache and other pains: an evaluative review. *Pain* 7:225–270, 1979.

127. Lichstein KL: *Clinical Relaxation Strategies.* New York, Wiley, 1988.

128. Marzuk P: Biofeedback for hypertension. *Ann Intern Med* 102:709–715, 1985.

129. Borgeat F, Elie R, Larouche LM: Pain response to voluntary muscle tension increases and biofeedback efficacy in tension headache. *Headache* 25(7):287–291, 1985.

130. Silver B, Blanchard E: Biofeedback or relaxation training in the treatment of psychophysiological disorders: or, are machines really necessary. *J Behav Med* 1:217–239, 1978.

131. Beiman I, Israel E, Johnson SA: During-training and post-training effects of live and taped extended progressive relaxation, self-relaxation, and electromyogram biofeedback. *J Consult Clin Psychol* 46:314–321, 1978.

132. Lacroix JM, Clark MA, Carson-Bock J, Doxey NC: Muscle-contraction headaches in multiple pain patients: treatment under worsening baseline conditions. *Arch Phys Med Rehabil* 67:14–18, 1986.

133. Sorbi M, Tellegen B: Differential effects of training in relaxation and stress-coping in patients with migraine. *Headache* 26:473–481, 1986.

134. Richter IL, et al: Cognitive and relaxation treatment of paediatric migraine. *Pain* 25:195–203, 1986.

135. Attanasio V, Andrasik F, Blanchard EB: Cognitive therapy and relaxation training in muscle contraction headache: efficacy and cost-effectiveness. *Headache* 27:254–260, 1987.

136. Peters RK, Bemson H, Parker D: Daily relaxation breaks in the working population: effects on self-reported measures of health, performance and well-being. *Am J Public Health* 67:946–959, 1977.

137. Benson H: *The Relaxation Response.* New York, Morrow, 1975.

138. West MA: Meditation and somatic arousal reduction. *Am Psychol* 40:717–719, 1985.

139. Jacobsen E: *Progressive Relaxation.* Chicago, University of Chicago Press, 1938.

140. Jacobsen E: Neuromuscular controls in man: methods of self direction in health and disease. *Am J Psychol* 68:549–561, 1955.

141. Schultz JH, Luthe W: *Autogenic Training.* New York, Grune & Stratton, 1959.

142. Burrow T: Kymograph studies of physiological concomitants in two types of attentional adaptation. *Nature* 142:142–156, 1938.

143. Wolpe J: *Psychotherapy by Reciprocal Inhibition.* Stanford, CA, Stanford University Press, 1958.

144. Lazarus AA: *In the Mind's Eye: The Power of Imagery for Personal Enrichment.* New York, The Guilford Press, 1977.

145. Smith JC: Meditation as psychotherapy: a review of the literature. *Psychol Bull* 82:558–564, 1975.

146. Wallace RK: Physiological effects of transcendental meditation. *Science* 167:1751–1754, 1970.

147. Bradley LA, Young LD, Anderson KO, et al: Effects of cognitive behavioral therapy on rheumatoid arthritis pain: one year follow-up. In Dubner R, Gebhart GF, Bonds MR (eds): *Proceedings of the Vth World Congess on Pain.* Amsterdam, Elsevier, 1988.

148. Sternbach RA: The psychology of pain. In Bonica JJ, Fassard DA (eds): *Advances in Pain Research and Therapy.* New York, Raven Press, 1976.

149. Weisenberg M: Understanding the pain phenomena. In Rachman S (ed): *Contributions to Medical Psychology.* London, Oxford Press, 1980.

150. Fordyce WE: Behavioral concepts in chronic pain and illness. In Davidson PO (ed): *The Behavioral Management of Anxiety, Depression and Pain.* New York, Brunner/Mazel, 1976.

151. Hockersmith VW: Biofeedback applications in chronic low back disability. Presented at the American Psychological Association meeting, Chicago, August 1975.

152. Turk DC, Meichenbaum D, Genest M: *Pain and Behavioral Medicine: A Cognitive-Behavioral Approach.* New York, Guilford Press, 1983.

153. Bernheim H: *Suggestive Therapeutics.* New York, GP Putnam's Sons, 1889.

154. Janet P: *Psychological Healing: A Historical and Clinical Study.* London, George Allen and Unwin, Ltd, vol 1, 1925.

155. Charcot JM: La foi qui guerit. As quoted in Janet P: *Psychological Healing.* London, George Allen and Unwin Ltd, vol 1, 1925.

156. Breuer J, Freud A: *Studies on Hysteria.* New York, Basic Books, 1957.

157. Hilgard ER: The pschophysiology of pain reduction through hypnosis. In Chertok L (ed): *Psychophysiological Mechanisms of Hypnosis: An International Symposium Sponsored by the International Brain Research Organization and the Centre de Recherceh, Institu de Psychiatrie La Rochefoucauld, Paris.* Berlin, Springer-Verlag, 1969.

158. Tart CT: *Altered States of Consciousness.* New York, Wiley, 1969.

159. Barber TX: *Hypnosis: A Scientific Approach.* New York, Van Nostrand Reinhold, 1969.

160. Barber TX: Hypnosuggestive procedures in the treatment of clinical pain: implications for theories of hypnosis and suggestive therapy. In Milton CJ, Meagher RB (eds): *Handbook of Health Care Clinical Psychology.* New York, Plenum, 1982.

161. Wall PD: The physiology of controls on sensory pathways with special reference to pain. In Chertok L (ed): *Psychophysiological Mechanisms of Hypnosis: An International Symposium Sponsored by the International Brain Research Organization and the Centre de Recherche, Institu de Psychiatrie La Rochefoucauld, Paris.* Berlin, Springer-Verlag, 1969.

162. McGlashan TH, Evans FJ, Orne MJ: The nature of hyp-

notic analgesia and placebo response to experimental pain. *Psychosom Med* 31:227–246, 1969.

163. Erickson M: An introduction to the study and application of hypnosis for pain control. Presented at the International Congress of Hypnosis and Psychosomatic Medicine, Paris, 1965.

164. Kihlstrom JF: The cognitive unconscious. *Science* 237:1455–1452, 1987.

165. Houle M, McGrath P, Moran G, Garrett OJ: The efficacy of hypnosis- and relaxation-induced analgesia on two dimensions of pain for cold pressor and electrical tooth pulp stimulation. *Pain* 28:30–35, 1988.

166. Carasso RL, Kleinhautz M, Peded O, Yehuda S: Treat-ment of cervical headache with hypnosis, suggestive therapy, and relaxation techniques. *Am J Clin Hypn* 27(4):216–218, 1985.

167. Bair JH: Development of voluntary control. *Psychol Rev* 8:474–501, 1901.

168. Baumel BS: Treatment of migraine. In *The Migraine Dilemma*. The Foundation for Research in Head Pain and Related Disorders, 1989, p 10.

169. Lake AE: Relaxation therapy and biofeedback in headache management. In Saper JR (ed): *Help for Headaches: A guide to Understanding Their Causes and Finding the Best Method of Treatment*. New York, Warner Books, 1987.

## 12

# ANALGESIC AND ANTI-INFLAMMATORY MEDICATION

*Glen D. Solomon*

## NONSTEROIDAL ANTI-INFLAMMATORY DRUGS

### HISTORY

The use of salicylates, in the form of extract of willow bark, for the treatment of pain and inflammation dates back to antiquity, with ancient physicians, including Hippocrates, recommending their use. In 1767, the Reverend Edward Stone wrote about his use of willow bark to treat fevers. The active agent, salicylin, was isolated in 1826, and salicylic acid was derived from salicylin in 1838 and synthesized in 1852. The modern use of salicylates began in the late 1800s when Mac-Lagan rediscovered the value of salicylates. It was accepted theory at that time that one should seek a medicine for a given disease by testing plants that had something in common with the disease. Since acute rheumatism (rheumatic fever) occurred in people exposed to damp environments, MacLagan resorted to the willow tree as a source of curative medicine since it grew in wet places. The salicin extracted from the willow bark proved effective in relieving the pain and fever of his patients, as he reported in *The Lancet* in 1876 (1).

Felix Hoffmann, a German chemist working for the Bayer Company in Germany, sought a preparation of salicylate to treat his father, who suffered with severe arthritis but developed dyspepsia from sodium salicylate and salicylic acid. He decided to try the synthetic salicylate preparation *acetylsalicylic acid*, which had originally been pre-

pared by the French chemist von Gerhardt in 1853. The Bayer Company introduced acetylsalicylic acid in 1899, coining the name "aspirin" from "a" for acetyl, "spir" for the *Spiraea* plant genus (salicylic acid was extracted from the flowers *Spiraea ulmaria*, or meadowsweet, rather than willow bark), and "in," which was added to improve the name. Aspirin was the drug that began the modern pharmaceutical industry (1).

It was 50 years before the next nonsteroidal anti-inflammatory drug (NSAID), phenylbutazone, was introduced in 1949. The fenamates and indomethacin were introduced in the early 1960s, followed by ibuprofen in 1969 and naproxen in 1970. Since then, over 30 additional NSAIDs have been developed (Table 12.1).

### PHARMACOLOGY

The NSAIDs are considered peripherally acting analgesics, implying activity at the site of pain origin by inhibition of the pathways that form prostaglandins and related autocoids (2). All NSAIDs inhibit the enzyme cyclo-oxygenase, thereby reducing tissue levels of prostaglandins. Prostaglandins act as mediators of inflammation and in the amplification of nociceptive pain (2).

NSAIDs appear to have both peripheral and central analgesic actions. While the anti-inflammatory effect of NSAIDs is mediated by the action on prostaglandins, the significant disproportion of analgesia and anti-inflammation noted with

168

**Table 12.1.**
**Major Classes of Nonsteroidal Anti-inflammatory Drugs[a]**

| Salicylates | Acetic Acids | Propionic Acids | Fenamic Acids | Pyrazoles | Oxicams |
|---|---|---|---|---|---|
| Aspirin | Indomethacin | Ibuprofen | Meclofenamate | Phenylbutazone | Piroxicam |
| Diflunisal | Sulindac | Naproxen | Mefenamic acid | | |
| | Tolmetin | Fenoprofen | | | |
| | Diclofenac | Ketoprofen | | | |
| | | Flurbiprofen | | | |

[a]Data from Buchanan and Keane (1) and Halpern (2).

certain agents suggests that other mechanisms may be at work (3). In order to prove that mechanisms other than prostaglandins mediate analgesia, NSAIDs were given to animals that cannot synthesize prostaglandins as a result of diets lacking in essential fatty acids. NSAIDs were effective analgesics in this model (1). Direct effects of salicylates on the central nervous system (CNS) have been observed and suggest a hypothalamic site for both analgesic and antipyretic effects (4). Salicylates do not appear to affect the reticular activating system (4).

Unlike the opiate drugs, the analgesia produced by NSAIDs is characterized by a ceiling dose, defined as a dose beyond which additional drug produces no further analgesia (3). The ceiling dose varies among individuals, as does dose-related toxicity (3). The analgesia generated by NSAIDs causes neither physical dependency nor tolerance.

All currently available NSAIDs are weak acids with $pK_a$ values of 3.5–5 and thus demonstrate either hydrophilic (in the ionized state) or lipophilic (nonionized state) properties, dependent upon the pH of the surrounding milieu. All are highly bound to plasma proteins, especially albumin, and their analgesic and anti-inflammatory activity directly correlates with the degree of albumin binding. This differs from many drugs in which the free drug is active while the bound drug is inactive (1). The individual responses of NSAIDs cannot be attributed to plasma concentration or pharmacokinetic behavior. The duration of analgesic action exceeds the plasma half-life, possibly as a result of tissue accumulation. Some evidence suggests that circadian rhythms may be important in determining the clinical efficacy of nonsteroidal drugs (1).

All currently available NSAIDs are principally administered via the gastrointestinal (GI) tract by the oral route. Additionally, indomethacin is available in rectal suppositories, diclofenac can be ad-

ministered intramuscularly, and flurbiprofen can be absorbed through the buccal mucosa. NSAIDs are weak acids and can be absorbed through the stomach by passive diffusion, although the large surface area of the small intestine usually makes it the major absorptive site (1). When administered with food, several NSAIDs have a reduced maximum concentration (aspirin, flurbiprofen, and diflunisal), whereas others have a reduced time to maximal concentration (ibuprofen, naproxen, sulindac, diclofenac, indomethacin, and piroxicam), but these differences are not clinically significant. The concomitant use of antacids or type 2 histamine receptor inhibitors does not inhibit absorption by the small intestine, and therefore does not alter the clinical efficacy of the NSAIDs (1).

The distribution and metabolism of NSAIDs may be altered by advancing age. In elderly patients, plasma volume, lean body mass, and serum albumin are all decreased. Since NSAIDs are predominantly bound to albumin, and since renal function, hepatic blood flow, and cardiac output are also decreased in the elderly, it is likely that more unbound drug will be in equilibrium with the tissues. This may explain some of the increased toxicity seen with NSAIDs in elderly patients. Benoxaprofen was removed from the market in 1982 after liver damage was found to occur in the elderly, and phenylbutazone was found to cause aplastic anemia and agranulocytosis predominantly in elderly patients.

## SIDE EFFECTS

Toxic effects from NSAIDs are common, and constitute over one quarter of the total adverse drug reactions reported in the United Kingdom (5). Several of these drugs have been withdrawn because of an unacceptably high prevalence of adverse effects, including benoxaprofen, which caused fatal cholestatic jaundice; zomepirac, which caused fatal anaphylactoid reactions; and

**Table 12.2.**
**Approximate Ratings of Side Effects**[a]

| Drug | Upper GI Ulceration | Other GI | Skin | CNS | Heme | Liver | Renal |
|---|---|---|---|---|---|---|---|
| Aspirin | 3+[b] | 4+ | + | + | + | + | + |
| Ibuprofen | 2+ | 3+ | + | + | + | 0 | 0 |
| Naproxen | + | 2+ | + | 2+ | | 0 | 0 |
| Fenoprofen | 3+ | 4+ | + | 3 | 0 | 0 | + |
| Ketoprofen | 2+ | 3+ | + | 0 | 0 | 0 | 0 |
| Flurbiprofen | 2+ | 3+ | 0 | 2+ | + | 0 | 0 |
| Diclofenac | 2+ | 2+ | + | + | +/− | +/− | 0 |
| Meclofenamic acid | 2+ | 3+ | | | | | |
| Mefenamic acid | + | 2+ | 3+ | 0 | 0 | | |
| Indomethacin | 3+ | 4+ | + | 2+ | + | 0 | + |
| Sulindac | + | 3+ | 2+ | + | + | +/− | + |
| Tolmetin | + | + | + | | | | |
| Diflunisal | 2+ | 2+ | + | + | | | |
| Piroxicam | 3+ | 4+ | 0 | 3+ | 0 | 0 | 0 |
| Phenylbutazone | + | 4+ | | | 3+ | + | + |

[a]Data from Rainsford (5).
[b]Incidence of the individual side effects:
+/− = 0.1%
    + = 0.1–5%
  2+ = 5–10%
  3+ = 10–15%
  4+ = 20%

suprofen, which caused flank pain and renal disease.

The most frequent side effects from NSAIDs are GI reactions, including dyspepsia, heartburn, nausea, vomiting, diarrhea, constipation, and generalized abdominal pain (Table 12.2). Gastrointestinal ulceration and hemorrhage are much less common, and their occurrence is poorly correlated with the symptoms of abdominal pain (5). Most NSAIDs cause bleeding in the upper GI tract, but those drugs with significant enterohepatic recirculation (indomethacin) or with slow-release formulations may cause lower intestinal lesions. Patients with inflammatory bowel disease may have exacerbations or hemorrhage following the use of these drugs.

The frequency of GI ulceration and hemorrhage can vary considerably between different NSAIDs. The potency of prostaglandin synthesis inhibition appears to correspond to the frequency of GI side effects. Drugs such as aspirin, indomethacin, piroxicam and fenoprofen have the greatest propensity to cause ulceration, whereas naproxen, ibuprofen, sulindac, and tolmetin have the least propensity to cause peptic ulceration (5).

Another GI side effect from NSAIDs is esophageal irritation. This is caused by direct chemical irritation in patients with prolonged esophageal transit time, such as elderly patients who take the tablets with small amounts of water immediately before retiring to bed. Pancreatitis is a rare complication of NSAID use, but has been reported with sulindac, indomethacin, and mefenamic acid (5).

Dermatologic side effects from NSAIDs are second in frequency to GI complaints. Skin rashes and photosensitivity reactions are the most common dermatologic side effects, and are particularly frequent with indomethacin and piroxicam. These problems are generally mild. Severe and potentially fatal skin reactions such as Stevens-Johnson syndrome, toxic epidermal necrolysis, and erythema multiforme are rare, but can occur with phenylbutazone, piroxicam, sulindac, and meclofenamate (5).

Renal effects of NSAIDs are of great clinical significance in the elderly patient, the hypertensive patient, or the patient taking diuretics, and have been reviewed in several major review articles (6–8). Prostaglandins serve an important role in maintaining renal vasodilation and ensuring adequate renal blood flow. Under normal conditions, prostaglandins do not have a major role in maintaining renal blood flow (6). Under conditions of acute hypotension, salt depletion, general anesthesia, heart failure, or cirrhosis, prostaglandin production increases to autoregulate renal blood flow and glomerular filtration (8). This autoregulatory effect is inhibited by NSAID therapy, causing a decrease in renal blood flow and glomerular filtration rate (GFR). A decrease in GFR leads to increased water and electrolyte reabsorption in the proximal tubule. Inhibition of prostaglandin $E_2$ allows increased transport of chloride and sodium in the ascending limb of the loop of Henle. Therefore, prostaglandin inhibition by NSAIDs may result in increased sodium, chloride, and water retention.

NSAIDs can block the renal relase of renin via the inhibition of vasodilating prostaglandins. The inhibition of renin release can, in turn, decrease the release of aldosterone, leading to hyperkalemia. The hyperkalemia occasionally reported with NSAIDs is thought to be due to this inhibition of renin and aldosterone release.

The most common cause of drug-induced chronic renal failure is "analgesic nephropathy," characterized by interstitial nephritis and papillary necrosis. While phenacetin is frequently thought to be the major drug responsible for analgesic nephropathy, aspirin and virtually all NSAIDs can produce papillary necrosis (7). Actual cases resulting from NSAIDs have been infrequent. Data suggest that it is the combination of acetaminophen (or phenacetin) with aspirin that leads to direct tissue damage at the renal papillary tip, and that the individual agents alone are not particularly nephrotoxic (9). Patients with diabetes mellitus and sickle cell anemia, who have an inherent risk of developing papillary necrosis, may be more prone to this potential complication of nonsteroidal therapy (7).

Acute renal failure following the administration of NSAIDs has been reported. Clinical risk factors include advanced age, use of diuretic drugs, and evidence of renovascular disease (longstanding hypertension, diabetes, or atherosclerotic cardiovascular disease) (10). Several cases of reversible acute renal failure have occurred from the combination of indomethacin and triamterene, including four cases in healthy, young medical students (11). In addition to the drug interaction with triamterene, some NSAIDs may antagonize the antihypertensive effects of betablockers, thiazide diuretics, and spironolactone (7).

When acute renal failure develops from NSAIDs, its onset is usually within 24 h of the initiation of nonsteroidal therapy, and is often associated with a marked diminution in urine output.

The microscopic urinalysis remains unchanged, but serum potassium levels may rise to high levels. Renal failure will usually reverse rapidly after withdrawal of the nonsteroidal agent (7).

The most nephrotoxic NSAIDs are fenoprofen (6) and indomethacin (7). Of all the NSAID-induced renal disease reported in the medical literature as of 1985, fenoprofen was responsible for 50% of the cases of nephrotic syndrome, 30% of the cases of acute tubular necrosis, and 28% of the cases of acute interstitial nephritis (6). Sulindac appears to cause little nephrotoxicity, and has been safely used when other NSAIDs have caused acute renal insufficiency (12). Sulindac is absorbed as the inactive drug and converted to the active sulfide form by the liver. The active sulfide form inhibits extrarenal cyclo-oxygenase activity, but has no effect on renal prostaglandins (6). Although acute tubular necrosis is unlikely with sulindac, the risk of immune-mediated renal diseases does exist.

The most common CNS side effect of NSAIDs is a nonspecific headache. Indomethacin causes the greatest incidence of headache. Salicylates cause a reversible hearing loss and tinnitus, which usually can be eliminated by reducing the dosage. Aseptic meningitis has occurred in patients taking ibuprofen, sulindac, and tolmetin, and appears to occur most frequently in patients with systemic lupus erythematosus who have taken ibuprofen (5).

Hematologic toxicity, including fatal aplastic anemia and granulocytopenia, has occurred from the use of phenylbutazone. Because of the risk of aplastic anemia, the duration of use of phenylbutazone should be limited to no more than 1 week (4). Aplastic anemia has also occurred with many other NSAIDs, including aspirin, indomethacin, ibuprofen, diclofenac, fenoprofen, naproxen, sulindac, and piroxicam (5).

## DRUGS

### Acetaminophen

Although it is not characterized as a NSAID, acetaminophen is used as an alternative to aspirin for its analgesic and antipyretic uses. Acetaminophen is the primary metabolite of phenacetin, metabolized primarily by the hepatic microsomal enzymes. Some other metabolites of phenacetin are responsible for methemoglobin formation and lysis of red blood cells.

Like aspirin, acetaminophen relieves pain of

moderate intensity. Phenacetin, unlike aspirin or acetaminophen, can cause drowsiness, euphoria, stimulation, and relaxation. When discontinued after chronic overuse, phenacetin can cause restlessness and excitability for 3 or 4 days.

The mechanism of analgesia of acetaminophen is unknown. It is an active inhibitor of prostaglandin synthetase of the brain, but has little effect on prostaglandin synthesis elsewhere. With its lack of synovial prostaglandin inhibition, acetaminophen has no efficacy as an antirheumatic agent.

In recommended doses, acetaminophen is usually well tolerated. Even the most common adverse effect, skin rash, is rare. It does not cause GI bleeding or gastric irritation. The nephrotoxicity of phenacetin or acetaminophen in combination with NSAIDs (analgesic nephropathy) was discussed earlier. Hematologic reactions have been rarely reported with acetaminophen, and include thrombocytopenia and pancytopenia. Unlike aspirin, acetaminophen does not affect platelet aggregation. Phenacetin has been associated with hemolytic anemia and methemoglobinemia, usually as a consequence of chronic overdose.

The most serious adverse effect of acetaminophen and phenacetin is dose-dependent and potentially fatal hepatic necrosis. Hepatotoxicity may occur after 10–15 g of acetaminophen, while 25 g or more is potentially fatal. Self-poisoning with large doses of acetaminophen is a common method of suicide in Great Britain. Acetylcysteine, given within 10 hr of acetaminophen ingestion, may reduce the severity of liver injury. At usual doses, acetaminophen does not cause liver injury.

The major therapeutic use of acetaminophen is for moderate analgesia in patients with peptic ulcer disease, coagulopathy, or thrombocytopenia, or who are taking medications that contraindicate the use of NSAIDs. It is particularly valuable for occasional mild analgesic or antipyretic use in patients already on chronic nonsteroidal therapy. The chronic use of acetaminophen with a NSAID should be avoided because of the risk of analgesic nephropathy.

## Aspirin

Introduced in 1899, aspirin is the oldest of the salicylates still in use. Salicylates are available in hundreds of forms and combinations, with an annual consumption of pills in the billions.

The absorption of aspirin does not differ greatly from that of NSAIDs in general. The serum level of salicylate (the primary metabolite of aspirin) is poorly related to the dose ingested. A small increase in dose may lead to a profound increase in serum level. The half-life of salicylate is many hours, and is directly proportional to the serum level. Therefore, the higher the serum level the slower the disappearance of the drug from serum. The two major determinants of serum levels of salicylate are urinary pH and the rate of conjugation to glycine.

Concomitant ingestion of antacids facilitates absorption of the drug by accelerating gastric emptying, and also facilitates excretion by the kidney. Accordingly, withdrawal of antacids can cause a sudden rise in serum salicylate levels. Since some aspirin products are marketed as combination drugs with antacids (i.e., Bufferin, Ascriptin), a change in brand may lead to significant changes in serum level.

Aspirin is an effective analgesic for various kinds of pain. Several double-blind studies have confirmed that aspirin is a more effective analgesic than placebo. Aspirin is classified as a mild analgesic, equivalent to moderate doses of codeine and less potent than full doses of narcotic analgesics, but more effective than narcotics against inflammatory pain. Aspirin's dose-response curve for analgesia is not known. A maximum response is usually reached with a dose of 600–625 mg in an adult. As with other NSAIDs, the analgesia provided by aspirin is characterized by a ceiling dose above which additional dosage produces no further analgesia.

The major indications for aspirin are inflammation, pain, and fever. The antipyretic and analgesic actions require only modest doses of one or two tablets, four to six times a day. This generally yields a serum salicylate level of 5 mg/dl. Anti-inflammatory doses of aspirin require a salicylate level of between 20 and 30 mg/dl, which may require eight to 20 tablets a day.

Drug interactions between the coumarin family of anticoagulants and aspirin are important because of the wide use of aspirin products. Aspirin may have some minor effects on prothrombin time, and may reduce the amount of anticoagulant needed to maintain a given prothrombin time. Of more importance is the inhibition of platelet aggregation and the increased risk of bleeding when aspirin is used in conjunction with oral anticoagulants.

In low doses, aspirin raises serum uric acid levels; at higher doses it may lower uric acid levels. Aspirin, in any dose, can block the uricosuric action of both probenecid and sulfinpyrazone and should not be used together with them.

Other notable drug interactions with aspirin include the potentiation of hypoglycemic effects of the sulfonylurea drugs, the enhancement of the bone marrow suppressive effects of methotrexate, and the augmentation of the gastric irritant effect of alcoholic beverages.

While all drugs are best avoided during pregnancy, for some patients the use of a nonsteroidal drug is necessary. Aspirin does not appear to increase the risk of congenital malformation, but does add some risk of prolonged gestation and labor and an increase in maternal perinatal bleeding. Neither hypoglycemia nor bleeding problems are more common in babies born of mothers taking salicylates.

Salicylate toxicity or overdose in adults may be manifest by dyspnea, confusion, ataxia, oliguria, or renal insufficiency. Elderly patients are the usual victims of salicylate intoxication, usually when a supervening event causes acidosis and alters the metabolism of aspirin to cause a rise in serum levels. Salicylate intoxication can be initially marked by hyperventilation and respiratory alkalosis, compensated with renal excretion of bicarbonate and a drop in plasma bicarbonate levels. With severe toxicity metabolic acidosis ensues, characterized by a low plasma bicarbonate concentration, decreased blood pH, and normal plasma $P_{CO_2}$. Respiratory depression occurs with toxic doses of salicylate, producing a respiratory acidosis in the setting of a true metabolic acidosis.

## Ibuprofen

Ibuprofen is the prototype of the propionic acid nonsteroidal drugs. Originally introduced as a prescription drug in the United States in 1974, its widespread use and safety profile allowed it to be released as a lower dose over-the-counter preparation several years later.

Ibuprofen is well absorbed and reaches peak serum levels in 1–2 hr. It has a half-life of 2 hr and does not accumulate in tissues that are not in equilibrium with the plasma. It is metabolized in the liver into two pharmacologically inactive metabolites, and is completely excreted in the urine within 24 hr (13). A dose of 2400 mg/day of ibuprofen is equivalent to 4000 mg/day of aspirin in anti-inflammatory effect (2).

Ibuprofen is analgesic in low doses, with its anti-inflammatory effect occurring at higher, more prolonged dosages (13). A single 400-mg dose has analgesic effect in dental pain, postpartum pain, soft tissue injuries, and dysmenorrhea. In the acute treatment of migraine headache, ibuprofen was superior to acetaminophen in reducing the severity and duration of headache (14).

Drug interactions with ibuprofen are uncommon and probably of no clinical significance. There is a slight reduction in peak serum levels when given with aspirin or naproxen, although there may actually be increased clinical effect. Ibuprofen may slightly raise plasma digoxin levels, but not to a clinically relevant degree. Unlike aspirin, ibuprofen does not interact with coumarin anticoagulants nor change prothrombin time (13). The anti-platelet aggregation effect of ibuprofen may still create a problem for a patient on oral anticoagulants, however.

While all NSAIDs can cause GI ulceration and bleeding, ibuprofen has only between one fifth and one half the gastric irritant capacity of aspirin. This makes ibuprofen among the best tolerated of NSAIDs. Renal and hematopoietic adverse effects from this agent are rare. Sterile meningitis has been reported in patients with systemic lupus erythematosus treated with ibuprofen.

Among nonsteroidal drugs, propionic acid derivatives appear to have the greatest analgesic effect with comparable anti-inflammatory effect. Ibuprofen has the advantage of being a safe and well-tolerated propionic acid derivative NSAID, and should be considered, along with naproxen, to be the anti-inflammatory drug of choice.

## Naproxen

Naproxen is a propionic acid derivative NSAID available commercially as both naproxen and naproxen sodium. With a long half-life of 12–15 hr, naproxen has the advantage of a twice daily dosing regimen. The absorption of naproxen is delayed if it is prescribed with food or antacids (except sodium hydroxide, which enhances its absorption). Naproxen is well absorbed and reaches peak plasma levels in 1 hr; naproxen sodium has the advantage of reaching peak plasma levels in 20 min, with concomitant rapid onset of analgesic effect. The rapidity with which the drug reaches peak plasma levels has little importance when the drug is used chronically for anti-inflammatory effect. In addition to tablets, naproxen is available as a suspension. A dose of 750 mg/day of naproxen is equivalent to 4000 mg/day of aspirin or 2400 mg/day of ibuprofen (2).

Like aspirin, naproxen prolongs prothrombin time and should not be used in patients on coumarin anticoagulants (2). There are no other clinically significant drug interactions specific to naproxen.

Naproxen has been widely prescribed and appears to be as free from adverse effects as ibuprofen. Dyspepsia is the most common adverse effect. The incidence of gastrointestinal bleeding with naproxen is low, but slightly greater than with ibuprofen, fenoprofen, and tolmetin (5).

Naproxen (15) and naproxen sodium (16) have both been proven to prevent migraine attacks. Additionally, naproxen and naproxen sodium have been used to treat acute migraine attacks and have been found to be more effective than ergotamine tartrate in reducing the severity of the attack (14). Since these drugs do not act as vasoconstrictors, they are particularly valuable in migraine sufferers with concomitant heart disease, peripheral vascular disease, or hypertension.

## Fenoprofen

Fenoprofen is well absorbed orally, reaching peak plasma levels in 2 hr. The plasma half-life is 2 hr, with metabolism by glucuronidation in the liver. It is more tightly bound to plasma proteins than any NSAID except phenylbutazone. This binding to plasma proteins may be problematic for elderly patients, those on concurrent drug therapy, or patients with hepatic dysfunction. Fenoprofen will interact with other protein-bound drugs such as oral antidiabetic or anticoagulant drugs (17). Fenoprofen appears to be the most nephrotoxic of the NSAIDs (6), possibly because of the tight protein binding. A fenoprofen dose of 2400–3200 mg/day compares with 4000 mg/day of aspirin in anti-inflammatory effect (2).

Like naproxen, fenoprofen was significantly better than placebo in reducing the frequency of migraine attacks. A dosage of 1800 mg/day was superior to 600 mg/day (18).

## Ketoprofen

Ketoprofen has been used in Europe since 1973, and was released for use in the United States in 1986. Peak plasma levels are reached in 1–2 hr, with a plasma half-life of 6–8 hr. The drug is metabolized by the liver and does not accumulate with multiple doses. Like indomethacin, ketoprofen blood levels fall off rapidly while synovial fluid levels rise slowly and exceed plasma levels after 6 hr.

In Europe, alternate dosing forms of ketoprofen are available. Parenteral ketoprofen has been used for postoperative pain, renal colic, and acute inflammatory conditions (19). Ketoprofen suppositories and slow-release oral forms are also available.

Ketoprofen, like ibuprofen and naproxen sodium, has been approved by the Food and Drug Administration for analgesia as well as arthritis indications. A 75-mg dose is slightly superior to 400 mg of ibuprofen for dysmenorrhea (20). It is generally well tolerated, and comparable in safety with ibuprofen (20). Dyspepsia is the most common side effect.

## Flurbiprofen

Flurbiprofen is well absorbed from the GI tract, metabolized by the liver, and excreted in the urine and in the bile. It is also absorbed topically and through the buccal mucosa, although no such formulations are currently available. An ophthalmic preparation is available in the United States.

Flurbiprofen is an effective anti-inflammatory with beneficial effects on rheumatoid and degenerative arthritis, ankylosing spondylitis, acute gout, and dysmenorrhea. It has been shown to be an effective analgesic in several pain models (21). One study found that 100 mg of flurbiprofen was effective in the acute treatment of migraine (22).

Studies in several models have shown flurbiprofen to inhibit bone loss in periodontal disease. This effect is not seen with other NSAIDs in clinically used doses.

## Diclofenac

Diclofenac is the sodium salt of aminophenylacetic acid, a NSAID with anti-inflammatory, analgesic, and antipyretic properties. It is completely absorbed following oral or intravenous administration, and excreted primarily in metabolized form in the urine and bile. Age and renal or hepatic impairment do not significantly affect plasma concentration. Aspirin administration decreases the plasma diclofenac level. Diclofenac can increase the plasma concentrations of digoxin, methotrexate, and lithium. It does not interact with oral anticoagulants, although it does inhibit platelet aggregation (comparable to most other NSAIDs).

In clinical trials, diclofenac was effective for the

treatment of rheumatoid and osteoarthritis and ankylosing spondylitis. For analgesic uses, the potassium salt of diclofenac has been found superior to diclofenac sodium in a preliminary study, and is being evaluated in clinical trials.

Intramuscular diclofenac sodium (not available in the United States), in a dose of 75 mg, was found to be more effective than placebo for the acute treatment of migraine attacks (23). In addition to the oral and intramuscular forms, diclofenac suppositories are also available in Europe.

Adverse effects from diclofenac are primarily GI discomfort and CNS symptoms such as dizziness and headache.

## The Fenamates

Mefenamic acid is comparable to aspirin as an analgesic, but is a relatively weak anti-inflammatory agent. A dose of 500 mg three times daily is comparable to 2400 mg of aspirin daily. It is metabolized by the liver and has a plasma half-life of 4–6 hr. It is widely promoted for the treatment of dysmenorrhea; however, it is no more effective than several other less toxic NSAIDs.

Meclofenamate has a half-life of 2–3 hr and reaches peak plasma levels in 30–60 min. There is no evidence of drug accumulation with either meclofenamate or mefanamic acid.

Adverse reactions limit the clinical utility of the fenamates. Diarrhea occurs in about 15% of patients within the first 4 weeks of treatment. This resolves if the drug is discontinued, but it recurs if the drugs are restarted. Dyspepsia may be somewhat less frequent with the fenamates (particularly mefenamic acid), but skin rashes, hemolytic anemia, and blood dyscrasias have been observed (24).

## Indomethacin

Indomethacin is rapidly absorbed following oral or rectal administration, reaching peak plasma levels in 1–2 hr. The plasma half-life is less than 2 hr, with 60% of the drug excreted in the urine. The plasma half-life is prolonged in patients with obstructive jaundice, but is not affected by moderately severe degrees of renal insufficiency. Indomethacin is available in 25- and 50-mg capsules, 75-mg sustained-release capsules, and 100-mg suppositories.

Indomethacin is not uricosuric and does not interfere with other uricosuric drugs. When used for the treatment of acute gout, a large loading dose (100 mg) is used, followed by doses adjusted to the rate of symptom relief.

It has been clinically observed that only certain patients will respond to indomethacin. Those who fail to respond or who develop intolerable side effects will usually do so in the first few weeks of therapy. Those patients who show an early response without significant side effects can usually continue to take it successfully for several years (17).

In patients with rheumatoid arthritis, indomethacin at bedtime has been shown to reduce the severity and duration of morning stiffness, reduce pain at night and in the morning, and improve the quality of sleep.

There are several rare forms of headache that are extremely responsive to treatment with indomethacin but fail to respond to other therapies, including other NSAIDs. These headaches include chronic persistent hemicrania, hemicrania continua, and cluster headache variant, sometimes grouped together as indomethacin-responsive headaches.

Primarily GI and neurologic side effects with indomethacin are common. Dyspepsia, nausea, and abdominal pain occur in 10–20% of patients, regardless of dose, and usually occur soon after the initiation of treatment. Gastric ulceration and hemorrhage can occur. Central nervous system effects can occur in up to 20% of patients, and include headache, loss of concentration, drowsiness, tremor, light-headedness, vertigo, dizziness, confusion, and depression (17). The CNS symptoms are attributed to the decreased cerebral blood flow induced by indomethacin. Uncommon side effects include toxic hepatitis, marrow aplasia, ocular problems, reduced host defense against infection, and skin rash (17). Indomethacin can cause fluid retention and precipitate congestive heart failure in the elderly.

Drug interactions with indomethacin are notable. When given with triamterene-containing diuretics, it may produce a reversible acute renal failure. It may reduce the natriuretic effect of furosemide and the antihypertensive effect of angiotensin-converting enzyme inhibitors. Indomethacin can increase plasma lithium levels, leading to toxicity. It increases the anticoagulant effect of warfarin (5).

## Sulindac

Sulindac is an indene derivative of indomethacin. The drug is given orally as a prodrug that is reduced in the liver to an active sulfide derivative within an 18-hr half-life. Sulindac is loosely bound to plasma proteins, and does not affect anticoagulant or antidiabetic drugs. It is not uricosuric, does not affect platelet function, and does not produce significant GI blood loss. A dose of 400 mg/day is equivalent to 4000 mg/day of aspirin.

Sulindac causes somewhat more epigastric discomfort and dyspepsia than the propionic acid derivatives, but far less than aspirin. Skin rashes have sometimes been reported. Although chemically similar to indomethacin, sulindac does not cause headache or CNS symptoms. One particular advantage of sulindac is the relative absence of nephrotoxicity (6). Sulindac does not block renal prostaglandins and should not impair renal blood flow. Sulindac may be the NSAID of choice in patients with renal disease, with concurrent diuretic or antihypertensive therapy, or with congestive heart failure.

## Tolmetin

Tolmetin is an acetic acid derivative similar to indomethacin. The drug is well absorbed and has a short plasma half-life of 60–90 min, requiring frequent dosing. It is effective in rheumatoid arthritis and juvenile rheumatoid arthritis.

Side effects are more common with tolmetin than with propionic acid derivatives, with GI upset occurring in up to 30% of patients (17). As many as 15% of patients complain of headache or dizziness.

## Diflunisal

Diflunisal is a phenylcarboxylic acid derivative of acetylsalicylic acid, which is rapidly absorbed after oral administration, reaches peak plasma levels in 2 hr, and has a half-life of 5–6 hr. Absorption is reduced by aluminum-based antacids, and elimination is impaired by renal insufficiency. It is uricosuric and does not affect platelet aggregability.

Diflunisal is an effective analgesic and has been used in osteoarthritis in a dose of 250 mg twice daily. Its major toxicity is GI upset, but several cases of Stevens-Johnson syndrome have been reported with its use.

## Piroxicam

Piroxicam was the first oxicam-class NSAID clinically available. It is notable for its extended half-life of 45 hr and its once-daily dosage. It is rapidly absorbed after oral administration, reaching peak plasma levels in 1–2 hr.

Like most other NSAIDs, piroxicam is effective in the treatment of rheumatoid and osteoarthritis, ankylosing spondylitis, and dysmenorrhea.

Piroxicam has been widely used worldwide since its introduction. Upper GI bleeding and ulceration have been much more common with piroxicam than with the propionic acid derivatives. The frequency of these problems is twentyfold greater with this drug than with ibuprofen or fenoprofen. Piroxicam is particularly toxic in elderly patients, with 92% of ulcers occurring in patients older than 50 years [compared with naproxen (53%), ibuprofen (57%), and sulindac (84%)] (5). Dermatologic problems such as phototoxicity and skin reactions have been reported, as have headaches and dizziness.

In the clinical use of piroxicam, the lack of dosage flexibility and frequency of GI side effects, particularly in the elderly, offsets the advantage of once-daily dosage.

## Phenylbutazone

Phenylbutazone is the oldest nonaspirin NSAID, introduced in 1949. It is slowly absorbed, and has a long half-life of 20 hr. It is very slowly eliminated, with drug still detectable in urine as long as 2 weeks after withdrawal. It is this prolonged serum steady state that leads to the potentially fatal adverse effects of agranulocytosis and aplastic anemia.

Phenylbutazone is a highly effective anti-inflammatory agent with efficacy in ankylosing spondylitis, rheumatoid arthritis, and gout. However, its effectiveness is overshadowed by a high incidence of adverse effects, including GI disturbances in 10–20% of patients, fluid retention and cardiac failure (particularly in the elderly), hepatitis, and lymphadenopathy. Aplastic anemia is rare, but tends to occur in elderly patients after prolonged treatment. Agranulocytosis may appear in young patients after a brief exposure. The hematologic side effects cause an appreciable mortality (17).

With so many effective and safer alternative NSAIDs available, it is difficult to justify the use of phenylbutazone.

## GUIDELINES FOR NSAID DRUG SELECTION

Reasonable guidelines for the selection of NSAIDs in pain management were developed by Portenoy (3), and include:

1. *Choose an appropriate drug.* NSAIDs are most useful for the treatment of mild to moderate pain, particularly if associated with an inflammatory lesion. A favorable previous experience with a specific drug should be an important consideration. The individual response to different NSAIDs can vary dramatically.

   In patients requiring a nonsteroidal drug who have a relatively mild bleeding or ulcer diathesis, including some patients with thrombocytopenia, coagulopathy, history of peptic ulcer disease, or concurrent use of ulcerogenic medications, the NSAIDs of choice are those that do not significantly affect platelet aggregation or the gastric mucosa. These drugs include acetaminophen, salicylate, and choline magnesium trisalicylate.

   Since NSAIDs are generally expensive drugs, cost may be a factor in drug selection. Over-the-counter drugs such as aspirin, acetaminophen, and ibuprofen may be less expensive than prescription drugs. Large doses of name-brand aspirin or ibuprofen, however, may approach the cost of prescription drugs.

   Certain NSAIDs appear to be less toxic than others. The propionic acid derivatives, particularly ibuprofen and naproxen, are generally well tolerated. Phenylbutazone is significantly more toxic than other NSAIDs and should be avoided except in unusual situations.

2. *Explore the dose-response relationship.* Since the individual response to a NSAID is variable, it is reasonable to begin with a low dose and increase the dosage as needed to find the ceiling dose for a given patient. Since toxicity is dose related, a maximal dose based on clinical experience, customary use, or 1.5 to 2 times the usual starting dose is appropriate, except for piroxicam, the dosage of which is fixed at 20 mg/day.

3. *Continue drugs for an adequate duration.* A trial of 2–3 weeks is the minimum duration needed to determine the efficacy of a NSAID. If there is partial benefit, consider a longer trial or increasing the dose. Data in press suggest the need for 10-week trials for anti-inflammatory effects to be maximized.

4. *Switch drugs if they are ineffective.* It is common for patients to respond poorly to one NSAID and very well to another. It is generally suggested that patients who fail to respond to one NSAID be switched to a drug in an alternate class (e.g., salicylate to propionic acid derivative).

## NARCOTIC ANALGESICS

### HISTORY

The term "opioid" refers to any natural or synthetic drug that binds to opiate receptors and has agonist actions (i.e., morphine-like pharmacologic actions). It is synonymous with "narcotic analgesic."

Knowledge of the effects of opium dates back at least to 4000 BC to the ancient Sumerians, whose ideograph for the poppy *(Papaver somniferum)* was "joy plants." Undisputed reference to the juice of the poppy is found in the writing of Theophrastus in the third century BC. The word "opium" is derived from the Greek name for juice (the drug being derived from the juice of the poppy capsule). Arabian physicians were noted for their prescription of opium. Arabian traders introduced the drug to the Orient, where it was used mostly to control dysentery. By the middle of the 16th century, opium was used for analgesia in Europe. In 1680, Sydenham wrote, "Among the remedies which it has pleased Almighty God to give to man to relieve his sufferings, none is so universal and so efficacious as opium." Three centuries later, this statement remains valid.

In 1803, the German pharmacist Serturner isolated the opium alkaloid that he named "morphine," after the Greek god of sleep, Morpheus. It is morphine that gives opium its analgesic action. In 1838, Robiquet discovered the opium alkaloid codeine. In 1848, Merck discovered another opium alkaloid, papaverine. By the middle of the 19th century, pure alkaloids had succeeded the use of crude opium extracts in the medical world.

Recreational use of opium began in the 18th century when opium smoking became popular in the Orient. In Europe, the problem of "opium eating" (drinking laudanum) existed, but never became as serious or widespread as alcohol abuse. In the United States, the immigration of opium-smoking Chinese laborers, the widespread use of morphine among wounded Civil War veterans, and the unrestricted availability of opium until the early 1900s led to an increasing problem with opiate use (25). Even to this day, the illicit use of opiates, such as heroin, plagues American society.

## PHARMACOLOGY

In order to understand the variety of actions of various opioids, it is valuable to review the subtypes of opiate receptors. There are a variety of opioid receptors differing in ligand specificity and location in the nervous system, and these receptors mediate different functions (26) (Table 12.3).

Mu receptors are divided into $mu_1$ and $mu_2$ receptors. $Mu_1$ receptors mediate supraspinal analgesia and temperature control, and $mu_2$ receptors cause respiratory depression, constipation, and growth hormone release. High concentrations of

**Table 12.3.**
**Receptor Subtypes**[a]

| Receptor | Agonist | Antagonist | Physiologic Actions | Pharmacologic Effects |
|---|---|---|---|---|
| Mu$_1$ | Normorphine | Naloxone | Analgesia, temperature control | |
| Mu$_2$ | Morphine Sufentanil | Naloxone | Respiratory depression, constipation, growth hormone release | Miosis, bradycardia, hypothermia, indifference to environment |
| Delta | Enkephalins | | Euphoria, brain reward | |
| Kappa | Metenkephalin $\beta$-endorphin Dynorphin | | Stimulation, ataxia, locomotor activity | Miosis, sedation |
| Epsilon | $\beta$-endorphin | | Heat-related antinociception | |
| Sigma | Pentazocine Phencyclidine Ketamine | Haloperidol | Psychomimetic effects | Mydriasis, respiratory stimulation, tachycardia, delirium |

[a]Data from Brown et al. (26).

mu receptors are located in the periaqueductal grey and substantia gelatinosa of the spinal cord (27). Agonists for these receptors include morphine, sufentanil, and dihydromorphine, and antagonists include naloxone. Physiologic effects of mu receptor stimulation include miosis of the pupils, bradycardia, hypothermia, indifference to environmental stimuli, and a decrease in spinal and supraspinal nociceptive reflexes (28).

Delta receptors mediate euphoria and brain reward. Enkephalins appear to be the primary agonists for these receptors (26). Delta agonists act antinociceptively at the spinal level against thermal stimuli (27).

Kappa receptors mediate stimulation, ataxia, and locomotor activity (26). Spinal kappa receptors mediate antinociception against nonthermal noxious input, such as pressure (27). Agonists for the kappa receptors include dynorphin, metenkephalin, and $\beta$-endorphin. Physiologic effects of kappa stimulation include miosis of the pupils, sedation, and a decrease in spinal nociceptive reflexes (28).

Epsilon receptors are not well defined, but appear to be stimulated by $\beta$-endorphin. The possible role of epsilon receptors is control of heat-related antinociception (27).

Sigma receptors mediate psychomimetic effects, including hallucinations, dysphoria, and excitation (2, 26). It is unlikely that sigma receptors play a significant role in nociception. Sigma receptor agonists include pentazocine, phencyclidine (PCP), and possibly ketamine. The receptor can be antagonized by haloperidol (26). Physiologic effects of sigma stimulation include mydriasis, res-

piratory stimulation, tachycardia, delirium, and a slight effect on nociceptive reflexes (28).

Based on their relative agonism or antagonism at one or more opioid receptor sites, the opioids can be divided into the pure agonist class (morphine, hydromorphone, methadone, levorphanol, meperidine, oxycodone) and the agonist-antagonist class (pentazocine, nalbuphine, butorphanol). Buprenorphine is unique, serving as a partial agonist of the mu receptor, without true mixed agonist-antagonist properties (see below).

The clinical utility of the opioid agents is in three areas—analgesic, antitussive, and antidiarrheal. Many narcotics are potent suppressors of the cough reflex, usually at lower doses than required for analgesia (e.g., 15 mg of codeine orally). The constipating effects of narcotics can be used therapeutically either in treating patients after ileostomy or colostomy, or in treating exhausting diarrhea or certain dysenteries. Extreme care must be used in prescribing these agents for long-term treatment of diarrhea because of the risk of physical and psychological dependence. These agents should be used with great caution in patients with inflammatory bowel disease or toxic diarrhea because of the risk of toxic megacolon or systemic bacteremia. As with the antitussive effect, the dose of opioid required to produce constipation is much lower than is needed for analgesia.

The primary use of the opioids is analgesia. The mechanism of action in producing pain relief is uncertain, but may be related to reduced sensation, reduced recognition of stimuli, and altered sensory discrimination, memory of past pain events, or judgment that follows recognition (2). The pain relief can be described in terms of the organization of the opioid system and the multiplicity of sites at which opioids, either endogenous or exogenous/pharmacologic, might potentially modify nociception (27).

First, peripheral nerve endings are accessible to opioids in systemic circulation, such as β-endorphin and proenkephalin A. Second, the dorsal horn of the spinal cord is the primary processing site of primary afferent nociceptive information. It is rich in dynorphin and enkephalin. Third, the midbrain, brainstem, and thalamus are relay stations for nociceptive information ascending to the cerebral cortex. These structures are rich in dynorphin and enkephalin, and receive β-endorphin innervation from the hypothalamus. Fourth, the limbic system and the cortex produce the emotional dimension of pain, and are very rich in dynorphin and enkephalin neurons and have β-endorphin input (27).

## DRUGS

### Pure Agonist Analgesics

**Morphine.** Morphine is the prototype opioid, and produces analgesia, drowsiness, changes in mood, and mental clouding. This analgesia occurs without loss of consciousness. The relief of pain is selective; other sensory modalities such as touch and vibration are not altered. At therapeutic levels, the painful stimulus may still be recognized but it may not be perceived as painful (25). Continuous dull pain is better relieved than intermittent sharp pain, although with high enough doses even severe pain is controlled.

Unlike NSAIDs, morphine and the other opioids (except pentazocine) do not have a ceiling dose above which further analgesia does not occur (3). This is because pain is a natural antagonist to the action of opiates. The stronger the pain the more opiate is required to relieve it (3).

The analgesic effectiveness of 10 mg of morphine intramuscularly has become the standard against which all other drugs are compared (Table 12.4). A single oral dose of 60 mg is required to produce the same degree of analgesia as 10 mg intramuscularly. With repeated dosing, biotransformation inactivates about two thirds of the oral dose of morphine, and the oral dose must be three times larger (30 mg) than the parenteral dose (3). Although the oral dosage is higher, the ultimate

**Table 12.4.**
**Morphine Equivalent Dose of Opioids[a]**

| Drug | Dose (mg) i.m. | Dose (mg) p.o. | Duration (hr) |
|------|------|------|------|
| Morphine | 10 | 30 | 4–5 |
| Hydromorphone | 1.5 | 7.5 | 4–5 |
| Codeine | 130 | 200 | 4–6 |
| Hydrocodone | — | 5–10 | 4–8 |
| Methadone | 10 | 20 | 4–5 |
| Levorphanol | 2 | 4 | 4–5 |
| Oxycodone | 15 | 30 | 4–5 |
| Oxymorphone | 1 | 6 | 4–5 |
| Meperidine | 75 | 300 | 1–3 |
| Pentazocine | 60 | 180 | |
| Nalbuphine | 10 | — | |
| Butorphanol | 2 | — | |
| Buprenorphine | 0.4 | 0.3 (s.l.) | |

[a]Data from Halpern (2) and Portenoy (3).

dose reaching the opiate receptors in the CNS will be the same as with the smaller parenteral dose, and have identical analgesic, respiratory depressant, and addictive effects.

Morphine can be given intravenously for cardiac pain, pulmonary edema, and severe pain. The usual dose is 4–10 mg. The analgesic effect begins immediately and peaks in 20 min. Maximal respiratory depression is manifest within 10 min (25). Because of its respiratory depressant effect and inhibition of respiratory response to carbon dioxide, morphine and other narcotics should be used with caution, if at all, in patients with chronic obstructive pulmonary disease. Since morphine increases cerebrospinal fluid pressure, patients with suspected CNS disease should not receive opiates.

The half-life of morphine is 2–4 hr, and the drug must be administered at least every 4 hr. Recently developed sustained-release morphine products [MS Contin (Purdue Frederick) and Roxanol SR (Roxane)] have a long half-life and produce stable plasma levels with every-8-hr to every-12-hr dosing. Patients should initially be titrated to analgesia with short-acting morphine, then switched to an equivalent milligram dosage of the sustained-release preparation, divided into two equal doses at 12-hr intervals (3).

**Hydromorphone.** Hydromorphone is a congener of morphine with rapid onset of action, and duration of action similar to morphine. It has a short half-life of 2–3 hr, therefore causing less drug accumulation in the elderly or in patients with renal or hepatic insufficiency. It is available in parenteral, oral, and suppository formulations. An intramuscular dose of 1.5 mg, or an oral dose of 7.5 mg, is equipotent to 10 mg of morphine intramuscularly.

**Levorphanol.** Levorphanol is a highly potent narcotic with a long duration of action and a half-life of 12–16 hr. It is available in parenteral and oral formulations. An intramuscular dose of 2 mg, or an oral dose of 4 mg, is equipotent to 10 mg of morphine.

**Codeine.** In prescribed doses large enough to provide prolonged analgesia, codeine, an opium alkaloid, has limited utility because of its side effects of nausea, vomiting, constipation, and dizziness. When given parenterally, 120 mg of codeine is equipotent to 10 mg of morphine. The major use of codeine is as an oral analgesic. An oral dose of 32 mg of codeine is equivalent to 325–600 mg of aspirin; when combined with aspirin or acetaminophen the analgesic effect equals or exceeds that of 65 mg of codeine. The variability of analgesic response at this dosage level is considerable (25). The abuse potential of codeine is less than with other morphine congeners because side effects tend to predominate with high doses and prolonged usage. Withdrawal symptoms are less intense than, although qualitatively similar to, morphine withdrawal syndrome.

**Oxycodone.** Oxycodone is a short-acting oral narcotic analgesic available in combination with either aspirin or acetaminophen. An oral dose of 30 mg is equipotent to 10 mg of morphine intramuscularly. Physical dependence on oxycodone is common in chronic nonmalignant pain syndromes because of its morphine-like potency (2). Special caution should be given to prevent excessive use of this drug with its corresponding habituation. At higher doses, toxicity from the aspirin or acetaminophen in the mixture can occur.

**Meperidine.** Meperidine is a synthetic opioid with an onset of analgesic action within 10 min of intramuscular injection, peak analgesia at 90 min, and a duration of action of 2–3 hr (2). The short duration of action requires that meperidine be given at frequent (2–3 hr) dosing intervals, rather than the customary 4–6 hr. An intramuscular meperidine dose of 75–100 mg is equipotent to 10 mg of morphine. An oral dose of 200–300 mg of meperidine is required for comparable analgesia. Meperidine is metabolized to normeperidine, a product with a half-life four times longer than the parent compound and whose accumulation is associated with CNS excitation, myoclonus, tremulousness, and seizures. This most commonly oc-

curs in patients with renal failure and in those with prolonged use of the oral drug at high doses (3). Meperidine is not useful for cough or diarrhea. Because it has less smooth muscle effect than morphine, it is often selected for patients with biliary colic or pancreatitis.

When administered to patients taking monamine oxidase inhibitors, meperidene may cause a severe reaction characterized by excitation, delirium, hyperpyrexia, convulsions, severe respiratory depression, and death. This reaction does not occur with morphine. When meperidine is given concurrently with phenothiazines, there may be an exaggeration of the respiratory depression. Meperidine-induced respiratory depression may also be enhanced by tricyclic antidepressants (25).

**Methadone.** Methadone is a synthetic opioid with the longest half-life of any opioid, 15–57 hr. In a single dose methadone is comparable with morphine in potency and duration of action; however, after 4 days of regular dosing at fixed time intervals the drug provides long periods of analgesia (2). Because of the long half-life, gradual accumulation of the drug can occur for a week or longer when dosing is instituted or the dose increased, resulting in serious toxicity (3). The long half-life of methadone makes it one of the drugs of choice in chronic cancer pain because its use may avoid periodic abstinence effects and the prolonged analgesia reduces the anticipation of pain common with short-duration narcotics (2). Methadone given orally is about half as potent as the parenteral form; 20 mg orally is equivalent to 10 mg intramuscularly and is equipotent to morphine 10 mg intramuscularly.

Although the overall abuse potential of methadone is comparable to morphine, withdrawal from methadone develops more slowly and is more prolonged and generally less intense (25). The abstinence syndrome causes no symptoms until 24–48 hr after the last dose of methadone. At high doses, methadone blocks heroin-induced euphoria. It is frequently used for the treatment of heroin withdrawal.

**Propoxyphene.** Propoxyphene is a stereoisomer of methadone with limited analgesic potency. With oral use, 32 mg of propoxyphene is no better than placebo and 90–120 mg have equivalent analgesic effects to 60 mg codeine or 600 mg aspirin (25). Combinations of propoxyphene with aspirin or acetaminophen provide better analgesia than either agent alone. The abuse liability of propoxyphene is lower than that of codeine, and the abstinence syndrome caused by abrupt withdrawal is generally mild. As with the oral codeine preparations, toxicity at high doses of propoxyphene may be from the aspirin or acetaminophen used in combination.

## Agonist-Antagonist Analgesics

**Buprenorphine.** Buprenorphine is a semisynthetic derivative of thebaine that binds strongly to mu receptors. It is 20–30 times as potent as morphine intramuscularly. Like morphine, its onset of action is in 15–60 min, but its duration of action averages over 8 hr (2).

Buprenorphine has minimal effects on the cardiovascular system. Respiratory depression occurs after 3 hr and lasts for 7 hr after a single dose, but is only partially reversible with naloxone.

Buprenorphine can induce abstinence syndrome in patients dependent on narcotics. It is classified as a drug with low abuse potential. Tolerance to the analgesic effect was not reported after months of use. Abrupt withdrawal after prolonged use resulted in a mild-to-moderate abstinence syndrome, peaking 2 weeks after discontinuation and lasting for 1 week.

The usual dose of buprenorphine is 0.3–0.8 mg every 6–8 hr, given either parenterally or sublingually. The primary side effects include sedation, nausea, constipation, diaphoresis, and respiratory depression.

**Pentazocine.** Pentazocine has both weak agonist and antagonist activity. A dose of 50 mg intramuscularly is equipotent to 10 mg of morphine. Like all agonist-antagonist agents, it can precipitate abstinence syndrome in narcotic-dependent patients (2). Tolerance and physical dependency have been seen with pentazocine, although less commonly than with the opiates. The predominant side effect is sedation, followed by diaphoresis and dizziness (25).

**Nalbuphine.** Nalbuphine is an agonist-antagonist that is equipotent to morphine, but respiratory depression appears to plateau at a 10-mg dose. It has a half-life of 5 hr, but should be given every 3–4 hr for analgesic effect. It can be administered intravenously, intramuscularly, or subcutaneously (2).

**Butorphanol.** Butorphanol is an agonist-antagonist that is three to five times as potent as morphine. It should be given in a dose of 2–4 mg every 3–4 hr. It is currently available for parenteral administration, but sublingual and intranasal dosage forms are in development. The major problem with butorphanol is the frequency of psychomimetic reactions. There is a correlation between these reactions and cumulative dose used (2).

## GUIDELINES FOR OPIATE DRUG SELECTION

As with NSAID selection, Portenoy (3) has devised guidelines for the use of opioids in the patient with chronic pain. Although these guidelines were designed for patients with cancer pain, the basic concepts are valuable for all chronic uncontrollable pain.

1. *Choose an appropriate drug.* Since all narcotics, with the exception of pentazocine, have no ceiling dose for analgesia, the division of narcotics into weak and strong categories is based largely on dose-related toxicity (e.g., seizures from meperidine or propoxyphene, psychomimetic effects from pentazocine or butorphanol); more frequent side effects at higher doses (e.g., GI upset with codeine); potential for toxicity of the coanalgesics aspirin or acetaminophen; or prescribing tradition.

   Agonist-antagonist drugs cannot be given to patients already dependent on opioids without inducing abstinence syndrome; therefore they can only be used as first-line agents. Since there are no currently available oral preparations of these agents, their utility as first-line agents is limited. When it becomes available, sublingual buprenorphine, with its 8-hr duration of action, may prove to be of value as an initial narcotic agent.

   The use of meperidine is limited by its short duration of action and the accumulation of its long half-life metabolite. Accumulation of normeperidine can lead to CNS excitation and seizures.

   There is only a loose relationship between plasma half-life and duration of analgesic effect after a dose. Drugs like morphine and hydromorphone must be administered at least every 4 hr, meperidine at least every 3 hr, and methadone every 6 hr. The sustained-release oral morphine products can be given from every 8 to every 12 hr.

2. *Start with the lowest dose that produces analgesia.* A usual starting dose for a patient with severe pain is 5–10 mg of morphine intramuscularly or its equivalent. Patients who are switched to an alternative opioid after prolonged exposure to an opioid should be started at one half to two thirds of the equianalgesic dose of the current medication. Elderly patients, or those with renal or hepatic impairment, should be started at lower doses.

3. *Titrate the dose to the favorable effects or to the appearance of intolerable and unmanageable side effects.* A useful approach to dose titration involves the concurrent administration of fixed dosage at a set schedule

(usually every 4 hr) and a rescue dose, every 2 hr as needed, for pain control. This will determine the need for upward titration of the fixed dose. The rescue drug should be the same as the fixed-dose agent, except when the fixed-dose agent has a prolonged half-life and potential for accumulation (methadone or levorphanol).

4. *Use as-needed dosing selectively.* Routine administration of narcotics to chronic pain patients should be on a fixed basis.

5. *Use an appropriate route of administration.* Whenever feasible, the oral route is preferred.

6. *Be aware of equianalgesic doses* (Table 12.4).

7. *Use a combination of drugs.* The addition of a NSAID to a narcotic may provide greatly improved analgesia.

8. *Anticipate and manage side effects.* Constipation is so common with chronic opioid use that concurrent treatment should be given in most patients. Nausea can usually be managed with the addition of an antiemetic. Respiratory depression is rarely a problem because of the rapid development of tolerance.

9. *Be aware of tolerance.* Tolerance typically presents as a reduction in the duration of analgesia after a dose. There is no limit to tolerance, and doses can become enormous in an effort to maintain analgesia.

10. *Understand the distinction between physical and psychological dependence.* Psychological dependence in a patient with no prior history of drug abuse who is administered opioid drugs for the management of intractable pain is extremely rare.

While the above guidelines are appropriate for patients with cancer pain, or for the short-term treatment of patients with acute pain states, it is important to note that chronic narcotic therapy is inappropriate for patients with chronic, nonmalignant pain. In addition to the problems of tolerance and addiction with long-term narcotic use, narcotics will worsen the depression that is typical of patients with chronic nonmalignant pain (29). These chronic pain states are better treated with tricyclic antidepressants, NSAIDs, physical modalities, and psychotherapy.

## REFERENCES

1. Buchanan WW, Kean WF: Current nonsteroidal anti-inflammatory drug therapy in rheumatoid arthritis, with emphasis on use in the elderly. In Lewis AJ, Furst DE (eds): *Nonsteroidal Anti-inflammatory Drugs.* New York, Marcel Dekker, 1987, pp 9–30.

2. Halpern LM: Analgesic and anti-inflammatory medications. In Tollison CD (ed): *Handbook of Chronic Pain Managment.* Baltimore, Williams & Wilkins, 1989, pp 54–68.

3. Portenoy RK: Practical aspects of pain control in the patient with cancer. *CA* 38:327–352, 1988.

4. Woodbury DM, Fingl E: Analgesic-antipyretics, anti-inflammatory agents, and drugs employed in the therapy of gout. In Goodman LS, Gilman A (eds): *The Pharmacologic Basis of Therapeutics,* ed 5. New York, Macmillan, 1975, pp 325–358.

5. Rainsford KD: Toxicity of currently used anti-inflammatory and antirheumatic drugs. In Lewis AJ, Furst DE (eds): *Nonsteroidal Anti-inflammatory Drugs.* New York, Marcel Dekker, 1987, pp 215–244.

6. Carmichael J, Shankel SW: Effects of nonsteroidal anti-inflammatory drugs on prostaglandins and renal function. *Am J Med* 78:992–1000, 1985.

7. Garella S, Matarese RA: Renal effects of prostaglandins and clinical adverse effects of nonsteroidal anti-inflammatory agents. *Medicine* 63:165–181, 1984.

8. Clive DM, Stoff JS: Renal syndromes associated with nonsteroidal anti-inflammatory drugs. *N Engl J Med* 310:563–572, 1984.

9. Goldberg M: Analgesic nephropathy in 1981: which drug is responsible? *JAMA* 247:64–65, 1982.

10. Blackshear JL, Davidman M, Stillman T: Identification of risk for renal insufficiency from nonsteroidal anti-inflammatory drugs. *Arch Intern Med* 143:1130–1134, 1983.

11. Favre L, Glasson P, Vallotton MB: Reversible acute renal failure from combined triamterene and indomethacin. *Ann Intern Med* 96:317–320, 1982.

12. Bunning RD, Barth WF: Sulindac—a potentially renal-sparing nonsteroidal anti-inflammatory drug. *JAMA* 248:2864–2867, 1982.

13. Kantor TG: Ibuprofen. *Ann Intern Med* 91:877–882, 1979.

14. Pradalier A, Clapin A, Dry J: Treatment Review: nonsteroidal anti-inflammatory drugs in the treatment and long-term prevention of migraine attacks. *Headache* 28:550–557, 1988.

15. Lindegaard KF, Ovrelio L, Sjaastad O: Naproxen in the prevention of migraine attacks. A double-blind placebo-controlled cross-over study. *Headache* 20:96–98, 1980.

16. Welch KMA, Ellis DJ, Keena PA: Successful migraine prophylaxis with naproxen sodium. *Neurology* 35:1304–1310, 1985.

17. Dick WC, De Ceulaer K: Nonsteroidal antirheumatic drugs. In Kelley WN, Harris ED, Ruddy S, Sledge CB, (eds): *Textbook of Rheumatology.* Philadelphia, WB Saunders, 1981, pp 768–784.

18. Diamond S, Solomon GD, Freitag F, Mehta ND: Fenoprofen in prophylaxis of migraine: a double-blind, placebo controlled study. *Headache* 27:246–249, 1987.

19. Avouac B, Teule M: Ketoprofen: the European experience. *J Clin Pharmacol* 28:S2–S7, 1988.

20. Vavra I: Ketoprofen. In Lewis AJ, Furst DE (eds): *Nonsteroidal Anti-inflammatory Drugs.* New York, Marcel Dekker, 1987, pp 419–437.

21. Smith RJ, Lomen PL, Kaiser DG: Flurbiprofen. In Lewis AJ, Furst DE (eds): *Nonsteroidal Anti-inflammatory Drugs.* New York, Marcel Dekker, 1987, pp 393–418.

22. Awidi AS: Efficacy of flurbiprofen in the treatment of acute migraine attacks: a double-blind placebo-controlled cross-over study. *Curr Ther Res* 32:492–497, 1982.

23. Del Bene E, Poggioni M, Garagiola U, Meresca V: Intramuscular treatment of migraine attacks using diclofenac sodium: a crossover clinical trial. *J Int Med Res* 15:44–48, 1987.

24. Huskisson EC: Antiinflammatory drugs. *Semin Arthritis Rheum* 7:1–20, 1977.

25. Jaffe JH, Martin WR: Narcotic analgesics and antagonists. In Goodman LS, Gilman A (eds): *The Pharmacologic Basis of Therapeutics,* ed 5. New York, Macmillan, 1975, pp 245–283.

26. Brown RM, Clouet DH, Freidman DP (eds): *Opiate Receptor Subtypes and Brain Function.* NIDA Research Monograph Series, Rockville, MD, NIDA, 1986.

27. Milan MJ: Multiple opioid systems and pain. *Pain* 27:303–347, 1986.

28. Offermeier J, Van Rooyen JM: Opioid drugs and their receptors. *S Afr Med J* 66:299–305, 1984.

29. Gildenberg PL, DeVaul RA: *The Chronic Pain Patient.* Basel, Karger, 1985, p 97.

# 13

# MUSCLE RELAXANT MEDICATIONS

*R. Michael Gallagher*

Complex neurologic mechanisms are involved in the maintenance of muscle tone. Any malfunction of this system can result in sustained abnormal muscle contraction, which can produce significant stiffness and discomfort. This muscle contraction can stem from various precipitants, such as injury, inflammation, or anxiety.

Muscles of the neck are particularly prone to spasm from a variety of causes. The most frequently encountered cause is injury, often the result of motor vehicle accidents, falls, work and athletic injuries, or overstretching. Other causes include inflammatory disease states and prolonged anxiety or stress.

Neck pain persisting for any length of time can be a frustrating experience for both the patient and the clinician. Complicating the problem further is a potential "muscle spasm–pain–anxiety cycle" that is self-perpetuating.

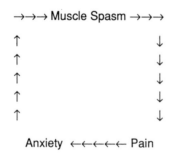

## THERAPY

The usual therapeutic approach for patients suffering with acute musculoskeletal disorders such as neck strain or sprain is comprehensive. It includes rest, physical therapy, mild analgesics, and muscle relaxants. The inclusion of muscle relaxants as adjunctive therapy is accepted by most clinicians, although well-controlled efficacy studies are few.

A group of pharmacologic agents commonly used in the treatment of acute musculoskeletal neck pain are the central-acting skeletal muscle relaxants (Table 13.1). These agents have no direct effect on muscle, the myoneural junction, or motor nerves. Muscle relaxation is produced by a depression of the central nerve pathway and possibly through the effect on higher centers.

Because the central-acting muscle relaxants exert effects on higher brain centers, they are sometimes used as anxiolytics and analgesics. The muscular pain is reduced through a modification of central perception without interfering with

**Table 13.1.**
**Central-Acting Skeletal Muscle Relaxants**

| Drug | Brand Name |
| --- | --- |
| Carisoprodol | Soma |
| Chlorzoxazone | Parafon Forte DSC, Paraflex |
| Cyclobenzeprine HCl | Flexeril |
| Diazepam | Valium |
| Metaxalone | Skelaxin |
| Methocarbamol | Robaxin |
| Orphenadrine citrate | Norflex, Norgesic, Orphengesic |
| Chlorphenesin carbamate | Maolate |

normal peripheral pain reflexes or motor activity. As a group, they are well tolerated and have a low toxicity profile.

## CENTRAL-ACTING SKELETAL MUSCLE RELAXANTS

### CARISOPRODOL

Carisoprodol (Soma) is a central nervous system depressant with a structure similar to that of meprobamate. It is reported to have analgesic properties (1) and to reduce local muscle spasm without significantly interfering with muscle or neuromuscular function. The exact mechanism of action is not completely understood, but is thought to involve a depression of polysynaptic transmission in interneuronal pools at the supraspinal level in the brainstem reticular formation. In addition, the muscle relaxation effect may, in part, be due to its sedative qualities.

Cullen (2) studied 65 patients with a variety of acute musculoskeletal conditions treated with carisoprodol or placebo. Forty-two patients were treated with 350 mg of carisoprodol or placebo, four times daily, over a 10-day period. Carisoprodol was significantly more effective than placebo in the relief of muscle spasm, pain, and stiffness. The conditions treated included sprains and strains of the cervical, thoracic, lumbar, and sacroiliac regions.

Various studies have compared carisoprodol to other muscle relaxants, analgesics, and sedatives. Hindle (3) studied 48 patients with back pain who were treated with carisoprodol, butabarbital, or placebo. In this double-blind study, carisoprodol was shown to be significantly more effective. Baratta (4) showed that carisoprodol was significantly more effective than propoxyphene or placebo in the treatment of low back syndrome in 94 patients. A multicenter study involving 71 patients with thoracic strain or sprain showed carisoprodol to be slightly more effective than diazepam in reducing muscular spasm (5).

Carisoprodol is a relatively short-acting drug with minimal cumulative effect. Peak blood levels are achieved in 1–2 hr after ingestion, and the duration of effect is about 4–6 hr. It is generally well tolerated and its potential for organ toxicity is extremely low. Metabolization takes place in the liver with excretion through the kidney. Drug interactions are an additive sedative effect when taken with central nervous system depressants such as alcohol or antihistamines.

### Dosage

The adult oral dose of carisoprodol is 350 mg three to four times daily. It is usually recommended for adult use, but its use in the pediatric age groups is not uncommon. Baird and Menta (6) studied 29 children ages 5 months to 14 years with minimal adverse effects. The suggested dosage for children above 5 years is 25 mg/kg four times daily (7). Carisoprodol should be used with caution in children.

Carisoprodol is not recommended during pregnancy or in nursing women.

Carisoprodol (200 mg) is combined with aspirin (325 mg) (Soma Compound) or aspirin (325 mg) and codeine (16 mg) (Soma Compound with Codeine) for those patients experiencing significant pain. The rationale for this combination is to add an anti-inflammatory and additional analgesic effect. Soma Compound and Soma Compound with Codeine are given in a dose of one or two tablets four times daily. The usual aspirin and codeine prescribing precautions should be followed.

### Side Effects

Untoward side effects are usually transient and occur within the first several days of use. These include drowsiness, dizziness, vertigo, ataxia, tremor, agitation, irritability, headache, depression, syncope, and insomnia. Side effects that do not resolve within 48–72 hr may do so with a reduction in dose. Allergic or idiosyncratic reactions, although rare, can occur and are usually evident within the first several doses.

### CHLORZOXAZONE

Chlorzoxazone (Paraflex, Parafon Forte DSC) is a central-acting skeletal muscle relaxant with sedative qualities. The mode of its action has not been clearly identified. It acts at the spinal cord level and subcortical areas of the brain, inhibiting reflex arcs involved in producing and maintaining muscle spasm. Until recently, chlorzoxazone was commonly prescribed in combination with acetaminophen for musculoskeletal disorders.

Vernon (8) studied 59 patients treated with chlorzoxazone or placebo for musculoskeletal back conditions. Patients received 750 mg of chlorzoxazone or placebo four times daily over 6–8 days. By day 2, those treated with chlorzoxazone reported a reduction in symptoms of spasm, pain, tenderness, and restricted range of motion. At completion of the study, 97% of the chlorzoxazone group experienced complete remission of symptoms as opposed to 39% of the placebo group.

Scheiner (9) reported on 53 patients treated with chlorzoxazone (300 mg) and diazepam (20 mg) for muscular spasm in a controlled double-blind study. In this study, chlorzoxazone was shown to be significantly more effective and to have fewer side effects than diazepam. Gready (10) studied 49 patients treated with chlorzoxazone in combination with acetaminophen, methocarbamol in combination with aspirin, or placebo for various musculoskeletal disorders, including cervical sprains. In this study, the chlorzoxazone combination was shown to be the most effective.

Chlorozoxazone is rapidly absorbed, with an onset of action in 1 hr after ingestion. Peak blood levels are attained in 3–4 hr and its duration of action is approximately 3–4 hr. Chlorzoxazone is rapidly metabolized in the liver and excreted in the urine.

## Dosage

Chlorzoxazone is administered orally and is available in 250-mg and 500-mg tablets. The usual initial adult dosage is 750–2000 mg daily in three to four divided doses. In unresponsive patients, the daily dosage can be increased to 3000 mg and then lowered as improvement occurs.

Chlorzoxazone can be administered to children. The daily dosage is 375–1000 mg in three to four divided doses. Dosage should take into account the age and weight of the child. As with many other medications, chlorzoxazone should be administered only when clearly necessary.

The safe usage of chlorzoxazone during pregnancy has not been established, and therefore this drug is not recommended in pregnant women. Chlorzoxazone should be used with caution in those patients with liver or renal impairment.

## Side Effects

Chlorzoxazone is generally well tolerated and undesirable side effects are not common. Side effects include gastrointestinal disturbances, drowsiness, dizziness, light-headedness, overstimulation, and allergic skin rash. Serious reactions such as angioneurotic edema or anaphylaxis are extremely rare.

## CYCLOBENZEPRINE

Cyclobenzeprine (Flexeril) is a central-acting muscle relaxant similar to the tricyclic antidepressants. It is believed to relieve skeletal muscle spasm within the central nervous system at the brainstem level (as opposed to the spinal cord level), although it may have an effect at the spinal cord level (11). It was initially studied for psychotherapeutic use with limited benefit (12) and is more widely used for the relief of muscle spasm. Cyclobenzeprine can be sedating, but does not appear to interfere with muscle function 13).

Basmajian (12) studied 55 patients treated with cyclobenzeprine or placebo for chronic neck spasm. The active treatment period was preceded by a 5–7 day washout to screen for placebo responders. Those patients treated with cyclobenzeprine received 30–50 mg/day for approximately 14 days. The cyclobenzeprine group showed significantly more reduction in muscle spasm and pain.

Rollings et al. (14) reported on 78 patients treated with cyclobenzeprine or carisoprodol for acute thoracolumbar strain and sprain. The cyclobenzeprine and carisoprodol were equally effective in relieving spasm and pain. Brown and Womble (15) studied 49 patients treated with cyclobenzeprine, diazepam, or placebo for long-term cervical and lumbar pain and skeletal muscle spasm. The cyclobenzeprine and diazepam groups showed significantly more improvement than the placebo group, with cyclobenzeprine being the most effective.

Cyclobenzeprine is relatively long-acting as compared to other central-acting skeletal muscle relaxants. The onset of action is within 1 hr after ingestion, with plasma therapeutic levels being attained in 3–8 hr. Its duration of action is 12–24 hr and its elimination half-life is 1–3 days.

## Dosage

Cyclobenzeprine is administered orally. The usual daily dosage is 20–40 mg in two to four divided doses. Prescribing information often recommends a treatment period of 2–3 weeks. However, a postmarket surveillance study of 6311 patients by Nibbelink and Strickland (16) showed no unexpected adverse effects after as long as 237 days of therapy. Cyclobenzeprine is excreted in the urine as inactive metabolites and in the feces as unchanged drug. It is extensively metabolized and its metabolites may undergo enterohepatic recycling.

Cyclobenzeprine is not recommended in children under 15 years of age or in nursing women. Reproductive studies involving rats, mice, and rabbits using comparatively high doses have revealed no fetal abnormalities. However, cyclobenzeprine should be used in pregnant women when absolutely necessary and only with extreme caution.

## Side Effects

Drowsiness is a common side effect and may occur in as many as 40% of treated persons. This symptom often lessens with time. For this reason, this author sometimes recommends that the total daily dose be taken at bedtime, as with the tricyclic antidepressants. Dry mouth and dizziness also are commonly experienced. Other possible side effects include nausea, constipation dyspepsia, unpleasant taste, headache, nervousness, confusion, syncope, tachycardia, arrythmia, hypotension, vomiting, anorexia, edema of the tongue, abnormal liver function, jaundice, tremors, depressed mood, sweating, and urinary retention.

Because of its anticholinergic properties, cyclobenzeprine should be used with caution in patients with angle-closure glaucoma or prostatic enlargement.

## DIAZEPAM

Diazepam is a benzodiazepine commonly used as a sedative. The effects of the benzodiazepines, as a group, are the result of their action on the central nervous system. Their most significant clinical effects are sedation, hypnosis, decreased anxiety, anticonvulsant activity, and muscle relaxation. The effects are believed to be from a potentiation of $\gamma$-aminobutyric acid (GABA) on neurons at all levels (17). In addition, muscle relaxation may in part be due to the interruption of the muscle spasm–pain–anxiety cycle through the anxiolytic effect. Other benzodiazepines, such as clonazepam, chlordiazepoxide, or meprobamate, are sometimes prescribed.

Basmajian (18) studied 40 patients treated with diazepam, phenobarbital, or placebo over 4 days for cervical muscle spasm. The muscle spasm symptoms were due to trauma, nervous tension, cold weather, degenerative joint disease, overexertion, and unknown causes (7 patients). Patients treated with diazepam showed a statistically sig-

nificant improvement over those treated with phenobarbital or placebo. Boyles et al. (5) showed diazepam to be of benefit in skeletal muscle spasm in a comparison study with carisoprodol.

Diazepam is rapidly absorbed, with peak blood levels being attained at 1 hr in adults and as soon as 15 min after ingestion in children. Secondary peak blood levels can occur at 6–12 hr, most likely as a result of enterohepatic recirculation. Diazepam is metabolized in the liver and excreted in the urine, and has an elimination half-life of 30–60 hr.

Diazepam and other benzodiazepines should be used with caution because tolerance and dependency can occur. Careful surveillance of amounts of the drug prescribed is mandatory. In patients who may be prone to addiction, such as those with histories of alcoholism or previous addiction, benzodiazepines should be used only when absolutely necessary.

## Dosage

Diazepam can be administered orally or by injection. The oral route is preferred except for the most serious cases of cervical muscle spasm. The usual adult daily dosage of diazepam is 6–40 mg in three to four divided doses. The pediatric daily dosage is 1–2.5 mg in three to four divided doses.

When parenteral diazepam is necessary, 5–10 mg can be injected intramuscularly. The dose can be repeated as necessary at 4–6-hr intervals and changed to the oral form when improvement begins. Patients should be monitored for possible undesirable effects for 4–6 hr after administration of the injectable form.

## Side Effects

The most commonly reported side effect is drowsiness. Ataxia, dizziness, confusion, headache, gastrointestinal disturbances, rash, and chills can occur, but are infrequent. There may be an increased risk of congenital malformations associated with minor tranquilizers during the first trimester of pregnancy. Diazepam is not recommended during pregnancy.

## METAXALONE

Metaxalone (Skelaxin) is a central-acting skeletal muscle relaxant that is chemically similar to mephenoxalone, a mild tranquilizer. Its mode of action is unclear, but it is thought to induce muscle relaxation through central nervous system depression. It has been used clinically as adjunctive therapy in acute musculoskeletal disorders for many years.

Dent and Ervin (19) reported a multicenter study involving 228 patients suffering from acute musculoskeletal disorders. Patients received 1600–3200 mg of metaxalone or placebo for 7–9 days. Those treated with metaxalone showed a significantly greater improvement of spasm and pain symptoms as compared to those treated with placebo.

Fathie (20) studied 100 patients treated with metaxalone or placebo for low back muscular pain. A medically significant improvement was observed in 69% of the metaxalone group as compared to 17% of the placebo group. The entire double-blind study of 100 patients was repeated. In this second series, a medically significant improvement was observed in 75% of the metaxalone group as compared to 28% of the placebo group. Diamond (21) conducted a similar study involving 100 patients and found near-equal improvement with metaxalone and placebo (52% and 46%, respectively).

Metaxalone is absorbed rapidly, with an onset of action in approximately 1 hr after ingestion. Peak blood levels are attained in approximately 2 hr and its duration of action is 4–6 hr. Its metabolites are excreted in the urine.

## Dosage

Metaxalone is administered orally and is available in 400-mg tablets. The usual adult daily dosage is 2400–3200 mg in divided doses. It should be administered with caution in patients with impaired liver function. Metaxalone is contraindicated in patients with significant renal or liver disease and in those with a history of drug-induced anemias. It is not recommended in children under 12 years of age.

Reproductive studies in rats have revealed no evidence of reduced fertility or fetal injury as a result of metaxalone. However, because safety has not been established, it is not recommended in pregnancy. It is not known whether metaxalone is secreted in human milk and, therefore, it is not advised to be taken by nursing mothers.

## Side Effects

Metaxalone is generally well tolerated. Side effects include nausea, vomiting, gastrointestinal upset, drowsiness, dizziness, headache, nervousness and irritability, rash, and pruritis. Leukopenia, jaundice or hemolytic anemia can occur but are extremely rare.

## METHOCARBAMOL

Methocarbamol (Robaxin) is a central-acting skeletal muscle relaxant with a structure similar to that of mephenesin. It has been available in the United States for over 30 years and has been used with success in the treatment of acute musculoskeletal conditions. The mechanism of action is yet to be established. It has no apparent direct effect on striated muscle itself or the myoneural junction. In animals, it inhibits nerve transmissions in the internuncial neurons of the spinal cord and blocks polysynaptic reflexes.

In a double-blind parallel study of methocarbamol and placebo (22), methocarbamol was shown to be effective in the treatment of acute musculoskeletal disorders of traumatic and inflammatory origin. A total of 180 patients participated and results were analyzed at 2 days and 9 days. Methocarbamol was significantly more effective (80%) than placebo (45%) after 2 days. After 9 days, methocarbamol continued to be more effective but to a much lesser degree. This difference in effectiveness at 9 days may be due to the self-limiting nature of many musculoskeletal disorders.

Few thorough comparison studies involving methocarbamol have been conducted by investigators. Preston et al. (23) concluded that methocarbamol was slightly more effective than cyclobenzaprine and significantly more effective than placebo in the treatment of 227 patients. Stearn (24) studied 200 patients treated with methocarbamol, chlorpenesin, carisoprodol, and placebo and concluded that the three active medicaments were superior to placebo. Other studies establishing the efficacy of methocarbamol were reported by Feinberg et al. (25), Valtonen (26), and Dent and Ervin (27).

Methocarbamol is a short-acting drug. In the oral form its onset of action is 30 min after ingestion. Peak blood levels are attained in about 2 hr and its duration of action is approximately 4–6 hr. Its inactive metabolites are predominantly excreted in the urine, with a small amount excreted in the feces.

## Dosage

Methocarbamol is available in both oral and injectable forms. Oral tablets are available in 500-mg and 750-mg strengths, and in combination with 325 mg of aspirin (Robaxisal). The injectable form is usually used in hospitalized patients and contains 100 mg/ml.

The average starting daily oral dosage of methocarbamol is 6 g in four divided doses; this is then decreased to 4.0–4.5 g for maintenance. The combination methocarbamol and aspirin tablets are given two tablets four times daily. In severely suffering patients, three tablets can be given four times daily as tolerated for several days. Methocarbamol is not recommended in children under 12 years of age or in pregnant or lactating women.

The injectable form of methocarbamol can be administered intramuscularly, by intravenous push, or by slow intravenous drip. It should not be administered subcutaneously. Intramuscularly 200–500 mg (2–5 ml) can be injected into each gluteal region, and this dose can be repeated at 8-hr intervals as necessary. As soon as improvement occurs, the patient can be switched to the oral form.

As much as 3000 mg (30 ml) of methocarbamol can be given by the intravenous route in divided doses daily for up to 3 days. For intravenous drip, methocarbamol is mixed with up to 250 ml of sodium chloride or 5% dextrose solution. By direct intravenous push it can be administered at a maximum rate of 300 mg (3 ml) over 1–2 min. Patients receiving intravenous methocarbamol should be in the recumbent position during administration and for at least 15 min after treatment.

## Side Effects

Methocarbamol is generally well tolerated by most patients. Many of the reported side effects occur early in treatment and improve with time. Reported side effects include light-headedness, dizziness, vertigo, headache, mild muscular incoordination, blurred vision, urticaria, rash, flushing, gastrointestinal upset, nasal congestion, fever, and a metallic taste in the mouth (with injectable). The most significant adverse effects with parenteral use are syncope and light-headedness.

## ORPHENADRINE CITRATE

Orphenadrine (Norgesic, Norflex, Orphengesic) is a central-acting skeletal muscle relaxant with anticholinergic properties. It is presumed to relax skeletal muscle by blocking neuronal circuits whose hyperactivity may be implicated in hypertonia and spasm.

Gold (28) studied 40 patients treated with orphenadrine or placebo intravenously for painful muscle spasm. The patients treated with orphenadrine showed a statistically significant improvement in overall clinical progress and acute painful muscle spasm. Bakris et al. (29) studied 38 patients treated with orphenadrine, diazepam, or placebo for prolonged headache resulting from continuous muscle spasm. Orphenadrine and diazepam were equally effective in relieving muscle spasm and pain as compared to placebo.

Orphenadrine is relatively rapid acting, with peak blood levels being attained within 2 hr after ingestion. Its duration of action is 4–6 hr. In the sustained-release form, absorption takes place over 8–10 hr and peak blood levels are attained within 8 hr after ingestion. Orphenadrine is extensively metabolized and its metabolites are excreted in the urine. A small amount is excreted unchanged in the urine.

## Dosage

Orphenadrine can be administered in both injectable and oral forms. Parenteral orphenadrine contains 30 mg/ml in aqueous solution. Two milliliters (60 mg) is administered intramuscularly or intravenously twice daily. When improvement occurs, parenteral therapy can be changed to oral tablets.

Orphenadrine is available in three oral tablet forms: 100 mg in a sustained-release formulation, 25 mg in combination with 30 mg caffeine and 365 mg aspirin, and 50 mg in combination with 60 mg caffeine and 770 mg aspirin. The 100-mg tablet is administered twice daily. One or two of the 25-mg combination tablets are administered three to four times daily, and one half or one of the 50-mg combination tablets is administered three to four times daily.

The safety of orphenadrine has not been established in children or in pregnant women and, therefore, it is not recommended in these patients. Because of its anticholinergic effects, it should not be taken by patients with glaucoma, achalasia, prostatic enlargement, or bladder outlet obstruction. The usual aspirin guidelines should be followed when prescribing the orphenadrine combination products.

## Side Effects

Many of the reported side effects that do occur are related to orphenadrine's anticholinergic effects and are dose related. Possible side effects include tachycardia, palpitations, urinary retention, dry mouth, blurred vision, increased intraocular pressure, weakness, nausea, vomiting, headache, dizziness, constipation, and drowsiness. Although rare, confusion, excitation, hallucinations, and syncope have been reported.

## CHLORPHENESIN CARBAMATE

Chlorphenesin carbamate (Maolate) is a central-acting skeletal muscle relaxant structurally and pharmacologically similar to methocarbamol. The precise mechanism of action is not known. Its direct muscle relaxation effects are minimal and benefit is probably related to its sedative effects. In animals, chlorphenesin appears to modify central pain reception.

Chlorphenesin is rapidly absorbed, with peak blood levels being attained at 1–3 hr. It is partially metabolized in the liver and excreted in the urine.

### Dosage

Chlorphenesin is administered orally in 400-mg tablets. The usual adult daily dosage is 1600 mg in divided doses. In more difficult cases, dosage can be begun at 800 mg three times daily and lowered as improvement occurs. Chlorphenesin should not be administered for more than 8 weeks.

Chlorphenesin is not recommended in children under 12 years of age or in pregnant or lactating women. It should be used with caution in patients with hepatic dysfunction.

### Side Effects

The most commonly reported side effects from chlorphenesin are drowsiness and dizziness. Other side effects include confusion, paradoxical stimulation, insomnia, headache, nausea, and epigastric distress. Rash, pruritis, fever, or anaphylaxis are rare.

## TRICYCLIC ANTIDEPRESSANTS

In practice, the tricyclic antidepressants are sometimes utilized in the treatment of musculoskeletal spasm and pain. Their precise mechanism of action is not known, but may be related to their analgesic effects (30). These effects may be independent of their antidepressant effects (30, 31). In addition, the sedative and anxiolytic effects (32) of the tricyclic antidepressants may contribute to the reduction of symptoms through an interruption of the muscle spasm–pain–anxiety cycle.

The tricyclics most often used in the treatment of cervical spasm and pain are the tertiary amines, amitriptyline (Elavil, Endep), nortriptyline (Aventyl, Pamelor), imipramine (Tofranil), and doxepin (Adapin, Sinequan). Dosage is generally less than that used for depression, ranging from 25 to 100 mg/day. Common side effects of the tricyclic compounds include weakness, drowsiness, dry mouth, weight gain, and constipation. The usual prescribing guidelines should be followed.

## CONCLUSION

Reflex cervical muscle spasm and pain are a common occurrence in our active society. The symptoms are usually a result of overexertion, sudden and unusual movements, injury, overwork, poor posture, and sometimes prolonged stressful states. The pain is often accompanied by limitation of motion, which may represent a protective response to the acute muscle spasm. It is important to institute therapy as soon as possible after symptoms develop. Early intervention will aid in restoring mobility, reduce symptoms, and interrupt the muscle spasm–pain–anxiety cycle. Muscle relaxants have been shown to be useful as part of a comprehensive program for the treatment of acute cervical muscle spasm and pain.

## REFERENCES

1. Bergen FM, Kletztein M, Ludwig BJ, Margolin S: History, chemistry and pharmacology of carisoprodol. *Ann NY Acad Sci* 86:90–107, 1960.
2. Cullen AP: Carisoprodol (Soma) in acute back conditions. *Curr Ther Res* 20:556–562, 1976.
3. Hindle TH: Comparison of carisoprodol, butabarbital and placebo in treatment of the low back syndrome. *Calif Med* 117:7–11, 1972.
4. Baratta RR: A double-blind comparative study of carisprodol, propoxyphene and placebo in the management of low back syndrome. *Curr Ther Res* 20:233–239, 1976.
5. Boyles WF, Glassman JM, Soyka MD: Management of acute musculoskeletal condition. *Today Ther Trend* 1:1–16, 1983.
6. Baird HW, Menta DA: Preliminary observations on the use of carisoprodol in infants and children. In Miller EG (ed): *Pharmacology and Clinical Use of Carisoprodol.* Detroit, Wayne State University Press, 1959, pp 85–96.
7. McEvoy GK (ed): Autonomic drugs. in *Drugs Info 85.* Bethesda, MD, American Society of Hospital Pharmacists, 1985, pp 417–548.
8. Vernon WG: A double-blind evaluation of Parafon Forte in the treatment of musculo-skeletal back conditions. *Curr Ther Res* 14(12):801–806, 1972.
9. Scheiner JJ: Muscle relaxants: chlorzoxazone compared with diazepam (a double-blind study). *Curr Ther Res* 19(1):51–57, 1976.
10. Gready DM: Parafon Forte vs Robaxisal in skeletal muscle disorders: a double-blind study. *Curr Ther Res* 20(5):666–673, 1976.
11. Share NN, McFarlane CS: Cyclobenzeprine: a novel cen-

trally acting skeletal muscle relaxant. *Neuropharmacology* 4:675, 1975.

12. Basmajian JV: Cyclobenzeprine HCL effect on skeletal muscle spasm in the lumbar region and neck: two double-blind controlled clinical and laboratory studies. *Arch Phys Med Rehabil* 59:58–63, 1978.

13. Nibbelink DW: Flexeril (cyclobenzeprine HCL/MSD). Review of clinical double-blind evaluations of efficacy and tolerability. *Postgrad Med Commun* May:19–24, 1978.

14. Rollings HE, Glassman JM, Soyka JP: Management of acute musculoskeletal conditions—thoracolumbar strain and sprain; a double-blind evaluation comparing the efficacy and safety of carisoprodol with cyclobenzeprine. *Curr Ther Res* 34(6):917–928, 1983.

15. Brown BR, Womble J: Cyclobenzeprine in intractable pain syndromes with muscle spasm. *JAMA* 240(11):1151–1152, 1978.

16. Nibbelink DW, Strickland SC: Cyclobenzeprine (Flexeril): report of a post marketing surveillance program. *Curr Ther Res* 28(6):894–903, 1980.

17. Harvey CH: Hypnotics and sedatives. In Gilman AG, Goodman LS, Rall TW, Murad F (eds): *Pharmacological Basis of Therapeutics*. New York, Macmillan, 1985, p 345.

18. Basmajian JV: Reflex cervical muscle spasm: treatment by diazepam, phenobarbital or placebo. *Arch Phys Med Rehabil* 64:121–124, 1983.

19. Dent RW, Ervin MS: Study of metaxalon (Skelaxin) vs placebo in acute musculoskeletal disorders: a comparative study. *Curr Ther Res* 18(3):433–440, 1975.

20. Fathie K: Second look at a skeletal muscle relaxant: a double-blind study of metaxalone. *Curr Ther Res* 6(11):677–683, 1964.

21. Diamond S: Double-blind study of metaxalone. *JAMA* 195(6):479–480, 1966.

22. Tisdale SA, Ervin DK: A controlled study of methocarbamol (Robaxin) in acute painful musculoskeletal conditions. *Curr Ther Res* 17:524–530, 1975.

23. Preston EJ, Miller CB, Herbertson RK: A double-blind, multicenter trial of methocarbamol (Robaxin) and cyclobenzaprine (Flexeril) in acute musculoskeletal conditions. *Today Ther Trends* 1(4):1–11, 1984.

24. Stern TH: A controlled comparison of three muscle relaxant agents. *Clin Med* Feb:367–372, 1961.

25. Feinberg I, Carey J, Hussussien J, Arias B: Treatment of painful skeletal muscle disorders: a report of a double-blind study of methocarbamol, aspirin, and placebo. *Am J Orthop* Nov:280–282, 1962.

26. Valtonen EJ: A double-blind trial of methocarbamol vs placebo in painful muscle spasm. *Curr Med Res Opin* 3:382–385, 1975.

27. Dent RW, Ervin MS: Relief of acute musculoskeletal symptoms with intravenous methocarbamol (Robaxin injectable): a placebo-controlled study. *Curr Ther Res* 20(5):661–665, 1976.

28. Gold RH: Orphenadrine citrate in low-back pain. *Clin Trial J* 15(5):145–149, 1978.

29. Bakris GL, Mulopulos GP, Subhash T, Franklin C: Orphenedrine citrate: an effective alternative for muscle contraction headaches. *Ill Med J* 161(2):106–108, 1982.

30. Spiegel K, Kalb R, Pasgernak GW: Analgesic activity of tricyclic antidepressants. *Ann Neurol* 13:462–465, 1983.

31. Norman TR, Burrows GD: Antidepressants: inpatient drugs in the analgesic pharmocopeia. *Curr Ther* Nov:63–72, 1986.

32. Headler N: Anatomy and psychopharmacology of chronic pain. *J Clin Psychopharmacol* 43:8(2):15–21, 1982.

## 14

# PSYCHOTROPIC MEDICATIONS

### J. Hampton Atkinson, Jr., and Mark A. Slater

For over 30 years psychotropic drugs have been used as analgesics, as adjunctive agents to enhance conventional analgesics, and as primary treatment for psychiatric symptoms or disorders associated with pain. This chapter reviews the therapeutic efficacy of the major psychiatric medications (i.e., the antidepressant agents, neuroleptics, antianxiety drugs, and psychostimulants) in acute and chronic pain syndromes, and applies these findings to the rehabilitative treatment of patients with painful cervical trauma.

One issue must be addressed in critically evaluating the role of these drugs in cervical pain syndromes: few studies directly address groups of patients with cervical pain. The results from studies of the treatment of the *psychiatric* complications (e.g., depression and anxiety) of noncervical pain syndromes probably can be generalized to patients with cervical pain. It is not certain, however, that these data apply to the treatment of *pain* itself, since the etiology of pain from cervical trauma may differ from pain syndromes documented to respond to psychotropics.

This chapter is divided into two sections. The first section critically assesses drug therapy outcomes, mainly from controlled studies. It reviews each major class of psychopharmacologic agent. Since accurate medical and psychiatric diagnosis is essential, drug efficacy is discussed in relation to specific pain and psychiatric diagnoses. Finally, acute pain is differentiated from chronic pain. The second section offers some clinical guidelines for using psychoactive drugs. It describes selecting a drug, preparing and evaluating patients for treatment, and conducting initial and longer term

pharmacotherapy. Thus, a clinician considering drug treatment of patients with cervical pain syndromes can review the evidence for drug efficacy in various pain syndromes in part one. Part two suggests an approach to applying these agents in specific clinical situations. Much of this material is discussed in greater detail in our chapters in companion volumes in this series (1, 2).

## STUDIES OF EFFICACY

### ANTIDEPRESSANT AGENTS

Each of the three major classes of antidepressant drugs—the tricyclic antidepressants (TCAs), monoamine oxidase inhibitors (MAOIs), and lithium carbonate—has been used as primary or adjunctive agents in pain management. There are four major clinical questions with regard to antidepressants in acute and chronic pain:

1. Are some antidepressants analgesic, and if so, are they applicable to the kinds of pain syndromes associated with cervical trauma?
2. Is this analgesia independent of an antidepressant effect?
3. Do antidepressants potentiate narcotic or nonnarcotic analgesics in a clinically relevant manner?
4. Do antidepressants relieve depression associated with chronic pain?

To begin to answer these four questions one must define what is meant by "depression" and distinguish depressive syndromes from symptoms often associated with chronic pain.

The term "depression" can be used to describe a mood, a symptom, and a syndrome or disorder.

192

Saddened or discouraged mood, or unhappiness as a reaction to life events or physical limitations, is not a disorder. A diagnosis of a major depressive disorder, as described by the third revised edition of the *Diagnostic and Statistical Manual of Mental Disorders* (DSM III-R) (3), requires the presence of an inability to experience pleasure, reduced interest in the environment, and reduced energy. A major depressive episode is thus defined as a period lasting at least 2 weeks that may be marked by a dysphoric mood and is often accompanied by a disorder of sleep and appetite, loss of energy, loss of interest, self-reproach, difficulty concentrating, and thoughts of death or suicide. Major depression differs from depressive symptoms in that the above problems are persistent, *interfere with function,* and are not explained better by other illness (3). Dysthymic disorder is defined as a chronically depressed mood for most of each day, on more days than not, for at least 2 years. This disturbance of mood must be associated with some symptoms of alteration either in appetite, sleep, energy, self-esteem, or ability to concentrate. Interference in everyday functioning generally is related to chronicity rather than severity of symptoms. Some symptoms of chronic pain (e.g., fatigue, withdrawal, or insomnia) can overlap with depressive symptoms, and may complicate the diagnosis of major depression. Generally patients are able to relate a distinct or progressive change in overall function, or report an increased severity of such symptoms, which helps to define the onset of a depressive episode and to distinguish it from their usual experience. Perhaps 25% or more of patients with chronic pain suffer a major depressive episode at some point in their pain career (4), and its detection is extremely important.

## Tricyclic Antidepressants

Tricyclic antidepressants (TCAs) have been administered to patients suffering many kinds of pain syndromes. The agents tested include amitriptyline (Elavil), desipramine (Norpramin), imipramine (Tofranil), and doxepin (Sinequan, Adapin). The data most clearly support their efficacy for neurologic (deafferentation) pain and headache syndromes. Their effectiveness in other chronic pain syndromes, such as arthritic disorders and musculoskeletal pain—which may well represent the diagnosis for which the drugs are most commonly employed—is less certain and varies by diagnosis of the underlying disorder impeding rehabilitation.

**Acute Pain.** Studies using animal models demonstrate that TCAs provide species-specific analgesia in experimentally induced acute pain, raising the questions of whether these agents have a role in managing the early phases of cervical pain. Unfortunately the data supporting an analgesic effect in humans are inconsistent. One study of experimentally induced pain (5) suggested that doxepin had no analgesic efficacy, whereas another (6) noted that imipramine outperformed placebo. A double-blind, placebo-controlled investigation studying patients with pain after dental extraction reported no efficacy for either amitriptyline or desipramine (Norpramin, Pertofrane) (7). Thus, there is little convincing evidence that these compounds are likely to relieve acute pain in the individual with cervical trauma, although no known studies directly address this question. Several studies of chronic pain document a role for TCAs in selected syndromes, however, and results in several of these conditions may be applicable to the patient with chronic cervical pain.

**Chronic Back Pain.** Neck and back pain frequently coexist. Further, similar mechanisms may be producing neck and back pain, particularly in musculoskeletal and posttraumatic pain. Therefore, results obtained in studies of TCAs in back pain may also apply to the treatment of cervical pain. Two basic groups of chronic low back pain patients have been studied. The first includes those with rigorously diagnosed major depressive disorders (unipolar depression or dysthymic disorder) that either precede or are secondary to pain. The second includes patients with depressive symptoms who do not meet criteria for a diagnosable depressive disorder. Efficacy of antidepressants depends on the diagnostic group considered.

Back pain patients with a major affective disorder respond well to tricyclic antidepressants. Ward and coworkers (8, 9) noted that both doxepin and desipramine significantly reduced self-reported and objective ratings of depression and anxiety, pain severity, and percentage of day in pain. Over half of the patients achieved 30% or greater reduction in pain intensity and 40% reduction in severity of depressive symptoms (9). Clinical pain relief and clinical depression relief were significantly related. The doses achieved were within the usual antidepressant range (3 mg/kg, or at least 150 mg daily for either agent), and the onset of maximum therapeutic response occurred after 3–4 weeks. These factors indicate that therapeutic response most likely was related to an antidepressant effect. The best clinical predictor of response was a shorter duration of pain complaint; age, number of surgeries, employment status, and orthopaedic ratings of the amount of physical impairment did not predict outcome (9).

Mixed effects are reported in back pain patients without diagnosed major affective disorder. Alcoff et al. (10) described a sample of chronic back pain patients, 10% of whom had documented depressive symptoms. After 6 weeks of treatment, the group given imipramine (150 mg daily) showed significantly higher activity levels and work capacity than those on placebo, but did not differ in pain severity, analgesic use, or degree of change in Beck depression scores. This study is particularly informative because the groups were well matched for pain chronicity, prior surgery, and depressive symptoms. Plasma antidepressant concentrations did not correlate with change in depressive symptoms or pain intensity in the subgroup of patients with higher depression scores.

In another controlled study of back pain patients with documented depressive symptoms, Hameroff et al. (11) reported that doxepin (2.5 mg/kg daily) was clearly superior to placebo for improving mood and sleep and reducing muscle tension and the percentage of time patients reported being in pain. Pain intensity, level of activity, and analgesic consumption did not respond to the antidepressant.

In a crossover study of amitriptyline, Pilowsky et al. (12) used a pain clinic sample comprised mostly of chronic back pain patients without significant organic pathology. These investigators reported that the treated group had significantly less pain than the placebo group at weeks 2 and 4, but that pain ratings became equivalent after 6 weeks of drug therapy. Overall, amitriptyline did not improve daily functioning or symptoms of anxiety and depression; nevertheless the subset of patients with clear-cut major depression did appear to improve with TCA therapy.

Finally, Pheasant et al. (13) reported a controlled, crossover trial of amitriptyline (50–150 mg daily) in patients with depressive *symptoms*. Analgesic consumption significantly decreased (by almost 50%) during treatment with amitriptyline, but mood and activity level were unaltered. A related finding from another controlled trial (14) was that chlorimipramine (Anafranil) (150 mg), an analogue of imipramine, significantly decreased verbal pain estimates in low back pain patients and increased tolerance to experimentally induced

pain after 2 weeks of therapy. The same study also showed, however, that the efficacy of amitriptyline (150 mg) did not differ from that of placebo. Studies using lower dosages of imipramine (75 mg) reported no significant differences between treatment and control groups in objective or self-reported mood, pain, or stiffness in patients with and without documented depressive symptoms (15).

One major problem in evaluating these studies is that questionnaires were used to rate depressive symptoms, but patients were not examined clinically for psychiatric diagnosis. It is possible that some of those patients had an undiagnosed major depression. A second problem is that follow-up is generally limited to 2–6 weeks, whereas the effect of these agents often may not appear within 6 weeks. Finally, given the clinical nature of most studies in this area, it is difficult to clearly establish the mechanisms of effects that were obtained.

In summary, it would appear that TCAs are especially effective in back pain complicated by major depression, and that dosages customarily used in treatment of major depressive disorders (2.5–3.0 mg/kg) are indicated. In patients not having major depression, symptoms such as insomnia or subjective muscle tension may lessen, but an improvement in functional activity and reduced analgesic consumption may not occur. Imipramine and desipramine may reduce pain intensity in nondepressed back pain, but this is not well established. The data, then, do not convincingly support use of these agents in the absence of major depressive disorder. A similar pattern of results may be expected in patients with pain following cervical trauma or disease, but no known studies singularly address this patient population.

**Arthritic Disorders.** Experimental models suggest that TCAs may have anti-inflammatory effects in chronic adjuvant-induced arthritic rats. These effects reduce the physical signs of arthritis itself, and increase mobility (16). Because cervical spine osteoarthritis may be associated with pain, this finding may have important therapeutic implications.

Studies have been conducted in heterogeneous groups of patients with arthritic disorders (rheumatoid arthritis, osteoarthritis, ankylosing spondylitis). In each study imipramine (75 mg) was added to a nonsteroidal anti-inflammatory drug regimen. One study (17) noted no significant drug effect, whereas another (18) showed significant improvement in pain, stiffness, and activity. In the third study (19) patients "preferred" the antidepressant to placebo, but specific dependent variables (mood, pain, grip strength, and physical function) were not assessed. Thus, imipramine may have therapeutic effects but more rigorous controlled studies are needed to establish its role in these arthritic disorders.

**Neurologic Disorders.** Arachnoiditis, thought to be due to injury or to an inflammatory response to radiopaque material used during myelography, may occur in a small proportion of patients with chronic cervical back complaints, and may represent a neuropathic pain syndrome. The etiology of such neuropathic or deafferentation pain is believed to be spontaneous neuronal hyperactivity or disturbed inhibition following injury to the central nervous system or to peripheral nerves. TCA medications may play a role in quieting this spontaneous neuronal hyperactivity. Neuropathic syndromes reported to respond to TCAs include postherpetic neuralgia, diabetic peripheral neuropathy, persistant postoperative scar pain, trigeminal neuralgia, thalamic pain, and neuralgias from lesions of plexus or peripheral nerves (e.g., postamputation stump pain) (20–24).

Treatment of these neuropathic pain states may be effective in depressed or nondepressed patients, and improvement appears to be independent of a primary antidepressant effect. Therapeutic serum TCA levels are below those usually associated with an antidepressant effect (18); dosage regimens generally are less than one half those used in major depression, and relief of pain generally occurs within 1–2 weeks (17, 18). Some authors reported that higher dosages produced increased pain in some patients, suggesting a "therapeutic window" for dosage. In patients with some syndromes (e.g., postherpetic neuralgia) there was a later decay of drug efficacy, casting doubts on the long-term benefits of treatment (18). Nevertheless, some patients discontinued therapy but maintained their improvement beyond 12 months.

We are not aware of controlled drug trials involving patients selected for arachnoiditis and pain. Yet to the extent that this disorder resembles neuropathic or deafferentation syndromes known to respond to tricyclic agents, then it may represent another indication for these antidepressants.

**Tricyclics as Adjuncts to Analgesics.** Amitriptyline (25), nortriptyline (Aventyl, Pamelor) (25), chlorimipramine (26), desipramine (27), and doxepin (28) are all reported to potentiate opiate analgesia in acute pain animal models, although the effect may not persist with chronic administration (29). In human acute clinical pain, chronic administration of desipramine (25–75 mg), but not amitriptyline, potentiates and prolongs morphine analgesia, resulting in 10–20% lower verbal estimates of pain intensity (7).

Reports on chronic back pain patients (30, 31) suggest that the combination of either doxepin or amitriptyline (25–75 mg daily) with a narcotic analgesic reduced pain intensity more than either an antidepressant or a narcotic agent alone. Since these patients also were enrolled in a comprehensive pain management program, the authors speculate that both the program itself and the tricyclics may have contributed to the efficacy and low maintenance dosages of narcotic.

The combination of TCAs with conventional analgesics may be a promising approach, but it remains unproven. Controlled trials assessing the efficacy of combination versus single-drug therapy on pain intensity, functional status (e.g., employment, exercise tolerance), and emotional state are needed to clarify this adjunctive use of TCAs.

**Mechanisms of Action.** Tricyclic antidepressants have several postulated actions, including (*a*) antidepressant effects, (*b*) "anticonvulsant" properties, (*c*) anti-inflammatory–like properties, (*d*) serotonergic and noradrenergic activity with augmentation of endogenous pain inhibitory mechanisms, and (*e*) central skeletal muscle relaxation. Some of these effects may apply in patients with pain following cervical trauma, depending upon the etiology of the pain syndrome. An antidepressant effect would be paramount in pain patients with coexisting major depressive illness. Improved mood is generally followed by increased activity and by more available psychological resources to cope with pain. If the patient has an arachnoiditis, stabilizing aberrantly conducting neurons or inhibiting their afferent transmission at the level of the spinal cord may be therapeutic. Here the putative anticonvulsant effects of TCAs (32, 33) may have a role, given the evidence of epileptiform activity in deafferentated neurons, the structural similarity of tricyclics to traditional anticonvulsants such as carbamazepine, and their ability to suppress firing in polysynaptic neurons (21, 32, 33).

Peripheral anti-inflammatory–like properties of TCAs may be prominent in other pathologic states. Possible mechanisms of action include: (*a*) altering the transport or activity of substances involved in inflammation, such as serotonin; (*b*) inhibiting prostaglandin synthetase, an enzyme crucial to inflammation and to activation of primary afferent nociceptors; and (*c*) modifying of protein binding capacity, another property tricyclic agents share with conventional anti-inflammatory drugs (16). Finally, amitriptyline has a chemical structure almost identical to that of cyclobenzeprine (e.g., Flexeril), a centrally acting skeletal muscle relaxant. The centrally acting skeletal muscle relaxants are sedatives and preferentially depress polysynaptic reflexes, without directly relaxing skeletal muscle or depressing neuronal conduction or muscle excitability. Amitriptyline potentially could act by sedative or neuronal mechanisms to provide symptomatic relief in selected disorders.

Of course, an augmentation of serotonergic or other endogenous pain-inhibitory neurotransmitter systems may be a fundamental therapeutic effect common to many of these sites of action. It must be noted, however, that the clinical syndrome most likely to respond to a TCA is a major depressive episode, and that there are only limited data supporting the use of these drugs in other conditions accompanying cervical pain.

## Monoamine Oxidase Inhibitors

Monoamine oxidase (MAO) is a term for intramitochondrial enzymes widely distributed throughout the body. Intraneuronal MAO deactivates biologically active amines potentially important in pain perception, including norepinephrine, 5-hydroxytryptamine (serotonin), and dopamine. Monoamine oxidase inhibitors (MAOIs) increase intraneuronal pools of these neurotransmitters by inhibiting their degradation. Phenelzine (Nardil) and tranylcypromine (Parnate) are the most commonly prescribed MAOIs, and have well-documented efficacy for treating major depression.

MAOIs do not appear to have analgesic properties in acute pain. MAOIs have been used to treat migraine headache (34) and facial pain (35). There are no known trials to evaluate their efficacy in patients with primary cervical pain states, with or without major depression.

Because of their documented efficacy in psychiatric patients with major depression, MAOIs would be expected to benefit cervical pain patients with major depression, although tricyclic

antidepressants would remain the drugs of first choice.

## Lithium Carbonate

Beyond its use in psychiatric disorders (bipolar mood disorder, recurrent major depression), lithium also has been employed for numerous medical and neurologic conditions (36). The rationale for its use in pain syndromes derives from its postulated effects on central nervous system dopaminergic and serotonergic systems, and its demonstrated efficacy in treating cyclic or recurrent disorders (e.g., bipolar mood disorder). Trials employing lithium for chronic pain have been confined to recurrent headache syndromes (e.g., refs. 37–39), and the drug has not been used systematically in the treatment of cervical trauma and pain. If the patient with cervical trauma develops a major depression, the TCAs are the agents of first choice, with the possible exception that patients with a frequently recurring major depression might be candidates for lithium.

**Mechanisms of Action.** The therapeutic mechanism of action of MAOIs and lithium in headache syndromes is unknown, but probably is not simply a primary antidepressant effect. Their widespread effects on serotonergic and noradrenergic neurotransmission may interact with endogenous pain modulating systems.

## Summary

Studies involving TCAs identify promising approaches to the rehabilitation of some patients with cervical trauma and pain. Patients with definite major depression are likely to benefit. Some symptoms associated with pain (e.g., insomnia, muscle tension) may respond in nondepressed patients, although this is not thoroughly established. Pain itself, if based on neuropathic mechanisms, may be relieved.

## NEUROLEPTIC DRUGS

Neuroleptics include the various classes of phenothiazines, butyrophenones, and other compounds used primarily as antipsychotic drugs or "major tranquilizers." Like opiates they inhibit gross motor activity, and act at higher centers to produce affective indifference and emotional quieting. Neuroleptics are used widely in combination with narcotics to treat postoperative pain and have been employed for chronic pain syndromes.

Recently, however, it has been recognized that there is very little evidence that neuroleptics have analgesic effects in acute pain or that they potentiate opiate analgesia, and a reassessment of their use is in order.

## Phenothiazines and Related Drugs

**Experimentally Induced and Clinical Acute Pain.** Most of the studies of neuroleptics have used experimentally induced pain. Dundee et al. (40–43) assessed the effect of 14 different phenothiazines on pain experimentally induced by pressure on the anterior surface of the tibia, using healthy patients admitted for minor surgical procedures. All phenothiazines tested increased sensitivity to pain at 20 min after injection. By 60 min after injection, however, the drugs differed in their action. Some agents demonstrated mild analgesic activity [e.g., chlorpromazine (Thorazine), promazine (Sparine), and propiomazine (Largon)] (40). Other agents moderately amplified pain reports [e.g., prochlorperazine (Compazine), perphenazine (Trilafon), and trifluoperazine (Stelazine)]. One agent [promethazine (Phenergan)] markedly increased pain report over baseline (40). Further observations suggested that the action of selected phenothiazines was biphasic—initially antianalgesic and hours later analgesic (40–43). Only one neuroleptic, methotrimeprazine (Levoprome), has clinically reliable analgesic properties in acute pain (44, 45). The agent is roughly equipotent with morphine on a milligram basis.

Later work (41), again using experimentally induced pain, explored the ability of phenothiazines to potentiate a narcotic analgesic [meperidine (Demerol)]. Promazine slightly but significantly increased the analgesic activity of meperidine at 60–90 min after injection. Other phenothiazine derivatives (propiomazine, trifluopromazine) had no effect on meperidine analgesia. An important finding was that perphenazine and promethazine were strongly antianalgesic and diminished the therapeutic effect of meperidine when given in combination with the narcotic.

**Chronic Pain.** Controlled studies using neuroleptic medications for chronic pain syndromes have studied tension headaches and neuropathic disorders rather than cervical trauma and pain. Despite some efficacy in these conditions, the use of neuroleptics to treat the chronic sequelae of cervical trauma probably is rarely indicated because of the risk of tardive dyskinesia (46). This

problem is discussed in detail later (see "Clinical Approaches and Guidelines").

**Neuroleptics as Adjuncts in Neurologic Disorders.** Several anecdotal reports suggest that phenothiazine or butyrophenone antipsychotic agents, when used in combination with TCAs, are effective for neuropathic or deafferentation syndromes (e.g., diabetic peripheral neuropathy, postherpetic neuralgia) (47, 48) when treatment with a tricyclic agent alone is ineffective (47, 49). Suggested combinations include amitriptyline (25–75 mg) plus fluphenazine (Prolixin) (1–3 mg) (47), or imipramine (25–75 mg) with haloperidol (Haldol) (1–3 mg) (22). The use of an antipsychotic agent alone is less likely to be helpful in these conditions. If painful arachnoiditis complicates cervical trauma and is not responsive to a TCA, a trial of combination therapy may be warranted. It should be noted, however, that evidence for the effectiveness of such combination therapy is limited to anecdotal reports and awaits evaluation in controlled studies.

**Neuroleptics as Adjuncts to Analgesics.** Data regarding the chronic use of neuroleptics to augment conventional narcotic and nonnarcotic analgesics come mainly from cancer populations. Neuroleptics have not improved pain control either in outpatients with mild to moderate cancer pain treated with aspirin (50) or in hospitalized patients with severe pain treated with morphine (51). It appears that these drugs have little use as meaningful adjuncts to the usual analgesic regimen of most cervical pain patients.

**Mechanism of Action.** The therapeutic mechanism of action of neuroleptic medications for pain syndromes is unclear. Antidopaminergic activity may explain the analgesic effects of methotrimeprazine in acute pain, although other neuroleptic agents with similar ability to block dopamine neurotransmission are not analgesic. The membrane-stabilizing properties of antipsychotic drugs may account for their therapeutic effects in some neuropathic or deafferentation syndromes (32, 33). Alternatively, the neuroleptic may simply increase serum concentrations of the tricyclic to a therapeutic range.

## ANTIANXIETY AND SEDATIVE AGENTS

Two classes of antianxiety drugs are used in pain syndromes. The most frequently used are the benzodiazepines [chlordiazepoxide (Librium), diazepam (Valium), clonazepam (Klonopin), and others]; less often employed are the diphenylmethane derivatives [hydroxyzine (Vistaril)]. The barbiturates (phenobarbital, secobarbital, and others) have been replaced by benzodiazepines in routine clinical care. Antianxiety agents are used to treat anxiety secondary to pain, or to alleviate skeletal muscle spasm and contraction associated with pain. The benzodiazepines also show promise in the treatment of neuralgias, perhaps by reducing neuron firing rates.

## Benzodiazepines and Hydroxyzine

**Experimentally Induced and Clinical Acute Pain.** Diazepam has no documented primary antinociceptive effects, nor does it potentiate the antinociceptive activity of narcotic analgesics in animal models (52, 53). Nevertheless, diazepam decreases the affective emotional response to pain and potentiates this property of opiates in animal paradigms (54) and in experimentally induced pain in humans (55, 56). Chapman and Feather (55) noted that diazepam (10 mg orally) prolonged tolerance to experimentally induced pain significantly more than did placebo and aspirin, and diminished pain-associated anxiety better than did placebo. Gracely et al. (56) confirmed that diazepam reduced the affective response to experimentally induced pain without altering sensory sensitivity. Surprisingly, the use of benzodiazepines as adjuvants for reducing acute clinical (e.g., postoperative or posttraumatic) pain, however, has not been thoroughly investigated. Clinical experience indicates that benzodiazepines are often useful in anxious postoperative or acutely injured patients, and that reduction of anxiety helps diminish pain complaints.

Hydroxyzine is a diphenylmethane derivative having antihistaminic, antiemetic, spasmolytic, and anxiolytic activity. Hydroxyzine, like the benzodiazepines, has minimal analgesic activity. It does not consistently enhance opiate analgesia in animal models of pain, but it potentiates opiate reduction of the affective component of pain (54).

Results of studies on clinical pain indicate that hydroxyzine has a very limited role, if any, in postoperative care. Oral hydroxyzine (100 mg) has not been shown to be superior to placebo in relieving postoperative pain, and does not potentiate oral meperidine (57) or alter meperidine pharmacokinetics or metabolism (58). Parenteral hydroxyzine (100 mg) is reported to be superior to placebo and equivalent to very low-dose morphine (8 mg) in patients suffering severe pain (59). Two studies indicate intramuscular hydroxyzine (100

mg) combined with morphine produced greater pain relief than did morphine alone (59, 60). Nevertheless, in these studies the addition of hydroxyzine to morphine did not increase the percentage of patients who reported better than 50% reduction in pain. The combination did, however, produce significantly greater drowsiness, which may have confounded pain reports.

Thus, hydroxyzine (75–100 mg parenterally) may have an analgesic effect equivalent to 8–10 mg of morphine. Hydroxyzine administration causes sedation and marked discomfort at the injection sites, and subcutaneous administration can produce severe tissue damage. Because of these liabilities and the limited data for therapeutic efficacy, the routine use of hydroxyzine to potentiate opiate analgesia in postoperative care cannot be recommended. Its use in acute phases of soft tissue injury of the neck has not been investigated.

**Chronic Musculoskeletal Pain.** Musculoskeletal pain is a very broad "diagnostic" term, but is often employed to describe discomfort resulting from soft tissue injury and perhaps compounded by chronic anxiety. Given the extensive use of benzodiazepines in the care of patients with chronic neck and back pain, it is surprising that there are so few rigorous studies of their efficacy, indications, and interactions with other treatments. While there is some evidence that benzodiazepines may be useful in short-term management of tension headaches, their role in chronic pain from soft tissue injury remains largely unexplored. Hollister et al. (61) suggested that diazepam produces extended relief in chronic pain from musculoskeletal disorders and is rarely associated with abuse. Others (62, 63) argue that conventional measures such as heat, rest, and nonnarcotic analgesics are as effective as diazepam, and that even high doses of this drug do not produce clinically detectable skeletal muscle relaxation (62). Furthermore, Hendler et al. (64) reported evidence of significantly more impairment in intellectual processes such as problem solving, speeded thinking, and motor performance in chronic pain patients receiving diazepam than in those receiving nonnarcotic or narcotic analgesics. This is especially important since intact problem-solving skills are associated with good outcome in rehabilitation programs.

Given the limited evidence for their effectiveness and the well-known risks associated with chronic administration, benzodiazepines appear to be vastly overused in chronic pain cases. These agents should be reserved for patients who manifest diagnosable episodes of anxiety, and should not be routinely prescribed as a general "aid" in helping patients cope with chronic pain.

**Mechanism of Action.** Benzodiazepines increase the ability of γ-aminobutyric acid (GABA) to inhibit brain and spinal cord neurotransmission; they also inhibit cholinergic and monoaminergic pathways (65). The anxiolytic effects may be mediated by GABAergic inhibitory effects on the limbic system. Since GABA is thought to mediate presynaptic and postsynaptic inhibition and facilitate recurrent inhibition (66), benzodiazepines might decrease the central transmission of ascending noxious stimuli, although this has not been associated with acute pain reduction in clinical samples.

## CENTRAL NERVOUS SYSTEM STIMULANTS

Central nervous system stimulants, such as the amphetamines [d,l-amphetamine (Benzedrine), d-amphetamine (Dexedrine), methamphetamine (Methedrine)], the related compound methylphenidate (Ritalin), cocaine, and caffeine, have selected roles in medical practice. The amphetamines and methylphenidate are used primarily for attention-deficit disorders and hyperactivity associated with minimal brain dysfunction in children, and in narcolepsy. Cocaine has traditional use as a local anesthetic, and caffeine appears in numerous combinations with analgesics.

### Amphetamines, Cocaine, and Caffeine

**Experimentally Induced and Clinical Acute Pain.** Psychostimulants lack primary analgesic properties (67). Amphetamines potentiate narcotic and nonnarcotic analgesia in animals (68, 69) and in man (70–72), presumably by catecholaminergic mechanisms (68). A single-dose study of postoperative patients concluded that the combination of dextroamphetamine (10 mg parenterally) and morphine (10 mg) was twice as potent as morphine alone, and a combination with 5 mg dextroamphetamine was 1.5 times as potent as a given dosage of morphine (72). There were minimal effects on blood pressure, pulse, and respiratory rate. Because of the study design, the effects of longer term use of amphetamine on mood, appetite, sensorium, and other aspects of postoperative convalescence could not be addressed.

Caffeine may augment pain relief obtained from nonsteroidal anti-inflammatory analgesics. In patients with mild to moderate postsurgical pain, caffeine (100–200 mg orally) increased the analgesic potency of aspirin and acetaminophen by 40% (73). Oral dosages up to 600 mg/day of caffeine cause few side effects. Thus caffeine may have some usefulness as an adjunct to analgesics used in the acute rehabilitation of patients with pain from cervical trauma who have undergone surgery.

**Chronic Pain.** Potent stimulants may have restricted use in patients undergoing rehabilitation from cervical injury. There is some evidence that psychostimulants are effective antidepressants in depressed medically ill subjects (74). Recent anecdotal reports from the psychiatric literature (75–77) suggest that dextroamphetamine (2–20 mg/day) and methylphenidate (up to 20 mg/day) may be effective antidepressants in hospitalized medically ill patients whose rehabilitation is delayed beyond expected limits, as well as in patients having a major depressive episode. Improved mood, reduced focus on pain, and renewed interest in participating in rehabilitation occurred in about 50% of patients within 2–7 days. The major side effect was confusion, which developed in demented patients. Most patients were successfully treated in about 1 week, although some required several months of treatment. Whether these agents generally might be useful in the rehabilitation of hospitalized and demoralized patients is speculative and awaits further data.

**Mechanism of Action.** The mechanism of action of psychostimulants is unclear. The therapeutic effects probably result from activation of monoamine systems important in pain suppression. Amphetamines exert their effects directly by stimulating adrenergic receptors, and indirectly by releasing catecholamines and inhibiting their degradation by the enzyme MAO. Caffeine has direct and indirect effects similar in kind to those of the amphetamines, but obviously less potent.

## SUMMARY

Because it focuses on controlled studies, this review presents a conservative summary and may overlook promising anecdotal reports of the use of psychotropic agents in pain syndromes relevant to cervical injury and rehabilitation. Given the available evidence, the TCAs have the most clearly documented efficacy in the rehabilitation of patients with cervical injury. The primary indication for TCAs is concurrent major depressive disorder and pain, although they may be helpful in pain associated with arachnoiditis. Other classes of antidepressants (MAOIs and lithium) may be employed if the depression is unresponsive to TCAs.

By contrast, the antipsychotic agents should be considered only as adjuncts to TCAs in the management of patients with neuropathic pain. The benzodiazepines are overprescribed in pain syndromes, and little documentation exists for their efficacy in treatment of chronic skeletal muscle contraction or chronic anxiety. The potent psychostimulants (e.g., amphetamines and methylphenidate) have no firmly established role as primary or adjunctive agents in the rehabilitation setting. Nevertheless, their short-term role in activating depressed or demoralized patients toward fruitful participation in rehabilitation awaits controlled investigation.

In the next section we describe psychopharmacologic treatment approaches for selected syndromes. This includes pretreatment evaluation, initial therapy, maintenance treatment, and alternative strategies for patients who fail to respond to first-line agents.

## CLINICAL APPROACHES AND GUIDELINES

### TRICYCLIC ANTIDEPRESSANT AGENTS

The indications for TCAs are described in Table 14.1. The compounds and dosages are listed in Table 14.2.

## Properties and Side Effects

Tricyclic antidepressants were derived from neuroleptics: imipramine, the first TCA introduced, represents a modification of chlorpromazine, and amitriptyline was derived from imipramine. More recently available drugs such as amoxapine (Asendin) are variations on the basic tricyclic structure and are pharmacologically and clinically similar to imipramine (78). TCAs increase serotonergic and/or noradrenergic tone by blockade of serotonin and norepinephrine reuptake at presynaptic nerve endings, may increase norepinephrine or serotonin receptor density or sensitivity, and may reduce $\beta$-adrenergic receptor sensitivity (65). The tricyclics also have strong anticholinergic properties, producing autonomic, cardiac, and central nervous system (CNS) side effects. Autonomic effects include dry mouth, blurred vision, constipation, ileus, and urinary retention. Cardiovascular effects include orthostatic hypotension, increased heart rate, and repolarization abnormalities on the electrocardiogram (Q-T interval prolongation and T wave inversion or flattening). Atrial and ventricular arrhythmias, as well as conduction delay with bundle-branch block, may occur. This results from prolongation of the H-V interval (the time from activation of the bundle of His to activation of ventricular myocardium). These effects resemble the properties of type I cardiac antiarrhythmics, such as quinidine and procainamide (66). The tricyclics also can depress myocardial contractility. CNS effects can include

**Table 14.1.**
**Indications for Psychotropic Drug Treatment in Cervical Pain Syndromes**[a]

| Treatment | Diagnosis and Clinical Efficacy | |
|---|---|---|
| | Relatively Well-Established Clinical Efficacy[b] | Possible Clinical Efficacy[c] |
| Tricyclic antidepressants | Chronic pain | Neuropathic pain (arachnoiditis) |
| | Primary major depression | |
| | Major depression secondary to chronic pain | Augment narcotics |
| MAO inhibitors | Primary major depression | |
| | Major depression secondary to chronic pain | |
| Lithium carbonate | Primary major depression | |
| Neuroleptics | | Neuropathic pain (arachnoiditis) |
| Antianxiety agents | | Chronic anxiety |
| | | Neuropathic syndromes |
| Stimulants | | Depression-pain syndromes |

[a]Adapted from Atkinson (1).
[b]Effectiveness established in controlled trials.
[c]Effectiveness reported in open label studies.

**Table 14.2.**
**Representative Antidepressants**[a]

| | Usual Daily Oral Dose (mg) | |
|---|---|---|
| | In Neuropathic Pain[b] | As Antidepressant |
| Tricyclics | | |
| Tertiary amines | | |
| Imipramine (Tofranil) | 10–75 | 150–250 |
| Amitriptyline (Elavil) | 10–75 | 150–250 |
| Doxepin (Sinequan) | 10–75 | 150–250 |
| Secondary amines | | |
| Desipramine (Norpramin) | 10–75 | 100–250 |
| Nortriptyline (Aventyl) | 10–75 | 100–150 |
| Maprotiline (Ludiomil) | c | 150–200 |
| Monoamine oxidase inhibitors | | |
| Tranylcypromine (Parnate) | 10–30 | 10–30 |
| Phenelzine (Nardil) | 15–90 | 45–90 |
| Lithium carbonate | 300–1200 | 900–2400 |

[a]Adapted from Atkinson (1).
[b]Potential neuropathic syndrome in cervical pain is arachnoiditis.
[c]Experience insufficient to determine usage. Probably below usual antidepressant dose.

agitated states (not uncommon in elderly patients, perhaps because there is less protein plasma binding of the drug in the elderly and higher plasma concentrations), and deliria caused by an anticholinergic brain syndrome. Other common side effects are weight gain, delayed ejaculation, and impotence. Extrapyramidal symptoms (tremor, increased muscle tone) are rare, but can develop.

## Selected Drug Interactions

**Sympathomimetic Amines.** Tricyclics potentiate the pressor response of direct-acting amines such as norepinephrine, epinephrine, and phenylephrine (79), with possible hypertensive crisis characterized by hypothermia, sweating, severe headache, and cerebrovascular accident.

**Neuroleptics.** Since tricyclics and neuroleptics compete for the same hepatic metabolic pathways, their anticholinergic and hypotensive properties may be additive or potentiated (80).

**Sedative-Hypnotics.** Tricyclics increase the CNS and respiratory depressant activity of barbiturates and related sedatives (80, 81) and increase the toxicity and potential lethality of these agents.

**Propranolol.** Tricyclics may potentiate propranolol-induced depression of myocardial contractility and hypotension from central vasomotor regulatory centers (82), and patients with mi-

graine headaches treated with these combinations should be monitored closely.

**Opiates.** Tricyclics potentiate meperidine-induced respiratory depression in animals (81), and increase the anticholinergic activity of opiates.

## Pretreatment Evaluation

Patients over the age of 50 or who have a history of cardiovascular disease (stroke, myocardial infarction, angina, congestive heart failure, syncope, or arrhythmias) should have an electrocardiogram and standing and supine blood pressure measurements before treatment. Careful assessment of the risk-benefit ratio and cardiology consultation are indicated in the presence of bradyarrhythmias, heart block, or prolonged Q-T intervals. Orthostatic blood pressure changes of over 10 mm Hg *before* drug treatment may be associated with pronounced postural changes during treatment, and patients with preexisting orthostatic changes should be carefully observed (83). A careful drug history should be obtained, both to assess possible drug interactions and to determine past response and reactions to TCAs. Additional laboratory investigation should include a complete blood count with differential and liver function tests.

Patients with cervical spinal cord injury require

meticulous assessment because of the effects of TCAs on the autonomic nervous system (84). Anticholinergic effects of TCAs and neuroleptic agents can disrupt reflex drainage of the neurogenic bladder by parasympatholytic effects; $\alpha$-adrenergic blockade of these drugs can lead to profound hypotension if the patient with quadriparesis and compromised sympathetic outflow is tilted into an upright position. In these instances, use of a TCA with fewer anticholinergic properties is indicated. The TCAs all have equivalent $\alpha$-adrenergic blocking properties and should be given at night, when cord-injured patients are supine (84). Starting doses should be low (e.g., desipramine 10 mg) and increases should be made cautiously (25–50 mg increments per week).

## Drug Selection

Amitriptyline, nortriptyline, imipramine, and desipramine all have approximately equivalent antidepressant efficacy. Additionally, these agents are probably equally effective in the back pain syndromes for which they are indicated. Drug selection therefore depends on side effects. In general, anticholinergic, cardiac, and CNS side effects are more common with tertiary amines (amitriptyline, imipramine, and doxepin) than with demethylated secondary amines (nortriptyline, desipramine, and others). Thus, desipramine is the least anticholinergic and sedating of the tricyclic drugs. Patients with agitation or insomnia may benefit more from sedating drugs. There is some evidence that nortriptyline is less likely to depress H-V conduction and less likely to produce orthostatic hypotension (at the serum concentrations usually employed to treat depression) than are other tricyclics (83). Nortriptyline may thus be preferred in patients with bradyarrhythmias, heart block, or prolonged Q-T interval. Doxepin is also thought to be relatively noncardiotoxic, but that is not well documented. All tricyclics will increase heart rate secondary to adrenergic and anticholinergic effects. Furthermore, imipramine suppresses ventricular arrhythmias (ectopy) and patients on quinidine may need their dosage of that agent revised.

Some second-generation antidepressants [e.g., trazodone (Desyrel)] are structurally unrelated to and exert their action through mechanisms different from tricyclic drugs. The efficacy of these agents for neuropathic syndromes has not been adequately assessed, but their antidepressant efficacy approaches that of the first-generation agents (amitriptyline and imipramine). Newly available agents with more specific and potent serotonergic effects [e.g., fluoxetine (Prozac)] may hold additional promise for management of chronic pain and associated depression. At this time, however, most patients with responsive neuropathic syndromes or depression should be treated initially with a first-generation drug. Claims of an improved safety record for second-generation antidepressants await documentation.

## Treatment Technique for Acute Pain

Because of the limited evidence of efficacy of TCA agents in alleviating acute pain, either alone or in combination with conventional analgesics, there is no indication for these drugs in the (nondepressed) patient with acute pain. Treatment of the patient with a major depressive episode who also happens to suffer from acute pain is the same as discussed below for the depressed chronic pain patient.

## Treatment Technique for Chronic Pain

**Considerations in Treatment of the Nondepressed Cervical Pain Patient.** Efficacy of TCA in nondepressed individuals depends upon the etiology of the pain syndrome: selected neuropathic pain and headache syndromes are likely to benefit, but evidence that pain from arthritic disorders responds is equivocal. No data indicate that the TCAs alleviate pain from intervertebral disc herniation, or from muscle, tendon, and ligament injury such as might occur in mild flexion-hyperextension ("whiplash") trauma. Painful cervical radiculopathy from nerve root lesions (e.g., from cervical vertebral osteophytes or disc herniation) theoretically might benefit, to the extent this represents one of the neuropathic phenomena known to respond to TCAs. Again, however, no data are available from trials using patients with cervical root lesions. Our own limited clinical experience using TCAs in such cervical neuropathies has yielded mixed results. Clinicians wishing to attempt treatment could proceed as follows:

Patients without evidence of complicating medical or psychiatric disorders are generally started on nortriptyline or imipramine at 10–25 mg at night, with 10–25-mg increases every 3 days to a maximum of 75 mg daily. The drug is usually given at bedtime to take advantage of any sedating effects, although doses initially may be divided if a single dose produces excessive side effects.

Elderly patients or those with cardiovascular disease should receive a 10–25-mg test dose and have orthostatic blood pressure determinations taken 1 hr later.

A therapeutic response to other neuropathic pain (e.g., diabetic peripheral neuropathy, postherpetic neuralgia) usually ensues within 2 weeks, often within 5–7 days. The physician should schedule follow-up appointments at least every week during the initial month of treatment, with orthostatic blood pressure determinations or electrocardiograms as warranted. Every-other-week appointments are useful in the next month of therapy to ensure compliance and monitor progress.

If no benefit appears within 3–4 weeks, or if side effects are unusually severe, a determination of the plasma concentration of the antidepressant is warranted. Plasma concentrations may be used to check compliance, improve efficacy, diminish toxicity, and detect unsuspected drug interactions (84). This allows the clinician to assess whether an alternative therapy is indicated, or if an increase or decrease in dose is necessary. Other indications for a plasma concentration determination include cardiovascular disease; these patients may warrant routine plasma monitoring because they are at increased risk for toxicity. The practitioner should have his or her own protocol for interpreting results from any particular laboratory.

The most effective plasma concentrations of antidepressants for pain syndromes generally are thought to be below those usually therapeutic for depression. Therapeutic levels for treating depression with amitriptyline are 200 ng/ml total tricyclic (amitriptyline plus nortriptyline); for nortriptyline there may be a therapeutic window of efficacy between 50 and 150 ng/ml. Concentrations below or above this interval may be ineffective for an antidepressant reponse. With imipramine, concentrations exceeding 225 ng/ml are therapeutic in depression; doxepin therapeutic concentrations are uncertain, but perhaps in the range of 150–250 ng/ml.

Blood samples drawn for plasma concentrations of antidepressants should reflect steady state levels, and a patient's dosage should have been stabilized for at least 1 week. Samples are obtained 10–16 hr after a single dose, or 2–5 hr after the morning dose if a divided dosage regimen is employed.

*Maintenance Treatment.* In patients with endocrine or postinfectious neuropathies a positive response warrants treatment for about 5–6 months.

The maintenance dose should be the minimum effective level after control is established. Attempts to discontinue the tricyclic should be made at least every 6 months. The TCA should be discontinued over a 2–3-week period, to avoid an abstinence syndrome. These guidelines may apply in posttraumatic neuropathies, but there is no good evidence at this time to guide treatment.

**Initial Treatment of the Depressed Pain Patient.** All depressed patients should be evaluated for suicidality and the need for hospitalization, and psychiatric consultation is warranted. If a diagnosis of major depression is made, treatment with a tricyclic agent at full antidepressant dosages is indicated. There is no evidence that these agents are effective in patients with depressed mood who do not qualify for a diagnosis of major depression or dysthymic disorder. If outpatient treatment is offered instead of hospitalization, caution must be exercised in the total amount of drug prescribed if suicide is a concern. TCA overdoses amounting to 1000 mg produce serious side effects and those of 2000 mg of any tricyclic commonly are lethal. In cases of major depression the target antidepressant dosages are the same as those indicated in psychiatric populations. We usually begin at a low initial dosage (e.g., imipramine 25 mg) with increases of 25–50 mg every 3 days to a final dose of 150–300 mg daily. Hospitalized patients may receive higher initial dosage with 50-mg increases daily up to the full amount.

An antidepressant effect is evidenced by improved activity, energy, and mood, and should appear within 3–8 weeks. Patients should be informed that these agents take time to exert their full effect, and not to expect immediate relief. Reduction of pain intensity may lag behind improvement in activity and mood by several weeks, and is not a target symptom. As above, plasma antidepressant concentrations should be obtained if a poor response is noted after 6 weeks of administration, or if severe side effects intervene.

*Maintenance Treatment.* A maintenance dose of a TCA is usually about 25% lower than the dosage used in the acute phase of treatment (78). Treatment is maintained for about 5 or 6 months (the usual length of an affective episode), and the antidepressant may then be discontinued (85). Again, tapering the tricyclic regimen over several weeks is indicated to avoid an abstinence syndrome. Over 40% of individuals hospitalized for major depression may experience chronic or fluctuating depressive symptoms on 2-year follow-up

(86, 87) and almost 25% may relapse within 3 months after full recovery from the index episode (87). For these reasons careful follow-up is essential.

*Treatment Nonresponse.* Treatment of the pain patient with major depression who does not respond to initial therapy is a complex topic beyond the scope of this chapter. Generally, treatment nonresponse indicates a need for consultation by an experienced psychiatrist to reevaluate the diagnosis and treatment regimen. If the treatment of depression is still required, the choices include: (*a*) adding L-triiodothyronine (Cytomel) (25–50 μg) to the tricyclic antidepressant; (*b*) switching to another antidepressant of a different class, with or without adding L-triiodothyronine; (*c*) considering electroconvulsive therapy; (*d*) switching to a MAOI; and (*e*) attempting combination therapy using lithium or a MAOI with a TCA (78).

## MONOAMINE OXIDASE INHIBITORS

The indications for MAOIs are described in Table 14.1. The compounds and doses are listed in Table 14.2.

### Properties and Side Effects

Monoamine oxidase inhibitors enhance the availability of CNS norepinephrine and serotonin in the brain by inhibiting their catabolism. Antidepressant activity may also be related to effects on noradrenergic and serotonergic postsynaptic receptor function or sensitivity.

The major indications for MAOIs are (*a*) agoraphobia with or without panic attacks, (*b*) the so-called atypical depressive disorders with "reversed" vegetative symptoms (increased sleep, weight gain, reactive mood), and (*c*) major depression that has not responded to trials of TCAs.

The MAOI side effect profile is similar to that of the TCAs but of a lesser degree, and includes postural hypotension, agitation, confusion, and mild anticholinergic symptoms: blurred vision, dry mouth, constipation, ileus, and urinary retention. The major issue in using these agents is the need to instruct patients to avoid foods or medications containing tyramine or other pressor amines. Proscribed foods include cheeses (except cottage cheese and cream cheese), pickled foods, beer and red wines, and fava beans (88). Because the MAOIs block metabolism of pressor amines contained in these foods, severe hypertension may develop abruptly after they are eaten.

### Selected Drug Interactions

**Sympathomimetic Agents.** All medication with sympathomimetic activity, including phenylephrine and ephedrine (found in over-the-counter cold tablets), can produce a hypertensive crisis.

**Narcotic Analgesics.** The so-called type I interaction is a potentiation of primary narcotic effects (including analgesia, hypotension, respiratory depression, and coma) as a result of MAOI inhibition of hepatic metabolism of narcotics (66, 89). Naloxone (Narcan) reverses this response. Phenelzine may be safer in this regard than other MAOIs.

The type II interaction is similar to that resulting from administration of sympathomimetic amines or tyramine to patients on MAOIs. The concurrent use of MAOIs and meperidine (90, 91) or dextromethorphan (92) produces agitation, excitement, restlessness, hypertension, headache, rigidity, and convulsions. The mechanism of this response is unknown but it may be mediated by increased brain serotonin release (93).

Codeine may be used safely in patients on MAOIs who require moderate analgesia (88). If other narcotics are mandatory only 20–25% of the usual therapeutic narcotic dose should be used and vital signs and level of consciousness should be observed carefully (88). Meperidine should never be used since its interaction with MAOIs is too unpredictable and life-threatening complications can occur rapidly.

**Sedative Hypnotics.** MAOI inhibition of microsomal enzymes prolongs the effects of sedative hypnotics, including barbiturates and chloral hydrate (94). Lower doses of sedative hypnotics and close monitoring are advised.

### Pretreatment Evaluation

The physical and laboratory evaluation is similar to that used for TCAs, with a special emphasis on drug and dietary history, the patient's ability to comply with the complex dietary restrictions, and cardiovascular status. There is little experience to guide use of MAOIs in patients with cervical spinal cord injury, and expert psychiatric consultation should be obtained when considering these patients for treatment.

### Drug Selection

Phenelzine and tranylcypromine are the most commonly prescribed agents. Tranylcypromine is sometimes preferred because it inhibits MAO activity for only about 24 hr after it is discontinued. Phenelzine inhibits MAO for over a week after it is discontinued.

## Treatment Technique for Chronic Pain

**Initial Treatment.** The principal use of an MAOI in cervical pain syndromes is in patients with major depression who are not candidates for TCAs or who have failed to respond to TCAs. Again, it is recommended that psychiatric consultations be obtained to reevaluate the patient's diagnosis before commencing treatment. Serious side effects from use of MAOIs are relatively rare, and their danger has probably been overstated, but relatively few clinicians are experienced in their use.

Proper dosage is crucial to antidepressant efficacy, and therapeutic failure is commonly due to undertreatment (88). The clinical endpoint for correct dosage is mild postural hypotension and muscle fasiculations after the second week of treatment. The usual dosage of phenelzine for initial treatment is up to 60–90 mg/day. A treatment protocol may begin with 15 mg on day 1, 30 mg on day 2, and 15 mg in the morning and 30 mg in the evening on day 3, if the patient is asymptomatic. Phenelzine is maintained at 45 mg daily until day 14 if there are no side effects, and then the dosage can be increased to 30 mg in the morning and 30 mg in the evening; on day 21 the dosage can be increased to 30 mg in the morning, 15 mg in the afternoon, and 30 mg in the evening; on day 28 the dosage can be increased to 30 mg three times daily if there are no side effects. After adequate or maximum dosage is achieved, the patient should be monitored weekly for another 4–6 weeks (88).

**Maintenance Treatment.** Guidelines for continuing treatment are the same as those established for psychiatric patients with major depression. Psychiatric patients with major depression may experience a relapse of symptoms at dosages below the initial optimal regimen (88). After approximately 6 months of successful therapy the MAOI can be slowly discontinued (by 15 mg every 1–3 weeks until the patient is off the drug) and the patient should be observed for relapse.

**Treatment Nonresponse.** Again, experienced psychiatric consultation is often indicated because treatment of refractory mood disorder is complex. Another MAOI may be used. MAOIs have been combined with various medications, including TCAs and L-tryptophan. It is difficult to

evaluate the efficacy of these combinations, and both tricyclics and tryptophan may provoke a hypertensive crisis.

## NEUROLEPTIC AGENTS

The neuroleptic drugs are described in Table 14.1, and the compounds and dosages are listed in Table 14.3. Neuroleptic agents have an extremely limited role in patients with cervical trauma and pain. They may be used to help sedate the delirious or severely agitated postoperative patient. Another use may be as adjunctive treatment in neuropathic pain associated with cervical pain.

## Properties and Side Effects

Neuroleptics inhibit dopaminergic transmission in the CNS. Blockade of the nigrostriatal system produces extrapyramidal symptoms (tremor, rigidity, bradykinesia, akathesia, and dystonia). Blockade at the chemoreceptor trigger zone of the hypothalamus produces antiemetic properties. Blockade in the limbic system and associated cortex produces antianxiety and antipsychotic effects (95).

Neuroleptics also have anti-α-adrenergic and anticholinergic effects. These properties are most prominent with the aliphatic agents (e.g., chlorpromazine) and less so with piperadine and piper-

**Table 14.3.**
**Representative Neuroleptics[a]**

| Class | Relative Potency | Usual Daily Oral Dose in Pain Treatment (mg) |
|---|---|---|
| Phenothiazines | | |
| Chlorpromazine (Thorazine) | Low | 10–50 |
| Methotrimeprazine (Levoprome) | Low | 10–50 |
| Thioridazine (Mellaril) | Low | 10–75 |
| Perphenazine (Trilafon) | High | 1–5 |
| Trifluoperazine (Stelazine) | High | 1–5 |
| Fluphenazine (Prolixin) | High | 1–3 |
| Butyrophenones | | |
| Haloperidol (Haldol) | High | 1–3 |

[a]Adapted from Atkinson (1).

azine agents and the butyrophenones. Cardiovascular effects include increased heart rate and postural hypotension. Repolarization abnormalities of the electrocardiogram include T wave abnormalities, prolonged PQ-T intervals, and S-T segment depression. Direct myocardial depressant effects may occur in patients with cardiovascular disease. Neuroleptic agents may alter conduction times and, rarely, induce potentially fatal ventricular arrhythmias.

Idiosyncratic allergic responses can occur with suppression of the hematopoietic system (leukopenia, anemia, or thrombocytopenia). These reactions usually occur within the first 6 weeks of treatment and their clinical hallmark is the sudden onset of painful pharyngitis and fever. An allergic hepatitis with mild increases in liver function tests can occur, and cholestatic jaundice has been reported.

Extrapyramidal symptoms, dystonias, and tardive dyskinesia are the most common side effects. Extrapyramidal symptoms can be managed with anti-Parkinson agents [benztropine mesylate (Cogentin), trihexyphenidyl (Artane)], diphenhydramine (Benadryl), or amantadine (Symmetrel). Nevertheless, anti-Parkinson drugs should not be given prophylactically, since extrapyramidal symptoms often do not occur at the low doses of neuroleptics prescribed for patients with cervical syndromes. If these agents are used, the usual daily dose is 1–6 mg benztropine mesylate daily or 2–10 mg trihexyphenidyl daily (95). If such symptoms are treated, it is recommended that these drugs be tapered or discontinued after 3 months.

Dystonia involves tonic contraction of muscles, usually of the head and neck, and produces grimaces, posturing, and torticollis. It rarely occurs at low dosages. Treatment is with 25–50 mg diphenhydramine intramuscularly. Akathesia (the perception of an inability to sit still) responds best to dose reduction of the offending drug (95), and would be rare at the low dosages employed for pain patients.

Tardive dyskinesia is a syndrome of involuntary choreiform movements that commence after prolonged treatment with neuroleptics and persist up to years after the neuroleptics are withdrawn. Symptoms can include periodic tongue protrusions, lip smacking, chewing movements of the mouth, athetoid movements of the fingers, and restless shifting from leg to leg. In their severe form such movements can be disabling. The mechanism for tardive dyskinesia is unknown but may involve dopaminergic receptor supersensitivity or excessive dopaminergic activity in the basal ganglia. Oftentimes treatment is not effective and the best approach is prevention (95). Dosages for the neuroleptics should be kept below 5 mg daily of the high-potency agents or the equivalent in the low-potency agents. Treatment should be limited to months rather than years.

## Selected Drug Interactions

**Nonnarcotic Analgesics.** There are no apparent adverse drug interactions between nonnarcotic analgesics and neuroleptics, although acetaminophen inhibits metabolism of some neuroleptics (e.g., chlorpromazine) and therefore augments their effects.

**Narcotic Analgesics.** Phenothiazines enhance and prolong the hypotensive and respiratory depressant effect of narcotics. Chlorpromazine also increases serum levels of the neurotoxic and cardiotoxic N-demethylated metabolites of meperidine, which are associated with neuromuscular irritability, seizures, bradycardia, and hypotension.

## Pretreatment Evaluation.

The medical evaluation is the same as that for candidates for TCAs, including electrocardiogram for patients over age 50 or those with preexisting heart disease, and genitourinary assessment for benign prostatic hypertrophy. These drugs are metabolized by the liver and patients with hepatic disease will need lower dosages. Laboratory assessment should include baseline complete blood count with differential and liver function tests.

## Drug Selection

Generally pain patients with neuropathic syndromes will be treated with a high-potency, low-dose agent, such as haloperidol or fluphenazine, in combination with a TCA. The side effect profile and therapeutic efficacy of these agents are equivalent, and the clinician need select only one or two neuroleptics in this classification and become thoroughly familiar with their properties and usage.

## Treatment Technique for Acute Pain

The antipsychotic drugs generally do not appear to have analgesic properties or to reliably augment narcotic analgesics. Therefore, for our purposes they are most likely to be used to sedate delirious or acutely agitated patients. A high-potency neuroleptic is usually chosen. For example, 0.5–5.0 mg haloperidol orally, intravenously, or intramuscularly may be administered every 30–60 minutes until sedation is achieved. The total dose needed to calm the patient is computed, and one half this total dose may be given 12 hr later to maintain sedation. Two to 3 days of treatment usually suffices, since by then metabolic or other abnormalities associated with the delirium can be corrected.

## Treatment Technique for Chronic Pain

**Initial and Maintenance Treatment.** Neuroleptics might be considered (rarely) for use as adjuncts to TCAs in treatment of painful neuropathic conditions associated with cervical trauma. Adjunctive treatment is used only if the tricyclic alone has produced unsatisfactory relief. The usual choice would be a high-potency neuroleptic, generally fluphenazine or haloperidol, added to the chosen TCA. The starting dose is 0.5–1 mg at night, with an increase to 1 mg twice daily after 3–5 days, or to 1 mg three times daily if there is no improvement after 10 days. Once the maximum dose of 3 mg daily is reached, this is given as a one-time dose at bedtime. There should be a response within 2 or 3 weeks. Some authorities employ low-potency/high-dose aliphatic agents such as methotrimeprazine, a congener of chlorpromazine. The usual dosage is 50 mg or less, given once daily at bedtime (96). The risk of tardive dyskinesia always must be kept in mind and may mitigate against using these drugs.

The patient should be carefully monitored for symptoms of tardive dyskinesia. After 3 months the drug should be tapered to the lowest therapeutic dosage. At no more than 6 months one should taper the patient off the neuroleptic and observe for an increase in pain. If continued treatment is needed the maintenance dosage should be at the lowest possible amounts, with periodic attempts to discontinue the neuroleptic.

**Treatment Nonresponse.** If tricyclics fail to improve neuropathic pain, one might employ clonazepam and avoid tricyclic-neuroleptic combinations altogether. The usual dosage range is 1–3 mg daily. A response should occur within 3 weeks. Experienced psychiatric consultation is essential when using these medications.

## ANTIANXIETY DRUGS

The indications for anxiolytic drugs are described in Table 14.1. The compounds and dosages are listed in Table 14.4.

### Benzodiazepines

**Properties and Side Effects.** The benzodiazepines enhance GABA-mediated presynaptic and postsynaptic inhibition in the spinal cord, brainstem, cerebellar cortex, cerebral cortex, and

**Table 14.4**
**Representative Antianxiety Agents**[a]

| | Usual Daily Oral Antianxiety Dose in Pain Treatment (mg) | Usual Oral Hypnotic Dose (mg) |
|---|---|---|
| Benzodiazepines | | |
| Long half-life | | |
| Clorazepate (Tranxene) | 3–15 | 15–30 |
| Flurazepam (Dalmane) | — | 15–30 |
| Intermediate half-life | | |
| Chlordiazepoxide (Librium) | 15–30 | 50 |
| Diazepam (Valium) | 2.5–15 | 15–30 |
| Short half-life | | |
| Alprazolam (Xanax) | 0.5–3.0 | — |
| Lorazepam (Ativan)[b] | 2–5 | — |
| Oxazepam (Serax)[b] | 10–50 | 30–60 |
| Other | | |
| Hydroxyzine (Vistaril) | 100–400 | — |

[a]Adapted from Atkinson (1).
[b]No active metabolites.

other structures. This activity may in part explain their antianxiety, anticonvulsant, and sedative effects, along with an ability to produce centrally induced muscle relaxation. Benzodiazepines have the potential to produce tolerance, psychological as well as physical dependence, and an abstinence syndrome upon withdrawal. Their effects are additive with those of other CNS depressants, and cross-tolerance and cross-dependence develop.

Abrupt discontinuation of benzodiazepines after 1–6 months of uninterrupted use can produce an abstinence syndrome consisting of insomnia, nausea, myalgia, muscle twitching, diaphoresis, and potentially major motor seizures. The probability of developing a withdrawal syndrome appears to vary with the length of treatment: patients treated for less than 4 months at the usual therapeutic dosage are unlikely to develop symptoms; about 5% of those treated for up to 1 year may develop symptoms, and those treated for over 1 year run a much higher risk (97).

CNS depressant side effects are sedation, ataxia, and dysarthria. In the elderly these agents may produce confusion and paradoxical excitement. Caution should be used in pregnant patients, since teratogenic effects (i.e., cleft palate) are postulated. Bradycardia and hypotension can occur. Allergic phenomena are also reported, and include neutropenia and jaundice.

**Drug Interactions.** The most important interactions involve additive effects with other CNS depressants. Cimetidine (Tagamet), disulfiram (Antabuse), and oral contraceptives can increase the half-life of benzodiazepines.

**Pretreatment Evaluation.** Acutely the major concern is for the patient's ability to tolerate the CNS-depressive effects of the drug. Chronically, the primary concern is misuse or abuse. Elderly patients are particularly at risk for falls resulting from intoxication, ataxia, and acute confusional episodes. Such side effects may occur at relatively low dosages because of the reduced rate of drug metabolism and reduced protein binding in the elderly. A cardiovascular history and electrocardiogram should be obtained as indicated: benzodiazepine withdrawal can precipitate angina, elevated blood pressure, or cardiac arrhythmias. Liver function tests should be obtained, and patients with liver disease may require a diminished dose.

**Drug Selection.** The benzodiazepines differ mainly in their elimination half-life and the presence of active metabolites. Those with the longest half-lives are chlorazepate (Tranxene), prazepam (Centrax), and halazepam (Paxipam). Moderately long-acting agents are diazepam (Valium) and chlordiazepoxide (Librium). The shortest acting are oxazepam (Serax), and lorazepam (Ativan). Because it is associated with a severe abstinence syndrome, and because drug tapering is difficult, many clinicians no longer prescribe alprazolam (Xanax). All these drugs have clinically important active metabolites except for oxazepam and lorazepam, and cumulative clinical effects occur with repeated dosage. If drug accumulation or prolonged effects are problems (as in elderly patients or those with hepatic disease), short-acting agents with no active metabolites may be preferred. The problems of drug accumulation also can be met by reducing the dosage of longer acting drugs. Although by themselves benzodiazepines are unlikely to be lethal in overdoses, their depressant effects are dangerous and potentially lethal if they are taken with alcohol, barbiturates, or other drugs that depress the CNS. Additionally, clinicians must be concerned with the possibility of benzodiazepines worsening clinical depression and increasing suicidal risk. Administration of these agents in depressed patients is therefore not recommended.

**Treatment Techniques for Acute and Chronic Pain.**

*Anxiety as a Special Problem.* Many patients with pain appear to be acutely or chronically anxious and may have diffuse neck or back pain, presumably related to painful muscular contraction. We rarely employ antianxiety agents for these patients and prefer to recommend progressive physical reconditioning, education about effects of pain, and perhaps biofeedback training when specific patterns of arousal and/or muscle activity are associated with pain. Nevertheless, if anxiety is a major source of disability in everyday activities, benzodiazepines may be indicated. Hollister (98) and others (99) have described guidelines for the proper use of benzodiazepines:

1. Use benzodiazepines only when there is interference in usual daily activities.
2. Use nondrug methods when possible.
3. Drug treatment should be brief and intermittent.
4. Doses should be titrated individually.
5. Efficacy should be assessed early.
6. Avoid benzodiazepines if a history of drug abuse is known.
7. Gradually discontinue the drug after chronic treatment (98).

To this list we would add the importance of combining pharmacologic agents with behavioral treatments aimed at mastery of stressors and anxiety response. This approach allows the physician to avoid the pitfall of overprescribing these agents. The nonpharmacologic measures described above for managing anxiety (e.g., exercise programs, relaxation training, and biofeedback) should still be considered the backbone of treating the anxious patient, and can be employed before, during, and after drug therapy.

Ideally benzodiazepine treatment is intermittent and brief. Most anxiety related to life stress is resolved within 1 month. Chronic anxiety and chronic pain waxes and wanes in intensity. Anxiolytics would be used only during exacerbations of the chronic disorder. Chronically anxious patients should not be treated indefinitely without periodically assessing the need for continuous treatment. Whether the patient is acutely or persistently anxious, a drug response generally occurs within the first 2 or 3 weeks of treatment (100). Therefore, if there is no improvement after several weeks on a proper regimen, benefit is unlikely with prolonged therapy and other avenues should be explored. Tolerance and/or dependence are avoided if the physician indicates that treatment will be brief, and that drug efficacy is best preserved by using medication only during exacerbations of pain or distress (98).

Hollister (98) described an effective protocol for use of benzodiazepines in treating anxiety. In this approach medication is given at night, 2–3 hr before normal bedtime. The minimum effective dose is determined as the amount required to produce restful sleep when taken 2–3 hr before bedtime. If the initial dose does not produce effective hypnosis the first night, twice the dose is given the second night, four times the dose is given the third night, and eight times the dose is given the fourth night. The patient can commence with 2.5 mg diazepam and then increase to 5, 10, or 20 mg. The usual minimum effective hypnotic dose is 10 mg or less. As a result, the patient achieves a good night's rest, unwanted oversedation is avoided during the daytime, and the anxiolytic effect is retained. If additional amounts are required during the day, usually one half or one third of the nighttime dose will suffice. This technique works best for long-acting benzodiazepines and is not suited for short-acting agents.

Failure to respond to treatment within 3 weeks may indicate an inadequate dosage regimen, or that another psychiatric diagnosis has been missed. For example, anxiety frequently masks depressive syndromes and an antidepressant would be required to successfully treat the depression. Alcohol abuse may also be present, and treatment with benzodiazepines may be undermined by the patient's tolerance to CNS depressants (98, 100). Indeed, some suggest that patients with histories of alcohol or other CNS depressant drug abuse be treated with agents less likely to be abused, such as hydroxyzine (100).

*Maintenance Treatment for Anxiety.* Occasionally chronically anxious patients may benefit from long-term treatment. In such cases the minimum effective dose should be used; reevaluation of the regimen should occur at least every 6 months. The clinician therefore should be alert that requests for escalating the dose may indicate misuse of the agent rather than tolerance. Patients who have been treated for more than 4 months with 20–40 mg diazepam daily (or the equivalent) should be withdrawn slowly, usually over 4–6 weeks or longer.

Buspirone (BuSpar) is an anxiolytic chemically and pharmacologically unrelated to the benzodiazepines. Since maximum benefit emerges only after 3–4 weeks of treatment, it has been advocated for treatment of chronic anxiety. Preliminary data indicate it has few CNS side effects. Its abuse potential is unknown.

## CENTRAL NERVOUS SYSTEM STIMULANTS

Indications for psychostimulants are described in Table 14.1, and the compounds and dosages are listed in Table 14.5. These drugs have a very restricted use in the treatment of any patient with pain, and are usually given only for primary treatment of attention deficit disorder in childhood, or for narcolepsy.

### Properties and Side Effects

Common preparations include *d*-amphetamine (Dexedrine), methylphenidate (Ritalin), and pem-

**Table 14.5.**
**Representative Psychostimulants**[a]

| | Usual Daily Antidepressant and Pain Management Dose (mg) |
|---|---|
| *d*-Amphetamine (Dexedrine) | 10–20 |
| Methylphenidate (Ritalin) | 15–20 |

[a]Adapted from Atkinson (1).

oline (Cylert). CNS stimulants are metabolized by hepatic oxidation and conjugating enzyme systems and also are excreted unchanged in the urine. They are postulated to produce CNS arousal by decreasing neuronal reuptake and deactivation of norepinephrine and dopamine. Physiologic dependence does not seem to occur in the same sense as with CNS depressants, although a withdrawal syndrome of inertia and depressed mood appears upon sudden withdrawal after high intake. Tolerance to euphoriant effects occurs rapidly (78). Side effects are those of anorexia plus sympathomimetic actions.

### Drug Interactions

The ability of psychostimulants to compete for hepatic enzymes reduces the metabolism of TCAs neuroleptics, antianxiety agents, and many other drugs. There are additive effects with other sympathomimetic drugs.

### Pretreatment Evaluation

Patients over age 50 years and those with a history of hypertension or cardiovascular disease are at increased risk for the drugs' sympathomimetic effects, and risk-benefit ratios must be carefully appraised. The elderly are particularly vulnerable to acute agitation or confusion. History of substance abuse must be elicited.

### Drug Selection

The stimulants are very similar in their side effect profiles. Because of its short half-life methylphenidate may be preferred in the elderly to reduce duration of any toxic effects.

### Treatment Techniques for Acute and Chronic Pain

**Initial and Maintenance Treatment.** While CNS psychostimulants augment narcotic analgesia acutely, there really seems to be little advantage to these drugs since simply increasing the dose of analgesic accomplishes the desired goal.

These agents are not used for first-line treatment of depression because of their limited efficacy (78). Some authorities describe successful use of these agents in depressed, hospitalized, medically ill individuals who have not progressed well in their rehabilitation (90). The initial dose of dextroamphetamine or methylphenidate is usu-

ally 5–10 mg each morning. Dextroamphetamine may be given once daily, whereas methylphenidate is administered in two divided doses at 8 AM and noon. If no response occurs after 2 days the dose is increased, but more than 20 mg daily is rarely required (77). A response should ensue by 7–10 days.

Maintenance treatment is not well described, and rarely extends beyond several weeks. Reports usually indicate that the agent is discontinued a few days after the patient becomes asymptomatic (77). Given the controversial nature of treatment with CNS stimulants the physician should carefully document his or her reasons for employing these drugs and the explanation to the patient of side effects and risk-benefit ratio. Treatment should be brief and there should be meticulous follow-up care.

### GENERAL COMMENTS AND CONCLUSIONS

Chronic cervical pain is a complex problem with biologic, psychological, and social aspects, which may disrupt multiple areas of the patient's life (e.g., work and household responsibilities, social and recreational pursuits, interpersonal relationships, moods and thoughts, sexual function, finances, and self-perception). Therefore, patients typically present not with pain in isolation, but rather with a constellation of symptoms, complaints, and complicating factors, such as impairment in everyday activity, emotional distress, medication misuse or abuse, and family problems. Obviously, psychopharmacologic treatment alone cannot be expected to "cure" all aspects of the problem (i.e., "suffering"), and thus should be considered as only one component of a comprehensive program of pain management and rehabilitation as described in this text. Although psychopharmacologic agents may play a significant role in comprehensive clinical care of patients with cervical pain, the importance of administering these drugs within the context of sound behavioral management principles and multidimensional treatments cannot be overemphasized.

### ACKNOWLEDGMENT

This work was supported in part by the Veterans Administration.

### REFERENCES

1. Atkinson JH: Psychopharmacologic agents in treatment of pain syndromes. In Tollison CD (ed): *Handbook of Chronic*

*Pain Management.* Baltimore, Williams & Wilkins, 1989, pp 69–103.

2. Atkinson JH, Slater MA: Interdisciplinary rehabilitation of low back pain: psychopharmacological Agents. In Tollison CD, Kriegel ML (eds): *Interdisciplinary Rehabilitation of Low Back Pain.* Baltimore, Williams & Wilkins, 1989, pp. 169–204.

3. American Psychiatric Association: *Diagnostic and Statistical Manual of Mental Disorders,* ed 3 (rev). Washington, DC, American Psychiatric Association, 1986.

4. Sternbach RA: *Pain Patients: Traits and Treatment.* New York, Academic Press, 1974.

5. Chapman CR, Butter SH: Effects of doxepin on perception of laboratory-induced pain in man. *Pain* 5:253–262, 1978.

6. Bromm B, Meier W, Scharein E: Imipramine reduces experimental pain. *Pain* 25:245–257, 1986.

7. Levine JD, Gordon NC, Smith R, McBryde R: Desipramine enhances opiate postoperative analgesia. *Pain* 27:45–49, 1986.

8. Ward NG, Bloom VL, Friedel RC: The effectiveness of tricyclic antidepressants in the treatment of coexisting pain and depression. *Pain* 7:331–341, 1979.

9. Ward NG: Tricyclic antidepressants for chronic low back pain. *Spine* 11:661–665, 1986.

10. Alcoff J, Jones E, Rust P, Newman R: Controlled trial of imipramine for chronic low back pain. *J Fam Pract* 14:841–846, 1982.

11. Hameroff SR, Cork RC, Scherer K, Crago BR, Neuman C, Womble JK, Davis TP: Doxepin effects on chronic pain, depression and plasma opioids. *J Clin Psychiatry* 43:22–27, 1982.

12. Pilowsky I, Hallett EC, Bassett DL, Thomas PG, Penhall RK: A controlled study of amitriptyline in the treatment of chronic pain. *Pain* 14:169–179, 1982.

13. Pheasant H, Bursk A, Goldfarb J, Azen SP, Weiss JN, Borelli L: Amitriptyline and chronic low back pain. *Spine* 8:552–557, 1983.

14. Sternbach RA, Janowsky DS, Huey LY, Segal DS: Effects of altering brain serotonin activity on human chronic pain. In Bonica JJ, Albe-Fessard D (eds): *Advances in Pain Research and Therapy.* New York, Raven Press, 1976, vol 1, pp 601–606.

15. Jenkins DG, Ebbutt AF, Evans CD: Tofranil in the treatment of low back pain. *J Int Med Res* 4(suppl 2):28–40, 1976.

16. Butler SH, Weil-Fugazza J, Godefoy F, Besson J-M: Reduction of arthritis and pain behavior following chronic administration of amitriptyline or imipramine in rats with adjuvant-induced arthritis. *Pain* 23:159–175, 1985.

17. MacNeill AL, Dick WC: Imipramine and rheumatoid factor. *J Int Med Res* 4(suppl 2):23–27, 1976.

18. Gringas M: A clinical trial of Tofranil in rheumatic pain in general practice. *J Int Med Res* 4(suppl 2):41–45, 1976.

19. McDonald Scott WA: The relief of pain with an antidepressant in arthritis. *Practitioner* 202:802–805, 1969.

20. Woodforde JM, Dwyer B, McEwen BW, DeWilde FW, Bleasel K, Connelley TJ, Ho CY: Treatment of post-herpetic neuralgia. *Med J Aust* 2:869–872, 1965.

21. Kvinesdal B, Molin J, Froland A, Gram LF: Imipramine treatment of painful diabetic neuropathy. *JAMA* 251:1727–1730, 1984.

22. Dalessio DJ: Chronic pain syndromes and disordered cortical inhibition: effects of tricyclic compounds. *Dis Nerv System* 28:325–328, 1967.

23. Kocher R: Use of psychotropic drugs for treatment of chronic severe pain. In Bonica JJ, Albe-Fessard D (eds): *Advances in Pain Research and Therapy.* New York, Raven Press, 1976, vol 1, pp 579–582.

24. Langohr HD, Stohr M, Petruch F: An open and double-blind cross-over study on the efficacy of clomipramine (Anafranil) in patients with painful mono- and polyneuropathies. *Eur Neurol* 21:309–317, 1982.

25. Malseed R, Goldstein FJ: Enhancement of morphine analgesia by tricyclic antidepressants. *Neuropharmacology* 18:827–829, 1979.

26. Lee RL, Spencer PSJ: The effect of clomipramine and other amine-uptake inhibitors on morphine analgesia in laboratory animals. *Postgrad Med J* 53:53–60, 1977.

27. Liu SJ, Wang RIH: Increased analgesia and alterations in distribution and metabolism of methadone by desipramine in rats. *J Pharmacol Exp Ther* 195:94–104, 1975.

28. Gonzalez JP, Sewell RDE, Spencer PSJ: Antinociceptive activity of opiates in the presence of the antidepressant agent nomifensine. *Neuropharmacology* 19:613–618, 1980.

29. Kellstein DE, Malseed R, Goldstein FJ: Contrasting effects of acute vs. chronic tricyclic antidepressant treatment on central morphine analgesia. *Pain* 20:323–334, 1984.

30. France RD, Urban BJ, Keefe FJ: Long-term use of narcotic analgesics in chronic pain. *Soc Sci Med* 19:1379–1382, 1984.

31. Urban BJ, France RD, Steinberger EK, Scott DL, Maltbie AA: Long-term use of narcotic/antidepressant medication in the management of phantom limb pain. *Pain* 24:191–196, 1986.

32. Anderson LS, Black RG, Abraham J, Ward AA: Neuronal hyperactivity in experimental trigeminal deafferentation. *J Neurosurg* 35:444–452, 1971.

33. Loeser JD, Ward AA, White LE: Chronic deafferentation of human spinal cord neurons. *J Neurosurg* 29:48–50, 1968.

34. Anthony M, Lance JW: Monoamine oxidase inhibitors in the treatment of migraine. *Arch Neurol* 21:263–268, 1969.

35. Lascelles RG: Atypical facial pain and depression. *Br J Psychiatry* 112:651–659, 1966.

36. Yung CY: A review of clinical trials of lithium in neurology. *Pharmacol Biochem Behav* 21(suppl 1):57–64, 1984.

37. Medina JL, Diamond S: Cyclical migraine. *Arch Neurol* 38:343–344, 1981.

38. Chazot G, Chauplannaz G, Biron A, Schott B: Migraines: treatment per lithium. *Nouv Presse Med* 8:2836–2837, 1979.

39. Kudrow L: Lithium prophylaxis for chronic cluster headache. *Headache* 17:15–18, 1977.

40. Moore J, Dundee JW: Alterations in response to somatic pain associated with anaesthesia, Part VII: the effects of nine phenothiazine derivatives. *Br J Anaesth* 33:422–431, 1961.

41. Dundee JW, Love WJ, Moore J: Alterations in response to somatic pain associated with anaesthesia, Part XV: further studies with phenothiazine derivatives and similar drugs. *Br J Anaesth* 35:597–609, 1963.

42. Moore J, Dundee JW: Alterations in response to somatic pain associated with anaesthesia, V: the effect of promethazine. *Br J Anaesth* 33:3–8, 1961.

43. Dundee JW, Moore J: Alterations in response to somatic pain associated with anaesthesia, I: an evaluation of a method of analgesimetry. *Br J Anaesth* 32:396–406, 1960.

44. Lasagna L, DeKornfeld TJ: Methotrimeprazine—a new phenothiazine derivative with analgesic properties. *JAMA* 178:887–890, 1961.

45. Minuck R: Postoperative analgesia—comparison of meth-

otrimeprazine and meperidine as postoperative analgesia agents. *Can Anaesth Soc J* 19:87–96, 1972.

46. Baldessarini RJ: Drugs in the treatment of psychiatric disorders. In Gilman AG, Goodman LS (eds): *The Pharmacological Basis of Therapeutics*, ed 7. New York, Macmillan, 1985, pp 387–445.

47. Taub A: Relief of post-herpetic neuralgia with psychotropic drugs. *J Neurosurg* 39:235–239, 1973.

48. Merskey H, Hester RA: The treatment of chronic pain with psychotropic drugs. *Postgrad Med J* 48:594–598, 1972.

49. Davis JL, Lewis SB, Gerich JE, Kaplan RA, Schultz TA, Wallen JD: Peripheral diabetic neuropathy treated with amitriptyline and fluphenazine. *JAMA* 238:2291–2292, 1977.

50. Moertel CG, Ahmann DL, Taylor WF, Schwartau N: Relief of pain by oral medications. *JAMA* 229:55–59, 1974.

51. Houde RW, Wallenstein SL: Analgesic power of chlorpromazine alone and in combination with morphine. *Fed Proc* 14:353, 1955.

52. Shannon HE, Holtzman SG, Davis DC: Interaction between narcotic analgesics and benzodiazepine derivatives on behavior in the mouse. *J Pharmacol Exp Ther* 199:387–399, 1976.

53. Weis J: Morphine antagonistic effect of chlordiazepoxide (Librium). *Experientia* 25:381, 1969.

54. Morichi R, Pepeu G: A study of the influence of hydroxyzine and diazepam on morphine antinociception in the rat. *Pain* 7:173–180, 1979.

55. Chapman CR, Feather BW: Effects of diazepam on human pain tolerance and pain sensitivity. *Psychosom Med* 35:330–340, 1973.

56. Gracely RH, McGrath P, Dubner R: Validity and sensitivity of sensory and affective verbal pain descriptors: manipulation of affect by diazepam. *Pain* 5:19–29, 1978.

57. Kantor TG, Steinburg FP: Studies of tranquillizing agents (hydroxyzine and meprobamate) and meperidine in clinical pain. In Bonica JJ, Albe-Fessard D (eds): *Advances in Pain Research and Therapy*. New York, Raven Press, 1976, vol 1, pp 507–572.

58. Stambaugh JE, Wainer IW: Metabolic studies of the interaction of meperidine and hydroxyzine in human subjects. In Bonica JJ, Albe-Fessard D (eds): *Advances in Pain Research and Therapy*. New York, Raven Press, 1976, vol 1, pp 559–565.

59. Beaver WT, Feise G: A comparison of the analgesic effects of morphine, hydroxyzine and their combination in patients with post-operative pain. In Bonica JJ, Albe-Fessard D (eds): *Advances in Pain Research and Therapy*. New York, Raven Press, 1976, vol 1, pp 553–557.

60. Hupert C, Yacoub M, Turgeon LR: Effect of hydroxyzine on morphine analgesia for the treatment of postoperative pain. *Anesth Analg* 59:690–696, 1980.

61. Hollister LE, Conley FK, Britt RH, Shuer L: Long-term use of diazepam. *JAMA* 246:1568–1570, 1981.

62. Yosselson-Superstine S, Lipman AG, Sanders SH: Adjunctive anti-anxiety agents in the management of chronic pain. *Israeli J Med Sci* 21:113–117, 1985.

63. Greenblatt DJ, Shader RI, Abernathy DR: Current status of benzodiazepines. *N Engl J Med* 309:410–416, 1983.

64. Hendler N, Cimi C, Terence MA, Long D: A comparison of cognitive impairment due to benzodiazepines and to narcotics. *Am J Psychiatry* 137:828–830, 1980.

65. Charney DS, Menkes DB, Heninger GR: Receptor sensitivity and the mechanism of action of antidepressant treatment: implications for the etiology and therapy of depression. *Arch Gen Psychiatry* 38:1160–1179, 1981.

66. Risch SC, Groom GP, Janowsky DS: Interfaces of psychopharmacology and cardiology, Parts I and II. *J Clin Psychiatry* 42:23–34, 47–59, 1981.

67. Goetzl FR, Burrill DY, Ivy AC: The analgesic effect of morphine alone and in combination with dextroamphetamines. *Proc Soc Exp Biol Med* 55:248–250, 1944.

68. Notl MW: Potentiation of morphine analgesia by cocaine in mice. *Eur J Pharmacol* 5:93–99, 1968.

69. Sigg EB, Capriob A, Schneider JA: Synergism of amines and antagonism of reserpine to morphine analgesia. *Proc Soc Exp Biol Med* 97:97–100, 1958.

70. Ivy AC, Goetzl FR, Burril DY: Morphine-dextroamphetamine analgesia. *War Med* 6:67–71, 1944.

71. Evans WO: The synergism of autonomic drugs on opiate or opioid-induced analgesia: a discussion of its potential utility. *Milt Med* 127:1000–1003, 1962.

72. Forest WH, Brown BW, Brown CR, Defalque R, Gold M, Gordon HE, James KE, Katz J, Mahler DL, Schraff P, Teutsch G: Dextroamphetamine with morphine for the treatment of post-operative pain. *N Engl J med* 296:712–715, 1977.

73. Laska EM, Sunshine A, Mueller F, Elvers WB, Siegel C, Rubin A: Caffeine as an analgesic adjuvant. *JAMA* 251:1711–1718, 1984.

74. Silverman EK, Reus VI, Jimerson DC: Heterogeneity of amphetamine response in depressed patients. *Am J Psychiatry* 138:1302–1306, 1981.

75. Katon W, Raskind M: Treatment of depression in the medically ill elderly with methylphenidate. *Am J Psychiatry* 137:963–965, 1980.

76. Kaufman MW, Murray GB, Cassem NH: Use of psychostimulants in medically ill depressed patients. *Psychosomatics* 23:817–819, 1982.

77. Woods SW, Tesar GE, Murray GB, Cassem NH: Psychostimulant treatment of depressive disorders secondary to medical illness. *J Clin Psychiatry* 47:12–15, 1986.

78. Baldessarini RJ: *Chemotherapy in Psychiatry: Principles and Practice*. Cambridge, MA, Harvard University Press, 1985.

79. Boakes AJ, Laurence DR, Teoh PC, Barar FSK, Benedikter LT, Prichard BNC: Interactions between sympathomimetic amines and antidepressant agents in man. *Br Med J* 1:311–315, 1973.

80. Thornton WE, Pray RJ: Combination drug therapy in psychopharmacology. *J Clin Pharmacol* 15:511–517, 1975.

81. Griffin JP, O'Arcy PF (eds): *A Manual of Adverse Drug Interactions*. Bristol, England, John and Sons Ltd, 1975.

82. Bigger JT, Kantor SJ, Glassman AH, Perel JM: Cardiovascular effects of tricyclic antidepressant drugs. In Lipton MA, DeMascio A, Killam KF (eds): *Psychopharmacology: A Generation of Progress*. New York, Raven Press, 1978.

83. Roose SP, Glassman AH, Giardina EG, Walsh TB, Woodring S, Bigger JT: Tricyclic antidepressants in depressed patients with cardiac conduction disease. *Arch Gen Psychiatry* 44:273–275, 1987.

84. Stewart TD: The spinal cord-injured patient. In Hackett TP, Cassen NH (eds): *Handbook of General Hospital Psychiatry*. St. Louis, CV Mosby, 1978, pp 415–428.

85. Risch SC, Kalin NH, Janowsky DS, Huey LY: Indications and guidelines for plasma tricyclic antidepressant concentration monitoring. *J Clin Psychopharmacol* 1:59–63, 1981.

86. Prien RF, Kupfer DJ: Continuation drug therapy for major depressive episode: how long should it be maintained? *Am J Psychiatry* 143:18–23, 1986.

87. Weissman MM, Prusoff BA, Klerman GL: Personality and the prediction of long term outcome of depression. *Am J Psychiatry* 135:797–800, 1978.

88. Keller MB, Klerman GL, Lavori PW, Coryell W, Endicott J, Taylor J: Long-term outcome of episodes of major depression. Clinical and public health significance. *JAMA* 252:788–792, 1984.

89. Sheehan DV, Claycomb JB, Kouretas N: Monoamine oxidase inhibitors: prescription and patient management. *Int J Psychiatr Med* 10:99–121, 1981.

90. Yeh SY, Mitchell CL: Potentiation and reduction of the analgesia of morphine in the rat by pargyline. *J Pharmacol Exp Ther* 179:642–651, 1971.

91. Palmer H: Potentiation of pethidine. *Br Med J* 2:944, 1960.

92. Shee JC: Dangerous potentiation of pethidine by iproniazid and its treatment. *Br Med J* 2:507–509, 1960.

93. Rivers N, Hornes P: Possible lethal reaction between nardil and dextromethorphan. *Can Med Assoc J* 103:85, 1970.

94. Roger KJ: Role of brain monoamines in the interaction between pethidine and tranylcypromine. *Eur J Pharmacol* 14:86–88, 1971.

95. Domino E, Sullivan TS, Luby ED: Barbiturate intoxication in a patient treated with a MAO inhibitor. *Am J Psychiatry* 118:941–943, 1962.

96. Taylor MA, Sierles FS, Abrams R: *General Hospital Psychiatry*. New York, The Free Press, 1985.

97. Monks R, Merskey H: Psychotropic drugs. In Wall PD, Melzack RD (eds): *Textbook of Pain*. London, Churchill Livingstone, 1984, pp 526–537.

98. Hollister LE: Principles of therapeutic applications of benzodiazepines. In Smith DE, Wesson DR (eds): *The Benzodiazepines. Current Standards for Medical Practice*. Lancaster, England, MTP Press Limited, 1985, pp 87–96.

99. Rickels K, Case WG, Diamond L: Issues in long-term treatment with diazepam therapy. *Psychopharmacol Bull* 18:38–41, 1982.

100. Marks J: Benzodiazepines—for good or evil. *Neuropsychobiology* 10:115–126, 1983.

## *15*

# ERGONOMIC CONSIDERATIONS AND INTERVENTIONS

*Elsayed Abdel-Moty, Tarek M. Khalil, Reneé S. Rosomoff, and Hubert L. Rosomoff*

"Ergonomics" is a term derived from two Greek words: *ergon* (work) and *nomos* (laws). Ergonomics is an interdisciplinary field of study that integrates psychology, physiology, physics, medicine, and engineering to address problems regarding the preservation of health and efficiency at work and in activities of daily living. Ergonomics is concerned with the study of people and their work or living surroundings, and how people interact with work, tools, and the environment in general. Ergonomists recognize that it may be easier to change the environment than to change people, thereby achieving a better fit of people to the environment.

Ergonomics helps people understand their abilities and limitations and teaches them how to perform safely, effectively, and comfortably within the environment. The principles of ergonomics apply universally and are relevant to jobs in every type and size of organization. They are also relevant to the rehabilitation and management of musculoskeletal injuries (1).

This chapter presents ergonomics considerations and intervention strategies in the rehabilitation and management of cervical trauma disorders.

## ERGONOMICS CONSIDERATIONS

The goal of the ergonomic approach is to eliminate and/or prevent stressful situations as well as take corrective actions. Implementation of ergo-nomic principles (as presented below) for the reduction of musculoskeletal stresses and accident prevention is the best approach to avoidance of injury and reduction of the individual's exposure to risk factors.

Methods and techniques in ergonomics call for a set of basic considerations and guidelines in the design of workplaces (or living environments) and in the manner in which tasks are carried out. The methods and techniques are the result of a wide range of extensive research and are delineated in simple "rules." The implementation of these rules is essential for the prevention of injury or reinjury. The basic considerations fall under three main categories (2): posture, engineering, and body mechanics.

## POSTURAL CONSIDERATIONS

The neck, which is the mechanical support system of the head, is vulnerable to pain and injury because of its great mobility and the stresses placed on it throughout life. The cervical region is a very common source of pain and suffering. Frequently, cervical injury with pain involves the arms and shoulders as well as the head. In order to reduce injuries and pain, musculoskeletal stresses on the cervical region need to be reduced. This requires a thorough analysis of the postures of the head and trunk as well as of the upper and lower extremities.

Good posture is achieved through the align-

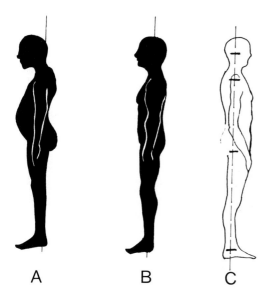

A          B          C

**Figure 15.1.** The key to good posture (*B*) is proper alignment of the head, shoulder, hip, knee, and ankle in one plane (*C*). Poor posture (*A*) should be corrected through exercise, awareness, and review of daily activities.

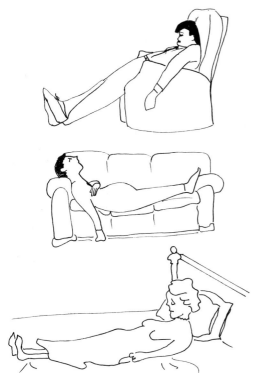

**Figure 15.2.** Faulty postures often feel comfortable. However, they can be a source of stress and should be corrected.

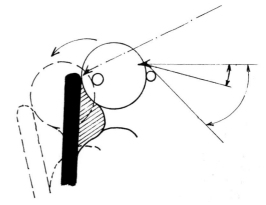

**Figure 15.3.** Flexible high back/head rest and neck support can benefit those who sit to work and prefer to recline. Proper visual area should be maintained.

ment of the musculoskeletal system in its neutral, balanced position (Fig. 15.1), wherein the head and spine are balanced in relation to the line of gravity. Poor or awkward postures cause fatigue, strain, and eventually pain, and should be corrected. Poor posture can also result in loss of stability, slips, falls, and other related accidents. Faulty postures and poor alignment of the musculoskeletal system develop slowly and do not induce an immediate feeling of discomfort (Fig. 15.2). Poor posture can develop as a result of obesity, weakened muscles, emotional tension, poor postural habits, and sometimes the improper design of task elements (tools and demands). Non-neutral postures of the neck and shoulders are known to contribute significantly to cervical trauma and pain, and should be avoided.

The primary requirement in proper head-neck posture is not to exceed a 20–30° angle between the head and neck (3). Another criterion for proper cervical posture is related to the eye's line of sight (Fig. 15.3). An easy, comfortable range of eye movement is within 15° below and above the normal line of sight—a total range of 30° (4). The line of sight 10–15° degrees below the horizontal plane is used the most. Continuous repetitive deviations from within this range can result in neck muscle fatigue, pain, and eventual health problems.

## Guidelines for Good Posture

**General Rules.** Basic requirements for good posture are:

1. Maintain the head, neck, and back as close to the same coronal and sagittal planes as possible.

2. Maintain the anatomic axis of the joints in a neutral position.
3. Avoid continuous pressure on sensitive body tissue, such as that under the thigh while sitting and that at the wrist joint while typing.
4. To prevent localization and concentration of stress on one side of the neck and to prevent fatigue, alternate sides.
5. When using the telephone, use a headset or support the elbow on the desktop to keep the neck aligned; alternate sides.
6. Identify what is causing pain and discomfort and correct it.
7. Practice correct body posture while standing, sitting, or moving.
8. Avoid awkward positioning of the head if wearing bifocals, trifocals, or "half-glasses." Position the glasses correctly to maximally utilize their reduced effective visual area (Fig. 15.4).
9. Do not favor one posture, which can lead to static muscle loading and fatigue. Allow for alternative movements.

**Sitting Posture.** Prolonged sitting is a major cause of poor postural habits, which are generally seen as forward neck, slumping, hunching over, slouching, or leaning to one side or the other. The individual assumes poor postures when static stresses on the muscles, joints, ligaments, and other musculoskeletal structures increase. Persistent static loading produces troublesome localized fatigue in the muscle involved, as well as chronic aches, and can build up to intolerable pain (4). The basic requirements in posture alignment while sitting are:

1. Maintain the knees at a level equal to, or slightly higher than, that of the hips. This enables the use of

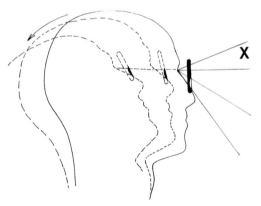

**Figure 15.4.** Use of bifocals reduces the "effective visual area." If an object (X) is positioned outside this area, the individual compensates by tilting the head backward, thus placing stress on cervical musculature.

a back rest and allows alignment of spinal structures while sitting.
2. Weight should be distributed uniformly under the thighs while sitting, to ensure proper balanced support of the spine, head, and shoulders.
3. Support the arms and the back while sitting.
4. Reclined postures are acceptable, provided that the chair gives adequate support to the head; the task must be adjustable within the viewing area.
5. Alternate between sitting and standing.

**Standing Posture.** The basic requirements for good posture in the standing position are:

1. Provide a balanced base of support at the feet while standing. If necessary, widen the stance.
2. Stand straight without slumping.
3. Avoid twisting and sudden turning of the head. Turn the body as a whole unit.

## BODY MECHANICS CONSIDERATIONS

Body mechanics (also known as posture in motion) is the safest way to sit, stand, lift, carry, squat, or climb stairs while performing activities of daily living. There are numerous advantages of using proper body mechanics in activities of daily living. Improper use of body mechanics taxes the neck and shoulder muscles, thus leading to poor alignment and faulty postures.

### Guidelines for Proper Body Mechanics

**Body Mechanics for Sitting.** The basic requirements for proper use of body mechanics while sitting are:

1. Reduce stress by moving and shifting weight. Do not sit in one place for long periods of time without moving or shifting weight.
2. Keep the back straight and do not hunch shoulders over the desk.
3. Do not develop the habit of slouching when reading in a chair. Sit with the back against the back support of the chair.
4. Elevate the knees to a level higher than that of the hips through adjustment of chair height or use of a footrest while keeping the work surface at its proper height.
5. Driving requires less effort when the driver is in the proper position. Poor posture while driving leads to neck pain. Sit with the shoulders level with the steering wheel. Adjust side and rearview mirrors so that the head need not be turned to use them. Seat angles and height should be adjusted for comfort and to allow the head to remain level and maintain the line of sight.

**Body Mechanics for Handling Objects.** The basic requirements for proper use of body mechanics while handling objects (lifting, carrying, pulling, pushing) are:

1. Test (size) the weight before handling it. If the object is heavy, ask for help. Use mechanical help (trolley) whenever possible (Fig. 15.5A).
2. When carrying or lifting, keep the load as close to the body as possible (Fig. 15.6).
3. When lifting, place the feet far enough apart with one foot slightly ahead of the other for stability and balance.
4. If a shoulder bag is used to carry weight, do not overload it. Redistribute the weight by using both sides or use a backpack.
5. Do not favor one shoulder or arm when carrying a heavy handbag or briefcase. When possible, use luggage wheels.
6. If possible, slide the load; do not lift or carry it.
7. When there is a choice of muscle groups to perform the same task, use the stronger and most fit.

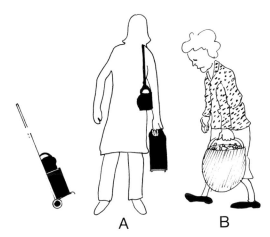

**Figure 15.5.** *A,* Mechanical aids are recommended whenever possible to reduce forceful exertions and concentration of stress. *B,* A combination of poor posture and unbalanced weight distribution are troublesome and should be corrected.

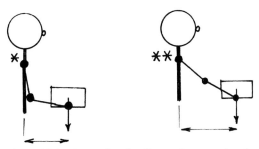

**Figure 15.6.** Increasing the distance between the object and the spinal support will increase the stress on the shoulders, neck, and back.

8. When pulling, alternate hands to avoid straining shoulder and neck muscles. When possible use two hands to pull, which will distribute the weight more evenly.

**Body Mechanics for Task Performance.** The basic requirements for proper use of body mechanics while performing various tasks are:

1. Get as close to the workbench or work area as possible, while maintaining proper posture and freedom of movement.
2. Work with good light within the viewing area.
3. Bring objects into an appropriate focus without crouching.
4. When using the telephone, rest the elbows at a level so that the receiver is at ear level. Do not prop the phone between the jaw and the shoulder (Fig. 15.7). Free hands for taking notes or dialing the telephone by using a speaker phone or headset, or install a padded shoulder rest.
5. Use both hands to work symmetrically and in smooth path motions.
6. Avoid twisting, sudden turning, and abrupt reflex movement. Turn the whole body as a unit by pointing both feet in the direction of movement.
7. Avoid repetitive forward flexion of the head.
8. Avoid repetitive movements of the head for extended periods of time.
9. Avoid working with the head tilted too far back or too far forward for extended periods of time, especially when reaching overhead.
10. Minimize overreaching as well as reaching behind the head. Keep forward reach short.
11. Use ballistic movements at the joints.
12. Avoid extreme pivotal movement of the head.
13. Motions of the head and neck should be kept within comfortable cervical ranges of motion.

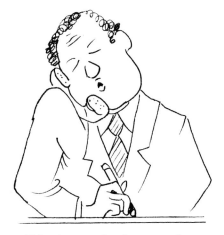

**Figure 15.7.** An example of a commonly seen poor static posture of the head and neck.

14. If neck pain is a problem, assess the bed, pillow, and sleeping habits or positions. Keep the head level and do not sleep on the stomach while using a thick pillow.
15. Avoid prolonged hyperextension and hyperflexion of the head and neck when performing activities such as showering, shaving, or drinking from a bottle (use a straw, for example).
16. Daily stretching maintains or improves ranges of motion, and strengthening exercises to extend endurance should be performed.

## ENGINEERING CONSIDERATIONS

Engineering considerations deal with the design and layout of the physical workplace (equipment, tools, and workstations) with special attention to human characteristics. Poorly designed workstations contribute to pain, trauma, and accidents by not allowing the operator either to assume good posture or use proper body mechanics. People working in ergonomically designed workplaces tire less quickly, are less stressed by poor environmental conditions, are less affected by overtaxing physical demands on the musculoskeletal system, are less likely to get injured, feel better, and work effectively.

Job tasks that require repetitive awkward movements create what is currently referred to as cumulative trauma disorders (CTDs), which include chronic soft tissue injuries of the musculoskeletal system. CTDs can be defined in terms of a cause (risk factors)–effect (consequences) relationship. Commonly cited risk factors that can contribute to potential tissue trauma include, but are not limited to:

1. Repetitive tasks—particularly when tasks are carried out with improper body mechanics.
2. Forceful exertions—during tasks requiring excessive muscular effort, and subsequent fatigue.
3. Stresses due to equipment design—sharp edges on desks and keyboards, improper chair and workstation design, location of work tools, and physical space available. A variety of CTDs can be caused by improper design of work tools (even when the tool is designed correctly, it can still produce stress by being used too frequently or improperly).
4. Environmental stresses—e.g., vibration.

The ergonomic approach to the control of CTDs consists of four basic components: (a) identification of the problem, (b) identification of the cause(s), (c) application of intervention strategies or control measures, and (d) evaluation of the effectiveness of the control program. The engineering considerations for the reduction of physical stresses on the musculoskeletal system deal with the "optimal" arrangement of facilities, tasks, and personnel to produce a safe environment. Optimization is of prime importance since this directly affects the quality and productivity of work.

There are three main areas in which ergonomics can be applied: (a) the design of equipment and furniture, (b) the arrangement of the work environment, and (c) the design of job tasks that can be easily and effectively performed by the workplace user. Although workstation design and task modification may be applicable to many occupations, there are other jobs and tasks that are difficult to alter. In the latter cases, ergonomics offers job placement testing, preemployment screening, and selection criteria programs for workers.

All jobs/tasks that require use of the upper extremities and upper back can constitute a source of stress that can produce cervical pain and discomfort. However, there are specific jobs that seem to be more easily identified as presenting a high risk of cervical trauma (Fig. 15.8). Maeda and associates (5) observed cervical disorders among keypunch operators, assembly plant workers, typists, cash register operators, and telephone operators. Complaints are also common among visual display terminal (VDT) (computer) operators (6). Secretaries, clerks, typists, and other office workers who type, do keypunching, write extensively, take notes, or answer the telephone are easy targets for cervical trauma.

Electricians and plumbers working overhead when installing tubing or wiring, especially in confined spaces, are also exposed to cervical stresses. Drywall installation and painting, especially where ceilings are involved, demand that the worker extend the neck and overreach with the arms for prolonged periods of times in a static fashion. Similar stresses are encountered by carpenters who work with kitchen cabinets, which involve reaching, installing, or remodeling, and by persons in professions that require constant repetitive turning of the head from one side to the other (e.g., drivers). Musicians, dentists, professional photographers, laboratory technicians, radiologists, teachers, and vibrating tool operators are but few examples of persons whose occupation places them at high risk of cervical trauma.

## Engineering Considerations in Seated Workplaces

Often called "desk neck," cervical pain has been always associated with sedentary-type jobs. However, almost all activities of daily living can cause

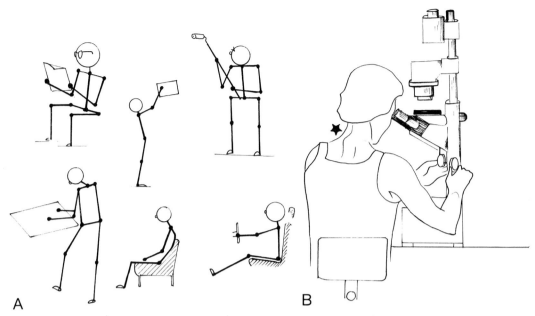

**Figure 15.8.** *A*, Examples of postures that might contribute to the onset or exacerbation of cervical trauma, especially when performed repetitively in a static fashion. *B*, Absence of elbow support and poor adjustment of the parameters of the microscope (angle, distance, height) can produce disabling cervical pain when working at the instrument for extended periods of time.

cervical distress if not performed properly. People spend a great deal of the 16 waking hours of every day sitting on chairs and using office or home furniture that is poorly designed or improperly adjusted. About three quarters of all operations in industrialized countries have sedentary jobs (4). There are many disadvantages to and drawbacks of sitting down to work. A poorly designed sitting environment can result in poor sitting habits, may place undue stresses on the musculoskeletal system and sensitive body tissues, can be hazardous to health, and consequently can affect productivity and the quality of life. Many studies have shown that, for people who already have pain, there is a risk of increased pain when they are required to sit for long periods of time. Mechanical stresses on the lumbar spine were found to be 40% higher when sitting unsupported than when standing (7).

Neck stress and upper back and shoulder pain may also develop if the head is too far forward or backward during desk activities (Fig. 15.9). Excessive bending, twisting, and reaching are related to the onset of pain and discomfort. Also, different types of work require different work surface heights for comfort and optimal performance. For example, light detailed work, such as writing, requires a work surface close to the elbow height of the seated person, provided there is enough

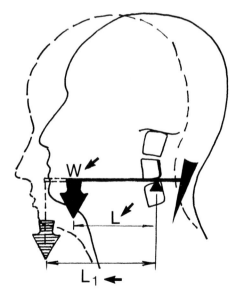

**Figure 15.9.** The weight of the head *(black arrow)* ($W$) is balanced by muscle force *(large black arrowhead)* in this first-class lever mechanical system. Forward tilting of the head (dashed outline) increases the distance ($L$) to the fulcrum *(black triangle)*, thus increasing muscle contraction force by ($W^*L_1 - W^*L$).

clearance under the work surface for the knees and legs.

Reach requirements of tasks that cause non-neutral postures can lead to discomfort. Severe deviation from neutral postures creates added stresses on joints. This occurs when work tools are placed outside comfortable reach.

The ability to achieve proper head and neck postures in a sitting workstation is largely determined by the interaction of several environmental, physical, and human characteristics (Fig. 15.10). Therefore, jobs resulting in significant postural stresses should be redesigned when feasible to encourage neutral positions. The process of redesigning or modifying the environment should address the individual's capability and limitations. If the environment cannot be modified then the worker must be made aware of methods to perform the task in the least stressful manner.

Ergonomics considerations for the design of workplaces are numerous because of the large number of human and environmental factors that are encountered. The multitude of these factors has led to the establishment of principles, guidelines, and norms for proper design of the workplace for maximum comfort and optimal performance (4, 8–11). The implementation of the following design guidelines has been proven to be very valuable as well as cost effective.

**Engineering Guidelines for Seated Workplaces.** The basic considerations in this category are:

1. It takes only a little forethought to make a workstation comfortable and less stressful.
2. Human capacities, capabilities, and limitations must be recognized and used as the focus of design.
3. Design for safety.
4. Design flexible offices that can adapt and change according to the postures and habits of different people.
5. Individualize the selection of appropriate seating to meet the dimensions of the individual and the demands of the task.
6. Lay out work areas within normal (horizontal as well as vertical) easy access reaches.
7. Have a special place to do each job so that equipment and supplies may always be kept for immediate use.
8. Locate control switches within easy reach.
9. The desk and tools should be positioned properly. All work tools should be placed within easy accessible reach of the individual and stored in a convenient location.
10. Design workplaces at which tasks can be conducted either sitting or standing.
11. Select work surface and chair heights appropriate for the individual and the task (Fig. 15.11). Take note of visual attributes of the individual. Inclined work surfaces are recommended for reading tasks (12).
12. Raise the work surface for fine or precise work and lower it if work is heavy.
13. Provide good light (intensity, quality, brightness, contrast) and good ventilation and control other environmental conditions.
14. Load stress (several tasks to perform) and speed stress (high work pace) are undesirable, particularly when combined with environmental stresses.

**Engineering Guidelines for the Design of VDT Workstations.** Visual display terminals are rapidly becoming a dominant piece of office equipment. Over the next few decades, the number of VDTs and people using them is expected to increase dramatically. The side effects of this new technology are slowly appearing. There has been a growing concern about musculoskeletal stresses caused by prolonged sitting and postural limitations due to the design characteristics of the VDT workstation. Computer operators are sometimes required to sit for long periods of time to perform tasks such as data entry, programming, and word processing. There are various elements in VDT workplaces and tasks that can place the VDT operator at risk of cervical trauma. This stress on the musculoskeletal system is primarily a result of:

1. Static loading (the muscles must overcome the gravity and limb weight in order to hold up the arms and head plus any external load).

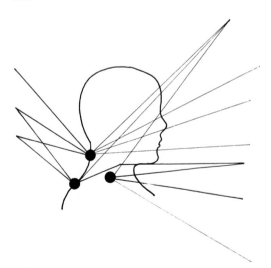

**Figure 15.10.** Musculoskeletal stresses can be caused by a multitude of factors. Ergonomics attempts to minimize the number of risk factors and their contribution to the severity of symptoms.

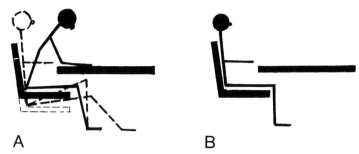

A          B

**Figure 15.11.** A tall person given a low table (A) will have to bend the neck over the work, causing trouble in the neck and back, or will have to lower the chair, which might be uncomfortable for the legs. Work surface height should allow the individual to sit comfortably and correctly (B).

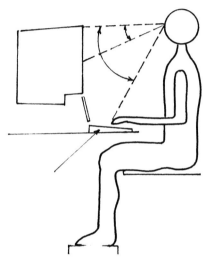

**Figure 15.12.** Placement of the VDT screen, source document, and keyboard within comfortable visual area reduces repetitive movement and static loading on the cervical musculoskeletal system.

2. Frequency of action (the greater the frequency the greater the risk, especially if posture is poor and load is high).
3. Work/rest regimens and poor pacing.

VDT-related stresses are usually experienced as vision strain, neck pain, headaches, upper and lower back discomfort, arm and shoulder muscle fatigue, leg pains and numbness, and wrist stress. Cervical discomfort is a common complaint. These stresses could be minimized or eliminated through proper engineering of the VDT workstation.

The guidelines and considerations for the design of VDT workstations are:

1. The operator must be able to scan—mainly within the range of vision and with minimum head and neck movement—the screen, the keyboard, and the source document (Fig. 15.12). This depends upon three interrelated factors: (a) the viewing distance, (b) the viewing angle, and (c) the "visual ability" of the operator. Eyeglasses may present additional problems if they alter head position.
2. The VDT screen should be within the optimal viewing angle of the eye (5–10° below the horizontal). This angle can be maintained for long periods of time with minimum discomfort and fatigue.
3. The entire primary viewing area (top of screen to keyboard to source material) should be less than 60° below the horizontal plane of the eyes (10).
4. The relative placement of the source documents, the keyboard, and a reflection-free screen should provide better eye-hand coordination and less strain on the neck, shoulders, and eyes.
5. The keyboard should fall directly below the hands with the elbows at about 90°.
6. An independent adjustable support surface for the keyboard is preferred. If the keyboard support is not adjustable, chair height should be adjusted so as not to violate the elbow height requirement (elbow angle about 90°).
7. If the job requires a combination of keypunching, answering the telephone, and/or writing, the different work elements should be placed within comfortable reach. Hand dominancy should be the primary consideration.
8. Gentle rest of the palms and forearms is recommended for long-term keyboard use to support the weight of the upper extremity and allow shoulder and neck muscles to be relaxed during work.
9. Having a stand for reference materials is essential to reduce neckache. By positioning the document holder at the screen level, one third of the movement is eliminated. This way the user can easily avoid unnecessary eye, neck, and head movement. The position of the document holder should be alternated from one side to the other in order to avoid lateralization of stress.
10. Avoid light reflection and glare on the VDT screen surface. Position the VDT screen adequately.

**Guidelines for Chair Selection.** With the advent of ergonomics, chairs are becoming precision sitting machines that are functionally correct and scientifically accurate for the specifics of the job. For individuals with cervical or neck pain, an adjustable chair should allow adequate, natural, comfortable, and flexible support and stability for body segments (elbows, lumbar region, legs, upper back, and head), as well as distribution of body weight and freedom of movement. A "good" chair may add as much as 40 productive minutes to the working day of each productive individual (13). Well-designed chairs are a prerequisite to safety and health of seated workers, including those with preexisting injury. A well-designed chair will favorably affect posture, circulation, the amount of effort required to maintain posture, and the amount of strain on the spine (14).

The basic engineering considerations in ergonomically designed chairs are:

1. The back and seat supports should be contoured to provide maximum support to the body.
2. The seat and back rest should have flexible tilt to allow for better support and give variety of movement while seated.
3. The seat and the back rest should be adjustable independently of one another. The angle between the seat and back rest should be more than 90° (10). A torso-to-thigh angle less than 90° leads to greater spinal stress and may lead to fatigue and discomfort (4). As this angle is increased work tasks and tools should be readjusted accordingly to avoid incorrect posture.
4. The chair should be upholstered with slightly porous, rough-textured material to dissipate heat, facilitate circulation, reduce static pressure, and support the body.
5. A high back rest is preferable for office work because most people often desire to lean back. A high back rest supports the trunk more than a small back rest.
6. The back rest should be angled about 10–15° from vertical. Back angle helps minimize stress on spinal structures and maintain the trunk-legs relationship. The height of the back rest should provide adequate support for the upper body. Depending on the task, the back rest should be concave to the front at its top to support the head.
7. The seat height should be easily adjustable to allow the feet to rest on the floor or on a stool while maintaining correct work surface height, knee angle, and support for the lower leg. If the seat is too high the legs will dangle, increasing pressure on the underside of the thigh and encouraging sliding. This will not allow the individual to use upper back support. If the seat is too low the elbows will be raised, in-

creasing static tension in cervical musculature. A footrest may be used to deal with the problem.
8. Seat depth should be adjustable to allow correct thigh support and proper knee clearance and avoid pressure on the back side of the lower leg.
9. Chair height that does not allow adequate support under the feet can result in cervical stresses caused by the individual's inability to use the back rest while sitting.
10. Seat width should allow the seated person to move about and assume various postures.
11. The weight of the arms is supported, in part, by the musculature of the neck and upper back. Prolonged sitting or standing to perform simple tasks while the elbows are unsupported imposes continuous static stresses on the cervical muscles, causing muscle fatigue and pain. Therefore, it is desirable to provide flexible support for the arms while not interfering with the individual's performance at the workstation or with musculoskeletal functions.
12. Depending on task demands and floor surface condition, casters on chairs are desirable and can give greater freedom of movement and permit the individual to get closer to the task.
14. A five-spur pedestal chair is recommended for stability, balance, safety, and ease of movement.
15. Swivel chairs are recommended to avoid excessive torsional moments in seated workplaces.
16. Chairs that provide a half-sitting–half-kneeling posture are no better than conventional chairs and could be worse than a well-designed office seat (4, 15).

## ERGONOMIC INTERVENTIONS

Ergonomics is both a science and technology, and when introduced into an organization it must be integrated into the formal organization and into the technical development of projects within that organization.

Ergonomics as a field of study and research has much to offer when applied to rehabilitation. Very few investigations in ergonomics have been devoted to postinjury management of painful conditions. This has always been thought to be the sole domain of medical and health care professionals. However, involvement in the injury evaluation and management program has proven to be quite successful (16, 17). Ergonomics reasoning has become an integral part of the multidisciplinary approach. It also permits an objective, quantitative assessment of the patient's ability to perform specific tasks. The pioneering approach utilized by the University of Miami Comprehensive Pain and Rehabilitation Center (17–19), in which ergonomists work jointly with physicians and professionals from other disciplines in a re-

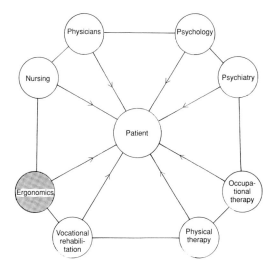

**Figure 15.13.** The integration of ergonomics in a multidisciplinary pain team has proven effectiveness and significance in all aspects of rehabilitation. Ergonomists work hand-in-hand with health care professionals for the well-being of the patient during and after rehabilitation.

habilitation environment, has provided an excellent intervention forum for recognizing and solving many complex problems related to pain and injury (Fig. 15.13). Examples of ergonomics intervention approaches are presented in this section.

## EVALUATION OF HUMAN PERFORMANCE

The effects of pain and injury on human performance may be measured either by asking the patients about their perception of how much they can or cannot do or by measuring the patient's abilities/limitations. It is recognized that there may be a potential discrepancy between these two different types of measures. Literature review has shown that there are many shortcomings associated with the self-report measures used to evaluate activity levels of pain patients. Self-report of activity levels in pain patients has been shown to lack reliability (repeatability), sensitivity (relation to treatment outcome), and validity (ability to predict performance in actual work situations). The recognized problems of self-report measures have led many practitioners to establish more standard and objective measures of function among injured persons.

In the area of measuring functional performance, it is important to examine the patients' ca-

pabilities and limitations. This can be achieved via a human performance profile (HPP). This profile includes measurements of strength, acceptable maximum effort (AME) (20), active ranges of motion, walking pace, psychomotor abilities such as reaction time and hand steadiness, squatting ability, and posture (Fig. 15.14).

These functional measures collectively establish a quantitative profile of muscular and mental performance abilities on each individual as a unit to determine his or her overall physical capacities and limitations at the time of the evaluation. The HPP profile is compared to profiles of healthy persons of equivalent age, sex, and work category. Evaluation occurs by comparing the patient's score on each measure to a set of "normative" data that presumably reflect ideal scores on those indicators. Treatment usually involves efforts to restore the individual to the target range of score values. Also, when combined with the medical, physical, and behavioral examinations, the HHP provides a sound basis for evaluation of rehabilitation outcome.

The functional capacity evaluation is also important to assist in the selection of jobs that match

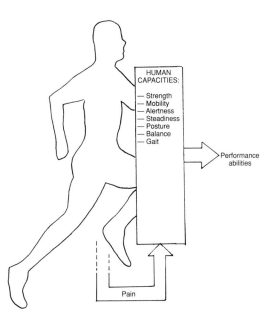

**Figure 15.14.** Accurate quantitative assessment of human performance (capacities as modified by pain perception) is an essential component in rehabilitation. Ergonomics uses recognized methods of human performance analysis to evaluate patient's capabilities and limitations.

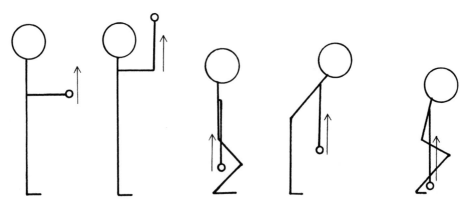

**Figure 15.15.** Schematic presentation of the five static strength testing positions employed by ergonomics for the evaluation of acceptable maximum effort (AME) of the arms, shoulders, legs, back, and composite postures in pain patients. The testing positions are representative of carrying and lifting activities encountered in daily tasks.

the measured functional capabilities of the rehabilitated persons. This approach presents an ideal strategy for prevention of further injury. Abilities and preferences are identified and compared to job demands, and special provisions are made for those at risk of reinjury.

### Evaluation of Strength

One example of a quantitative assessment of strength is to use static strength testing regimens. In this assessment, individuals perform static tasks similar in nature to those encountered in their daily activities and in their work environment (20). The positions are chosen on the basis of their high degree of applicability to lifting positions required of most people (21). The five postures selected (Fig. 15.15) allow for the assessments of the arm, shoulder, back, leg, and total body (composite) strengths. There are also some dynamic strength testing regimens that could be used as patient condition permits.

However, at the Comprehensive Pain and Rehabilitation Center, a psychophysical static measuring approach is used that focuses specifically on the assessment of strength in patients with chronic pain and/or injury. This approach is based on the concept of AME (20). For evaluating strength in persons with chronic pain, AME refers to the maximum level of voluntary effort that the person can achieve without an intolerable level of pain or discomfort. It defines the highest functional level that can be attained within the bounds of acceptable pain. This psychophysical measure of strength, which was proven to be safe and reliable, takes into account not only the patient's physical capabilities but also the perceptual fac-

tors related to pain status. Although it provides a method for improved quantification of functional abilities, the AME measure must be used in conjunction with other clinical measures of function evaluated by physicians and other health professionals.

Quantitative methods such as the ones described in this section can provide clinicians and researchers alike a vehicle by which evaluation of functional abilities of pain patients becomes standardized (20). Currently, it is nearly impossible to compare results from different studies on treatment outcome in rehabilitation in view of the widely divergent methods used to measure progress. Quantitative methods for assessing functional ability based on ergonomic principles have been used successfully in industry to standardize evaluations of workers' physical abilities relative to the demands of the work environment. While greater attention must be given to pain-related perceptual factors than is used in industry evaluations, such a quantitative approach needs to be adopted for the assessment of functional ability of pain patients.

### COMPUTER-AIDED WORKPLACE DESIGN

In order to facilitate the implementation of ergonomics principles and guidelines in workplace design, several researchers have used artificial intelligence and computer-aided approaches (22–24). Artificial intelligence is concerned with designing computer systems that exhibit characteristics associated with human intelligence (25). Artificial intelligence technology is being used to help people solve problems, increase efficiency, and decrease workload (26). An expert system is a

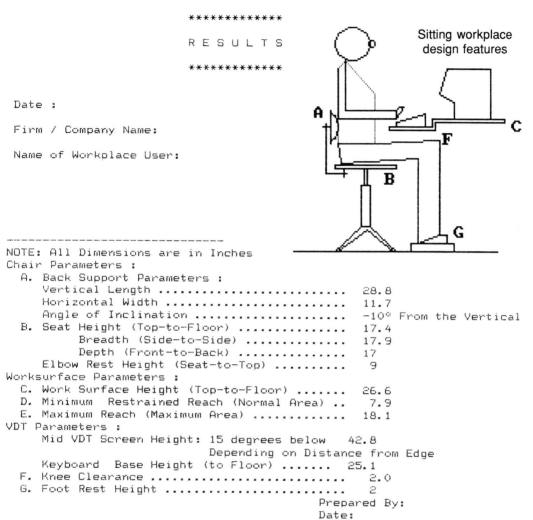

SWAD

Sitting Workplace Analysis and Design

```
                    *************

                    R E S U L T S           Sitting workplace
                                            design features
                    *************


Date :

Firm / Company Name:

Name of Workplace User:




-------------------------------------
NOTE: All Dimensions are in Inches
Chair Parameters :
  A.  Back Support Parameters :
      Vertical Length ...........................   28.8
      Horizontal Width ..........................   11.7
      Angle of Inclination ......................   -10° From the Vertical
  B.  Seat Height (Top-to-Floor) ...............   17.4
          Breadth (Side-to-Side) ..............   17.9
          Depth (Front-to-Back) ...............   17
      Elbow Rest Height (Seat-to-Top) ..........    9
Worksurface Parameters :
  C.  Work Surface Height (Top-to-Floor) .......   26.6
  D.  Minimum  Restrained Reach (Normal Area) ..    7.9
  E.  Maximum Reach (Maximum Area) .............   18.1
VDT Parameters :
      Mid VDT Screen Height: 15 degrees below    42.8
                          Depending on Distance from Edge
      Keyboard  Base Height (to Floor) .......   25.1
  F.  Knee Clearance ...........................    2.0
  G.  Foot Rest Height .........................    2
                              Prepared By:
                              Date:
```

**Figure 15.16.** Workplace design features screen output from SWAD. Results are based on the anthropometric dimensions and task demands of a 32-year-old female who is a VDT operator.

form of artificial intelligence in which intelligent software uses knowledge and inference procedures to solve problems that require human expertise.

Computer-aided design represents a new direction in the implementation of ergonomics knowledge through the use of microcomputer and expert systems technology. With computer aided design and expert systems, workplaces are designed and/or analyzed and proper seating devices are determined for the "individual" who is using the workplace in a very simple, yet professional, manner. Expert systems make ergonomics

guidelines for the design of sitting workplaces available to the consumer and interested groups.

SWAD (for Sitting Workplace Analysis and Design) is an example of such expert system technology applied to ergonomics and workplace design (27–29). The computer algorithm combines input static and functional anthropometric data of the individual with ergonomics principles and considerations to produce an optimal sitting workplace (Fig. 15.16). Information about the environment is combined with task parameters, postural adjustments, electromyographic activity of key muscles, force distribution, and goniometric data to provide a precise analysis of the working arrangement tailored to the specifics of the job and the capabilities of the individual.

## JOB/TASK SIMULATION AND ANALYSIS

In this area, ergonomics intervenes to develop realistic job simulations during rehabilitation to permit patients to simulate job tasks under supervision. Most often this type of activity should be performed as a joint effort between ergonomics, occupational therapy, vocational rehabilitation, and biofeedback. The patient is taught to review work activities and execute his or her job tasks properly, receives suggestions for modifications or adjustments, and learns to implement recommendations in the simulated environment, which in turn assures that he or she is capable of carrying out these recommendations upon returning to the actual work site.

## BIOMECHANICAL MODELING AND ELECTROMYOGRAPHIC TECHNIQUES

Overexertion and repetitive stress have been recognized as major sources of injuries. Computerized biomechanical models present a useful tool to predict safe levels of exertion and the severity of the stresses associated with specific tasks (30). Biomechanical models use information concerning body segment parameters (weight, lengths, mass, center of gravity) and body posture parameters (angles between links) to check stress forces and limits. These models examine the body as a series of rigid links joined at articulations and moved by the musculature (Fig. 15.17).

Tasks are analyzed biomechanically through determination of forces, angles, velocities, and acceleration at each joint. Estimates of inertial forces and reactive moments can also be calculated. The result of this computer-based analysis is a model of the body's response to the task being performed, which can be used to identify the stresses imposed upon the musculoskeletal system. Such biomechanical models are appropriate for nonfatigue states of performance. When fatigue becomes a factor, biomechanical models must be combined with electromyographic techniques (31) and measurements of other physiologic responses (e.g., heart rate) that are better predictors of endurance and fatigue.

Ergonomics extends the domain of biomechanical modeling from a study of internal characteristics of the human body to the forces exerted while the human is interacting with the environment. Electromyographic methodologies are used frequently for accurate evaluation of body mechanics in order to determine the level of neck muscle activity and stress during various tasks (Figs. 15.18 and 15.19). This approach is used to train patients, through electromyographic and postural feedback (32), in proper ways to perform certain tasks.

## PATIENT EDUCATION

Ergonomics contributes to the development of patient education programs rationalized by biomechanical concepts in order to increase the patient's awareness of the ergonomics consideration. Patients are taught to recognize their physical capabilities and limitations. Prevention

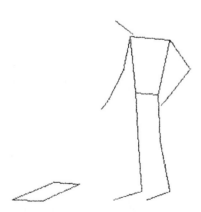
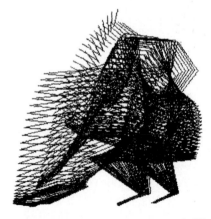

**Figure 15.17.**   Example of a multiple-link biomechanical model developed to predict static (*A*) and dynamic (*B*) stress on the musculoskeletal system during lifting tasks.

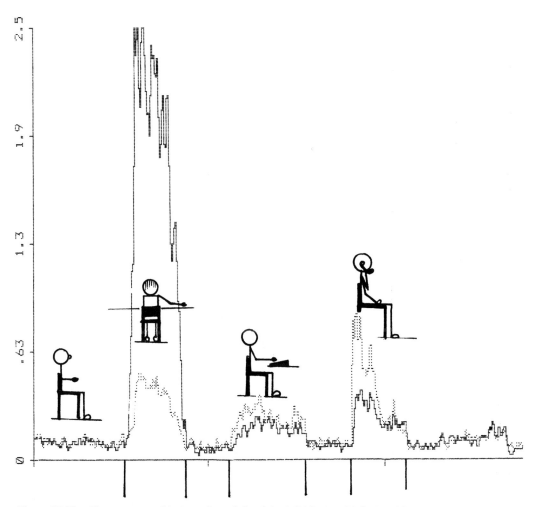

**Figure 15.18.** Electromyographic recording of the right *(solid line)* and left *(dotted line)* trapezius muscles during selected desk activities. Deviation from the neutral position, frequent overreaching, and static loading all impose serious stress on the muscles.

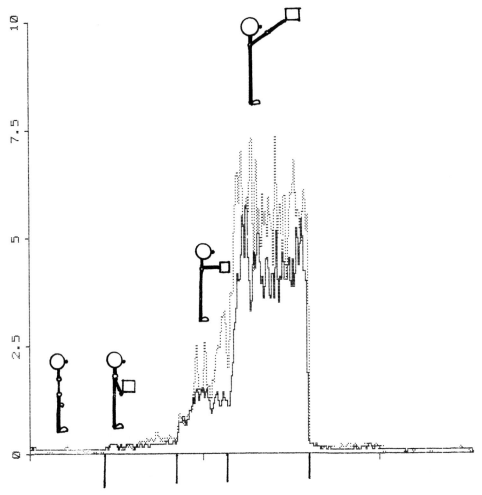

**Figure 15.19.** Electromyographic recording of the right *(solid line)* and left *(dotted line)* trapezius muscle activity while carrying a 4.5-kg object at different reach levels. The farther the weight is from the body the more stress on the muscular system.

and control of cervical reinjury through education and training should be individualized for the person, with a sufficient degree of flexibility to accommodate methods of working. Patients are taught to incorporate these concepts when performing home or recreational activities, and they should become an integral part of daily activities.

## CONCLUDING REMARKS

The role of ergonomics is integral to the analysis and control of stresses imposed on the musculoskeletal system. Ergonomics contributions to injury prevention and pain management have proven to be most valuable. Application of ergo-

nomics guidelines for proper posture, task performance, and workplace design can lead to significant reduction or prevention of trauma and pain. This can contribute significantly to the reduction of medical and compensation costs. Ergonomics intervention methods in clinical settings are effective and valuable to the comprehensive rehabilitation of chronic pain patients. The intervention strategies presented in this chapter are but a few examples of the potential contributions of ergonomics to the management of traumatic disorders. The inclusion of human engineering concepts following treatment is needed, especially where the return to gainful employment and a productive life-style become primary rehabilitation objectives.

## REFERENCES

1. Khalil TM, Asfour SS, Abdel-Moty E, Rosomoff RS, Rosomoff HL: Ergonomics contribution to low back pain rehabilitation. *Pain Management* Sep/Oct:225–230, 1988.
2. Abdel-Moty E, Khalil T, Asfour SS, Rosomoff RS, Rosomoff H: Ergonomics considerations for the reduction of physical task demands of low back pain patients. In Aghazadeh F (ed): *Trends in Ergonomics/Human Factors V.* Amsterdam, Elsevier Science Publishing BV, 1988, pp 959–967.
3. Chaffin DB, Andersson G: *Occupational Biomechanics.* New York, John Wiley, 1984.
4. Grandjean E: *Fitting the Task to the Man. A Text Book of Occupational Ergonomics,* ed 4. London, Taylor & Francis, 1988.
5. Maeda K, Horiguchi S, Hosokawa M: History of the studies of occupational cervicobrachial disorders in Japan and remaining problems. *J Hum Ergol* 11:17–29, 1982.
6. Nishiyama K, Nakaseko N, Uehata T: Health aspects of VDT operators in the newspaper industry. In Grandjean E (ed): *Ergonomics and Health in Modern Offices.* London, Taylor & Francis, 1984.
7. Nachemson A, Elfstrom G: Intravital dynamic pressure measurement in lumbar discs. *Scand J Rehab Med [Suppl]* 1, 1970.
8. Barnes RM: *Motion and Time Study Design and Measurement of Work,* ed 7. New York, John Wiley & Sons, 1980.
9. McCormick EJ, Sanders MS: *Human Factors in Engineering and Design,* ed 5. New York, McGraw-Hill Book Co, 1982.
10. American National Standards Institute: *American National Standard for Human Factors Engineering of VDT Workstations.* Santa Monica, CA, Human Factors Society, Inc, 1988.
11. Woodson WE: *Human Factors Design Handbook.* New York, McGraw-Hill Book Co, 1981.
12. Bendix T, Hagberg M: Trunk posture and load on the trapezius muscle while sitting at sloping desks. *Ergonomics* 27:873–882, 1984.
13. Tichaur ER: *The Biomechanical Basis of Ergonomics.* New York, John Wiley & Sons, Inc, 1978.
14. Andersson GBJ, Chaffin DB, Pope MH: Occupational biomechanics of the lumbar spine. In Pope MH, Frymore JW, Andersson GBJ (eds): *Occupational Low Back Pain.* New York, Praeger, 1984, pp 39–70.
15. Drury CG, Francher M: Evaluation of forward sloping chair. *Appl Ergonomics* 16:41–47, 1985.
16. Khalil TM, Asfour SS, Moty EA: New horizons for ergonomics research in low back pain. In Eberts RE, Eberts CG (eds): *Trends in Ergonomics/Human Factors.* Amsterdam: Elsevier Science Publishers BV, 1985, pp 591–598.
17. Khalil TM, Asfour SS, Moty EA, Steele R, Rosomoff HL: The management of low back pain: a comprehensive approach. In *Proceedings of the Annual Industrial Engineering Conference,* Louisville, KY. Institute of Industrial Engineers, 1983, pp 199–204.
18. Rosomoff HL, Green C, Silbert M, Steele R: Pain and low back rehabilitation program at the University of Miami School of Medicine. In Lorenzo KY (ed): *New Approaches to Treatment of Chronic Pain: A Review of Multidisciplinary Pain Clinics and Pain Centers.* NIDA Research Monograph No. 36. Washington, DC, US Department of Health and Human Services, 1981.
19. Rosomoff HL: Comprehensive pain center approach to the treatment of low back pain. In *Low Back Pain.* Report of a workshop at the Rehab Research and Training Center, Department of Orthopedic Rehabilitation, University of Virginia. Charlottesville, University of Virginia Press, 1987, pp 78–85.
20. Khalil TM, Goldberg ML, Asfour SS, Moty EA, Steele R, Rosomoff HL: Acceptable maximum effort (AME): a psychophysical measure of strength in back pain patients. *Spine* 12:372–376, 1987.
21. Chaffin DB: Ergonomics guide for the assessment of human static strength. *Am Ind Hyg Assoc J* 36:505–510, 1975.
22. Bonney MC, Schofield NA, Roberts EA, Evershed DG, Hughes BJ, Vasilvskis A: Ergonomics in design using a computer man and conversational graphics. *Int J Product Res* 10:313–323, 1971.
23. Cushman WH, Pugsley RE: Workplace design. In *Ergonomics Design for People at Work.* Belmont, CA, Lifetime Learning Publications (Eastman Kodak Co), 1984, pp 12–52.
24. Kilpatrick KE: Computer aided work place design. *J Methods-Time Measur* 4:24–33, 1969.
25. Barr A, Feigenbaum E: *The Handbook of Artificial Intelligence.* Los Altos, CA, William Kaufmann Inc, 1981.
26. McGraw KL: Artificial intelligence: the competitive edge in integrated systems development. *Texas Instruments J* 3:12–16, 1986.
27. Abdel-Moty E, Khalil TM: Computer aided design of the sitting workplace. *Comput Ind Eng* 11(1–4):23–26, 1986.
28. Abdel-Moty E, Khalil TM: A computerized expert system for work simplification and workplace design. In Botton NA, Raz T (eds): *Expert Systems.* Norcross, GA, Industrial Engineering and Management Press, 1988, pp 221–226.
29. Abdel-Moty E, Khalil TM: Microcomputers in the design and analysis of the VDT sitting workplace. In Asfour SS (ed): *Trends in Ergonomics/Human Factors.* Amsterdam, Elsevier Science Publishing BV, 1987, pp 113–120.
30. Khalil TM, Ramadan MZ: Biomechanical evaluation of lifting tasks: a microcomputer-based model. *Comput Ind Eng* 14:1, 1987.
31. Abdel-Moty E, Khalil TM: Computerized signal processing techniques for the quantification of muscular activity. *Comput Ind Eng* 12(3):193–203, 1987.
32. Goldberg ML, Orozco M, Arejano J, Khalil TM, et al: Use of electromyographic biofeedback in the rehabilitation of low back pain patients: body mechanics instruction. In *Proceedings of the 21st Annual Conference of the Human Factors Association of Canada,* Edmonton, Alberta. Mississauga, Ontario, Association Canadienne d'ergonomic, 1988.

## SUGGESTED READINGS

Davis HL, Rodgers SH: Ergonomics in industry. In *Ergonomics Design for People at Work.* Belmont, CA, Lifetime Learning Publications (Eastman Kodak Co, Human Factors Section), 1984, pp 3–11.

Khalil TM: Design tools and machines to fit the man. *Ind Eng* 1:32–35, 1972.

Kroemer KHE, Price DL: Ergonomics in the office: comfortable work stations allow maximum productivity. *Ind Eng* 7:24–32, 1983.

Oborne DJ: *Ergonomics at Work,* ed 2. Bath, England, Bath Press Ltd, 1987.

Putz-Anderson V: *Cumulative Trauma Disorders: A Manual for Musculoskeletal Diseases of the Upper Extremity.* New York, Taylor and Francis Ltd, 1988.

## 16

# THE COMPREHENSIVE PAIN PROGRAM APPROACH

*Benjamin L. Crue, Jr.*

One should very seldom begin a presentation with an apology, or even an explanation. However, I have found this assignment to write a chapter on the comprehensive pain program approach for a book on cervical trauma to be an overwhelming task indeed. There is just too much material. There are innumerable posttraumatic syndromes related to the cervical spine. Furthermore, to present the concepts of all the comprehensive pain program approaches is also an overwhelming task. There are now well over 1000 pain clinics and pain centers in the United States, most of which have some type of team treatment program, and so far experience has taught that probably no two of them are exactly alike.

I have written for a number of years on chronic pain syndromes and, in more recent years, in the health care delivery field regarding pain treatment for patients with chronic pain. It is absolutely impossible, in a chapter that will fit into this multifaceted cervical trauma book, to do justice to everyone's ideas concerning comprehensive pain therapy. Therefore, since I am now in my 32nd consecutive year as a medical and program director for either a pain clinic or a pain center (26 years in southern California, and the last 6 years in Durango, Colorado), I am going to be unabashedly personal about this chapter. I hope the reader will not think me too egotistical if the presentation is limited to my beliefs about chronic pain, and how I would recommend that a comprehensive pain team treatment center should be organized to deliver therapy to those suffering from chronic pain after cervical injury. I will include as references only some of the articles that I myself have written or coauthored. (I hope that in past publications I have always given due credit to those who came before; those readers interested can follow up by referring to the articles cited.)

### THE CHRONIC PAIN SYNDROME

The remarks in this chapter are limited to the treatment of *chronic* pain syndromes after cervical trauma. Pain following cervical injury starts as *somatopsychic acute pain* with nociceptive input from the injured site. Many posttraumatic cervical pain syndromes can then develop that may persist for a considerable length of time. Many are recurrent acute pain states; for example, there may be chronic residual osteoarthritic changes, perhaps with a spur at the joint of Luschka that with motion "irritates" an entering or exiting sensory fiber, giving a cervical radiculoneuritis with pain referred down the arm. There is still much discussion as to exactly how the so-called irritation (perhaps, on occasion, with recurrent intermittent compression) may cause inflammation in the nerve root leading to swelling and edema and producing a radiculoneuritis with its typical dermatomal sensory pattern and motor electromyographic changes (1). As this syndrome waxes and wanes, it can often be called chronic.

As I have written repeatedly, the pathologic arthritic changes are chronic, but the pain is a recurrent acute pain (2–8) with presumed sensory nociceptive input from the pathologic nerve root. Treatment of these patients usually does not require a "pain team approach," although with pain syndromes with this type of recurrent acute pain

230

there is often psychological "functional overlay," so that, just as in some cancer pain patients, the "team" approach (or at least a multidisciplinary or interdisciplinary approach) may well be indicated (beyond the therapeutic abilities or time available of any one individual treater) (9, 10). Sometimes, such radiculoneuritis pain after neck trauma may well seem to be entirely organic, and may respond to such simple treatments as adding neck flexion to the oft-used cervical traction (11, 12).

## OTHER CERVICAL SYNDROMES

Many other pain syndromes that are often considered among the chronic pain syndromes may well have a large cervical component. For example, the osteopaths and chiropractors (while I believe them incorrect in their views of the underlying pain mechanism) have often been ahead of many physicians in their emphasis on the clinical importance of the cervical spine in many of the syndromes with pain referred elsewhere, especially to the head (13). For example, in greater occipital neuralgia the pathology may be in the lower cervical spine (not in any entrapment of the posterior primary division of C2 itself), and then, with anxiety (and not with muscle tension), the pain (or numbness) is referred to the back of the head. Many cases of atypical facial neuralgia, and even subjective blurred vision and tinnitus (14, 15), may be due to underlying cervical pathology. Even in primary trigeminal neuralgia the individual central connections in the descending trigeminal tract and nucleus, where they are continuous with the substantia gelatinosa of Rolando and Lissauer's tract, may involve a cervical location anatomically (16, 17). This is all too speculative and too complicated to discuss further here.

## PSYCHOSOMATIC AS CENTRAL

I believe that *all chronic pain is always all psychosomatic.* It may have started as a *somatopsychic* input from the site of injury, but in that particular individual at that time with that particular injury, either the chronic pain syndrome that is established becomes entirely central, or it should not be referred to as *chronic pain.* If the pain continues but there is good clinical reason to suspect that there is continued nociceptive input from the periphery that might be amenable to treatment by various modalities aimed at stopping the presumed input, then the condition should not be classified as a

chronic pain syndrome but, rather, as a *chronic pathologic condition with recurrent acute pain with nociceptive input.* This oft-repeated declaration may appear too pedantic, but really is basic to an understanding of the underlying rationale of the treatment of patients with chronic pain syndromes. If there *is* continued nociceptive input, then such things as anti-inflammatory agents, nerve blocks, neurosurgical operations, peripherally acting analgesics, and centrally acting narcotics are all appropriate. However, if we are dealing with a chronic pain that is presumed to be all centralized, then almost by definition the treatment called for is psychotherapy. This problem is not just one of taxonomy, but leads into basically different concepts of the underlying pain mechanisms, regardless of the fact that the *etiology* is the known cervical trauma. It leads to what has been called the peripheralist versus centralist concept of chronic pain (2, 3, 10, 18–37).

## PERIPHERALIST VERSUS CENTRALIST

### PERIPHERALIST POSITION

The peripheralist believes that chronic pain can be viewed basically as a continuation of nociceptive input, as in the acute pain medical model, when for "some" reason the original cause of the pain, which started with the nociceptive input, continues "longer than expected," "longer than usual," or even "longer than seems reasonable." This situation might be due to continuing pathophysiologic change in the periphery at the site of the original cervical injury (or subsequent operation, or inflammation). Thus, there is a belief by peripheralists that there is presumed continued peripheral input, not only in *neuritis* but in *neuropathy* and perhaps even in *neuralgia.* This is thought to be possible because the peripheral pathology may not yet have healed correctly, or may not have been fixed correctly by the surgeon, or perhaps the continued nociceptive input originates in the inevitable "scar." This is the classic teaching in the discipline, and it appears to make good sense. Was it not the original injury that started the pain syndrome, and does it not still hurt out there in the periphery? Still, most experienced peripheralists do admit that with the passage of time there is, in addition, some considerable psychological central "functional overlay." Peripheralists do not claim, in general, that chronic pain is all due to continued peripheral nociceptive input.

## CENTRALIST POSITION

The centralist, in contrast, may seem more dogmatic in stating that with any tissue damage and acute pain there is established some type of central "memory" of pain that can hypothetically be conceptualized as a "reverberating circuit," an "internuncial pool," or "repetitive epileptiform firing" in the sensory networks of the central nervous system. Under appropriate conditions, the patient's brain itself can generate and continue to signal pain even further upward to the "alarm bell" in the patient's *mind* (which is referred to as the "conscious awareness of self" portion of central nervous system function). The pain thus becomes *chronic*, and can occur after only a few days or may take months. After the etiologic peripheral posttraumatic pathologic condition heals, there is then no need (and there is no neurophysiologic evidence) for postulated continued peripheral nociceptive input. The centralist believes that this input now exists only in the treating peripheralist activist physician's imagination! Thus, neuralgia becomes a central pain that is referred back to the periphery, to that part of the body image from which the initial etiologic nociceptive input occurred, often initiating and then utilizing the mechanism referred to as memory, or "learned pain" (34).

## POSSIBLE COEXISTENCE OF THE MECHANISMS

Of course, both possible mechanisms exist, and they may be acting together in any one case of continued human pain. However, the dogmatic centralist would then point out that, if there is any continued nociceptive input from the periphery, it should not be labeled chronic pain, no matter how long it has lasted clinically. The term "chronic pain" should be reserved for pain generated within the central nervous system, as well as perceived in consciousness within the brain, in patients in whom there is no evidence of any continued nociceptive input. This does not mean, however, that in chronic pain patients there may not, on occasion, be clinical exacerbation of the amplitude or severity of the central pain by many types of sensory input, whether it be from touch, noise, light, or the like. This admittedly becomes a tautologic classification in which *chronic* pain is equated with *central* pain.

## PAIN CLINICS AND PAIN CENTERS

It has been the failures experienced when treating patients with chronic pain on the part of most physicians utilizing the acute pain nociceptive input model that has led to a new phenomenon in this country—the *evolution* of pain clinics and pain centers. Gerald Aronoff, M.D., refers to these pain centers as a *revolution* in health care (6).

Over the last three decades there has been a development in the field of pain treatment that should be of interest to all. This is the organization of specialized pain clinics and pain centers. While the impetus at the beginning was a *demonstrated failure* of current medical and surgical treatment for the problems of patients with chronic pain, there was also a *concomitant belief* that the alternative of therapy at a pain center by a multidisciplinary trained team might have something additional to offer. Many such multidisciplinary and later interdisciplinary pain teams evolved when outpatient pain clinics found that they were failing in their mission, and pain clinic directors became dissatisfied with what they were personally able to do for many chronic pain syndrome patients utilizing previously learned techniques based on blocking nociceptive input, whether by nerve block or mutilating neurosurgical operations.

I am using the term pain "clinic" to mean a specialized facility that treats patients with chronic pain on an *outpatient* basis. The word "clinic" means outpatient care rather than free care, as was once true in England and in many parts of the United States. As these pain teams were assembled, they evolved in many different directions. Often nonmedical members were added, and the term "interdisciplinary" was obviously appropriate. These teams often included physical and occupational therapists for the reconditioning of the chronic pain patient's body, which was atrophied through disuse. They may have included a psychologist or, more rarely, a psychiatrist for the treatment of the recognized central or functional aspects of the chronic pain complaints. As these teams developed they usually mirrored the beliefs, training, and specialties of the original pain clinic directors, as well as the referral patterns, and the needs, of the individual host institution.

The pain clinic may have then evolved into a pain center in a cancer hospital, in a university or general hospital setting, or on an orthopaedic, rheumatologic, or dental service. As more and more physicians were assembled, first as consultants and then as members of pain teams, the program became multidisciplinary. Then, when inpatient services were added, the pain clinics became known as pain centers, and were often truly comprehensive interdisciplinary, multidisciplinary, interdepartmental pain centers, although the number of institutions that could truly be called comprehensive pain centers has remained relatively small.

## WHAT IS A PAIN CENTER?

I suggested several years ago (38) that a comprehensive pain center should include at least

1. An *outpatient pain clinic* for triage, diagnosis, and treatment.
2. An independent *inpatient pain service* of whatever specialty (i.e., neurology, neurosurgery, orthopedics, rheumatology) for those patients who could not be treated optimally for their pain on an outpatient basis.
3. A *specialized pain unit* for both inpatient and outpatient treatment of chronic pain syndromes believed to be psychosomatic, where a psychiatrist or psychologist was in charge.

It was my belief then, and is an even stronger belief today, that the treatment in a pain center is best organized on a *group* psychotherapy model. It was also believed that, in addition to the three components listed above, a comprehensive pain treatment center should include facilities for clinical and basic research and a component for teaching, either through a medical school affiliation or by having approved pain fellowships in this new field of chronic pain treatment and patient management, which has now come to be known as the specialty of "algology."

In 1979, after 19 years of evolution, we published our third book on the treatment of pain patients from the City of Hope National Medical Center in Duarte, California. As the medical director, and as a neurosurgeon, I wrote a chapter that both described the role of a neurosurgeon in the pain clinic and stated my beliefs in the primacy of psychotherapy as the therapeutic tool in the treatment of all patients with chronic pain syndromes (39). Furthermore, it was my and Dr. Jack Pinsky's belief at that time, and remains so today, that the most therapeutically effective, as well as the most cost effective, manner of delivering psychotherapy to chronic pain patients was in the group psychotherapy model (32, 33, 40, 41).

## EVOLUTION OF DIFFERENT TYPES OF COMPREHENSIVE APPROACHES

The main change over the last decade has been brought about by the fact that the socioeconomic times have led me to change from an inpatient model to an outpatient model for the treatment of the majority of patients with chronic pain syndromes. As expected, the cost assessment of a team outpatient program (rivaling in intensity our previous inpatient model) shows that we can usually deliver the same type of treatment in the same length of time at approximately 40–55% of the cost of inpatient therapy in many hospitals. This switch to an outpatient model has led to a profound change in the makeup of our patient mix within at least my own pain center, and, quite frankly, in a large percentage of those that I have also had a chance to see as a CARF surveyor. In general, there is a much larger percentage of compensation-covered cases, with more males, in outpatient clinics. The various state compensation laws covering injured workers have been the economic driving engine of many developing new pain clinics, as results have proven "cost-effective." Unfortunately, many private patients with only inpatient hospital insurance have been left to "fall between the cracks"!

There is no question but that we lose some intensity, and some control over the patient's management, by going from an inpatient to an outpatient model. However, in the outpatient setting we are able to better emphasize the "wellness" role in chronic pain patients, who in general are not "sick." We should have foreseen that the present structure of the insurance coverage programs in America would have had a profound effect on the type of patients that we would be able to accept within our outpatient treatment team regimen for economic reasons. When we switched from an inpatient to an outpatient model we gave up the routine standard hospital insurance programs (and most of our "private" patients). In the past we had excluded workers injured on the job who had compensation coverage as having obvious secondary gain involved. We had done so with a clear conscience, because there were other pain centers that would accept patients with workmen's compensation insurance coverage—for example, those of Dr. Joel Seres in Portland, Oregon, or Dr. Steve Brena in Atlanta, Georgia. We now found that for economic survival on an outpatient basis we *had* to accept workmen's compensation cases, in spite of the secondary gain issues, strictly for economic survival.

Much to our surprise and delight, we found that Dr. Brena and Dr. Stan Chapman were correct in that, when dealing with the basic psychodynamic mechanisms causing continued pain in patients with chronic pain syndromes, in most instances the secondary gain economic issues paled into insignificance and in only a few instances were they an insurmountable obstacle. However, it is true that the pain center administrator and medical director had to become much more proficient in their interface with attorneys, vocational rehabilitation counselors, claim adjusters, compensation insurance carriers, and, most recently in the state of Colorado, with the Colorado Foundation for Medical Care, which, while presented as a quality assurance mechanism, is quite obviously, in the opinion of many physicians, largely a governmental cost-containing mechanism at the state level.

We have continued to find that, if we are going to have an intense "therapeutic milieu," we must have a trained and experienced, cohesive and congruent pain team treatment program within a very structured framework. The patient must be subjected to a psychotherapeutic "crisis intervention" model if we are going to attempt to reverse within a reasonable time frame the pain syndrome in most of our chronic pain patients, many with on-the-job cervical injury. We have been able, over the course of 30 years, to reduce our structured program from 8 weeks of an inpatient model to 4 weeks (5 days a week, 8 hr a day) on an outpatient basis. This has proved sufficient for the vast majority of chronic pain patients, in spite of their secondary gain problems from on-the-job cervical injury.

## PATIENT EVALUATION

In an attempt to get off to a "running start," all of the patients who enter our pain center have been evaluated by this neurosurgeon on an outpatient basis, after referral either for a neurosurgery consultation or as a potential pain center candidate. This allows the patient to interact with me as a neurosurgeon in a medical context, and patients are often relieved when no further surgery or operative intervention is proffered. The patients are often seen several times on an outpatient basis, and perhaps put on a trial of antidepressant medication, mild peripherally acting analgesics, and, on occasion, even a short course of centrally acting oral narcotics in an attempt to alleviate the pain on a dyadic neurosurgical outpatient basis, without need for referral to the pain team at the pain center. Only when the patient's usually constant pain syndrome, which has often been present for several years, continues in spite of this type of approach is he or she recommended for admission to the outpatient structured 4-week team pain unit program.

## WRITTEN "BLUE BOOKS"

For some 20 years now we have supplied the patient who is being offered team therapy in the comprehensive structured pain program our so-called blue book (because of its blue cover) containing patient information regarding our program. Patients are asked to read the pamphlet and to bring it with them when they enter the program. We believe this instructive pamphlet is so important to successful treatment in an outpatient 4-week program that the patients are instructed that only after they have read it will their further questions about the pain center and its treatment program be answered by the appointed members of the pain team. From a practical standpoint, this also saves the referring neurosurgeon a considerable amount of time in trying to explain to the individual patient just what treatment he or she will receive when referred to the structured pain program at the pain rehabilitation center.

As the years have gone by, this blue book has been repeatedly revised, we hope refined, and (believe it or not) shortened. I consider it such an important part of the comprehensive treatment program of the patients with chronic pain that I am including it as an appendix to this chapter. We have found over the years that numerous pain clinics and pain centers around the world have either adopted our blue book or have developed ones of their own. It is well recognized now that some type of preadmission instruction saves much valuable time for the patient after entering the program, and I frankly cannot envision running our outpatient pain rehabilitation center program without such a "blue book."

## EVOLUTION OF PRESENT TEAM BY ECONOMIC NECESSITY

I in no way wish to denigrate the efforts of each and every member of the pain team in treating patients when they do finally enter the structured program. However, it is of interest that there has been a second big change brought about by socioeconomic pressures, which two decades ago I would have not found acceptable—a slowly evolving lowering in the level of formal education of pain team staff members around the country. Originally at the City of Hope I had seven M.D. and Ph.D. team members on a full-time basis, when we usually averaged about eight patients at a time in our inpatient structured pain unit program. This, in the 1980s, proved to be an insurmountable economic burden. Consequently, while we still have a multidisciplinary, interdisciplinary team, we are able at this time to accomplish our objectives for patient care with a primarily part-time staff.

The only full-time people in the entire program are the administrator, who takes care of the business (and also doubles as a part-time nutritionist in the pain team), and the pain center secretary. I function as a part-time medical director. If any other physicians are needed to make this truly a multidisciplinary program, we invite them in as consultants on a case-by-case basis as seems indicated; after 32 years' experience, this has rarely proven to be necessary. Our clinical psychologist supervisor at a Ph.D. level is on a part-time basis also. The rest of the team is made up of part-time therapists, in general at a master's degree level. They are paid on a reasonable, but not competitive, scale with private practitioners in their disciplines in the area, and they are paid only when they work. For example, while all patients receive physical therapy after initial evaluation by the registered physical therapist, their ongoing daily therapy is supplied by exercise therapists, because frankly a registered physical therapist is too expensive.

Thus, while the physical therapist may be in charge of the exercise therapist, and while the clinical psychologist may be supervising the master's level psychotherapists, from a practical standpoint the vast majority of the work of the team is carried out by people below the doctorate level. Quite frankly, the lowering in the level of formal education of the members of the pain team has not resulted, in my opinion, in any lowering of the quality of the therapy that the patient gets. The quality of the treatment depends on the expertise as well as the training of the individual therapists, and the internal congruence of the pain team. This approach to the treatment of patients with chronic pain fits very well with the beliefs of Dr. Jack Pinsky, who long ago taught me that in pain team therapy it is the *caring* of the treaters that is much more important than their academic degrees. In our pain team therapy, the treaters, including the exercise therapist and the nutritionist and the physical therapist and the occupational therapist, are all psychotherapists first and treaters of the soma second. This has on occasion been a difficult role for some individuals to learn and accept, but when the team is working together with the acceptance of the centralist approach to the treatment of chronic pain, frankly it is beautiful to behold.

## TYPES OF PAIN SYNDROMES TREATED AT PAIN CENTERS

The reader may have noticed that in the last few paragraphs I have said almost nothing that limits the treatment at a pain center to patients with chronic pain syndromes after cervical trauma. The reason for this is that if our conceptualization and belief about the underlying mechanisms of chronic pain are indeed correct, then we are among the "lumpers" rather than the "splitters." To paraphrase Gertrude Stein, "A pain is a pain is a pain."

In general, we have more "failed backs" than "failed necks," but the patients with chronic pain syndromes following lumbar injury (and often failed lumbar surgery) are usually very similar to patients with chronic pain from cervical injury. There are differences, but they are usually minor. The same cannot be said as precisely about some of the other chronic pain syndromes, such as chronic headache that started with migraine, or poststroke Dejerine-Roussy "thalamic" pain. For the purpose of this chapter, the comprehensive pain center team treatment of chronic cervical pain is considered to be similar to the treatment of all chronic pain syndromes. The major differences are the differences between the individual human patients.

## THE TREATMENT APPROACH: INSIGHT THERAPY

Unlike many chronic pain treatment centers run by psychologists, where the psychotherapy is based upon modern operant conditioning (or behavior modification) in the belief that the brain's modulation of presumed continued nociceptive input must be changed, we have purposely structured our psychotherapeutic program to be based on *insight* psychotherapy. While originally our therapeutic approach was perhaps more in the "psychoanalytical model," it does appear that treatment comes down to *cognitive therapy*, in that it appears largely to be based on *learning theory*, regardless of one's conceptualization of just what this means. While the caring therapeutic milieu is of tremendous importance, the changes we attempt to bring about in the life of the chronic pain patients under our therapy are much more profound than merely reducing their pain. Furthermore, we are horrified by the often-heard statement that "chronic pain centers teach patients to learn to live with their pain." While it may be true that after therapy chronic pain patients are able to enjoy life more, and perhaps return to work in spite of residual pain, this is a secondary goal. The goal of the pain center team remains primarily the reduction of the patient's subjective suffering.

## OUTLINE OF PATIENT INSTRUCTION

Our patients in general are treated as patients, but in many ways they are students. We follow an outline of instructions, very informally (39).

**First.** The patients are *first* gradually led to understand that they *perceive pain* in their *brain*.

**Second.** The patients are informed that modern science accepts the mind, both conscious and unconscious (the latter a contradiction in terms) as a function of the brain.

**Third.** The patients are then told that yes, we do believe that their chronic pain is "all in their minds." They are informed that yes, the main thrust of treatment within the pain program is to ascertain what the patients can learn to do about their own pain and suffering experience. They must not rely on what any of us on the pain team can do to or for them. Considerable time is spent in determining just what the implication is for each of them when they are told that their pain is all in their mind. To many it implies that "The doctor doesn't believe me; he thinks I am faking or malingering, but I know my pain is real." Many, if not almost all, of the chronic pain patients begin to discuss this concept and, in spite of any alexithymia, will finally verbalize that yes, they have often wondered "Am I going crazy?"

**Fourth.** We spend considerable time explaining to patients the difference between *acute pain* with *peripheral* nociceptive input and their *chronic suffering* process. Their chronic pain is not only perceived within that portion of brain function known as the conscious mind, but is generated and potentiated (not in the sense of continued peripheral input) by a central mechanism that refers it to consciousness. The pain from the original cervical injury, which *was* somatopsychic, is then perceived as a continuation of the original peripheral pain by referring it to the original site of injury, when in reality it has indeed become psychosomatic and is all central. We often use the illustration of the patient with "phantom limb" pain, where we point out that obviously the consciously perceived pain in the absent limb cannot

be from continued peripheral input, because there is no periphery.

The patients begin to ask "Are you telling us we are different?" Our answer is—yes! The majority of people who have neck injuries (or surgeries) promptly get over their pain. Approximately 85–90% of cervical laminectomy patients have good outcomes and go back to work, and the pain subsides relatively soon.

Much necessary time is spent on semantics. The patients are often familiar with terms such as "neuritis," "neuropathy," and "neuralgia" (3, 7, 39). Our explanations of the difference in these terms from the centralist point of view is surprisingly, and almost uniformly, understood by the patients, and seems to play a significant role in their cognitive therapy program.

**Fifth.** The patients are then asked to consider what may be wrong in their particular case, when there is nothing in the periphery (in the region of the painful previously injured cervical spine) that needs fixing. Since their injuries have long since healed, why are they different from other patients who have stopped hurting after a similar injury?

**Sixth.** It is then suggested to the patients that perhaps the answer lies in a subconscious or unconscious *need* to continue to hurt. This statement always engenders considerable immediate discussion. We spend considerable time discussing the difference between *wants* and *needs,* and the fact that many of our needs are at an unconscious level, and we have no knowledge of them. It is possible, without a doubt, that dysphoric defense mechanisms can cause their pain to continue without mental awareness on their parts that any such process is going on.

The problem of the *control* issue is usually discussed in depth. The fact that many chronic pain patients are *alexithymic* (and have trouble with imagery and regression therapy in attempting to get in touch with painful regressed emotional conflicts that they have "locked in the closet" years before) is dwelt on at length. It is often appropriate to point out the fact that many chronic pain patients are caretakers (and field directed). There are often angry disclaimers when we discuss the fact that the patient as a human being (that the team believes has his or her own "free will") must bear responsibility for receiving multiple orthopaedic or neurosurgical operations (when they were referred to an orthopaedist or a neurosurgeon). They must each accept some responsibility for past therapy.

**Seventh.** Most of the patients who still remain

fixed in the acute medical model are then the subject of discussion about how emotions can trigger the severity of their pains. By direct questioning, often the patients will admit that, while they do not like to think of their chronic pain syndrome as a psychosomatic illness, they have long since noticed that on many occasions it is psychological stress, not just physical stress, that triggers the amplitude of their suffering. The illustration of the elderly widow with atypical facial neuralgia (and cervical arthritis and perhaps recent dental trauma) is used. The cause is "lonesomeness" and the treatment is "love." This is usually very effective, especially if we have a neuralgic pain patient within the group, or if any of the pain patients have had such an individual in their families.

Most chronic pain patients, while at times seeming depressed, have not responded to antidepressive medication. They are more discouraged, and in fact often demoralized, than they are chemically depressed.

**Eighth.** Finally, the patients are asked to list what they think might be some of their unconscious, unresolved emotional conflicts that have led their unconscious brain mechanisms to emotionally continue the potentiation of the memory of chronic pain. What is it that keeps that alarm bell of pain ringing in their conscious mind and prolongs their suffering? It is absolutely amazing to me how many times the patients will catch on quickly to what we are suggesting when we say that chronic pain is always psychosomatic, and that we believe there is an unconscious need to continue to hurt, because of underlying unconscious unresolved emotional conflicts leading to dysphoric defense mechanisms and the continuation of the individual patient's chronic suffering.

## USUAL CAUSES OF UNRESOLVED EMOTIONAL CONFLICT

We teach our patients that there are six common causes of unresolved emotional conflicts that can lead to the continuation of chronic pain (Table 16.1). By far the most common is *unresolved grief.* This usually is over loss of a parent, a spouse, or a child; but often results from the loss of economic status or the physiologic decay of the body with aging. In all ages and both sexes, grief, in my opinion, is by far the most common problem. This is especially true of the older chronic pain patients, and perhaps women more than men.

The second common cause is anger, often unexpressed *anger* or repressed *rage.* Surpris-

**Table 16.1.**

**Common Emotional Causes of Continued Chronic Pain**[a]

Unresolved GRIEF—usually involving loss.
ANGER—often unexpressed or repressed rage.
DEPRESSION—anger turned inward.
FEAR—anxiety in civilized terms.
GUILT—sins of omission or commission.
SHAME—fear others will know about the guilt.

[a]Chronic pain is always psychosomatic. It is due to an unconscious *need* to continue to hurt, because of underlying unconscious unresolved emotional conflicts leading to dysphoric defense mechanisms—the continuation of suffering.

ingly, the patient may radiate anger and hostility and yet sincerely deny being angry at anyone. In our practice injured workers are still predominantly male. In the young injured male worker, anger appears to be the most common cause of unresolved emotional conflict.

The third common cause of unresolved emotional conflict is anger turned inward, which psychodynamically leads to *depression.* (We are not discussing other psychosomatic illnesses here, such as duodenal ulcers or high blood pressure.) The chronic pain patient with true depression in whom antidepressants have not stopped the suffering almost always turns out to have been severely angry over a long period of time. The patient has been unable to turn this anger outward (for catharsis), but has instead turned the anger inward and has become depressed.

*Fear* is another cause of unresolved emotional conflict, predominantly among our male patients. Many males are afraid, but because of the American "macho" image (and, in our location in the Colorado Four Corners area, that of the Hispanic culture as well), enabling a young male with a cervical injury to admit fear often requires considerable rapport and patience on the part of the staff. Many times the patients will talk about "anxiety," and admit being "anxious," but will be unwilling to accept the fact that fear underlies the anxiety.

A fifth cause of unresolved emotional conflict is a sense of *guilt*—the so-called *sins* of omission or commission. I use the words "sins" knowingly, not because this is the pain team's judgment of the patient, but because it is the individual chronic pain patient's moral self-judgment. These patients believe that they have done something that they *should* not have, or have not done something they know they *should* have. The fear in these often field-directed chronic pain patients that others may find out about the misdeed causing the guilt often leads to a sense of *shame*, yet another common cause of unresolved emotional conflict.

As Dr. Richard Sternbach has said, there are often "multifaceted" aspects to chronic pain. We often find that the patients have not just one but as many as all six of these types of unresolved emotional conflict impinging on their lives. They may not be able to resolve them all, they may never have the "Ah-ha" experience during imagery, regression, or hypnosis, but the fact that they can begin to get in touch with their feelings, and overcome some of their alexithymia, often leads to improvement—not only in reducing the patient's chronic pain following cervical injury, but in their increased enjoyment of all the aspects of living. This improvement includes family relationships, return to work, and increased feelings of self-worth. While in 4 weeks it is impossible to do more in most cases than "round the corner," we do believe that ongoing outpatient weekly psychotherapy in a "continuing care group" is indicated for many of our patients, and is so recommended (whether authorized by the compensation insurance carrier or not). This often leads to further improvement in the chronic pain and suffering state of these individuals.

## OUTCOME AND OUTLOOK

In my opinion, and at our pain center, the psychotherapeutic approach to the treatment of chronic pain following cervical trauma has led to a very satisfactory success rate. Over the years we have found, unfortunately, that 14–15% of the patients who enter the structured pain program find that the psychotherapeutic process is so distasteful and stressful (increasing their pain or the like) that they sign out against medical advice. We have long since gotten over our surprise when this happens. This does not produce anger but sadness in the pain team members. Of the approximately 86% of patients who finish the structured program, well over 90% have less pain, are leading more satisfactory lives, and are thankful and grateful for the pain team approach to their cervical chronic pain problem. After 32 years, and after having been trained as an operating neurosurgeon, I find this type of success ever surprising, but am very grateful that the psychotherapeutic approach does seem to work for the majority of patients with chronic pain.

## REFERENCES

1. Crue BL, Pudenz RH, Shelden, CH: Observations on the value of clinical electromyography. *J Bone Joint Surg* 39:492–500, 1957.
2. Crue BL: The centralist concept of chronic pain. *Semin Neurol* 3:331–339, 1983.
3. Crue BL: Neuritis, neuropathy and neuralgia. *Curr Concepts Pain* 1:3–10, 1983.
4. Brena S, Crue BL, Stieg R: Comments on the classification of chronic pain: its clinical significance. *Bull Clin Neurosci* 49:67–81, 1984.
5. Crue BL: Outpatient management of acute and chronic pain. In Wolcott MW (ed): *Ambulatory Surgery*, ed 2. Philadelphia, JB Lippincott Co, 1988, pp 144–154.
6. Crue BL: Foreward. In Aronoff G (ed): *Pain Centers in the U.S.A., A Revolution in Health Care.* New York, Raven Press, 1988, pp xii–xvii.
7. Crue BL: Management of painful neuropathies. In Tollison CD (ed): *Handbook of Chronic Pain Management.* Baltimore, Williams & Wilkins Co, 1989, pp 365–372.
8. Crue BL: Central vs. peripheral philosophies of pain. *Pain Management*, 1:218–222, 1988.
9. Crue BL, Felsoory A, Agnew D, Kamdar MD, Randle W, Griffin S, Sherman R, Menard P, Pinsky JJ: The team concept in the management of pain in patients with cancer. *Bull LA Neurol Soc* 44:70, 1979.
10. Crue BL: Multidisciplinary pain treatment programs—current status. *J Clin Pain* 1:31–38, 1985.
11. Crue BL: Importance of flexion in cervical traction for radiculitis. *US Armed Forces Med J* 8:374–380, 1957.
12. Crue BL, Todd EM: The importance of flexion in cervical halter traction. *Bull LA Neurol Soc* 30:95–98, 1965.
13. Crue BL, Todd EM, Carregal EJA: Observations on the present status of the compression procedure in trigeminal neuralgia. In Crue BL (ed): *Pain and Suffering—Selected Aspects.* Springfield, IL, Charles C Thomas, 1970, pp 47–63.
14. Crue BL, Carregal EA, Todd EM: Neuralgia: consideration of central mechanisms. *Bull LA Neurol Soc* 29:107–132, 1964.
15. Crue BL, Saltzberg B: Dynamic pain. *Bull LA Neurol Soc* 44:127, 1979.
16. Crue BL, Shelden CH, Pudenz RH, Freshwater DB: Observations on the pain and trigger mechanism in trigeminal neuralgia. *Neurology* 6:196–207, 1956.
17. Crue BL, Sutin J: Delayed action potentials in the trigeminal system of cats. *J Neurosurg* 16:477–502, 1959.
18. Shelden CH, Crue BL, Coulter JA: Surgical treatment of trigeminal neuralgia and discussion of compression operation. *Postgrad Med* 27:595–601, 1960.
19. Crue BL, Carregal E: Neuralgia as central pain. Paper presented at the Excerpta Medica Second International Congress of Neurological Surgery (ICS #36), Washington, DC, October 14–20, 1961.
20. Carregal E, Crue BL, Todd EM: Further observations of trigeminal antidromic potentials. *J Neurosurg* 20:277–288, 1963.
21. Todd EM, Crue BL, Vergadama M: Conservative treatment of post-herpetic neuralgia. *Bull LA Neurol Soc* 30:148–152, 1965.
22. Crue BL, Kilham OW, Carregal EJA, Todd EM: Peripheral trigeminal potentials. *Bull LA Neurol Soc* 32:17–29, 1967.
23. Crue BL, Todd EM, Carregal EJA: Cranial neuralgia—neurophysiological considerations. In Vinken PJ, Bruyn GW (eds): *Handbook of Neurology.* Amsterdam, North Holland Pub. Co., 1968, vol 5, pp 281–295.

24. Crue BL, Todd EM: Vagal neuralgia. In Vinken PJ, Bruyn GW (eds): *Handbook of Neurology*. Amsterdam, North Holland Pub. Co., 1968, vol 5.

25. Crue BL, Carregal EJA: Pain begins in the dorsal horn—with a proposed classification of the primary senses. In Crue BL (ed): *Pain Research and Treatment*. New York, Academic Press, 1975, pp 35–68.

26. Crue BL, Kenton B, Carregal EJA: Speculation concerning the possibility of a unitary peripheral cutaneous input system for pressure, hot-cold, and tissue damage: discussion of relationship to pain. *Bull LA Neurol Soc* 41:13–42, 1976.

27. Nashold B, Crue BL: Stereotaxic mesencephalic and trigeminal tractotomy. In Yowmans JR (ed): *Neurosurgery*, ed 2. Philadelphia, WB Saunders, 1982, pp 3702–3716.

28. Crue BL, Kenton B, Carregal EJA, Pinsky JJ: The continuing crisis in pain research. In Crue BL (ed): *Chronic Pain*. New York, Spectrum Publications, 1979, pp 545–561. (Also appears in Smith WL, Merskey H, Gross SC (eds): *Pain, Meaning and Management*. New York, Spectrum Publications, 1980, pp 1–20.)

29. Crue BL: A physiological view of the psychology of pain. *Bull LA Neurol Soc* 44:1, 1979.

30. Crue BL: Neurophysiology and taxonomy of pain. In Brena S, Chapman S (eds): *Management of Patients with Chronic Pain*. New York, Spectrum Publications, 1983, pp 21–32.

31. Crue BL: Causalgia and the deafferentiation syndromes. In Brena S, Chapman S (eds): *Management of Patients with Chronic Pain*. New York, Spectrum Publications, 1983, pp 33–46.

32. Pinsky JJ, Crue BL, Griffin S: Why a pain unit? In Crue BL (ed): *Chronic Pain*. New York, Spectrum Publications, 1979, pp 361–372.

33. Pinsky JJ, Crue BL: Intensive Group Psychotherapy. In Wall PD, Melzack R (eds): *Textbook of Pain*. New York, Churchill Livingstone, 1984, pp 823–831.

34. Crue BL: Foreward. In Aronoff GM (ed): *Evaluation and Treatment of Chronic Pain*. Baltimore, Urban & Schwarzenberg, 1985, pp xv–xxii.

35. Crue BL: Defining the chronic pain syndrome. In Long DM (ed): *Current Therapy in Neurosurgery*. Toronto, BC Decker Co, 1985, pp 205–208.

36. Crue BL: Pain research still ignores pain in absence of continuing nociceptive input [book review]. *J Pain Symptom Management* 2:172–173, 1987.

37. Crue BL: Historical perspectives. In Ghia JN (ed): *The Multidisciplinary Pain Center*. Boston, Kluwer Academic Pub, 1988, pp 1–20.

38. Crue BL, Pinsky JJ Agnew DC, Malyon AK, Felsoory A, Kenton B, Apuzzo M: What is a pain center? *Bull LA Neurol Soc* 41:160–167, 1976.

39. Crue BL: A role for a neurosurgeon on the pain unit. In Crue BL (ed): *Chronic Pain*. New York, Spectrum Publications, 1979, pp 397–412.

40. Crue BL, Pinsky JJ: An approach to chronic pain of nonmalignant origin. *Postgrad Med J* 60:30–36, 1984.

41. Crue BL, Pinsky JJ: Chronic pain syndrome—four aspects of the problem: New Hope Pain Center and Pain Research Foundation. In Ng LKY (ed) *New Approaches to Treatment of Chronic Pain* (Research Monograph Series, No. 36). Washington, DC, National Institute on Drug Abuse, 1981, pp 137–168.

*APPENDIX*

# Information for Patients with Chronic Pain Entering Treatment at the Durango Pain Rehabilitation Center

**WHAT IS CHRONIC PAIN?**

Pain in the "chronic intractable benign pain syndrome" (CIBPS) is an ongoing problem with pain that is not due to cancer. Generally, past medical and surgical approaches have been ineffective; and, there are often psychosocial dysfunctions that accompany the pain problem. The chronic pain has become intractable with no end in sight.

Another type of pain treated in our program is recurrent acute pain in which the cause is often more specifically known, such as the several types of arthritis, migraine headaches, or premenstrual syndrome.

Cancer pain is also treated at the Durango Pain Rehabilitation Center, but in a different part of the pain center. (This brochure is not meant for patients with pain from terminal malignancy.)

**WHAT IS AN INTERDISCIPLINARY PAIN REHABILITATION CENTER?**

An interdisciplinary pain rehabilitation center is composed of a team of specialists who provide a broad variety of therapies in one location. At Durango Pain Rehabilitation Center (DPRC), we utilize three main components that work together to provide a well-rounded approach to chronic pain relief. These components are medical, psychological and physical therapy units. The medical specialists are multidisciplinary (usually neurosurgery or neurology); and, the other interdisciplinary specialists include psychologists, psychotherapists, exercise therapists, and a nurse and nutritionist.

**HOW ARE PATIENTS EVALUATED?**

Patients are most often referred to DPRC by their personal physicians, or by a vocational rehab counselor, or by an insurance company. After referral, our initial evaluation screening consists of a medical history, physical examination and review of all pertinent prior medical records and x-rays, conducted by our medical director, Dr. Benjamin L. Crue, Jr., at his neurosurgery and algology office. Before, or at the time of, entrance to the pain program, a detailed psychosocial history and a psychological interview and evaluation will be obtained. A battery of psychological tests are given, including an MMPI, the McGill Pain Inventory, as well as several others. The patient is then evaluated by a physical therapist. On the basis of these evaluations, an individual treatment plan is designed and implemented for each patient with chronic pain.

**WHAT THERAPIES ARE GIVEN?**

Therapies may include as indicated: biofeedback training, nutritional counseling, physical therapy, therapeutic exercise, hydrotherapy, individual counseling, group psychotherapy, family therapy, assertiveness training, relaxation and visualization training, hypnotherapy, regression therapy, stress management, occupational therapy, and work hardening.

**WHAT IS PAIN MANAGEMENT?**

Pain management is an educational process that enables people to take charge of their pain and to progress with their lives. Techniques are taught to decrease the level of pain and/or to decrease the frequency of pain. Patients may still have some residual pain when they complete the program; however, they usually gain the ability to manage their pain. The goal of the treatment program is to decrease the patient's pain and suffering, and not just "to teach the patient how to learn to live with pain."

**WHAT GOALS MAY BE ACHIEVED?**

Goals may include reduction of pain severity, reduction of medication usage, increase in self esteem, increase in coping skills, increase in social activity, and improved quality of life. Work hardening program and vocational rehabilitation for return to work, or training for a new occupation, are an integral part of the pain therapeutic process.

**WHY IS MOTIVATION IMPORTANT?**

For the person with chronic pain, discomfort has become a part of a behavioral lifestyle, which not only affects the person, but also the family. We encourage as much family participation as possible. The center is of greatest benefit to those who are willing to deal with their pain and the related behaviors in an open manner. The more a person wants to make a change, the higher the chance for success in our pain treatment program.

**WHAT PROGRAMS ARE OFFERED?**

Possible programs are: intensive four-week pain management program; full program taken part-time over several months; selective therapies by physician prescription only; and, follow-up programs (for those who have completed programs at DPRC or elsewhere, which is known as our "continuing care" program).

**WHAT IS DURANGO PAIN REHABILITATION CENTER?**

The Durango Pain Rehabilitation Center is a non-profit team-oriented center designed to facilitate patients in learning the skills to decrease pain and be more self-directive in their personal lives.

**WHO IS DPRC?**

Rather than list the team members here, we refer you to the second pamphlet that is given along with this brochure to everyone who is recommended for admission to the pain treatment center. For specific clinical questions, refer to Jason Vance, who is not only the patient care coordinator, but is the patient case manager for each individual patient, and will act as your advocate and ombudsman. For specific medical questions, ask the medical director, Ben Crue. For general information or financial information, please ask one of the pain center secretaries, Carol Caruso or Gayle Ann Williams, or the administrator Pat Blair. For readings relating to pain therapy, although they are aimed at the professional rather than the patient population, we refer you to the references listed on the back of the accompanying brochure; and, we maintain an up-to-date "pain library" at the center.

**I. INTRODUCTION: AT REFERRAL**

After the brief introduction you have already been given, we would like to point out that the Durango Pain Rehabilitation Center has Dr. Benjamin L. Crue, Jr. as its medical director. He is now in his 28th consecutive year as a pain clinic or pain center medical director. He has been the medical director of a pain clinic or pain center here in Durango since January 1, 1986.

We would now like to continue the introduction, to help clarify the sequence of procedures that is beginning for you, the entering patient suffering from chronic pain. You were referred to the Durango Pain Rehabilitation Center for evaluation and possible treatment for your ongoing chronic pain program. The fact that you have been given this booklet that describes the outpatient pain unit indicates that the results of the medical examination so far suggests that it is not advisable, at this time, to treat your pain either surgically, or simply with a change of medication. Instead, you are being referred to determine if treatment in the specialized outpatient pain rehabilitation unit is indicated for you.

The Durango Pain Rehabilitation Center offers the most comprehensive forms of treatment for the problem of ongoing pain. The outpatient rehabilitation unit for patients with pain is outlined in the pages which follow.

## II. ASSESSMENT PROCESS

We welcome you to the Durango Pain Rehabilitation Center and look forward to the possibility of being able to help you. You are starting now an assessment process, which will allow us to determine whether or not this program is an appropriate treatment for you. This assessment in itself is rather time-consuming, and involves a commitment, not only on the staff's part, but on your part, as the patient. We will ask you to write up your life history in an autobiography of any length you choose; but, we would appreciate that, in general, the more detailed, the better. It enables us to get to know you. You will be having a psychological interview; and, a detailed psychosocial history will be taken. In addition, you will be given a whole battery of tests. Many of them at the outset will not seem to you to have much, if any, relationship to your particular problem with pain, which may well have started with a severe injury, (for example, while working on the job); and, the questions in many of these tests seem to have no direct relationship to your problem. We only can ask for your forebearance, and please take these tests seriously and answer them the best you can. We hope that you will, in the future, see that they may very well have a considerable relationship, not only to your pain problem, but also to the successful outcome of the pain team treatment. It is necessary that you have a rather complete understanding of the goals and the methods of this pain treatment program before the final decision (both on your part, and the pain team staff's part) is made regarding your final admission.

We are very aware that being referred to this pain unit may raise many questions for you. The referral almost always causes patients to wonder if their pain "is being taken seriously?" Frequently patients conclude that the referral to the pain unit means that their pain is being viewed as imaginary. This is definitely not the case. All patients referred for pain treatment at the outpatient pain rehabilitation center have real pains, and every member of the treating team knows and understands this.

We would like to state at the outset that pain is a perception that occurs in the central nervous system (brain and spinal cord), but this in no way implies that your pain is imaginary. Quite the opposite, your pain is real; and, we fully appreciate the many difficulties and limitations it has placed on you, the patient, as well as your family in many instances. We hope that this descriptive material will help to clarify the meaning of the referral to the pain unit. The preadmission assessment interviews will give you an opportunity to ask questions that you may have concerning your pain or this treatment process. We hope that this will result in your decision that will enable us to assist you in favorably altering your pain experience and longstanding suffering.

## III. ORGANIZATION OF THE PAIN CENTER

The Durango Pain Rehabilitation Center usually consists initially of referral to the outpatient neurosurgical and algology office of its medical director, Ben Crue, Jr., M.D. Many patients are handled by this individual physician, or by his medical partners, on an outpatient basis; and, no further referral for team therapy is indicated. In many ways, their office practice can be considered as an outpatient pain clinic. The hospital inpatient pain service consists of admitting patients, on Dr. Crue's neurosurgical service, to either Community Hospital or Mercy Hospital here in Durango for specific evaluation, drug detoxification, or perhaps surgical intervention (if, indeed, a neurosurgical pain-relieving procedure is indicated). Patients with cancer pain are often admitted for inpatient therapy and pain-relieving neurosurgical procedures. This part of the pain center therapy must not be confused with the outpatient pain rehabilitation unit in the team model that makes up the part of the pain center program that is under consideration here, and for which reason you have been given this brochure to study.

The initial pain clinic serves the following functions: outpatient diagnosis, treatment and further referral. Any person who is referred to the pain center is first evaluated by the medical director in an outpatient clinic setting. After the outpatient diagnostic procedures and evaluations are concluded, it is then determined if the patient should be accepted for further care in the pain center and referral to the structured outpatient pain rehabilitation unit for team therapy as indicated in this introductory brochure. This brochure is designed to describe the outpatient pain unit (or structured pain team chronic pain rehabilitation program here at the pain center).

This portion of the pain center is for the treatment of persons with intractable non-cancer pain problems; that is, ongoing and severe pain disorders. The program is organized to treat patients with pain problems for which further standard medical treatment (for example, surgery or more analgesic or narcotic medications) is not recommended. Patients in this program must be ambulatory, capable of self-care, and not in need of hospitalization. This is an outpatient program. If the patient comes from a distance so far removed from the pain treatment center here in Durango that they cannot stay at home, and either travel safely or conveniently drive here and back each day, facilities are provided for the patients and their families, either to stay in a nearby motel in Durango, or in the pain center rehabilitation rooms as available at the La Plata Community Hospital.

## IV. INTRACTABLE PAIN: ITS NATURE AND TREATMENT

Pain is always an individual and private experience. While there are still many unanswered questions regarding the exact neurophysiological mechanisms and processes that are involved in the perception of pain, it is known that it is an experience that takes place within the central nervous system; that is, within the brain or spinal cord. Because of this, most of the effective procedures for control of pain result in changes in central nervous system processes. In the past, these changes have most frequently been accomplished through various surgical procedures, or by the use of medications. It is now known, however, that there are many other ways to effectively alter central nervous system events. The treatment program of the outpatient pain unit of the Durango Pain Rehabilitation Center has been developed and organized to bring about a beginning of certain central nervous system changes, so that the pain experience can favorably be altered. The specific procedures which are utilized to help these changes occur will be described in this brochure.

Before proceeding, however, it should be pointed out that, while the presence of chronic and intractable pain (that is, continuing pain which has not responded favorably to standard medical treatment) is not a medical emergency, it is a complicated problem that results in immense human suffering. Its treatment is time-consuming, complex, and expensive. Successful resolution of the problem requires an extraordinary degree of effort, cooperation and involvement by both patient and family. It is desirable, therefore, that each potential outpatient pain unit patient be fully aware of the procedures and requirements of the program. We urge you to read and study this information carefully, so that you will be prepared to commit yourself fully to the program, if it is determined that our treatment program is appropriate for you. It should be noted that receipt of these descriptive materials does not mean that you have been finally accepted at (or that you have finally accepted) the pain treatment program. Rather, this information is only to inform you of the various aspects and goals of the outpatient pain program offered. If our treatment program is appropriate for your pain problem, this will be determined only after your full consultation with, and evaluation by, various members of the pain center team.

## V. GENERAL FOCUS AND GOALS OF THE OUTPATIENT PAIN PROGRAM

This treatment program focuses on both the ongoing pain and on the many disruptive and undesirable effects it has on people's lives. Admission to this program requires that you agree to participate fully in all parts of the treatment program. Once you have been accepted into the program, it is not the patient's prerogative to decline any specific portion of the program. Failure to fully cooperate with the pain team staff may, on occasion, lead to the prompt dismissal of the the patient with chronic pain from the treatment program. However, it is hoped that all of the pain team staff members will be able to offer explanations and advice so that the individual patient with chronic pain will understand and accept all of the individual modalities offered within the treatment program. It should be recorded that each patient has the right to leave the program at any time, although it will usually then be "against medical advice."

A fundamental aim of the treatment program is to enable each individual to return to normal and meaningful daily functioning. It has been found that chronic pain almost always results in a steady decrease in those activities, interests and concerns which are essential to the normal process of healthy, happy living. And, when these processes are disrupted, the result is usually a feeling of despair and uselessness. This further complicates and intensifies the pain experience.

Another goal of the outpatient pain treatment program is to increase the individual's ability to enjoy life, even if there is some continuing pain. For example, individuals may experience some degree of their chronic pain after successful completion of the treatment program. Many of our patients have found that it has not been necessary for pain to be entirely absent in order for them to derive increased meaning, satisfaction and enjoyment from life. However, what usually occurs is that the pain is perceived as both less constant and less severe. Almost always, these changes are substantial; and, they often result in a significant overall improvement in the quality of the individual patient's life.

## VI. TREATMENT PROCEDURES

Improvement in your pain experience will primarily be your own responsibility. This is stated, not because the staff wants to inform you ahead of time that it will not accept responsibility for your involvement in the program, but it is a fact that the staff just cannot do so. If the physicians or other staff members knew how to "fix you" (in what we refer to as the acute pain medical model)(with continued nociceptive or pain inpulse input into your central nervous system) then they, or someone else, would have long since done so, before the necessity for admitting you to such a pain treatment program as you now face. However, this new program you are being offered will be shared with you by many full time members of the pain center treatment team, whose responsibility it is to provide specialized treatment, as well as general support, and to guide and facilitate your own individual efforts as the pain patient. The program is designed to provide you with treatment, information, experience and opportunities that will enable you to begin the process of changing your own pain experience.

## 1. MEDICAL TREATMENT

Admission to the outpatient pain program means that further major reliance on standard medical or surgical procedures for control of your particular chronic pain is no longer advisable. However, the medical coverage provided in our program is ongoing, and is regarded as an actual part of the treatment process. Each patient receives a complete medical examination by one of the pain center physicians prior to being referred to the program, and is under the direct medical care of this attending physician, either a neurosurgeon or neurologist, while the patient is in the outpatient program. The purpose of this medical supervision is to make certain that no unknown health problems or appropriate standard medical treatment methods for the pain have been overlooked, as well as to allow the patients to settle any unanswered personal uncertainties about their pain problem and how it relates to their overall state of health.

It must be pointed out, however, that this is an outpatient program, and that the patients remain responsible for their own and their families health, whether at home, in the rooms provided within the Community Hospital, or in the motel available here in Durango near the pain center. This means that if the patients, for example, are taking their own heart medicines, thyroid medications, hormones, or other type of medications that are not directly related to the pain problem, they are expected to continue these on their own, and not through the staff at the pain center. Further, while we have a nurse and physician available almost all of the time for true emergencies of the patients with chronic pain undergoing therapy in our program, it is not the responsibility of the pain team staff to treat such problems as intercurrent respiratory infections, urine infections, dermatitis reactions, etc., etc. This treatment can be rendered or continued by the patient's own individual family or referring physician; or, if truly an intercurrent emergency, medical care is available through either the Emergency Room at La Plata Community Hospital or at Mercy Medical Center here in Durango.

## 2. MEDICATIONS

Medications frequently have become a problem for the individual who has an intractable pain problem. Not only do medications almost always fail to adequately relieve chronic pain, but they also often result in some or all of the following unwanted side effects: lethargy or tiredness, slurred speech, difficulty in thinking quickly and effectively, poor communication with others, changes in sexual functioning, problems in remembering, occasional confusion and disorientation, and "not feeling like oneself." In addition, pain medication may result in drug dependency and all of its attendant difficulties. There is also evidence that, for some patients, prolonged use of some pain medications actually may cause continued, or increased pain or discomfort.

Any individual who is admitted to the outpatient pain unit has had pain for a long time and has probably used many different kinds and combinations of medications in search for pain relief. Because medications are rarely effective in the control of chronic pain, and because prolonged medication use almost always creates many and serious difficulties for the individual who suffers from intractable pain, medication management and education is a basic part of the outpatient pain treatment program. A description of this aspect of the program follows.

*A. It is medically important for the patient to be truthful and accurate about reporting to the attending physician and pain program pharmacist the amount of all medications used prior to admission.*

*B. All medications that are used for pain relief, as well as all antidepressants, antianxiety tranquilizers, sleeping medications, muscle relaxants and anticonvulsants, are reconstitued in our pharmacy and given in the form of 4 capsules at 4 designated times a day; ususally 9 a.m., noon, 5 p.m., and bedtime. Those patients who have not used any of the above medications recently will still receive 4 capsules 4 times each day. No experimental or dangerous medications (or medications to which the patient by history has been allergic in the past) will be utilized. It is expected that all patients will demonstrate  trust in the pain center staff and take these "single blind" medications.*

*C. Other kinds of medications such as hormones, vitamins, etc., will be taken by the patients from their own supplies in the same way that they were used at home.*

*D. The amount of each medication in the special capsules described above will be changed by the attending physician without consulting the patient. This is called the "single blind" method of medication. These changes will take place without harm or serious discomfort to the patient, as far as is humanly possible. Specifically, we will see to it that as the medications are decreased there will be  no withdrawl symptoms of any severity.*

*E. All patients receive medications in this manner, even though the amount and type of medications contained in each capsule is different for each patient. This is done so that comparisons, along with discussions and anxiety that would accompany them, do not need to occur. We have found this procedure for giving medications is helpful to patients with chronic pain.*

*F. Medications are to be given only four specific times during the day at approximately 9 a.m., 12 p.m., 5 p.m., and again at bedtime. Patients will be taking capsules at the four specific times, and will be on their own concerning other medications for other medical problems. All medications must be made known, however, to both the physician and the pharmacist within the pain program. The patients will be given individually labeled packets of capsules to be taken when they are not actually on the pain center premises in the evenings, or, for example, on holidays or weekends. Patients must not take any other pain or sleep medications on their own.*

*Experience has shown that dispensing medications in an unidentified form (that is, in a plain capsule in which the type of medication and dosage level is not known to the patient) and at specified times only (rather than in direct response to the complaint of pain) makes the medication change process relatively easy for the patient. Furthermore, this procedure has the effect of diminishing the association between pain and medication, thereby making it less likely that problems with medication for pain will resume after discharge. Therefore, no medications for chronic pain problem will be given on any other schedule than that stated above. The patients must not take any of the included pain treatment medication on their own schedule. They must also agree not to use any medications available from other sources, such as prior physicians, but instead should report any increase in their pain severity to one of the pain team staff members so that appropriate changes can be made in the single blind medications by the physician and pharmacist.*

*Prior to discharge, you will be told exactly what medications you have been taking, and when any changes in your medications scheduled actually took place.*

### 3. GROUP PSYCHOTHERAPY

The major emphasis on the outpatient pain program is on medical psychology, because ongoing and intractable pain is almost always related to an individual's way of psychological functioning. That is, it has been found that there are significant emotional factors involved in all patients with chronic pain. Furthermore, the ever present stress that accompanies severe and chronic problems of any sort, including pain, almost always result in related psychologically based difficulties such as depression, anxiety, feelings of inadequacy, unsatisfactory sexual functioning, and a multitude of family and interpersonal problems. These difficulties often become major features in an individual's pain experience, and they frequently complicate and interfere with a resolution of the pain problem itself.

Group psychotherapy with other patients who suffer with pain has been found to be the most effective way of working with the psychological aspects of chronic and intractable pain. The sharing of life experiences and personal outlooks among people who have pain and suffering as a prominent feature of their lives is of major importance. When this is done in a manner that brings more understanding to this life process, it becomes a valuable way to begin to make constructive life changes which often result in less pain and suffering.

It should be noted that psychotherapy of any sort requires a very special kind of effort and commitment on the part of the patient. This means that one must be willing to engage in discussions and experiences that highlight the needs, motivations and conflicts which influence the way a patient thinks, feels and behaves. It is not unusual for an individual to experience some anxiety and increased pain during the course of initial psychotherapy. This discomfort, of course, decreases as the problems are resolved. We mention the fact that temporary discomfort may occur during the course of psychotherapy, in order to help you evaluate your own willingness to engage in such an effort.

All patients with pain under such a treatment program must agree to respect the confidentiality of the other patients with chronic pain. Our experience has shown that those individuals who are willing and fully able to participate in the group psychotherapy increase their chance to change their pain experience for the better. We look forward to your joining us in this mutual effort.

## 4. INDIVIDUAL PSYCHOTHERAPY

Each patient will receive some individual psychotherapy during the program; and, in addition, each patient may request an individual therapy session from any therapist member of the pain team. The frequency and duration of these sessions are determined on the basis of individual needs after evaluation of each patient with chronic pain. This scheduling should be arranged through the secretary of the pain program. They may also be scheduled by talking to your case manager, Jason Vance.

## 5. COUPLES GROUP PSYCHOTHERAPY

These therapy sessions are held for the purpose of including and opening meaningful exchanges between the patients and the significant other people in their lives. Strains in relationships almost always exist when there has been a continuing pain problem - both for the patient and for the family and/or close friends. These sessions have the potential for increasing understanding about how to make changes which will lead to a better quality of life. Also, as changes in the pain experience occur for the patient, all those involved must learn to adapt to these changes. In other words, improvement in the pain for the patient, believe it or not, may often be a threat to other members in the patient's family. In these sessions, patients and their other significant people meet as one group.

## 6. CONJOINT PSYCHOTHERAPY AND FAMILY THERAPY

Individual therapy sessions with the individual patient and their spouse or closest significant other may be requested by either the therapist or the patient. These meetings are held to help identify and clarify specific problems in the relationships and to suggest directions to take for their resolution. Prior to the patient requesting a therapy session, the patient should discuss the request with the other person involved, who, of course, must agree to the appointment. However, it is expected that the pain patient's family members will cooperate, when so requested by the staff. Failure to arrange for such family cooperation may result in the patient's discharge from the program.

Family therapy is often recommended when it is believed necesary or desireable for other members of the family unit to join in the session with the patient and his or her significant other. Staff members are always willing to help explain to other family members why they should make the effort often required to attend such family sessions.

## 7. BIOFEEDBACK

This is a relatively old, but only recently widely utilized, technique to try to alleviate chronic and intractable pain. It is a procedure by which an individual attempts to learn methods for controlling or altering certain bodily or physiological states (for example, electrical activity from tension in the muscles; or, temperature of the skin). The clinical importance of this is that it has been found that regulations of certain of these bodily functions can be accompanied by a reduction in pain in certain patients.

**8.    RELAXATION THERAPY; IMAGERY; AUTOGENIC TRAINING; AND, PROGRESSIVE MUSCULAR RELAXATION**

Medical evidence indicates that both the duration and severity of pain can be related to levels of skeletal muscle tension. Specifically, it has been found that even chronic pain can be more prolonged and made more severe by feeling states that are accompanied by increased tension and/or anxiety. Patients are taught to recognize generalized muscle tension, as well as tension in specific muscle groups. This learned skill can often be helpful in maintaining a state of decreased pain.

**9. PHYSICAL THERAPY; EXERCISE AND MOVEMENT THERAPY**

This treatment involves training and teaching of various body movement routines and exercise to facilitate general physical rehabilitation. It is an essential part of the program. Originally the evaluation by our registered physical therapist affiliated with the pain program will help in the evaluation and the establishment of the exercise needs of the individual patient with chronic pain. Most of the treatment within the program, however, is under the direction of our exercise and movement therapists, as well as a number of sessions for pool therapy and "Flugeling." Although most of the physical therapy takes place in a group, an individual program is designed for the specific needs for each patient, including a take home program at the end of the treatment period. We discuss openly with each patient any concerns about the potential risks from activities in the recommended physical therapy or exercise regime. Often patients are urged to participate in exercises that they may well have in the past been told by others, including previous treating physicians, that they probably should never do. This will be discussed with each patient in an open manner when such problems arise.

**10. OCCUPATIONAL THERAPY; RECREATIONAL THERAPY; AND, VOCATIONAL REHAB COUNSELING.**

Patients often need to extend their skills in various hobby and leisure activities, so that they can be productive as well as pleasurable. Oftentimes instruction in proper pacing, time management and body mechanics is a necessity. This is necessary for the program for the reduction of the pain experience. It is also appropriate that any occupational therapy should coordinate with the individual's vocational training and needs. Vocational rehab counseling will be provided for the individual patient with pain, when necessary to help plan for his ongoing life, including his future work plans and individual requirements.

**11. NUTRITION**

Many patients with chronic pain have poor diets. Often chronic pain patients are overweight; and, occasionally, undernourished. Nutritional instruction is given by Pat Blair. During lunch, the patients gain practice in food preparation, and further their interpersonal reactions under the supervision of the nutritionist and/or occupational therapist.

## 12. PHARMACEUTICAL INSTRUCTION

The attending physician assesses and records all pertinent data concerning preadmission medication. However, the outpatient pain unit pharmacist also interviews the patient and gets a drug history, and doublechecks on possible allergies before he compounds and packages all the daily medications given out in capsule form. In addition, the pharmacist will meet regularly with the patients to provide information about their medications, and medications in general, which are commonly used to attempt to control chronic intractable pain. While peripherally acting analgesics and centrally acting narcotics often help in acute or cancer pain, they usually do not, and often make symptoms worse, in chronic pain. The point will be stressed that if medication were a satisfactory answer, the patient with chronic pain would not need to be in this program. It must also be remembered that neither the pharmacist or the physician will indicate to the individual patient prior to the conclusion of the program exactly what medications (and what dosage) are in the four capsules given out four times a day.

## 13. DISCHARGE PLANNING

Plans for return to a desired level of activity begin at the start of the pain treatment program and continue throughout the course of treatment. Each patient has the opportunity to discuss individual social and vocational needs with any of the team members, as well as in group therapy. At time of discharge, appropriate referrals are provided to provide private or community agencies, depending on the patient's individual situation. These may include recommendations for further ongoing and continuing outpatient physical therapy, psychotherapy, marital counseling, etc., at other locations nearer home, or continued at the Durango Pain Rehabilitation Center in our "continuing care" program.

## VII. SOME SPECIFICS CONCERNING THE PROGRAM AND ITS ORGANIZATION

## 1. ADMISSION

As you begin your first week of active treatment in the outpatient pain program, your more general medical evaluation will be completed, and you will be medically cleared for full participation. You will be given a schedule of appointments and group activities, and this will continue to be modified weekly as necessary. It must be understood prior to your admission that attendance at scheduled activities is mandatory, and not optional, for any individual patient in the program. The usual length of stay is for four weeks, and begins, in general, on a Monday morning, and ends on a Friday afternoon of the last week. Occasionally a patient will have special needs which necessitates a somewhat longer stay or a shorter stay. Occasionally a patient may be admitted on a day other than Monday, and a patient may go home in the middle of the week, especially if they have had emergencies or intercurrent illnesses, so that they have missed time in the program; and, their usual four week authorized program may thus end on a day other than Friday (after the "make up" days).

## 2. LODGING

An important part of the program is the support, encouragement and group feeling that develops among the patients. We wish that all patients, even in the outpatient setting, could room together, spend their eveinings and weekends together, etc. For practical purposes, this is not ususally possible. But, for this reason, persons admitted to the program are, in general, lodged together in a motel close to the pain center, as well as close to recreational facilities, the City Market, etc. Pool exercises take place under a contract arrangement with a motel in the area, as at the present time the rehabilitation department at La Plata Community Hospital does not have available its own pool on campus. Breakfast and dinner are the patient's own responsibility to obtain before and after attending the outpatient program. For some specific patients (for example, on therapy under worker's comp rules and regulations) the motel as well as the meals will be provided, or the charges reimbursed. This should be discussed with the pain clinic administrator prior to admission.

The individual patient will be presented to the weekly 8 a.m. Thursday treatment staff meeting on the first week in the program, so that the patient may ask questions about what lies ahead; and, again on the Thursday before discharge, so that the staff may find out from the patient ideas concerning the program; and, to ascertain the patient's input concerning ongoing treatment after discharge, before the patient's treatment team makes its final recommendations. Following discharge, the responsibility for medical care is usually transferred back to the patient and their own family or referring physician. On occasion, by mutual agreement of all those involved, the patient may wish to continue under the outpatient medical supervision of the pain center neurosurgeons or neurologists. This will be arranged, with the concurrence of the entire treating team; and, of course with the agreement of the patient and his referring physician.

### 3. GENERAL PROCEDURES
*Dress:*
Street clothes are worn for all scheduled program activities. All patients, male and female, are requested to bring clothing appropriate for the season and the physical therapy program, and for outings to include arranged scheduled pool therapy sessions. Specifically, this often means shorts, sweatpants, slacks, comfortable walking and exercising footwear, etc. You will also need a bathing suit for the exercises in the pool.

*Meals:*
Morning and evening meals will be at the motel, or at adjacent restaurants. Lunch will be at the pain center, and will be part of your nutrition counseling supervised by the nutritionist.

*Medications:*
Medications will be issued to you on a daily basis for the four times, as stated before, by the pain unit secretary after they have been delivered daily from the pharmacist. Be prepared to use your own medications for the first few days in the program, so as to give the physicians and pharmacist time to initiate the program of single blind four times a day/four capsule routine, which usually takes one to two days to arrange. All medications will be individually containerized and appropriately labeled with name, date, day and hour, with appropriate labeled instructions.

*Visitors:*
You will be too busy with activities to entertain visitors during the treatment day, but they are certainly welcome to visit you at the motel in the evenings, on weekends, or when your schedule is occasionally open. Furthermore, family members are encouraged, when practical, to stay with the patient in the motel when the pain patient is from out of town.

*Self Care:*
Since you will be staying in a motel rather then a hospital as an inpatient, you will be expected to be independent regarding your own personal care. Opportunities will be made for you to do laundry, go shopping, etc.

## VIII. CRITERIA FOR ADMISSION

The following critieria for admission are being recorded, so that the patient will know, many times for the first time, the standards to which he has been subject, prior to the recommendation for admission. These following criteria have been carefully derived from the experience that has been gained through working with people who suffer with the problem of chronic intractable pain. They have been adopted as prerequisites for admission, because they have been shown to have a significant effect on the outcome of treatment.

### 1. PRE-ADMISSION EVALUATION PHASE
The first requirement for admission is that each prospective patient and his or her spouse or significant other complete the preadmission evaluation as required.

A. Interviews and evaluations will be scheduled by, and with, the pain team members. You will be contacted by phone or mail concerning specific times and dates.

B. The evaluation of all your medications currently being taken, as well as those in the past, will be obtained, and you will discuss this with either the pain treatment physician or the pharmacist, either before or at admission. Please bring all medications with you and report your daily intake of each accurately.

C. During this preadmission evaluation, you will be asked to fill out standard pencil and paper psychological questionnaires, which may take several hours to complete. These are the most widely used tests of their kind and are a routine part of your evaluation. Additional questionnaires will be given to you and your spouse during the first part of the program. Finally, you will be asked to complete some test questionnaires during the last phase of your treatment. If you need reading glasses, etc., please bring them with you for all appointments. Many of our patients within the pain program have Spanish as their native language, and English as a second language. Although familiarity and ability to converse in English is a necessary prerequisite for inclusion in the treatment program, the Durango Pain Rehabilitation Center is fortunate in having one of its therapists, John Baca, who is fluent bilingually in Spanish and English; and, we are thus able to take patients whom otherwise would have been excluded from the program.

D. The final part of the preadmission evaluation is your interview with the patient case manager, who is Jason Vance. Jason Vance will be your spokesman while you are within the program, and as the patient case manager, will also ascertain that the proper testing has been done, that the medical work-up has been completed, that the pharmacy interview will be carried out as promised, etc. If you have any problems within the program, either notify promptly Jason Vance or the pain center secretary, Carol Caruso or Gayle Ann Williams.

### 2. AMBULATION
All patients who are admitted to the outpatient program must be ambulatory; that is, they must be able to move about without wheelchair or walker, although many patients are accepted who initially start out using a cane, wearing braces, etc.

### 3. MEDICATIONS
All patients who are admitted to the pain unit must accept having their medications regulated in the manner described. Any use of alcohol or medicines not known and approved by the pain center physician may not only be injurious, but be a sufficient reason for discharge from the treatment program.

## 4. PARTICIPATION IN THE TREATMENT PROGRAM

Again, it must be pointed out, so there can be no mistake about this, that all patients admitted to the pain unit must agree to participate fully in all aspects of the program. The patient may not select which treatment modalities he will or will not choose to attend. The patient will not be asked to participate in any activity that we could possibly anticipate to be medically harmful.

## 5. FAMILY INVOLVEMENT

Spouses of married patients admitted to the pain unit are expected to participate in the program. It may also be necessary to arrange for other family members (children, parents, siblings, etc.) to come to the clinic for Family Therapy, when so recommended by the therapists.

## 6. AUTOBIOGRAPHICAL DATA

All pain unit patients will be requested to write an autobiographical record of all their significant life events. This is a personal life history; it does not need to include the medical history, which will be reviewed separately. Please write it in any style that is comfortable for you, and bring it in with you when you are admitted to the program.

## 7. FOLLOW-UP REQUIREMENT

All pain patients are asked to agree to cooperate fully with follow-up assessment requirements. These assessments will occur after discharge, and will span at least a five year period of time.

## 8. MOTIVATION FOR SELF-EXAMINATION

This final admission criteria is the most difficult to describe, yet it is probably the most important. To benefit adequately from the treatment program, all patients need to be willing to examine and deal with the possible psychological aspects of their intractable pain disorder. These parts of the ongoing pain process are often difficult to recognize, and dealing with them may be extremely difficult for any patient. Despite the discomfort that may accompany this aspect of treatment, it has shown itself repeatedly to be the most basic and significant dimension of the pain unit program. All individuals seriously considering admission to the program should carefully think over their willingness and ability to participate in this aspect of treatment. The program will be of greatest benefit to you when you come to realize that continuing chronic pain is strongly related to psychological and emotional experiences and processes.

In conclusion, it should be re-emphasized that the fundamental goal of the pain treatment program is to assist individuals to produce a favorable change in their chronic pain experience. The program aims at relieving the pain itself, as well as assisting each patient to derive increased satisfaction and meaning from life, whether or not there is still some residual remaining pain. The program is a demanding one, and we deeply appreciate and fully understand the discomfort that it may temporarily bring. Many patients hurt more at the end of their first week in the program than they do on admission! This shoud be known ahead of time. We know, however, that those individuals who actively participate in the program can expect to derive significant benefit from it. The entire pain treatment staff wants to help each individual to reach his or her treatment goals. We sincerely hope that we will have an opportunity to work with you.

## FINAL NOTES

If you are admitted to the pain program, please bring the following items, in addition to the clothing and the personal articles with you on the day of admission:

1. This pamphlet, so you may refer to it for questions that may arise once you begin the program. It also includes your individual treatment contract that you will be asked to sign.

2. Your written or typed autobiography.

3. All medications which you are currently taking. These will be kept in the pain center pharmacy, unless they are returned to you to take yourself, while living in your motel room or at home.

4. Your swimming suit.

We wish you well. If it is decided by you and by us that together this program offers potential help for you, we will enthusiastically work together with you, so that you may discover for yourself a way out of your life of pain and suffering.

**AUTHORIZATION AND RELEASE FOR TELEVISION, STILL PHOTOGRAPHS, VIDEOTAPED RE-
CORDINGS AND WRITTEN RESEARCH REPORTS**

To the pain center physicians; to the administrator, agents and employees of the Durango Pain
Rehabilitation Center; and to their licensees, assigns and successors:

In order to assist in the furtherance of knowledge and understanding of the health sciences by use of
communication media, the undersigned, a patient, student, or employee at the above-named institution, or the
authorized legel representative of such a patient, student, or employee, does hereby authorize and consent to the
use of the image, voice, psychological data, name and biography of said patient, student, or employee and, both
personally and on behalf of the heirs, representatives and successors of said patient, title and interest in any tape,
film, recording or written document produced, and does hereby agree to hold the above-named organization and
persons harmless from any and all liability whether known or unknown arising out of the use of such tapes, films,
recordings or written documents.

With the duly signed approval of the Director of the Pain Center, it is specifically understood that the
above-named organization and entities may use the said voice, image, name, biography, or psychological data
on tapes, films or recordings in connection with any professional or research activities of such organizations and
may use, copy, edit, alter, and revise said media for telecasts, films or recordings in connection with any
*educational, scientific, or informational* purpose whatsoever, except for commercially sponsored uses. Any
patient, student, or employee is free to withdraw this consent for authorization and release at any time. Such
a retraction will have a retroactive effect so that it will include any material not released before this retraction
is officially made by the undersigned.

In the accumulation and disposition of the material herein stated, the subject's privacy will be protected
at all times.

I hereby give my consent to participation in this study, with the understanding that by so doing I am
affording the Pain Research Team an opportunity to obtain a better understanding of pain mechanics in me and
other patients. I understand that I may choose not to participate in this without in any way interfering with my
treatment.


Patient_____     Date_____


_____     Date_____
Pain Center Administrator

## CONTRACT

This is a contract between _____ , called the patient, and the Durango Pain Rehabilitation Center (D.P.R.C.).

Read this agreement carefully and sign it at the bottom of the page to show that you have read and understand this agreement.

If you have any questions about this agreement, please discuss it with the Pain Center Administrator, Pat Blair.

The D.P.R.C. agrees to provide you with the following:
1. A variety of forms of training in pain mangement which are designed to help you learn to reduce and/ or better cope with your pain problem. (We do not claim that you will always be able to totally eliminate your pain.)
2. A program based on the sound principles of self-responsibility.
3. A program that is individually tailored to your needs at the time.
4. Access to 24 hour medical coverage through the La Plata Community Hospital.
5. The right to refuse any therapy. (However, if we feel that we are unable to provide you with adequate assistance because of the omitted component(s), we may choose to discontinue your program as explained previously in the brochure.)
6. The opportunity to discuss with your personal case manager any complaints or problems you may have with the staff; or, if not resolvable there, with the Pain Center Administrator or Medical Director.

In return, you agree to each of the following:
1. That you will attend the full program.
2. That you will attend each of the therapy sessions scheduled for you and give each of the therapies a fair chance.
3. That you will be punctual in attendance regardless of your pain level at the time. (Unless stated otherwise by your physician, the pain center is the best place for you to be when you are in pain.)
4. That you will abide by the regulations concerning your medications and abstain from the use of alcohol while in the program.
5. That you will speak with your case manager as soon as possible if you have any problem with the staff or program.
6. That you will not smoke in the center.
7. That you will respect the privacy of all other patients participating at the center, and under no circumstance will you discuss the names nor any specifics relating to the patients outside this center.
8. That you will participate in the continuing care program as recommended by the therapeutic staff.
9. That you will participate in the full research follow-up component of our program, which consists of approximately three return visits or reports during the five year period following your four week session at the center.


Patient_____     Date_____


Pain Center Administrator_____     Date_____

**PATIENT RIGHTS POLICY**
We recognize the basic right of a human being to maintain independence of expression, decision, and action, and to be treated with dignity.  The following are considered the basic rights and responsibilities of our patients.

1. ACCESS TO CARE
   You have a right to treatment and services that are available and medically indicated regardless of race, creed, sex, religion, and/or national origin.

   You have the responsibility to provide accurate and complete information about your name, address, insurance coverage, employer and other admitting information. Be sure you understand anything you sign. Ask questions if you are not sure.

2. RESPECT AND DIGNITY
   You have the right to considerate and respectful treatment at all times.

   You have the responsiblity to be courteous and cooperative with center staff.  Consideration must be given to other patients and their property.  Rules regarding smoking must be followed.

3. PRIVACY AND CONFIDENTIALITY
   You have the right to have all physical exams, interviews, and discussions to take place privately except for scheduled group or family sessions.  You have the right to have privileged communications and records regarding your health care be handled confidentially.  All medical records related to medical or health care will be handled in accordance with the center's policies and procedures.  No information related to your medical record will be released unless authorized by  you.  You should know that in work injury related chronic pain that the compensation carrier requires copies of all records.  You have the responsibility to be discreet when discussing your health care with anyone other than those responsible for your care.

4. INFORMATION RIGHTS
   You have the right to know the identity and status of individuals providing you service.  You have the right to know which physician is primarily responsible for your care while you are at the clinic.  You have the right to complete and current information regarding your diagnosis, prognosis, and treatment plan in terms you can reasonably expect to understand.

   You have the responsibility to understand what you are told about your present symptoms and the treatment proposed.  You are expected to provide the physician with **ALL** medical information, including any treatments and medications by other physicians.  You have the responsibility to ask questions about anything regarding your stay at the center and treatment you do not understand.

5. PARTICIPATION IN DECISIONS
   You have the right to consent to or refuse any or all tests or treatments, although such refusal may mean dismissal from the pain treatment program.  You have the right to ask for another physician's opinion and to request discharge at any time under most conditions.  You have the right to be provided with information regarding research, experimental, or educational projects that are related to your care.

You have the responsibility to cooperate and follow instructions in any test or treatments, either routine or experimental, to which you consent. You are responsible for your actions if you refuse treatment or leave the center against medical advice.

6. MEDICAL RECORD

You have the responsibility to make arrangements according to the center's policies and procedures for review of your medical record.

7. PAYMENT OF BILLS

You have the right to an itemized and detailed explanation of your total bill, regardless of the source of payment. You have the right to timely notice prior to termination of your eligibility for reimbursement by any third party payer for the cost of your care.

You are responsible for paying your bill within the time limit specified by the center. Arrangements should be made with the business office regarding insurance coverage, payment plans, etc. You are responsible for questioning your bill within the time limit set by the business office.

8. PROBLEMS

You have the right to discuss any problems and complaints with your case manager. The case manager will assist you in resolving complaints and following through with your suggestions or questions.

You are responsible for making grievances known as soon as possible so that they may be handled quickly and correctly.


Patient_____ Date _____


Pain Center Administrator_____ Date_____

# TREATMENT OF SELECTED DISORDERS

## *17*

# EMERGENCY MANAGEMENT OF STABLE AND UNSTABLE INJURIES

*Kim J. Burchiel*

Trauma is a major health and social problem that typically affects young individuals. The estimated cost for death, disability, and loss of productivity probably exceeds $284 million a day (1). Acute spine and spinal cord injuries are among the most common causes of severe disability and death following trauma. Spinal column trauma occurs at a rate of approximately 5 per 100,000 population. Of the roughly 5000 new cases of spinal cord injury occurring in the United States each year, 10% (or about 500) will result in the genesis of a quadriplegic patient (2). Unfortunately, the diagnosis of spinal injuries is often delayed, and the treatment is frequently unstandardized or inadequate, producing increasing problems with rehabilitation of the patient.

In this chapter I discuss some of the mechanisms, anatomy, and treatment of cervical spine injury. The acute care of these patients involves the combined expertise of emergency physicians, neurosurgeons, orthopaedic surgeons, urologists, physiatrists, specialized nurses, and others. This text is primarily directed to health care professionals who deal with chronic cervical pain of traumatic origin. Therefore, my purpose here is to provide an overview of some of the diagnostic and management principles that are relevant to the acute care of these patients. If necessary, more detailed descriptions of procedures can be accessed through other more detailed reviews of the subject (3–5).

## EPIDEMIOLOGY OF NECK INJURY

Most cervical spine injuries occur in the 15- to 30-year-old age range. Males outnumber females by a 3:1 ratio. At least 50% of these injuries result from vehicular accidents. Of the remainder, diving injuries are common in younger patients whereas falls account for the majority of injuries in older patients. Other causes include trauma from water sports (surfing, water skiing), snow skiing, and penetrating injuries such as gunshot wounds.

There is a spectrum of injury from simple myofascial strain, or "whiplash" injuries, to severe injuries resulting in fracture and dislocation of the spinal column caused by hyperflexion, hyperextension, and axial loading. The evolution of an injury is largely dependent on the baseline condition of the patient's cervical spine, the mechanism of injury, and the energy imparted to the head, neck, and associated structures at the time of the accident. More minor injuries typically result in stretching or tearing of the muscles and ligaments of the neck, and little or no bony injury. This type of injury will be discussed in detail in Chapter 19, and is not dealt with further here. The remainder of this chapter deals with the more serious end of the cervical spine injury continuum. However, lest the reader become complacent, the differentiation of minor from more serious injuries is often very difficult in the acute setting. In fact, in some instances as many as one third of patients

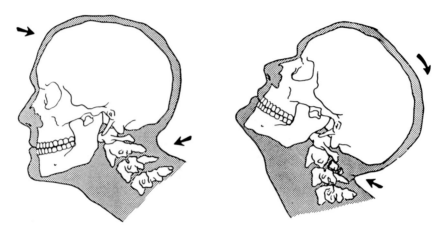

**Figure 17.1.** Forces involved in hyperextension injury of the neck. (From Yashon D: *Spinal Injury.* New York, Appleton-Century-Crofts, 1978.)

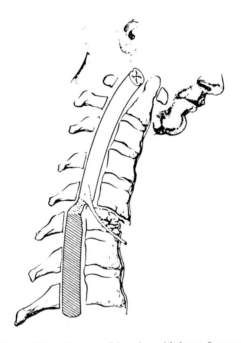

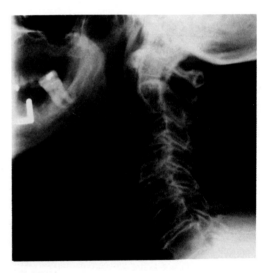

**Figure 17.3.** Lateral cervical spine radiograph showing severe spondylosis.

**Figure 17.2.** Fracture-dislocation with burst fracture at C5–6 resulting in spinal cord compression that is due to both the anterior fracture mass and the subluxation. (From Hoppenfeld S: *Orthopaedic Neurology.* Philadelphia, JB Lippincott, 1977.)

with later proven spinal injuries were missed on initial emergency department evaluation. The message is that patients suspected of having a cervical injury should be treated with great care and circumspection.

Approximately 80% of cervical spine injuries occur when the accelerating head strikes a stationary object. Sites of trauma, such as facial lacera-

tions, contusions, and facial fractures, give evidence of the energy imparted and the force vector of the injury. An acceleration extension mechanism accounts for most of the other cervical spinal injuries (6) (Fig. 17.1).

Approximately 60% of cervical spine injuries occur at the C5 and C6 segments, 30% at C4 and C7, and 10% above C4. These forces typically produce a fracture of the vertebral body, as well as disruption of the lateral and posterior elements. If any compromise of the spinal canal occurs it is usually anterior, although posterior compression can occur (Fig. 17.2). In patients with spinal cord injuries, fractures without dislocation occur in 15% of cases related to axial loading of the spine, but occur in only 5% of injuries from hyperexten-sion, hyperflexion, or rotational forces. In 10–15% of cervical injuries associated with spinal cord damage, no detectable fracture or disloca-tion can be found. This often occurs in elderly pa-tients with severe spondylosis and acquired cervi-cal spinal stenosis (Fig. 17.3; see also Fig. 17.5), typically from a hyperextension mechanism.

About 50% of patients with demonstrable cer-vical spine traumatic fracture-dislocation will have complete loss of motor and sensory function below the level of injury. Preservation of minimal function caudad to the injury can be demon-strated in approximately one third, leaving about 15–20% with useful sensory or motor function distal to the lesion. Thus, a reliable screening neu-rologic examination is critical in the early stages of the assessment of a patient with significant cervi-cal trauma.

## PATIENT EVALUATION

One of the most important messages of this chap-ter is that any patient who experiences trauma above the shoulders is at risk of sustaining a cer-vical spine injury (Fig. 17.4). Patients with an al-tered level of consciousness either from head in-jury or alcohol often cannot be adequately examined, and thus should be treated as if a cer-vical spinal injury is present until this is disproved by radiologic techniques (see below) and clinical exam.

The index of suspicion for a cervical spine in-jury is, of course, increased by the finding of bi-lateral impairment of motor and/or sensory func-tion. Other more subtle clues include abnormal or difficult respiration, vasomotor instability, brady-cardia, hypotension, or cardiac arrythmia. These latter findings can result from interruption of ac-cessory respiratory muscle function and normal sympathetic tone.

The complaint of acute neck pain from a reli-able, responsive patient is one of the most valu-able screening methods in patients with suspected neck injury. It is unusual for a patient with signif-icant bony and or ligamentous injury to *not* have pain on palpation or active range of motion of the neck. Cervical spine fractures and severe sprains are like similar injuries elsewhere in the body: They hurt! The presence of cervical pain or ten-derness on exam should signal the higher proba-bility of a significant injury. However, by the same token patients without pain should be treated cau-tiously until fracture-dislocation is positively ruled out radiographically.

In the emergency department a complete gen-eral examination is imperative, since multisystem injury is the rule rather than the exception in pa-tients with severe trauma, particularly that due to motor vehicle accidents. Alterations in the heart rate, blood pressure, and temperature may herald the presence of spinal cord injury. As with any emergent resuscitative effort, establishment of the airway and maintenance of the respiratory and

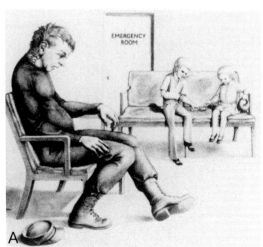 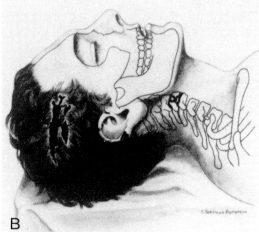

**Figure 17.4.** *A,* Patient sitting in emergency room with head and neck injury and associated lethargic level of con-sciousness. *B,* Patient in comatose level of consciousness with cervical fracture and scalp laceration. Since this patient will not complain of pain, cervical spine roentgenogram must be taken for diagnosis of neck injury. (From Bohlman JJ: The neck. In D'Ambrosia R (ed): *Musculo-skeletal Disorders.* Philadelphia, JB Lippincott, 1977.)

circulatory functions are of paramount importance. During this evaluation, specific attention should be directed to palpation of the posterior cervical spinous processes, as well as posterior and anterior cervical musculature. Tenderness in these locations is a harbinger of musculoligamentous and perhaps bony injury.

A detailed neurologic examination is also mandatory during the initial evaluation of the patient with neck injury. Neurologic assessment may occur concurrent with the general exam, but must remain a priority after initial stabilization of the patient. This exam should include detailed testing of the strength and tone of individual muscle groups in all four extremities. Strength is rated 5/5 for normal, 4/5 for movement against some resistance, 3/5 for antigravity movement only, 2/5 for nonantigravity movement only, 1/5 for contraction without movement, and 0/5 for no movement. Sensory testing should include an evaluation of pinprick or pain, light touch, proprioceptive, and vibratory sensations in all extremities. Deep tendon reflexes should be tested at the biceps, brachioradialis, triceps, knees, and ankles and recorded as absent (0/4), decreased (1/4), normal (2/4), increased (3/4), or spastic (4/4). Abdominal, cremasteric, anal wink, and Babinski reflexes should be tested and noted.

The functional anatomy of the cervical spinal cord has been reviewed in Chapter 1. To reiterate, the topographic arrangement of fibers in the corticospinal and lateral spinothalamic tracts are arranged such that the tracts destined for the most caudal segments (i.e., sacral) are located most peripherally in the spinal cord. Conversely, the cervical tracts are situated closest to the center of the cord. This general rule is true for most of the major pathways of the spinal cord, including the corticospinal, lateral spinothalamic (anterolateral system), and dorsal columns. Consequently, spinal cord injuries that produce central contusion fibers (Fig. 17.5) result in the clinical entity termed "sacral sparing," in which loss of function from cord injury is seen at and below the level of injury, with relative or even complete preservation of function in the sacral segments.

Other combinations of injury patterns in the cervical spinal cord may also be seen. Functional cord hemisection produces a picture of ipsilateral

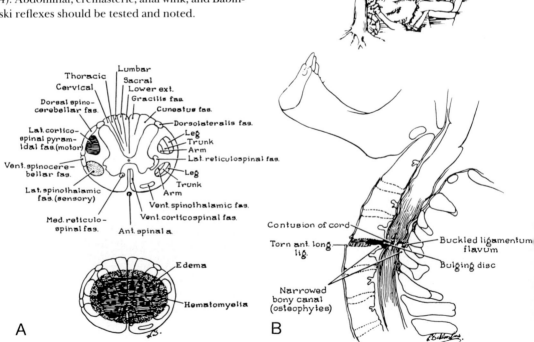

**Figure 17.5.** *A*, Schematic cross-section of cervical spinal cord showing laminations of the descending and ascending tracts, and central cord injury. *B*, Typical deceleration hyperextension mechanism of injury. Contusion of cord from hyperextension injury produced by narrowed bony canal, bulging disc, buckling of the ligamentum flavum, and ligamentous injury with minor subluxation. (From Bohlman JJ: The neck. In D'Ambrosia R (Ed): *Musculoskeletal Disorders*. Philadelphia, JB Lippincott, 1977.)

hemiplegia (corticospinal tract) and vibratory-proprioceptive loss (dorsal columns) with contralateral analgesia (lateral spinothalamic tract), the so-called Brown-Séquard syndrome. Suffice it to say that almost any pattern of neurologic injury can occur from cervical spinal cord injury. Early and accurate documentation of the neurologic status is therefore critical.

## RADIOLOGIC EVALUATION

In any severely injured patient, one of the initial radiographs taken should be a view of the lateral cervical spine. This film cannot be considered adequate unless the entire cervical spine from C1 to the C7–T1 interspace is imaged. Careful inspection of this film by an experienced radiologist, emergency department physician, neurosurgeon, or orthopaedist is required to evaluate soft tissue swelling, alignment, and possible fracture or dislocation. In practice, adequate lateral cervical spine radiography may not be possible in the emergency department in uncooperative patients, or those with short necks or muscular shoulders in whom the full extent of the cervical spine cannot be radiologically documented. In these cases specialized projections such as the swimmer's view, polytomography, or computed

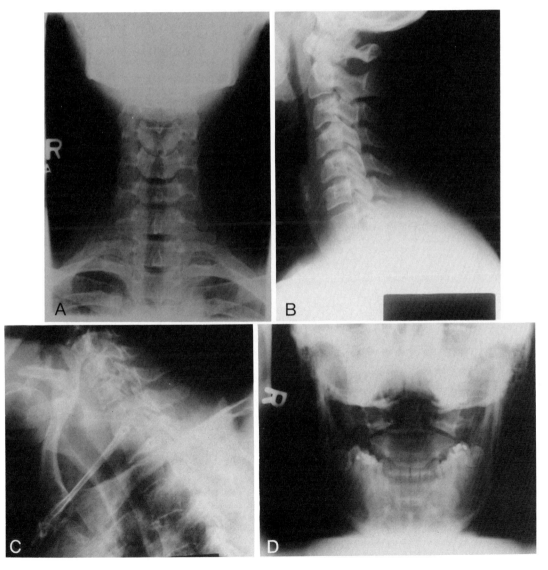

**Figure 17.6.** Plain cervical spine radiographs in (*A*) anteroposterior (AP), (*B*) lateral, (*C*) "swimmer's," and (*D*) open-mouth projections.

tomography (CT) must be pursued. In any case, plain radiography is typically completed by obtaining an anteroposterior (AP) view of the spine and an "open-mouth" view of the odontoid and C1–2 interface (Fig. 17.6).

CT is undoubtedly the best way to image the cervical spine in patients with severe injury (Fig. 17.7). Patients should remain in cervical immobilization or skeletal axial traction (see below) during this study to guard against inadvertent spinal cord injury.

If plain radiography is normal, a careful neurologic exam is performed. If this examination is normal but there is still cervical tenderness or other questions regarding the status of the cervical spine, active flexion and extension lateral radiographs can be obtained to rule out any ligamentous instability that might not be associated with bony injury (Fig. 17.8). The general criteria for instability are reviewed below, and apply to either bony or purely ligamentous injuries. Again, pain on range of motion of the cervical spine should signal the possibility of a significant bony or ligamentous injury.

In cases in which neurologic injury is well established, CT with intrathecal contrast enhancement or magnetic resonance (MR) imaging have replaced myelography as the procedures of choice. These modalities are rarely invoked in the acute setting, unless the patient has a documented course of progressive neurologic loss. In these rare instances, an epidural hematoma or ongoing bony compression of the spinal cord may warrant emergent diagnosis and surgical decompression.

Finally, even with the best available techniques and routine screening protocols, some injuries may be missed. The experienced clinician is watchful for the patient with persistent focal cervical pain or evolving neurologic complaints. In these cases occult fracture-dislocations or significant ligamentous injuries may eventually be revealed by repeat plain radiography or CT, sometimes days or even weeks following the traumatic event.

## STABILITY AND INSTABILITY

The assessment of the potential stability or instability of a cervical spine injury remains controversial. Until recently, and to some extent presently, stability has been largely a matter of opinion. Since one of the major functions of the cervical

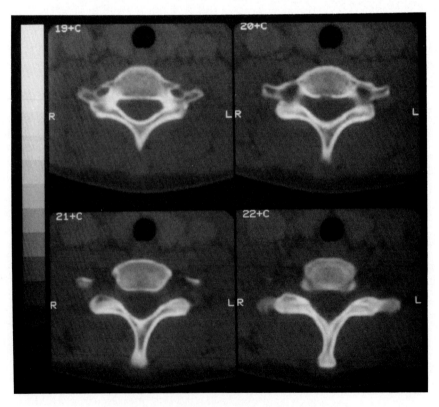

**Figure 17.7.**   CT scan of cervical spine in axial plane.

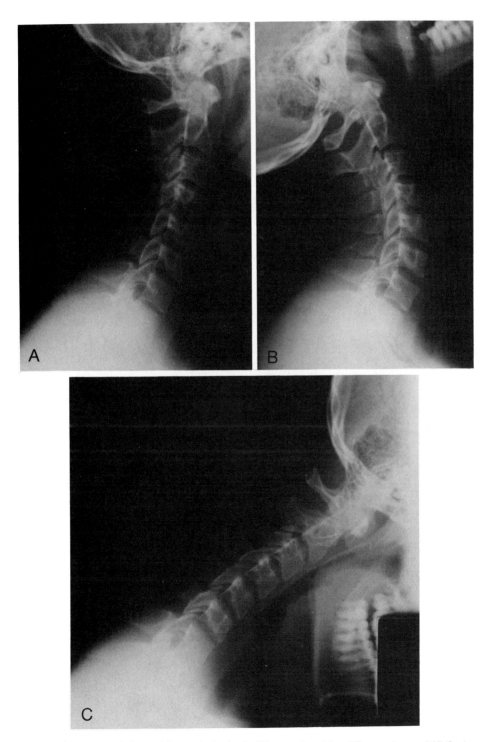

**Figure 17.8.** Lateral views of the cervical spine in (*A*) neutral position, (*B*) extension, and (*C*) flexion.

ANTERIOR

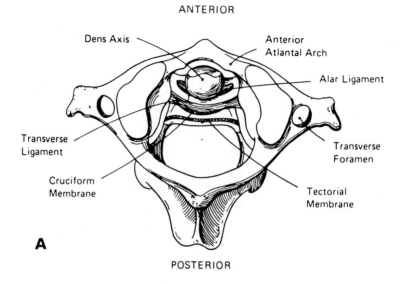

**A**

POSTERIOR

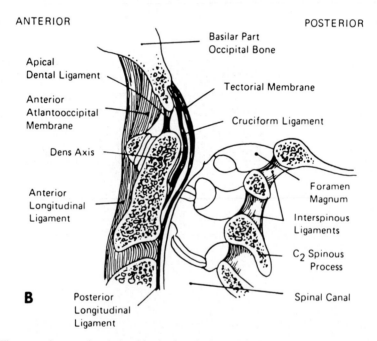

**B**

**Figure 17.9.** The normal anatomic relationships in the atlanto-occipital region. *A*, Superior view. *B*, Sagittal view. (From Schneider RC: High cervical spine injuries. In Wilkins RH, Rengachary SS (eds): *Neurosurgery.* New York, McGraw-Hill, 1985, pp 1701–1708.)

spine is to protect the spinal cord and nerve roots, theoretically any fracture in which damage to either of these structures is sustained is considered overtly unstable. Unfortunately, this definition is not universally applicable, since clinical situations commonly arise in which neurologic injury predicts future structural spinal failure. The problem is that no one definition seems to fit all circumstances.

To rationalize the debate, White and Panjabi (7) defined clinical instability as "the loss of the ability of the spine under physiologic loads to maintain relationships between vertebrae in such a way that there is neither damage nor subsequent irritation

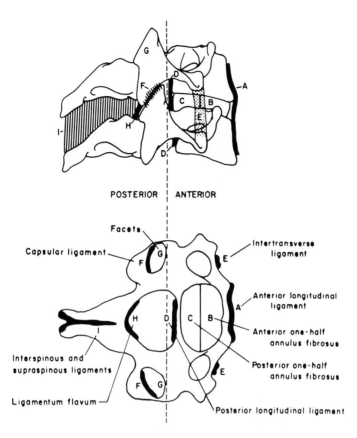

**Figure 17.10.** Schematic illustration of the ligamentous structures that stabilize the lower cervical spine. The ligaments are divided into *anterior* and *posterior* elements. (From White AA, Panjabi MM: *Clinical Biomechanics of the Spine.* Philadelphia, JB Lippincott, 1978.)

to the spinal cord or nerve roots, and in addition, there is no development of incapacitating deformity or pain due to structural changes." The normal ligamentous structures of the cervical spine are shown in Figures 17.9 and 17.10 for the upper and lower cervical spine, respectively. Instability has been defined biomechanically and tested by serially sectioning posterior and anterior ligaments in fresh cadaver specimens (8). By subjecting these specimens to physiologic loads, it was possible to measure abnormal motion occurring at the affected levels and relate this back to specific ligamentous injuries. By this means, stability of lower cervical spine fractures can be thus defined as "translatory displacement of two adjacent vertebrae greater than 3.5 mm, angulation of greater than 11 degrees between adjacent vertebrae, indicating a significant ligamentous disruption." White et al. (9) have developed a checklist for the diagnosis of clinical instability in the lower cervical spine (Table 17.1).

**Table 17.1.**
**Checklist for the Diagnosis of Clinical Instability in the Lower Cervical Spine**[a]

| Element | Point Value[b] |
|---|---|
| Anterior elements destroyed or unable to function | 2 |
| Posterior elements destroyed or unable to function | 2 |
| Relative sagittal plane translation >3.5 mm | 2 |
| Relative sagittal plane rotation >11 degrees | 2 |
| Positive stretch test | 2 |
| Spinal cord damage | 2 |
| Nerve root damage | 1 |
| Abnormal disc narrowing | 1 |
| Dangerous loading anticipated | 1 |

[a]From White AA, Southwick WO, Panjabi MM: Clinical instability in the lower cervical spine. A review of past and current concepts. *Spine* 1:15, 1976.
[b]Total of 5 or more = unstable.

The concept of functional instability is an important one. With the exception of active flexion/extension views, most of these criteria for instability are presumptive, based on experience in biomechanical cadaveric studies. Another strategy is to subject the cervical spine to a load and document the radiographic appearance of the spine with incremental addition of weight to axial traction applied by secure skeletal fixation (tongs) or halter traction. This is the so-called stretch test alluded to in Table 17.1. The application and interpretation of this test are beyond the scope of the present discussion, but it suffices to say that this is a further definition of "stability" that directly tests the functional integrity of the injured spinal motion segment.

By these generally accepted definitions, many other fractures can be tentatively defined as inherently unstable: (a) certain forms of C1 fracture (Jefferson); (b) atlantoaxial dislocation with an atlantodental interval of more than 3 mm in adults and 4 mm in children, indicative of rupture of the transverse ligament; (c) most odontoid fractures; (d) hangman's fractures (C2); and (e) bilateral locked facets at C3 through C7.

When examined in depth, the issue of spinal stability is both complex and confusing. In the daily management of acute cervical spine injuries, the determination of stability is still often a matter of some subjectivity. However, within a range we usually can classify injuries as "stable" or "unstable." The implications and treatment consequences for each of these judgments are discussed next.

## STABLE CERVICAL SPINE INJURIES

The reader is again directed to Chapter 19, which discusses in detail the pathophysiology, anatomy, and clinical syndromes of connective tissue and so-called whiplash injuries. The present comments are limited to injuries of the spinal motion segment proper, with definite evidence of focal ligamentous or bony injury but which do not fulfill the criteria for instability reviewed above.

In most cases a stable cervical spine injury can be satisfactorily treated with external bracing using a Philadelphia collar (Fig. 17.11), a SOMI brace, or a Yale orthosis (Fig. 17.12). Patients are treated with adequate analgesics, including narcotics if necessary; follow-up neurologic examinations are made and serial radiographs are obtained at regular intervals. Ligamentous healing typically takes approximately 1 month, whereas bony union is not well underway until about 3 months, at which time the rigid external orthosis

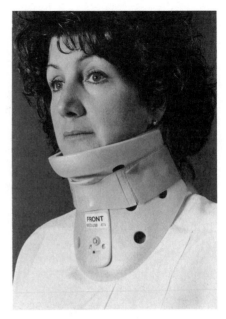

**Figure 17.11.** Philadelphia collar.

is usually removed. Radiographically evident bony healing and remodeling usually take up to 1 year after injury.

## HIGH CERVICAL INJURIES (OCCIPUT, ATLAS, AND AXIS)

Fracture-dislocations that involve the first two cervical vertebra are usually segregated from lower cervical spine (C3–7) injuries because of the highly specialized anatomy of these vertebra, and the forces and mechanisms that produce injury in this region (10, 11). About 40% of the normal motion of the cervical spine occurs at the atlantoaxial joint, so almost any abnormally great force that is applied to this joint can cause tearing of the supporting ligamentous structures. These include the tectorial membrane, the posterior atlanto-occipital membrane, and the apical and alar ligaments (Fig. 17.9).

Fractures of the upper cervical spine usually produce either instant high cervical cord dysfunction with quadriplegia and respiratory arrest or little to no deficit. Patients seen in emergency departments are almost always in the latter category. The vertebral arteries also have a close relationship to the first two cervical vertebrae, and occasionally fracture-dislocations in this area can result in injury to these structures with consequent neurologic sequelae in the territory of these arteries. These syndromes can include brainstem strokes, both bland and hemorrhagic (Fig. 17.13).

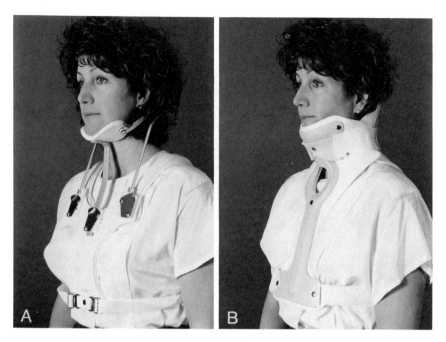

**Figure 17.12.** *A*, SOMI brace. *B*, Yale orthosis.

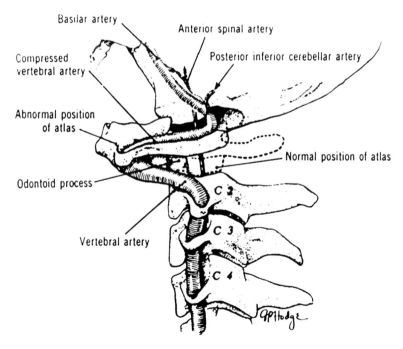

**Figure 17.13.** Normal and abnormal anatomy of upper cervical spine. Note stretching of vertebral artery in odontoid fracture. (From Schneider R, Crosby E: Vascular insufficiency of brain stem and spinal cord in spinal trauma. *Neurology* 9:643, 1959.)

## Jefferson Fracture (C1)

When viewed in the coronal (AP) plane, the lateral masses of the atlas, which are comprised mostly of the atlanto-occipital and atlantoaxial joints, form a wedge with its apex directed medially. Direct axial loading—for example, from a blow or impact to the vertex—produces an axial force vector against the lateral masses of the atlas. Because of the configuration of these joints this force is directed laterally, spreading and ultimately fracturing the ring of C1 (Fig. 17.14). Jefferson fractures are, in effect, burst fractures of C1 (Figs. 17.15 and 17.16).

Jefferson fractures are usually considered stable, and can be treated with external bracing. However, when a comminuted fracture of C1 shows bilateral overhang of the lateral masses that totals 7 mm or more on an AP radiograph, a rupture of the transverse ligament has probably occurred, rendering the spine unstable (Fig. 17.17).

## Odontoid Fractures and Atlantoaxial Dislocation (C1–C2)

The most common mechanism of injury at the atlantoaxial level is flexion, which may produce a fractured odontoid process or, much less commonly, traumatic disruption of the atlantoaxial supporting ligaments. This mechanism usually re-

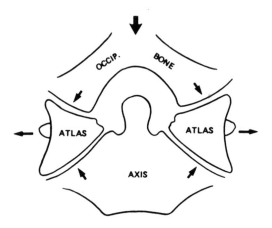

**Figure 17.14.** The mechanism of development of the Jefferson fracture. The top arrow indicates the downward thrust of the occipital bone, transmitting its force through the occipital condyles against the arches of the atlas, driving them outward with a "bursting" effect. (From Schneider RC: High cervical spine injuries. In Wilkins RH, Rengachary SS (eds): *Neurosurgery.* New York, McGraw-Hill, 1985, pp 1701–1708.)

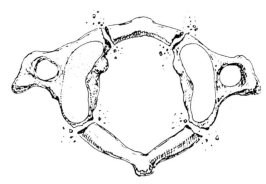

**Figure 17.15.** Jefferson fracture (From Hoppenfeld S: *Orthopaedic Neurology.* Philadelphia, JB Lippincott, 1977.)

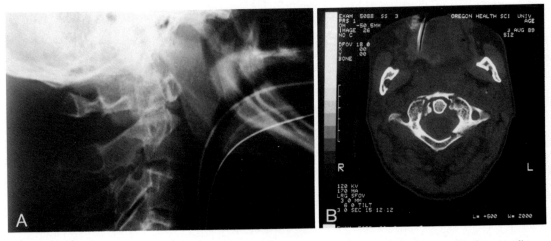

**Figure 17.16.** *A,* Lateral radiograph of Jefferson fracture. *B,* Axial CT scan through the fracture showing spreading and multiple fractures of C1.

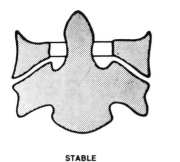 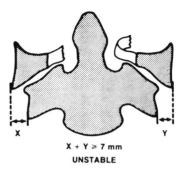

**STABLE**  **UNSTABLE**

X + Y ≥ 7 mm

**Figure 17.17.** Jefferson fractures. When a comminuted fracture of C1 shows bilateral overhang of the lateral masses that totals 7 mm or more, a rupture of the transverse ligament has probably occurred, rendering the spine unstable. (From White AA, Panjabi MM: *Clinical Biomechanics of the Spine.* Philadelphia, JB Lippincott, 1978.)

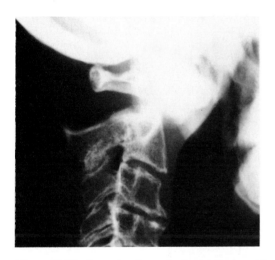

**Figure 17.18.** Lateral radiograph of a type 2 odontoid fracture. Note the anterior displacement of the dens.

sults in anterior displacement of the dens on C2 (Fig. 17.18). Extension injuries with posterior dislocation of the dens and rotatory injuries are much less common (Fig. 17.19).

Traumatic rupture of the atlantoaxial ligaments is unusual, but if lateral films demonstrate widening of the atlantodental interval of more than 3 mm in adults, and 4 mm in children, ligamentous damage should be suspected. If this interval increases abnormally with flexion, ligamentous rupture can be diagnosed (Fig. 17.20).

Odontoid fractures come in three varieties: type 1 are fractures of the tip of the odontoid; type 2 fractures, the most common, pass through the base of the dens (Fig. 17.19), and type 3 pass through the body of C2 (Fig. 17.21). These fractures are best seen on the open mouth view.

Nondisplaced type 1 or 2 fractures can usually be managed by external fixation in a halo vest (Fig. 17.22). Marked displacement or an elderly patient indicates an increased incidence of nonfusion and mitigates for surgical fusion of C1–2.

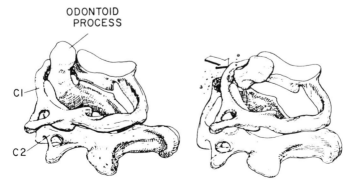

ODONTOID
PROCESS

C1

C2

**Figure 17.19.** Mechanism of a type 2 odontoid fracture with posterior displacement of the dens. (From Hoppenfeld S: *Orthopaedic Neurology.* Philadelphia, JB Lippincott, 1977.)

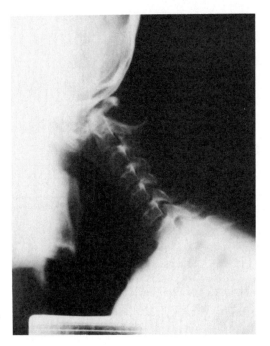

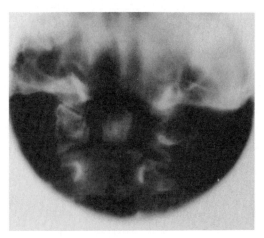

**Figure 17.21.** AP tomographic view of a type 3 odontoid fracture.

**Figure 17.20.** Lateral cervical spine radiograph of traumatic atlantoaxial instability without bony injury. Note the widened atlantoaxial interval on neck flexion.

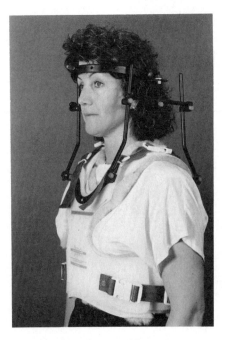

**Figure 17.22.** Halo vest.

## Hangman's Fracture (C2)

The so-called hangman's fracture is a bipedicle fracture of C2 produced by hyperextension of the neck (Fig. 17.23 and 17.24). It results in anterior displacement of C2 and C3 and is an unstable fracture. Fortunately, this displacement does not usually compromise the canal and neurologic deficit from a hangman's fracture is not common.

## LOWER CERVICAL INJURIES (C3–7)

The remaining cervical vertebrae and their supporting structures below C2 are similar enough

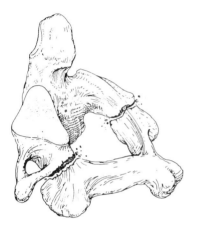

**Figure 17.23.** Hangman's fracture. (From Hoppenfeld S: *Orthopaedic Neurology.* Philadelphia, JB Lippincott, 1977.)

anatomically that fractures in this location can be dealt with as a group (11). The most frequent cervical injuries occur at C5 and C6 with fracture and dislocation. This relates to the fact that the maximal amount of cervical spine flexion and extension normally occurs at these levels, and these vertebrae are thus subjected to higher traumatic loads.

As with all traumatized patients, initial management should address airway control, respiratory status, and maintenance of the systemic circulation. This may mean ventilatory support, intravascular volume replacement, prevention of venous pooling in the legs by means of elastic stocking or MAST trousers, and vasopressors if necessary. Although high-dose corticosteroid medication has been advocated in the past, there is little current evidence that these agents improve neurologic outcome.

Injuries to the lower cervical spine can manifest as fractures of the body, pedicles, lateral masses (transverse processes and facet joints), laminae, and spinous processes. A full discussion of all the variants of injury is not pertinent to the aim of this chapter.

A special type of dislocation that is worthy of note is the "jumped" or "locked" facet. In this case the inferior articular process of the more superior vertebra becomes displaced and locked over the superior articular process of the more inferior vertebra, typically from a rotational force (Fig. 17.25). This can occur either unilaterally

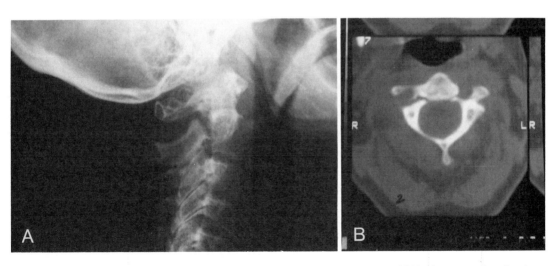

**Figure 17.24.** *A,* Lateral cervical radiograph of a hangman's fracture. *B,* Axial CT of C2 in the same patient showing a nondisplaced bipedicle fracture.

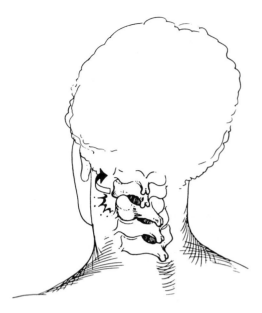

**Figure 17.25.** Rotational force mechanism of jumped facet. (From Hoppenfeld S: *Orthopaedic Neurology.* Philadelphia, JB Lippincott, 1977.)

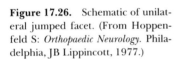

**Figure 17.26.** Schematic of unilateral jumped facet. (From Hoppenfeld S: *Orthopaedic Neurology.* Philadelphia, JB Lippincott, 1977.)

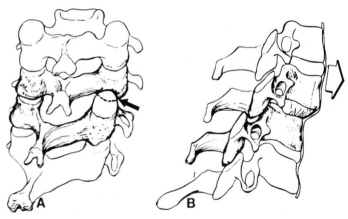

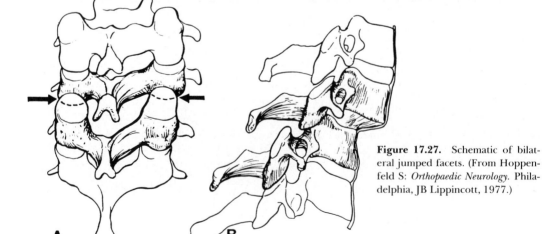

**Figure 17.27.** Schematic of bilateral jumped facets. (From Hoppenfeld S: *Orthopaedic Neurology.* Philadelphia, JB Lippincott, 1977.)

(Fig. 17.26) or bilaterally (Fig. 17.27). Sometimes this injury is associated with little bony injury, and simply rupture of the ligamentous structures of lateral mass. Cord compression can result from the subluxation and malalignment of the vertebra.

## MANAGEMENT OF UNSTABLE INJURIES

### EARLY MANAGEMENT

Appropriate management of cervical injuries begins at the accident site, obviously before a determination of stability is possible. For this reason, all patients who have apparent injury to the head or neck should be treated as having an unstable injury until proven otherwise. Early assessment of the patient is essential, and the principle of non-movement should be observed until proper equipment is available to immobilize the neck for transfer of the patient to a health care facility. If the patient is conscious, careful questioning regarding extremity movement, absence of feeling, and presence and location of pain may indicate the existence of a cervical spine or spinal cord injury (11).

The patient should be placed in situ in a cervical collar and carefully placed on a spine "backboard" while axial traction is continuously applied, if possible, to the head. The patient is fixed to the backboard to ensure immobility of the neck. Resuscitative efforts are initiated at the scene and continued during the transport process. Maintenance of the airway, respiration, and circulation are of primary importance, but after this the principle concern is avoidance of further injury to the nervous system.

### EMERGENCY DEPARTMENT MANAGEMENT

When a patient arrives at the emergency department immobilized in a collar and on a backboard, the status of the resuscitation and other injuries are assessed. Unless other life-saving procedures mandate violation of strict immobilization of the neck, the first two issues relevant to the potential cervical spine injury are (*a*) a brief neurologic exam and (*b*) a lateral cervical spine radiograph.

If an unstable cervical fracture-dislocation is identified radiographically, the patient is placed in skeletal traction, preferably with Gardner-Wells or similar skull tongs (Fig. 17.28). These tongs are easily placed under local anesthesia, usually at a point just above the root of the mastoid process, and do not require a scalp incision. The spring-loaded mechanism of the tongs permits a safe insertion without penetration of the inner table of the skull. Reduction of malalignment of the cervical spine is then attempted by se-

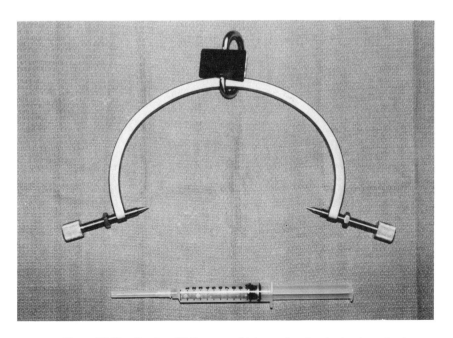

**Figure 17.28.** Gardner-Wells tongs, which are placed under local anesthesia.

quentially adding weight to the traction device in 5- or 10-pound increments. A general rule is to apply 5–7 pounds of traction for each vertebral level at or above the fracture site. A brief neurologic exam and plain lateral cervical spine radiographs are obtained after each addition of weight. Muscle spasms and pain can be treated acutely with intravenous diazepam in judicious doses.

A maximum of approximately 50 pounds can be applied safely to skeletal tong traction before the fracture can be declared irreducible by traction alone. Manipulation of the neck can also be attempted to reduce an unyielding dislocation, but only by a very experienced neurosurgeon or orthopaedist. Unilateral or bilateral locked facets can be particularly stubborn and may require both traction and some gentle manipulation to reduce. Surgical open reduction and internal fixation may be necessary where there is persistent spinal canal or neural foramen compromise despite maximal attempts at closed reduction.

The role of emergent decompressive surgery for patients with cervical spine fractures is still debated. Certainly patients with incomplete spinal cord injuries and persistent soft tissue (disc or hematoma) or bony cord compression should be considered for acute decompression and fusion (Fig. 17.29). The necessity for this is perhaps best evaluated by emergent CT scan of the level of injury after best possible reduction in traction (Figs. 17.30 through 17.32). Surgical decisions are based on the patient's neurologic status, the se-

verity of other traumatic injuries, and the evidence of continued cord compression. Most often traumatic spinal cord compression is from bony or other masses anterior to the cord, and surgery is undertaken from this direction. If the compression is posterior, decompression takes this route. Stabilization is most often performed posteriorly, but anterior fusion is also feasible in many cases, the general principle being to splint areas of ligamentous injury and preserve areas of ligamentous integrity.

## POSTACUTE MANAGEMENT

In the postacute phase, a myelogram with CT is used to assess cord compression in patients with stable, but incomplete, spinal cord dysfunction, or to assess foraminal compression of the nerve root in patients with signs of radiculopathy. As with more emergent decompression of patients with neurologically incomplete spinal cord injuries, later decompression of bony encroachment on the cord is controversial, but may in some cases result in improved outcome. More importantly, decompression of a nerve root that is adjacent to a functionally intact spinal cord may greatly improve a quadriplegic patient's functional status.

In patients with unstable injuries many surgeons favor early internal stabilization to permit early patient mobilization. Postoperatively, these patients are placed in a cervicothoracic support orthosis (Minerva brace) for 3 months to allow bony healing. Although there is no universally ac-

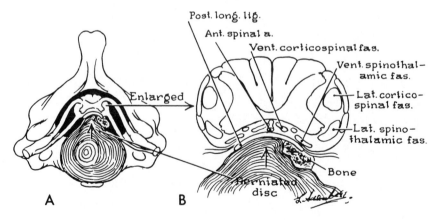

**Figure 17.29.** Diagram of spinal cord compression occurring after acute cervical trauma from herniated disc and bone fragments. (From Bohlman HH, Ducker TB, Lucas JT: Spine and spinal cord injuries. In Rothman RH, Simeone FA (eds): *The Spine.* Philadelphia, WB Saunders, 1982, pp 661–682.)

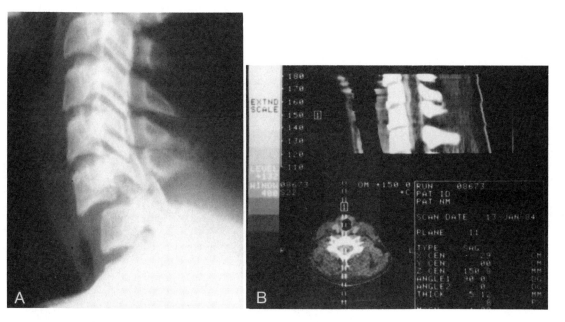

**Figure 17.30.** *A*, Lateral cervical spine radiograph showing bilateral jumped facets at C6–7. At this point the patient was quadriplegic. *B*, Sagittally reconstructed CT with intrathecal contrast (myelogram) after skull traction and reduction of the jumped facets. Note there is no residual cord compression. The patient made a full neurologic recovery.

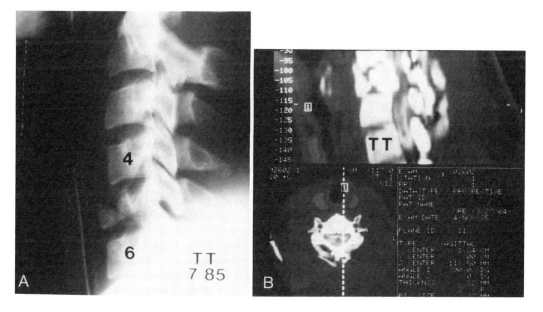

**Figure 17.31.** *A*, Lateral cervical spine radiograph showing burst fracture of C5 with concomitant quadriplegia. *B*, Sagittally reconstructed CT with intrathecal contrast showing residual cord compression due to bone fragments in the spinal canal at C5. Despite surgical cord decompression and stabilization of the spine, the patient made no neurologic recovery.

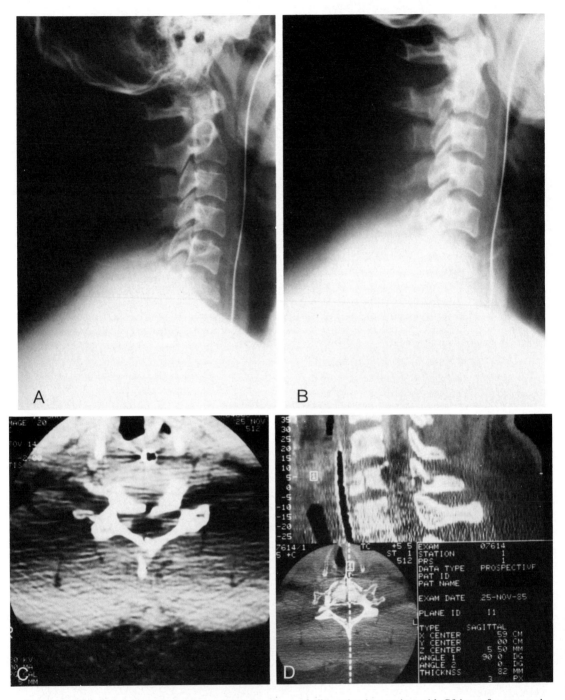

**Figure 17.32.** *A,* Lateral cervical spine radiograph prior to skull traction in a patient with C6 burst fracture and quadriparesis. *B,* After skull traction the fragments are more reduced and the canal is decompressed. *C,* Canal decompression at C6 with skull traction shown by axial CT with intrathecal contrast. *D,* Sagittally reconstructed CT after intrathecal contrast showing good restoration of the canal AP dimension.

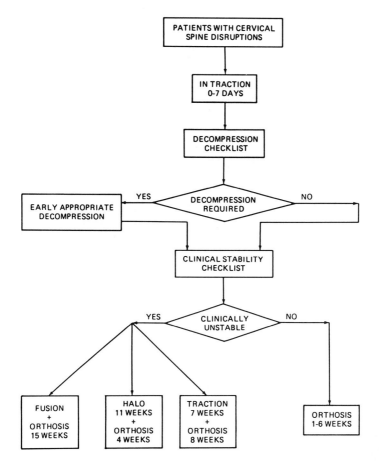

**Figure 17.33.** An algorithm for the management of patients with cervical spine injuries. (From White AA, Southwick WO, Panjabi MM: Clinical instability in the lower cervical spine. A review of past and current concepts. *Spine* 1:15, 1976.)

cepted protocol for the management of cervical spine injuries, one possible algorithm is shown in Figure 17.33.

## SUMMARY

A few basic rules epitomize the emergent management of cervical spine injuries:

1. All patients with injuries above the shoulders should be suspected of having a cervical spine injury.
2. All suspected cervical spine injuries should be treated as unstable until proven otherwise.
3. Pain is one of the hallmarks of significant cervical spine injury.
4. The differentiation of minor and major (unstable) neck injuries is often difficult in the acute setting and should be approached with care and circumspection.
5. Careful radiography of the entire cervical spine, and

in some cases CT, is essential in the evaluation of these patients.
6. Early involvement of a neurosurgeon or an orthopaedic surgeon is critical in patients with evidence of a major cervical injury.

### REFERENCES

1. Trunkey DD, Holcroft JW: Trauma: general survey and synopsis of management of specific injuries. In Hardy JD (ed): *Hardy's Textbook of Surgery*. Philadelphia, JB Lippincott, 1988, pp 145–175.
2. Weiss MH: Mid- and lower cervical spine injuries. In Wilkins RH, Rengachary SS (eds): *Neurosurgery*. New York, McGraw-Hill, 1985, pp 1708–1716.
3. Bohlman HH, Ducker TB, Lucas JT: Spine and spinal cord injuries. In Rothman RH, Simeone FA (eds): *The Spine*. Philadelphia, WB Saunders, 1982, pp 661–682.
4. Cloward RB: Acute cervical spine injuries. *CIBA Clin Symp* 32(1):2–32, 1980.
5. Piepmeier JH: Spinal disorders. In Long DM (ed): *Current*

*Therapy in Neurological Surgery.* St. Louis, Mosby, 1985, pp 135–138.

6. Hoppenfeld S: *Orthopaedic Neurology.* Philadelphia, JB Lippincott, 1977.

7. White AA, Panjabi MM: *Clinical Biomechanics of the Spine.* Philadelphia, JB Lippincott, 1978.

8. White AA, Johnson RM, Panjabi MM, Southwick WO: Biomechanical analysis of clinical stability in the cervical spine. *Clin Orthop* 109:85–96, 1975.

9. White AA, Southwick WO, Panjabi MM: Clinical instability in the lower cervical spine. A review of past and current concepts. *Spine* 1:15, 1976.

10. Schneider RC: High cervical spine injuries. In Wilkins RH, Rengachary SS (eds): *Neurosurgery.* New York, McGraw-Hill, 1985, pp 1701–1708.

11. Yashon D: *Spinal Injury.* New York, Appleton-Century-Crofts, 1978.

# *18*

# INDICATIONS FOR SURGICAL INTERVENTION IN CERVICAL SPINE TRAUMA

*John R. Cassidy and Richard B. North*

For any spinal disorder, there are only three indications for surgery: neurologic deficit, spinal instability, and intractable pain. These apply to the patient who has sustained cervical spine trauma. A simple algorithm may be applied by the primary care, rehabilitative, or emergency room physician to predict the need for surgical consultation.

The evaluating physician must answer the following three questions in the order presented:

1. Is there radiographic evidence of nerve root or spinal cord compression to account for the patient's symptoms or neurologic signs? If so, then the patient should be seen by a spinal surgeon; surgical intervention may be required to decompress the neural elements. If not, and if there is no evidence of radiculopathy or myelopathy:
2. Is the cervical spine unstable? If so, then the patient will require the attention of a spinal surgeon. If not:
3. Does the patient have intractable neck pain? If so, osteoligamentous disruption may be the cause of the patient's axial neck pain, and a surgical procedure may be beneficial. Intractable axial neck pain, however, constitutes the weakest indication for surgery, and the determination of which patients will actually benefit from an operation remains controversial. These issues are reviewed at the end of the chapter.

One point must be clarified as it pertains to the three questions outlined above: Surgical intervention for the purposes of spinal cord or nerve root decompression is distinct from surgical intervention to restore spinal stability. These are issues to be addressed separately and in the order presented. Operations directed at decompressing the neural elements can compromise stability of the cervical vertebral column. Since the decompressive operation is mandated by the neurologic compression, its implications for the stability of the cervical spine must be assessed.

Stated otherwise, an injury to the vertebral column that has resulted in displacement of bone, ligament, or disc against the spinal cord or nerve root does not necessarily result in an unstable cervical vertebral column. Surgery directed at removing the offending displaced bone, ligament, or disc may convert an injured, albeit stable, vertebral column to an unstable vertebral column. Consequently, surgery may be required not only to decompress the spinal cord but also to restore stability.

## CERVICAL SPINE TRAUMA WITH NEUROLOGIC DEFICIT

Patients with neurologic deficit following cervical spine trauma can be subdivided into three categories. First, there are quadriplegics. Second, there are patients with incomplete spinal cord injury. Third, there are patients in whom there is no evidence of spinal cord injury but who have signs or symptoms of radiculopathy.

## THE QUADRIPLEGIC PATIENT

A quadriplegic patient usually is not operated on with the intention of restoring spinal cord function distal to the level of the injury. It has been the experience of most surgeons that recovery of function is rare if not unheard of in instances of "complete" quadriplegia (1). Care must be taken in evaluating these patients to ascertain if there is any evidence of remaining distal function. If there is any distal motor function, sensation, or sacral sparing, the patient must be considered to have an incomplete spinal cord injury and should not be classified as a quadriplegic. The patient with incomplete spinal cord injury must always be assumed to have potential for recovery of spinal cord function.

Caution should also be exercised before declaring a spinal cord injury complete and unrecoverable if there is any chance that the patient is in spinal shock. Spinal shock can give the appearance of complete spinal cord injury, when in fact there is some function that has not yet been revealed. A patient is presumed to be in spinal shock, and therefore to have an incomplete spinal cord injury, as long as there has not yet been the return of normal spinal cord reflexes, and in particular the bulbocavernosus reflex, abdominal stretch reflexes, deep tendon reflexes, and the like.

Assuming that the possibility of spinal shock has been excluded, and the patient has been correctly labeled quadriplegic, the indications for decompressive surgery are limited to decompressing a nerve root or restoring spinal stability. Quadriplegic patients frequently have unstable cervical spines, requiring surgical stabilization. Consequently, although there may be little hope of drastically improving the patient's neurologic status, very little additional morbidity is incurred by performing a decompressive procedure when a fusion is necessary. Furthermore, as any rehabilitative physician will attest, every level of cervical function that can be restored will allow much greater activity in the affected patient. For example, a quadriplegic with C6 function can push a wheelchair, whereas a C5 quadriplegic cannot. Consequently, if there is any chance of restoring function to a compromised nerve root, then that root should be decompressed.

## PATIENTS WITH INCOMPLETE SPINAL CORD INJURY

The patient with an incomplete spinal cord injury and evidence of ongoing neural compression requires decompression. If the injury has resulted in radiologically demonstrable spinal cord compression, and there is clinical evidence of spinal cord injury, then the spinal cord must be decompressed. Dramatic recovery of spinal cord function has been reported by many authors, and in at least one series (Bohlman) significant improvement in neurologic function has been demonstrated even when the decompressive surgery has been deferred for great lengths of time (2). Again, instability is common; fusion may also be required.

The means by which the spinal cord is decompressed, however, do not always include an operation. In some cases only traction or manipulation may be required to restore spinal alignment. In many instances, immobilization with an external orthosis (halo or two-poster brace) allows natural healing of the fractured spine in its appropriately realigned position. Frequently, however, surgical stabilization and fusion with bone graft are necessary.

One of the more common incomplete spinal cord injuries is the central cord syndrome. These patients usually do not require surgery. The typical syndrome consists of profound weakness of the hands that is disproportionate to the weakness in the legs. The reflexes in the upper extremities can be either increased or decreased, depending upon whether injury to the corticospinal tracts or injury to the anterior horn cells predominates. The pain and temperature sensation usually is severely affected in the upper extremities as compared to the lower extremities. Position sense is usually better preserved. The usual mechanism of injury is hyperextension of the cervical spine that allows the buckled ligamentum flavum dorsally to pinch the spinal cord against ventral osteophytes (Fig. 18.1). The cervical spine radiographs are usually normal, and there is no evidence of cervical instability. As one might expect, the syndrome is more common in people who have congenitally narrow anteroposterior cervical spinal canal diameters (3).

There is a long history of cervical laminectomy performed acutely for this injury, but initial enthusiasm has since waned and most surgeons prefer only to immobilize the spine in a Philadelphia collar or two-poster brace for several weeks after the injury. Cervical decompression may still be considered if neurologic recovery has plateaued (4). We will consider for anterior cervical decompression and fusion a patient in whom a large ventral osteophyte or disc herniation can be implicated as the primary cause of the spinal cord injury. Persisting axial neck pain further pushes us toward surgery in these instances.

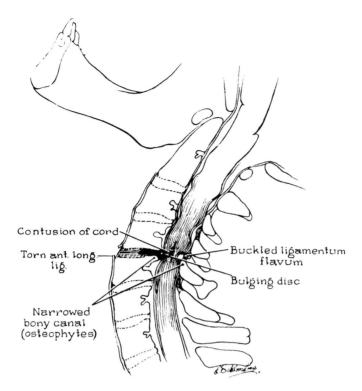

Contusion of cord

Torn ant. long. lig.

Buckled ligamentum flavum

Bulging disc

Narrowed bony canal (osteophytes)

**Figure 18.1.** Hyperextension of the neck in a patient with congenital stenosis of the cervical spine can cause the spinal cord to be pinched between an osteophyte anteriorly and the buckled ligamentum flavum posteriorly. The clinical result is a central cord syndrome. (From Bohlman HH, Ducker TB, Lucas JT: Spine and spinal cord injuries. In Rothman RM, Simeone FA (eds): *The Spine*, ed 2. Philadelphia, WB Saunders, 1982, pp. 661–756.)

One late complication of spinal cord injury is central cord pain. This syndrome occurs infrequently, but has proven to be notoriously refractory to treatment. At some point following injury, usually after several months, these patients begin to complain of dysesthetic sensations in their trunks or, less commonly, extremities (5). The onset of these symptoms should prompt reinvestigation of the injured region. The spinal cord may not have been adequately decompressed, or a posttraumatic syrinx may have developed, or arachnoiditis may be seen. A direct surgical approach to such lesions may prove successful. If one of these lesions cannot be demonstrated, the symptoms are treated medically or by functional neurosurgical procedures. Tricyclic antidepressants or carbamazepine are the preferred medications.

## RADICULOPATHY

Radicular pain is a common complaint following cervical spine trauma. This may reflect impingement upon individual nerve roots by displaced fractured bony fragments, herniated cervical discs, or osteophytic bars.

Unilateral facet dislocation and/or facet fracture can result in impingement upon a cervical nerve root within its foramen. This requires surgical decompression via a posterior approach. The nerve root can be exposed easily by performing a foramenotomy at the diseased level. Any offending fractured fragments can be removed. Furthermore, if intraoperative spinal realignment is to be attempted, this is best achieved via the posterior approach. Fusion, should it be required, is easily and reliably achieved as well. The prognosis for these patients is generally quite good.

The patient with an osteophytic bar probably represents the most frequent referral that a spinal surgeon sees with a history of traumatic cervical spine injury. These patients frequently complain of unremitting neck pain and cervical radiculopathy. Radiculopathy is often evidenced only by pain in the distribution of a cervical nerve root. Reflex changes or loss of power is not always apparent. The source of the neck pain is probably arthritic inflammation from the unaccustomed

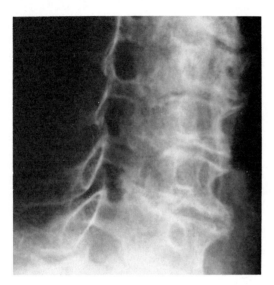

**Figure 18.2.** Four intervertebral foramina can be seen on this oblique projection. On the third intervertebral foramen from the top, one can easily see the extent to which a ventral osteophyte can compromise the exiting nerve root.

stress that has been placed on the uncovertebral and facet joints. The radiculopathy is presumed to be due to local nerve root injury at the level of the intervertebral foramen.

If one studies oblique views of cervical spine radiographs in patients with cervical spondylitic disease, it is easily seen how the osteophytic bar may impinge on the nerve root as it exits the intervertebral foramen (Fig. 18.2). Extreme flexion or extension can pinch the root at this point. The persistent and unremitting aspect of the pain may be attributable to subsequent nerve root swelling within the foramen. Normally, the cross-sectional area of the nerve root comprises approximately 80% of the cross-sectional area of the foramen. If one allows for swelling of the nerve root, and an increase in its size, it may become circumferentially constricted within the foramen. As a result, the swelling continues or worsens and the pain does not subside.

Clinically, this is treated with nonsteroidal anti-inflammatory agents or a short course of gluco-corticoids. We usually prescribe a two-poster brace to minimize motion of the joint and further trauma to the already inflamed root. These steps frequently will break the cycle of repeated nerve trauma and swelling and allow resolution of the syndrome without resorting to surgery. Should these treatments fail, we commonly recommend decompression of the nerve root by either posterior cervical foramenotomy or anterior cervical discectomy and Smith-Robinson fusion (6).

The herniation of a soft cervical disc into the neural foramen as a result of trauma is probably an overly recognized phenomenon. In many of these instances the disc herniation has surely been present prior to the trauma, and the trauma has contributed only marginally to the radiologic abnormality. Nevertheless, the cycle of trauma, swelling, and inflammation outlined above for osteophytic bars can probably also account for the persistence of these symptoms in the case of herniated cervical disc. As is customary, the initial treatment is conservative because the symptoms will frequently resolve without surgery. Several weeks of immobilization in a collar and treatment with anti-inflammatory medications are indicated before considering an operation. Should these treatments fail, anterior cervical discectomy and fusion or cervical foramenotomy and discectomy is warranted.

## CERVICAL SPINE TRAUMA WITH SPINAL INSTABILITY

The unstable cervical spine requires surgical intervention to achieve fusion and cervical stability. This is true regardless of the patient's neurologic status. The determination of which cervical spine injuries are stable and which are unstable is chiefly radiologic. Unfortunately, there is no universally applicable set of radiologic criteria for determining stability. To begin, spinal stability of the craniocervical junction is defined by an entirely different set of criteria than are used in evaluating mid- and lower cervical spine injuries. Consequently, these injuries are considered in separate categories.

## CRANIOCERVICAL INSTABILITY

Regardless of the patient's neurologic function, an unstable cervical spine requires stabilization and this frequently means surgical fusion. The craniocervical junction is defined as including the occiput, C1, and C2. Injuries to this region cause pain in the upper cervical spine and also occipital headache. Pain may be referred to the ears, the vertex of the head, or the lower cervical spine. The causes of craniocervical instability and the treatments required to restore stability are outlined briefly.

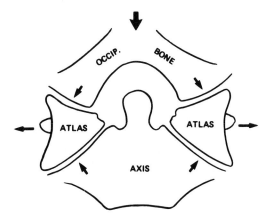

**Figure 18.3.** Forces exerted on the ring of C1 when a vertex injury is sustained. The superior articular processes of C2 and the occipital condyles combine to displace the lateral masses of C1 laterally. (From Schneider RC: High cervical spine injuries. In Wilkins RN, Rengachary SS (eds): *Neurosurgery*. New York, McGraw-Hill, 1985, pp 1701–1708.)

## Occipitocervical Dislocation

Separation and distraction of the occiput from C1 was at one time thought to be a uniformly fatal injury. Recent reports have shown that many patients, and in particular children, may sustain this injury without neurologic deficit. The dislocation is primarily due to ligamentous injury and not fracture. As a rule, disrupted ligaments do not heal with sufficient strength to restore stability. Consequently, these patients frequently require surgical fusion of the occiput to the upper cervical spine.

## Rotatory Dislocation of C1

Rotatory dislocation of C1 results from a strong rotational force being applied to the head. This is a very rare injury in which the lateral masses of C1 and their articulating facets are dislocated from either the superior articular processes of C2 or the occipital condyles. This injury results in a very painful torticollis with severe muscle spasm. Again, the disruption is primarily ligamentous, with no associated fracture; hence surgical fusion is required once the deformity has been reduced.

## Jefferson Fracture

In this injury, the ring of C1 is fractured in at least two places and splayed. The mechanism of injury is axial loading. The fracture is best seen on plain radiographs by the open-mouth odontoid view; the lateral masses of C1 are laterally displaced with respect to the superior articular processes of C2 (Fig. 18.3). Spence has determined that if the total displacement of the lateral masses exceeds 6.9 mm then the transverse ligament, which is responsible for virtually all the ligamentous stability of C1 on C2, has been disrupted (7, 8). Nevertheless, regardless of the degree of dislocation, halo immobilization for 12 weeks usually achieves primary union of the ring of C1 and stability of C1 with respect to C2. If after removal of the halo there is evidence of atlantoaxial instability, surgical fusion may be required.

## Fracture of C2 (Odontoid Fracture)

There are three types of odontoid fracture (Fig. 18.4). In the type I fracture the tip of the odontoid is avulsed. In the type II lesion the odontoid is fractured through its base. The type III fracture occurs within the body of C2 (9). Halo immobilization can be expected to result in fusion and stability in the majority of these injuries (10). The

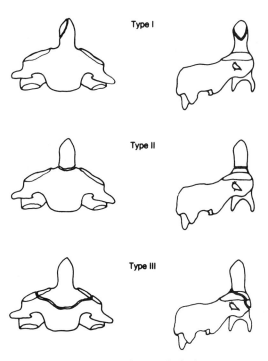

**Figure 18.4.** The type I fracture is the least common and most stable of the three odontoid fractures. The type II fracture is the most common and the most likely to require surgical intervention. The type III fracture will usually unite with halo immobilization alone.

most frequent exception to this rule is the displaced type II fracture. Surgical treatment may be recommended as the primary modality, because some surgeons have found a high incidence of nonunion in conservatively treated lesions (11).

## Os Odontoideum

An os odontoideum has the radiologic appearance of an old nonunited type II odontoid fracture, with smooth edges and cortical bone across the base (Fig. 18.5). There has been controversy in the past as to whether these are congenital or acquired lesions, but the bulk of evidence now supports unrecognized antecedent fracture as the cause (12). At the time of their discovery the patient is frequently asymptomatic, having had cervical spine radiographs obtained for a relatively minor incidental trauma. Many of these lesions will not require surgery, and we apply our usual two criteria in determining which patients are surgical candidates. First, if there is any history of neurologic deficit, or there is ongoing neurologic deficit, the neural tissues must be decompressed and the spine fused. If there is no deficit, prophy-

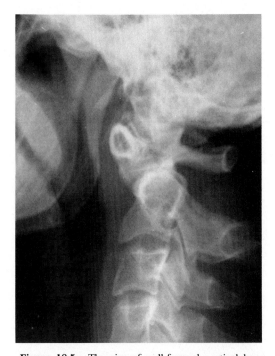

**Figure 18.5.** The rim of well-formed cortical bone seen at the base of the odontoid indicates that this injury is quite old. Most surgeons now believe that an os odontoideum actually represents a nonunited type II odontoid fracture.

lactic surgery can be recommended only if the atlantoaxial joint is unstable.

Instability of C1 on C2 is difficult to define. Most spine surgeons rely on the atlanto-dens interval as seen on the lateral cervical spine film to determine stability. An atlanto-dens interval of >4 mm is generally recognized to be abnormal, but many surgeons do not recommend fusion unless this distance is much greater. Application of this criterion to odontoid fractures, which may permit motion of the dens, is questionable. We prefer to judge instability less on the basis of the atlanto-dens interval than on the diameter of the spinal canal that remains when the dens is maximally displaced. As long as the canal diameter is >14 mm we believe that surgical fusion can generally be deferred.

## Atlantoaxial Subluxation

There are a number of disease processes in which ligamentous laxity results in atlantoaxial instability. This is most frequently seen in rheumatoid patients, Morquio dwarfs, and patients with Down's syndrome. The instability of the joint frequently causes intractable pain, but can also result in neurologic deficit if the spinal cord is compressed between the C1 lamina and the dens. As in the case of os odontoideum, we prefer to recommend fusion only when the canal diameter on a lateral radiograph is reduced to less than 14 mm, or there is evidence of severe basilar invagination of the dens into the basiocciput.

## Fracture of C2 (Hangman's Fracture)

The hangman's fracture is a traumatic spondylolisthesis of C2. In its most common form the fracture occurs bilaterally through the pedicle of C2 (Fig. 18.6). This fracture is unstable and requires treatment to restore stability. This can usually be achieved with halo immobilization for 12 weeks. Surgical fusion is rarely required.

## INSTABILITY OF C3–7

The vertebrae of the cervical spine from C3 to C7 are structurally similar. Consequently, fractures and dislocations of one vertebral body relative to another can be reviewed collectively.

Injury to the mid- and lower cervical spine causes axial neck pain. Injuries to the lower cervical spine may refer pain to the interscapular region. If the injury has resulted in nerve root im-

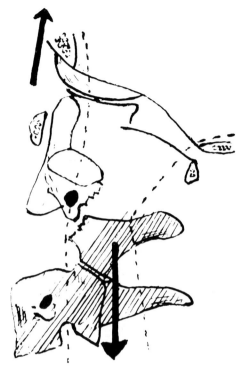

**Figure 18.6.** The most typical hangman's fracture is depicted. The axis is fractured through the pedicles. (From Schneider RC: High cervical spine injuries. In Wilkins RN, Rengachary SS (eds): *Neurosurgery.* New York, McGraw-Hill, 1985, pp. 1701–1708.)

pingement, radiculopathy will be superimposed on these symptoms.

Criteria for determining if one vertebra is unstable relative to its adjoining vertebrae have been defined by White et al. (13) (Fig. 18.7). These criteria are only applicable to adjacent vertebrae at the level of C3–7. Radiographically, if there is more than 11° of angulation of one motion segment with respect to the next, or if there is more than 3.5 mm of translation of one vertebra on another on flexion-extension views, then the segment is defined as unstable. It is our opinion that these findings alone warrant consultation by a spinal surgeon. However, clinical criteria will need to be considered by the surgeon before it is concluded that operative fusion is required. Individual examples of common injuries at the level of C3–7 are presented below.

## Unilateral Facet Fracture-Dislocation

This is a flexion injury with a rotational component. The superior articular process of the verte-

bra below is frequently fractured, and this fragment can remain in the intervertebral foramen, causing injury to the nerve root exiting that foramen. If the facet is dislocated, or "perched," there is a characteristic radiographic appearance. The most conspicuous finding is usually anterolisthesis of approximately 25% of the anteroposterior diameter of the upper vertebral body on the lower vertebral body on a lateral radiograph. On the same view, transition in the appearance of the facets to an oblique projection is seen at the level of injury (Fig. 18.8). On an anteroposterior radiograph the spinous processes may be offset, almost invariably by >4 mm of translation, and therefore this injury is unstable. Even when these injuries can be reduced in traction, surgical fusion is usually required, and a foraminotomy may be necessary to decompress the nerve root.

## Bilateral Facet Fracture-Dislocation

Again, this is a flexion injury. Bilateral facet fracture-dislocation usually results in severe spinal cord injury or quadriplegia. Because the spine is

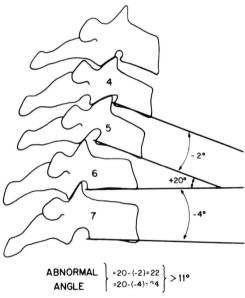

**Figure 18.7.** Lines drawn through the superior endplates of adjacent vertebrae are compared. The angle defined by adjacent lines is the angle of the motion segment. If the difference in the angle of one motion segment to its adjacent motion segment exceeds 11°, then there is a high likelihood that the spine is unstable. (From White AA III, Southwick WO, Panjabi MM: Clinical instability in the lower cervical spine: a review of past and current concepts. *Spine* 1:15, 1976.)

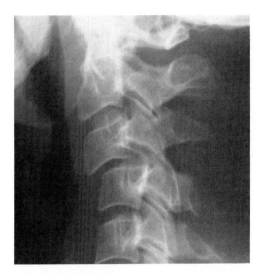

**Figure 18.8.** These facets have lost their normal shingled appearance. One can see that the superior articular process of the inferior vertebra has been displaced inferiorly and posteriorly such that the facets are "perched," or "locked."

unstable, the malalignment must be reduced, and surgical fusion usually is required. Failure to reduce and fuse this injury will likely result in chronic cervical pain and progressive flexion deformity of the cervical spine.

### Chip Fracture

Occasionally, an elderly patient with severe degenerative disc disease and osteophyte formation of the cervical spine will be found to have fractured a small portion of one of the anterior spondylitic bars. This is usually the result of an extension injury in which the osteophyte is avulsed by the stretched anterior longitudinal ligament (Fig. 18.9). This is a stable fracture, and hence in the absence of neurologic involvement no surgical intervention is required. These patients are usually placed in Philadelphia collars or soft collars for comfort. The most important point about this fracture is that it not be confused with a wedge compression fracture.

### Wedge Compression Fracture

This fracture usually occurs after severe axial loading or flexion. It must not be confused with a simple chip fracture, because it is an extremely unstable injury. Left unattended, there is great risk of progressive flexion deformity of the spine,

or retropulsion of bone or soft tissues against the spinal cord. These patients are usually placed in traction and ultimately immobilized in a halo. Surgery may also be necessary if posterior ligamentous disruption has rendered the spine unstable.

### Clay Shoveler's Fracture

Clay shoveler's fracture is the name given to a fracture of a spinous process of the lower cervical spine. If it occurs as an isolated bony injury, it is a stable fracture. The patients complain of local pain only. The pain frequently is more severe than in other forms of cervical spine trauma, and this may relate to the surrounding injury to the paraspinous muscles. The stability of the spinal cord and integrity of neural elements are not at risk. We prefer to place these patients in soft collars for their comfort, although more rigid external orthoses can be used as well.

## INTRACTABLE NECK PAIN

Persistent neck pain following cervical spine trauma is frequently referred to a spine specialist for surgical consideration. Unfortunately, in the absence of neurologic deficit or spinal instability, there are no established indications for surgery in

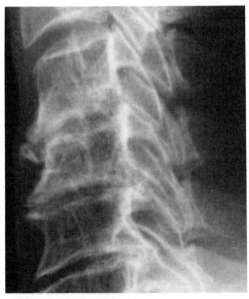

**Figure 18.9.** The small fragment of bone seen at the anterior and inferior aspect of the vertebral body is an osteophyte that has been avulsed by the anterior longitudinal ligament after a hyperextension injury.

these patients. Consequently, most surgeons are very selective in choosing patients from this category for operative treatment. Many of these patients have been treated conservatively for months or years prior to referral for surgery.

We will consider for surgery patients who have radiologic evidence of previous cervical spine trauma and whose spines are stable, yet who still have neck pain. Occasional patients will continue to experience pain after a facet fracture or compression fracture that has healed with a pseudarthrosis. Fusion across that joint will be likely to reduce their pain. Patients with purely ligamentous injuries are less reliably relieved of their pain by surgery; we are cautious in recommending surgery to them. Finally, a number of spine specialists feel that axial neck pain is due mostly to degenerative disc disease. These patients can be evaluated by discograms, and if their pain is reproducibly relieved by injection of a local anesthetic, they are considered candidates for surgery. Anterior cervical discectomy and interbody fusion is the preferred procedure.

Again, one must be very cautious before recommending an operation, and this is perhaps the most controversial indication upon which to base surgery. Most series report that these patients do not fare as well as those with radiculopathy (14, 15). Nevertheless, good results have been reported for anterior cervial fusion performed for discogenic pain only (16, 17).

## REFERENCES

1. Stauffer ES: Diagnosis and prognosis of acute cervical spinal cord injury. *Clin Orthop* 112:9, 1975.
2. Bohlman HH: Acute fractures and dislocations of the cervical spine: an analysis of 300 hospitalized patients and review of the literature. *J Bone Joint Surg [Am]* 61:1119, 1979.
3. Torg JS, Pavlov H, Genuario SE, et al: Neuropraxia of the cervical spinal cord with transient quadriplegia. *J Bone Joint Surg [Am]* 68:1354–1370, 1986.
4. Bose B, Northrup BE, Osterholm JL, Cotler JM, DiTunno JF: Reanalysis of central cervical cord injury management. *Neurosurgery* 15:367–372, 1984.
5. Melzack R, Loeser JD: Phantom body pain in paraplegics: evidence for a central "pattern generating mechanism" for pain. *Pain* 4:195–210, 1978.
6. Robinson RA, Smith GW: Anterior lateral cervical disc removal and interbody fusion for cervical disc syndrome. *Bull Johns Hopkins Hosp* 96:223–224, 1955.
7. Lipson SJ: Fractures of the atlas associated with fractures of the odontoid process and transverse ligament ruptures. *J Bone Joint Surg [Am]* 59:940, 1977.
8. Spence KF Jr, Decker S, Sell K: Bursting atlantal fracture associated with rupture of the transverse ligament. *J Bone Joint Surg [Am]* 52:543, 1970.
9. Anderson LD, D'Alonzo RT: Fractures of the odontoid process of the axis. *J Bone Joint Surg [Am]* 56:1663–1674, 1974.
10. Dickman CA, Hadley MN, Browner C, Sonntag VK: Neurosurgical management of acute atlas-axis combination fractures. A review of 25 cases. *J Neurosurg* 70(1):45–49, 1989.
11. Clark CR, White AA III: Fractures of the dens: a multicenter study. *J Bone Joint Surg [Am]* 67:1340–1348, 1985.
12. Fielding JW, Hensinger RN, Hawkins RJ: Os odontoideum. *J Bone Joint Surg [Am]* 62A:376–383, 1980.
13. White AA III, Southwick WO, Panjabi MM: Clinical instability in the lower cervical spine: a review of past and current concepts. *Spine* 1:15, 1976.
14. White AA III, Southwick WO, DePonte RJ, et al: Relief of pain by anterior cervical spine fusion for spondylosis: a report of sixty-five cases. *J Bone Joint Surg [Am]* 55:525, 1973.
15. Williams JL, Allen MD Jr, Harkess JW: Late results of cervical discectomy and interbody fusion: some factors influencing the results. *J Bone Joint Surg [Am]* 50:277, 1968.
16. Riley LH Jr, Robinson RA, Johnson KA, et al: The results of anterior interbody fusion of the cervical spine: review of ninety three consecutive cases. *J Neurosurg* 30:127, 1969.
17. Robinson RA, Walker AE, Ferlic DC, et al: The results of anterior interbody fusion of the cervical spine. *J Bone Joint Surg [Am]* 44:1569, 1962.

## *19*

# CLINICAL SPECTRUM AND MANAGEMENT OF WHIPLASH INJURIES

*Robert W. Teasell and Glenn A. McCain*

Whiplash injuries following motor vehicle accidents are an increasingly common yet poorly understood clinical entity. Also called cervical musculoligamentous sprain, flexion-extension injury, and acceleration-deceleration injury, the term refers to a sudden forced hyperextension-flexion injury of the cervical spine that results in cervical soft tissue injuries. The term "whiplash" is thought to have been first coined by Crowe (1) in 1928 but was first identified under the diagnostic label "railway spine" in individuals injured following train accidents. Erichsen (2) wrote in 1886: "I have often remarked that in railway accidents those passengers suffer most seriously from concussion of the nervous system who sit with their backs turned towards the end of the train which is struck. Thus when a train runs into an obstruction on the line, those who are sitting with their backs to the engine will probably suffer most; whilst if a train is run into from behind, those who are facing the engine will most frequently be the greatest sufferers." Just before the turn of the century "railway spine" was regarded as a medicolegal problem in much the same way as whiplash injuries are regarded today.

The last few decades have seen a growing epidemic of whiplash injuries occurring as a result of motor vehicle accidents, most commonly rear-end collisions. In 1971, the National Safety Council estimated that there were approximately 4 million rear-end collisions in the United States alone, resulting in as many as 1 million reported injuries

per year (3, 4). In that same year the Insurance Institute for Highway Safety reported an incidence of these injuries of 24% following rear-end collisions. Similarly, Macnab (5–9) has estimated that neck injury occurred in one fifth of all accidents involving rear-end collisions. Schutt and Dohan (10) in 1968 calculated the number of neck injuries sustained in automobile accidents to be 14.5 per 1000 industrial employees. This incidence is likely to have increased as the number of cars, and hence the likelihood of accidents, has increased. A reduction of "serious" injuries and death as a result of the current widespread use of seat belts might also be expected to contribute to an increased prevalence of this condition in medical practices. It seems reasonable, therefore, that physicians should have a better understanding of this common clinical condition.

Patients suffering whiplash injuries often present with subjective symptoms out of proportion to objective signs, psychological and behavioral sequelae of chronic pain, and a poor response to conventional therapeutic interventions. As a result patients are often misclassified as hysterics or malingerers such that many clinicians fail to regard whiplash as a legitimate injury. Nevertheless, experimental and clinical evidence leaves little doubt that the majority of whiplash injuries can be explained on firm physiologic grounds. This chapter focuses on the evidence for physiologic injury in these patients and discusses the mechanism of injury, clinical presentation, and preferred management of patients who suffer chronic cervical pain after such acceleration-deceleration–type injuries.

## THE WHIPLASH INJURY

## PATHOPHYSIOLOGY OF THE INJURY

The majority of whiplash injuries occur as a result of rear-end collisions. Typically the injured individual is the occupant of a stationary vehicle that is struck from behind (5–9, 11–14). Injury results because the neck is unable to adequately compensate for the rapidity of head and torso movement resulting from the acceleration forces generated at the time of impact. This is particularly true when the impact is unexpected and the victim is unable to brace for it. Interestingly, the biomechanics of whiplash injury were described over 40 years ago by Severy et al. (15), who conducted a series of rear-end collisions at a variety of impact speeds using anthropometric dummies and volunteer subjects. These initial experiments and others led to the following present understanding of the biomechanics of injury.

During impact the legs and pelvis of the occupant accelerate forward at approximately the same speed as the car. The torso is in contact with the seat, a situation reinforced by the shoulder belt. After a delay of 100 msec following the moment of impact, the torso and shoulders are accelerated forward by the back of the seat. The head and neck are unsupported at the time of impact and are therefore vulnerable to injury. The trunk is accelerated forward by the seat while the head, because of its mass, inertia, and lack of support, tends to lag behind. Thus, immediately following impact the head remains in its original position while the trunk accelerates forward beneath it. The head consequently falls back relative to the accelerating trunk and the neck is forced into extension (Fig. 19.1).

As the inertia of the head is overcome, it begins to accelerate forward and is catapulted into flexion (11). The neck and head characteristically attain acceleration levels over twofold greater in magnitude than the peak acceleration of the car. Severy et al. (15) showed that anthropometric dummies involved in a relatively slow 13 km/hr (8 mph) rear-end collision underwent a 5G acceleration of the head while the vehicle experienced a force of only 2G. The entire sequence of extension-flexion was completed within 0.5 sec of impact. Therefore, even low-speed rear-end collisions may generate substantial forces and result in significant injuries.

When the physiologic range of motion of the cervical spine is exceeded, damage and anatomic disruption of soft tissues of the neck, including muscles, ligaments, and joint capsules, may result. During impact, forward flexion is naturally limited as the chin strikes the chest or steering wheel. Similarly the shoulders limit undue lateral flexion of the head. However, neck extension is restrained only by the upper thorax, so that angulations of up to 120° may be attained, which are far beyond the physiologic maximum of 70°. According to McKenzie and Williams (16), damaging biomechanical forces during extension are focused primarily in the region of C6 and C7. However, although hyperextension is believed to be the cause of most major injuries, it is important to remember that there may also be some component of forced flexion that may contribute to the overall injury (17).

Soft tissue injuries to musculoligamentous structures occur frequently during motor vehicle accidents because neck movements (flexion-extension) occur with a speed and force that overwhelm normal protective cervical neuromuscular reflexes. Most abnormal and damaging movement is completed before the nervous system can react appropriately because the motor response may be delayed relative to the speed of neck movements.

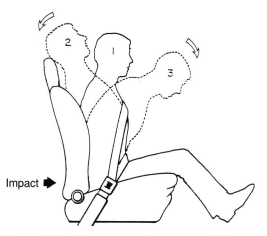

**Figure 19.1.** The sequence of movements of the car occupant following a rear-end collision. Beginning from position 1, the neck and head extend backward as the torso is accelerated forward (position 2). This is followed by the head and neck being catapulted into forward flexion as the inertia of the head is overcome (position 3).

This may aggravate impact forces, thus increasing the degree of soft tissue injury. For instance, the neck flexor muscles may contract forcefully to counter the sudden neck extension on impact. However, by the time they react, the neck may actually be moving into flexion such that muscle contraction may paradoxically augment forward force, throwing the spine into further flexion.

While the mechanism of injury is well understood, the **pathologic lesions** accounting for the whiplash syndrome remain poorly defined. Attempts have been made to delineate these lesions utilizing theoretical constructs as well as animal and human cadaver experiments (11). Animal experiments in which whiplash injuries are produced in a laboratory setting have offered the most important information about the pathology of whiplash injuries. This approach has obvious drawbacks since animals differ from humans both anatomically and physiologically and their pathologic lesions may not correlate well with human injuries. Human cadaver studies offer an anatomically better model. However, cadavers differ in their response to injury because of different tissue characteristics and because they lack the reflex responses seen in live subjects. Nevertheless theoretical predictions, animal experiments, human cadaver experiments, and clinical experiences provide us with a spectrum of possible pathologic lesions that may account for some or all of the symptoms of the whiplash syndrome (5–9, 11, 18).

Possible pathologic lesions following whiplash injuries are listed in Table 19.1. Most authors agree that injuries to the muscles of the neck, including stretching, tearing, and hemorrhaging of the longus colli, longus capitis, scalenes, and ster-

**Table 19.1.**
**Possible Pathologic Lesions in Whiplash Injuries**

Anterior longitudinal ligament strain or tear
Posterior longitudinal ligament strain or tear
Interspinous ligament sprain or tear
Intervertebral disc herniation
Spinous process fracture
Zygapophyseal joint sprain or fracture
Muscle strain or rupture
Concussion or minor head injury
Thoracic outlet syndrome
Temporomandibular joint dysfunction
Retropharyngeal hematoma
Esophageal hemorrhage
Sympathetic trunk injury
Vertebral artery ischemia

nocleidomastoids, commonly occur (19). Supporting structures around apophyseal and facet joints may also be sprained or suffer cartilaginous damage or fracture. In addition, anterior and posterior longitudinal spinal ligaments may undergo stretching and possible tearing. As expected, the anterior longitudinal ligament is more susceptible to injury during hyperextension of the neck. Esophageal and laryngeal damage as well as injury to the cervical sympathetic chain have also been documented. Finally, injuries to the brain, temporomandibular joints, and lower back following whiplash injuries have been reported but remain controversial.

## HEAD RESTRAINTS AND SEAT BELTS

The U.S. Department of Transportation recognized whiplash injuries as a major public health problem when they required all passenger cars manufactured after December 31, 1968 to be equipped with head restraints for front seat car occupants. Unfortunately, the results of this legislation aimed at preventing whiplash injuries have been controversial. Studies have noted that head restraints do reduce the incidence of neck extension injuries by as much as 18–24% (10, 21) but they still fail to prevent the majority of injuries.

There are several reasons for the apparent ineffectiveness of head restraints. Many head restraints are kept low in order to facilitate better rearview vision. Thus the head may hyperextend over the headrest, paradoxically producing greater hyperextension and more serious injury. Another reason is that most automobiles have backwardly inclined seats while motorists tend to sit upright or forward. Consequently, the headrest is rarely near the occiput but is generally some distance behind (Fig. 19.2). Under these circumstances the back of the seat may strike the trunk, accelerating it forward before the headrest contacts the occiput. The neck may then go into hyperextension before the head restraint is able to prevent this. Using a mathematical model, Fox and Williams (22) concluded that the head should be as close as possible to the restraint before impact and suggested 25 mm as a suitable distance. Head restraints are most useful when they come into contact with the head at the same time the seatback contacts the trunk during impact. An alternative explanation for the perceived ineffectiveness of head restraints may be related to underestimation of the importance of forced flexion

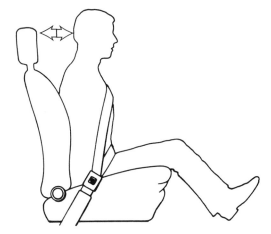

**Figure 19.2.**   Head restraints are often ineffective because most car occupants, particularly drivers, do not incline backward into the seat but tend to lean forward while driving. Car seats are often inclined backward at a slight angle for maximum comfort. The headrest-to-occiput distance is often too great to allow the headrest to function properly.

as a mechanism of injury (17). If injury occurs when the neck is catapulted into flexion, a head restraint would be largely ineffective.

There is some evidence that seat belts may place occupants at greater risk of suffering a whiplash injury. A slightly higher incidence of neck sprains has been reported in those individuals involved in rear-end collisions wearing seat belts compared to those not wearing seat belts (23–26). A possible explanation is that the trunk restrained by a shoulder belt is unable to dampen the rate of head acceleration, resulting in both greater extension and greater flexion movements compared to the forces generated on these structures when a shoulder belt is not worn.

## THE CLINICAL PICTURE OF WHIPLASH INJURIES

### THE WHIPLASH SYNDROME

The clinical picture of whiplash is dominated by head, neck, and upper thoracic pain and is often associated with a variety of poorly explained symptoms such as dizziness, tinnitus, or blurred vision. The symptom complex is remarkably consistent from patient to patient even though it may be complicated by anger, anxiety, depression, and pending litigation. Potential complications of whiplash injuries are listed in Table 19.2. In one

study Balla (27) reviewed 300 consecutive patients who had suffered isolated whiplash injuries after motor vehicle accidents. He described the "late whiplash syndrome," defined as persistence of symptoms greater than 6 months. Little difference was noted in the clinical picture of patients from 6 months to 2 years after injury. These patients suffered headache, neck ache and stiffness, arm pain, and tingling in the limbs as well as dizziness and blurring of vision. When pain persisted for more than 6 months, psychological symptoms of anxiety, irritability, and depression developed. A significant proportion of those individuals studied had difficulty with or were unable to perform their socially allocated tasks. The vast majority had sought multiple medical therapies and had litigation pending. This condition appeared to be most prevalent among women 21–40 years old. There was an absence of abnormal physical findings, apart from pain and tenderness in affected muscles, and poor correlation with radiologic abnormalities.

A delay in symptoms of several hours is characteristic of whiplash injuries. Most patients feel little or no pain for the first few hours following the injury, after which symptoms gradually intensify. During this time period findings on examination are generally minimal (28). However, after several hours, limitation of neck motion, tightness, muscle spasm and/or swelling, and tenderness of both anterior and posterior cervical struc-

**Table 19.2.**
**Potential Complications of Whiplash Injuries**

Neck and shoulder pain
Headache
Arm pain/paresthesias/weakness
Visual symptoms
Dizziness/vertigo
Tinnitus
Dysphagia
Low back pain
Temporomandibular joint symptoms
Depression
Anxiety
Anger and frustration
Hypochondriasis
Compensation neurosis
Posttraumatic syndrome
Chronic pain state
Loss of job and income
Marital and family disruption
Drug dependency

tures become apparent (28, 29). As pain becomes chronic, physical findings often do not correlate with areas of complaint and, generally, symptoms seem disproportionate to the extent of physical injury.

Females are reported to experience whiplash injuries more often than males. Women generally have a slimmer, less muscular neck that, theoretically, is less able to resist the damaging acceleration forces generated at the time of impact. Other possible reasons for the sex discrepancy are that women may be more likely to seek medical attention or be sent to a medical specialist for complaints of pain. At present the sex differential remains unexplained, but a biomechanical explanation would appear to be the most probable.

## Local Tenderness and Referred Pain

Local tenderness and pain referral to sites distant from the original injury are two hallmark features of the whiplash syndrome. The etiology of these two features remains enigmatic, but two explanations have been forwarded to try to explain their presence; they are myofascial and sclerotomal pain.

Myofascial pain is a poorly understood clinical entity despite the fact that it may account for the majority of persistent neck, head, and upper thoracic pain following whiplash injury. Confusion regarding this syndrome has resulted from controversy over objective physical findings and has been confounded by the usual psychological and behavioral sequelae that often accompany chronic pain. The "trigger point" is the characteristic feature of myofascial pain (Table 19.3).

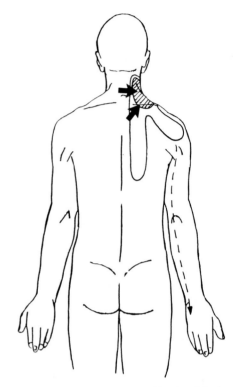

**Figure 19.3.** Trigger points within the right levator scapulae muscle are indicated by *arrows*. The main area of referred pain is shown as the *shaded area;* some pain may also refer down the medial border of the scapula and out into the posterior shoulder. Referral of pain may also occur down the medial aspect of the arm and into the fourth and fifth fingers. (Adapted from Travell and Simons (44).)

**Table 19.3.**
**Trigger Point Characteristics**

Sudden onset of pain with overload of the muscle (either during the accident or afterward)
Gradual onset with chronic overload of muscle
Hallmark is referred pain pattern characteristic of a specific muscle
Localized tender area in a firm band of muscle
Deep finger palpation evokes an alteration in pain and a "jump sign"
Muscle may be shortened (by about 10–20%), subjectively weaker, and more easily fatigued
Reproduction of patient's pain by pressure or trigger point needling

Myofascial trigger points are sharply circumscribed, 2–5 mm in diameter, self-sustaining, hyperirritable foci of tenderness reported to be located within a taut band of skeletal muscle or its associated fascia. Compressing this hyperirritable focus is locally painful and may give rise to characteristic referred pain, tenderness, and autonomic phenomena. The area of pain referral, which is surprisingly consistent, is termed the "zone of reference" (Figs. 19.3 and 19.4). Myofascial pain is thought to occur as a result of an acute muscle strain or "overload" that occurs at the time of impact. One hypothesis is that a small area of muscle contraction develops and becomes self-sustaining (Fig. 19.5). A tender point may then develop in this band of contracted muscle. There are certain factors that patients quickly recognize as aggravators or alleviators of the pain and discomfort caused by these myofascial pain

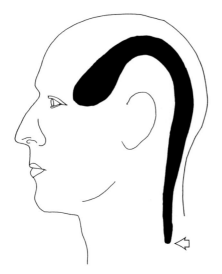

**Figure 19.4.** The trigger point in the upper trapezius muscle is indicated by the *open arrow*. The main area of referred pain is shown in *black*. (Adapted from Travell and Simons (44).)

accompainied by autonomic phenomena. This has obvious relevance to whiplash injuries and explains why pain is often delayed, is frequently referred in nonanatomic patterns, and may be unresponsive to nerve blocks.

Whiplash patients often complain of an achy discomfort in the posterior cervical region radiating into the trapezius ridge, down to the interscapular region, up to the occiput, and/or down the arms. The pattern of radiation of pain is often of little value in localizing the injured site. A deep aching discomfort is often associated with burning and stiffness, with the latter often being worse in the morning. Many patients describe a "cracking" or crepitus when they move their neck. This "cracking" sensation is particularly disconcerting to patients, who associate it with ongoing bony or articular damage. Tenderness is often present over the spinous prominence of the sixth cervical vertebra as well as the posterior paracervical mus-

syndromes (Table 19.4). Aggravating factors are usually related to activities or postures that cause contraction of involved muscles; alleviating factors generally are those that contribute to relaxation of the involved muscles.

An alternative explanation for local tenderness and pain referral is the concept of sclerotomal pain. In early embryologic development of the cervical spine, somites differentiate into a dermatome (area of skin), myotome (muscle), and sclerotome (skeleton) each representing one spinal cord segment. The cells that form these three tissue types migrate, each taking its nerve supply with it. Thus injury at one level of the cervical spine readily exhibits a wide distribution of signs and symptoms such that injury to ligament, tendon, capsule, or muscle may result in perception of pain throughout the entire somite (30). Pain arising from structures below the deep fascia (ligament, tendon, capsule, bone) therefore has certain characteristics that differ from pain arising in other structures (i.e., fascia or muscles). It often presents as an aching discomfort made worse with stretching or stressing the involved structures (31). Experimental mechanical irritation (31–34) of these deep tissues results in poorly localized aching or burning often associated with muscle soreness and tenderness over bony prominences (34). The referred pain, although often delayed in onset, is surprisingly consistent and may often be

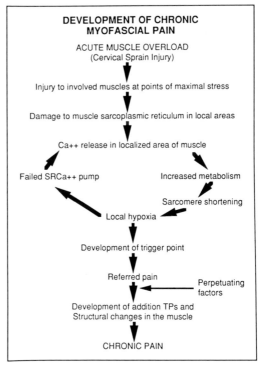

**Figure 19.5.** A proposed mechanism for development of chronic myofascial pain following whiplash injury. An acute muscle overload occurring at the time of impact results in damage to muscle fibers, which develop localized, self-sustaining areas of muscle contraction. Within these localized bands of muscles typical trigger points develop with the characteristic referred pain.

**Table 19.4.**
**Factors Influencing Myofascial Pain Following Whiplash Injuries**

**Aggravating factors**
Strenuous use of involved muscles, especially in shortened position (44) (i.e., heavy lifting, strenuous exercise)
Excessive rapid stretching of the involved muscles
Sustained or repeated contraction of the muscle (44) (i.e., working with arms above level of shoulder or repetitive arm work)
Placing the involved muscle in a shortened position for prolonged periods of time (44) (i.e., long car rides, reading, typing, sleeping)
Applying pressure to trigger point (44)
Cold drafts or cold, damp weather (44)
Periods of muscle tension (i.e., anxiety, anger)

**Alleviating factors**
Short period of rest following activity (44)
Slow, steady passive stretch of the involved muscles (44)
Ice (for less than 5 min) or moist heat applied over the trigger point
Short periods of light activity following prolonged posturing or rest (44)
Specific myofascial therapy (spray and stretch, local injections) (44)
Dry, hot weather

culature. Initially, there may be restricted range of motion of the cervical spine.

Radiographic studies of the cervical spine are generally unremarkable or reveal evidence of pre-existing degenerative changes. The most commonly reported abnormal radiographic finding in the acute phase is straightening of the normal cervical lordotic curve. Rarely, films may reveal evidence of bony injury such as posterior joint crush fractures or minimal subluxation (7). As a rule, however, radiologic investigations are of limited value in diagnosis and prognosis and their main use is in ruling out correctable anatomic injuries. Computed tomographic scanning and magnetic resonance imaging should be reserved for those cases in which cervical disc protrusion or spinal cord injury are suspected. Radionucleotide bone scanning is the most sensitive test for ruling out fractures and should be reserved for situations in which clinical suspicion is great.

## Headache

Headache is a common and disabling symptom. Within 24 hr of the accident, many patients complain of diffuse neck and head pain. The headache may be limited to the occipital area or may spread to involve the vertex, temporal, frontal, and retro-orbital areas (35). The pain may be a dull pressure or squeezing sensation that may include pounding and throbbing (migrainous) components (35, 36). Muscle contraction and vascular headaches often are present simultaneously (posttraumatic mixed headache). These patients may have nausea, vomiting, and photophobia. The frequency of these various forms of headache in patients with whiplash injuries is not known. However, the incidence of unspecified headache in a retrospective analysis of 300 cases was 97% (37).

Traditionally, tension and migraine headaches have been regarded as entirely separate entities, with differing characteristics, mechanisms, and treatment. However, the distinction may not be so apparent in clinical practice since there may be overlapping features between tension and migraine headaches. The clinical spectrum of benign, recurrent headache appears to include classic migraine at one end, the variations of common migraine and tension-vascular headache occupying the vast middle ground, and tension headache at the other end (38) (Fig. 19.6). In our experience common migraine headaches are not uncommon following whiplash injuries and often occur in individuals with no previous history of migraines. They sometimes respond to pharmacologic treatments directed at migrainous symptoms.

## Dysphagia

Dysphagia occurring early after whiplash injury may be the result of esophageal and pharyngeal trauma or a retropharyngeal hematoma. The early occurrence of dysphagia suggests a serious injury likely due to hematoma formation in retropharyngeal structures and is an important prognostic symptom (7). Hoarseness may also be reported but, like dysphagia, is usually seen only in the acute phase, rarely persisting over the long term.

## Visual Disturbances

Patients commonly complain of intermittent blurring of vision, which may cause them to change their glasses without improvement (39). Blurring of vision by itself is not considered to hold prognostic significance. If it is associated with severe damage to the cervical sympathetic trunk it may lead to a Horner's syndrome (7).

## Dizziness

Complaints of dizziness or vertigo-like symptoms are common following whiplash injuries. Many patients complain of suddenly "veering" to one side or feeling dizzy if they move their necks or change their posture too quickly. A variety of theories have been proposed to explain these features, including vertebral artery insufficiency, inner ear damage, injury to the cervical sympathetic chain, and an impaired neck righting reflex. One concept—known as the "reflex" or "neuromuscular" theory—proposes that interference with normal signals coming from the upper cervical joints, muscles, or nerves to the inner ear induces a feeling of ataxia (7, 40). This could explain the posture-related vertigo experienced by many of these patients. This symptom generally disappears as painless neck range of motion is restored.

## Tinnitus

Tinnitus may be due to vertebral artery insufficiency, injury to the cervical sympathetic chain, or inner ear damage. Tinnitus alone does not appear to carry any prognostic significance (7). Additional auditory complaints include decreased hearing and loudness recruitment. Electronystagmographic abnormalities have been reported in a number of whiplash victims (41, 42).

## Other Miscellaneous Symptoms

Anterior chest pain is sometimes seen in a variety of cervical syndromes, and whiplash is no exception. The pain may be mistaken for angina pectoris. It is usually an achy type of pain, made worse with exercise and neck movement and often associated with anterior chest wall tenderness. The electrocardiogram is normal unless there is coincidental cardiac disease. Paresthesias of the face, head, or tongue are occasionally present. Nausea and even vomiting are commonly seen in association with dizziness/vertigo, migrainous-type headaches, or intense unremitting pain. Fatigue and irritability are commonplace and are often associated with a restless, nonrestorative sleep pattern.

## ASSOCIATED DISORDERS

### Arm Pain and Thoracic Outlet Syndrome

Arm pain and paresthesias are reported frequently following whiplash injury. Early authors (43) attributed these symptoms to cervical nerve root compression and reported a high incidence of cervical disc herniation following whiplash injuries. However, modern imaging techniques have shown that disc herniation in association with whiplash injuries is uncommon. Symptoms have also been attributed to "thoracic outlet syndrome" with intermittent or transient compression of the brachial plexus. At present there is little evidence to implicate thoracic outlet syndrome as a sequela of this type of injury.

A common extracervical complaint among whiplash victims is numbness or a "pins and needles" sensation down the arm and into the ipsilateral hand. It is most commonly noted along the ulnar aspect of the forearm and hand. Macnab (7) speculated that symptoms along the ulnar aspect of the distal upper extremity may be the result of

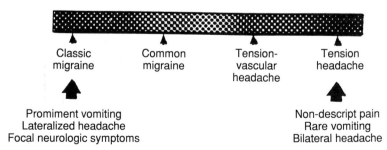

**Figure 19.6.**   Spectrum of benign recurrent headaches includes classical migraine and tension headaches at opposite ends of the spectrum, with common migraines and tension-vascular headaches occupying the middle ground. All of these are commonly seen following whiplash injuries with the exception of classical migraine, and all appear to have a cervicogenic origin. (Adapted from Raskin (38).)

spasm of the scalene muscles compressing the trunks of the brachial plexus. No data supporting this theory have emerged. Another theoretical cause is injury to the zygapophysial or facet joint, which may have been fractured or had its capsule injured at the time of the accident (11). In the acute stage, edema of the joint, or surrounding hemorrhage, may compromise the adjacent nerve roots posteriorly. In the chronic stage, organization of pericapsular exudates could result in nerve root fibrosis. Objective evidence of these various entities is also lacking.

Myofascial trigger points throughout the cervical and upper thoracic musculature are commonly seen following whiplash injury. Several of these trigger points, including those at the infraspinatus, supraspinatus, pectoralis major, scalenes, and serratus anterior, send referred pain and other symptoms down the ipsilateral arm (Fig. 19.3). These referred symptoms may be interpreted in some patients as pain and in others as paresthesias or numbness. Weakness often is present in the same arm and is due in part to lack of use as a result of habitual and instinctive avoidance of activities or movements that cause pain. "Give-way"–type weakness is common and represents an attempt by the patient to avoid excessive pain. Travell and Simons believe that the muscle itself tends to limit the force of its contraction below the trigger point pain threshold, resulting in clinical weakness (44).

In whiplash patients objective neurologic tests are usually normal, as are nerve conduction studies, F wave studies, and needle electromyographic studies. Too often the clinician who is eager to make a psychiatric diagnosis will interpret the nonanatomic numbness and pain as well as the give-way weakness as indications of hysteria or malingering. As discussed later, these symptoms occur with a consistency and frequency that makes a psychological etiology seem unlikely.

## Low Back Pain

The lumbar and thoracolumbar spine may be suddenly forced into extension or flexed forward as the torso moves in an arc over a fixed pelvis. Wiley et al. (37), in a study of 320 uncomplicated whiplash victims, reported a 60% incidence of low back pain. This was thought to result from a sprain or mechanical disruption of the supporting ligaments of the lumbar spine during sudden flexion-extension of the lower back. Braaf and Rosner (45) reported low back pain in 42% of their whip-

lash patients, with sciatic-like symptoms in 15%. Croft and Foreman (46) have reported low back pain in 57% of individuals with moderate to severe whiplash injuries arising from rear-end collisions. Seventy-one percent of patients involved in side-on collisions reported low back pain, prompting the authors to suggest that the lumbar spine was more vulnerable during lateral flexion than flexion-extension. A soft seatback and a lap seat belt with no shoulder strap would be expected to increase the risk of low back pain following motor vehicle accidents.

Like neck pain, low back pain is usually bilateral but may be unilateral or asymmetrical. The pain is typically myofascial, with multiple trigger points noted along the ischial crests, quadratus lumborum and paravertebral muscles, upper sacroliac joints, and sacrum (Fig. 19.7). Prolonged sitting, standing, and lying down all tend to worsen back pain. It is not uncommon for patients to ex-

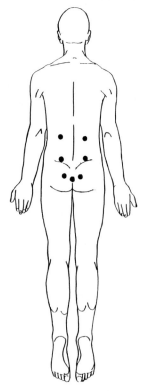

**Figure 19.7.** Some of the common trigger points seen in the lower back. Shown are points over the midsacrum, upper sacroiliac joint, iliac crest, and quadratus lumborum. It is of note that palpation of these areas can reproduce nonneurogenic sciatica, sometimes seen in whiplash patients.

perience paresthesias and referred pain down the leg, which is often mistaken for sciatica. Neurologic examination is invariably normal. Disc herniation does not appear to be a common complication of flexion-extension injuries. Low back pain usually resolves before the neck symptoms but in some cases may persist indefinitely and may even become the prominent persistent complaint.

A particularly confusing group of patients are those with low back pain with an onset several weeks or even months following the accident. Ameis (47) stated, "Back ache occurring for the first time several weeks post trauma probably reflects the effect of spasm and the chronic alteration of posture, anxiety, increased body weight and reduced fitness brought on by the indolence of a prolonged illness." Many patients in this category have no history of low back pain before the accident. One possible explanation is that less severe degrees of low back pain may be overshadowed by neck pain only to be "rediscovered" with natural improvement in neck pain as tissues heal and movement returns. As expected, preexisting low back pain may be aggravated by forced flexion or hyperextension during the accident, and this may account for a large number of individuals with this syndrome.

## Minor Head Injury

The presence of minor brain injury in association with whiplash has been postulated based on observed similarities between the "whiplash syndrome" and the "postconcussion syndrome." However, no convincing data supporting such an association are presently available. It has been proposed that rotational brain shear injuries occur as a result of sudden movement of the skull, especially sudden angular acceleration, resulting in surface trauma to the cerebral cortex and cerebellum. This theory posits that the brain lies relatively free within the skull. As the head moves, the brain, because of its inertia, tends to maintain its position within the vault. The moving skull may therefore concuss the brain either as it rotates backward or as it accelerates forward.

In support of this theory, Torres and Shapiro (48) reported significant electroencephalographic (EEG) abnormalities in 45 patients who had experienced whiplash injuries. Many demonstrated concomitant abnormal neurologic signs. The abnormal EEG findings were similar to those seen in closed head injuries. Similarly, Ommaya et al. (49) induced experimental whiplash injuries in rhesus monkeys and were able to demonstrate consistent brain damage without direct impact to the head. The authors speculated that rotational displacement or acceleration of the head accounted for the observed anatomic lesions. They estimated that, if a car was hit from behind causing it to move at a speed of 18 km/hr (10.8 mph), within 0.1 sec a 5G horizontal acceleration would result, leading to a 50% probability of cerebral contusion for the occupants. Gibbs (50) has also reported a variety of abnormal EEG changes among 178 cases of uncomplicated whiplash injury (see Chapter 26).

The postconcussion syndrome consists of a constellation of symptoms that resemble those seen in whiplash injuries. Alves et al. (51) reported that 6 months after injury the most common complaints in order of decreasing frequency were: headache, memory deficits, dizziness, tinnitus and hearing abnormalities, numbness, weakness, nauseas and diplopia. Many of the complaints lasted for over 1 year, with the majority of patients exhibiting at least one or two symptoms. Like postconcussion syndrome patients, many whiplash victims report feeling "dazed" or "in shock" immediately after trauma, and "whiplash amnesia" has been reported in the neurologic literature (52). Reports of dizziness, tinnitus, and memory and concentration problems are also common following whiplash injuries. Nevertheless, while evidence of an organic etiology for posttraumatic symptoms after concussion is accumulating, its presence after whiplash injuries remains largely speculative.

## Temporomandibular Joint Dysfunction

The diagnosis of temporomandibular joint (TMJ) disorders after whiplash injury has enjoyed increasing popularity. Frankel (53) reported that, following hyperextension injury, 15 of 40 patients had signs and symptoms consistent with damage in the area of the TMJ. However, the true incidence of TMJ disorders is unknown. Controversy regarding the proposed mechanisms of injury to the TMJ abounds. Much of this controversy is related to whether the pain is due to internal derangement of joint structures or is a consequence of myofascial pain involving the surrounding musculature. Making the distinction is important since internal derangement of the joint is often treated with invasive techniques, whereas myofascial pain yields to more conservative measures.

It is noteworthy that the architecture of the

TMJ may predispose to anatomic injury. The joint is a complex two-compartment hinge and gliding joint that has an articular disc interposed between the head of the condyle and the articular eminence. The attachments of this articular disc to the condylar poles are easily injured. Similarly, muscles acting on the joint may themselves be susceptible to injury. During the hyperextension phase of neck movement the mandible may lag behind until it forcibly comes to the limit of its anterior soft tissue attachments. Lack of a sturdy anterior capsule in the TMJ renders it susceptible to stretching with tearing of the (posterior) lateral pterygoid muscle attachment and adjacent synovial tissues in addition to loosening or tearing of the discal attachment to the medial and lateral condylar poles. After the hyperextension phase, the head and neck are snapped forward into hyperflexion at the cervical spine. The mandibular condyle may now be thrown posteriorly to the limit of its position in the glenoid fossa. There is potential for the posterior attachment tissues to be crushed between the mandibular condyle and glenoid fossa of the temporal bone.

The patient with TMJ dysfunction complains of a steady and gnawing pain in the region of the TMJ. It may be worse on arising in the morning, increase as the day progresses, and be exacerbated during periods of stress or in cold weather. Pain may radiate to the frontal temporal region, resulting in a headache. "Clicking" or jaw pain may occur with talking or chewing. The diagnosis is made clinically and radiographs may serve to rule out bony abnormalities. In very select patients, when internal derangement of the joint is suspected, arthrography or magnetic resonance imaging of the TMJ may be employed. Treatment remains controversial, and we opt for a conservative, nonsurgical approach in virtually every case. Treatment options are listed in Table 19.5.

## Fibromyalgia

Fibromyalgia is a painful condition characterized by chronic diffuse musculoskeletal aches, pains, and stiffness and associated with marked tenderness at characteristic anatomic locations known as fibrositic tender points. The clinical features of fibromyalgia are well described and are listed in Table 19.6. The prominent feature is widespread musculoskeletal pain, which is most prominent in the axial skeletal regions, including the neck, shoulders, lower back, and hips. The pain typically has a deep, aching quality. Other symptoms include a subjective feeling of swelling, numbness and paresthesias involving the extremities, fatigue, stiffness, nonrestorative sleep, anxiety, irritable bowel symptoms, and chronic headaches. Patients often have difficulty sleeping and awaken frequently. Most complain of awakening in the morning feeling poorly rested. Stiffness and fatigue on arising in the morning are very common. Symptoms are often worse during cold, damp weather and in women just before menstruation.

**Table 19.5.**
**Treatment Options for TMJ Disorders**

Reassurance
Soft diet
Anti-inflammatory medications
Physical therapy
Transcutaneous electrical nerve stimulation
Biofeedback and relaxation therapy
Psychotherapy
Orthotics (bite appliances)
Restorative dental treatment
Surgical procedures
Arthroscopy
Disc repositioning and plication
Discectomy with or without implants
Total joint replacement

**Table 19.6.**
**Clinical Manifestations of Fibromyalgia**

**Musculoskeletal symptoms**
   Diffuse aches and pains
   Diffuse stiffness
   Subjective soft tissue swelling
   Self-palpated tender spots
**Nonmusculoskeletal symptoms**
   Fatigue
   Nonrestorative sleep pattern
   Irritable bowel symptoms
   Muscle contraction (tension) headaches
   Painful menstruation
   Anxiety/stress
   Paresthesias
**Physical examination**
   Tender points at specific sites (usually more than
      four sites)
   Cutaneous hyperemia at sites of tender point
      palpation
   Skin roll tenderness
   Diffuse soft tissue swelling (commonly in hands)
   Abdominal tenderness (related to irritable bowel
      syndrome)

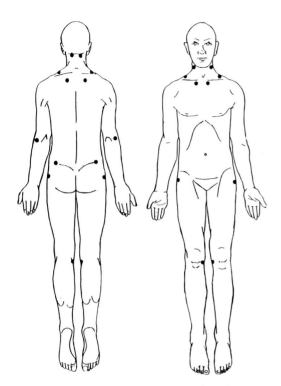

**Figure 19.8.**  Typical fibrositic tender points.

Physical examination shows normal joint and neurologic findings. However, fibromyalgia is characterized by many tender points at well-described sites that are consistently present. Laboratory tests are normal.

Fibromyalgia is a clinical diagnosis, and various criteria were recently subjected to validation by a group of North American rheumatologists headed by Wolfe (54). New criteria for the diagnosis of fibromyalgia include:

Widespread pain involving both the upper and lower parts of the skeleton in bilateral distribution.
Tenderness at 11 or more of 18 specified fibrositic tender points.

These criteria performed equally well in patients with and without other rheumatic conditions, with a sensitivity and specificity of 88.6% and 88.1%, respectively. The designated fibrositic tender points are shown in Figure 19.8. A particularly frustrating group of patients are those with a typical whiplash injury who, rather than gradually improving, actually seem to progressively develop a generalized chronic pain state identical to the fibromyalgia syndrome. Patients with severe whiplash injuries often meet established criteria for fi-

bromyalgia. This carries with it a generally poorer prognosis.

## PSYCHOSOCIAL PROBLEMS

In patients with chronic pain, psychosocial problems inevitably develop in response to unremitting discomfort and subsequent disability. Personality changes, depression, difficulty coping with everyday activities, anxiety, anger, frustration, preoccupation with somatic complaints, marital stress, financial pressures, and unemployment are common (Fig. 19.9). One difficulty encountered by clinicians is determining whether the patient's psychosocial problems experienced in response to pain are appropriate.

Unfortunately, the psychosocial sequelae of chronic pain are often misinterpreted, at least on initial assessment, as the source of, rather than the result of, pain. In other words persistent pain is

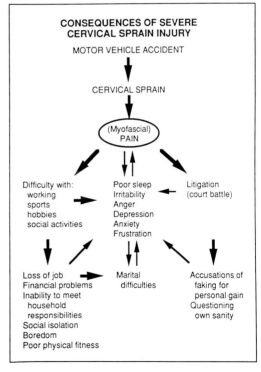

**Figure 19.9.**  Whiplash injuries can have far-reaching consequences that go beyond the pain itself and affect the individual psychosocially. After severe injuries chronic pain can completely dominate the individual's life. Unfortunately these psychosocial consequences interact with each other and eventually influence the pain itself.

seen as the result of an inadequate personality or primary psychiatric disorder. This belief has enjoyed remarkable popularity and has resulted in patients with chronic pain and disability secondary to whiplash injuries being labeled as hysterical, somatizers, hypochondriacs, "psychogenic pain" sufferers, and malingerers. Attribution of whiplash symptoms to a psychological etiology persists among many clinicians and is reinforced by the high selection bias of patients attending speciality practices. This section summarizes our current view of psychological difficulties experienced by these patients and provides an overview for management of these difficult problems.

## Stages of Chronic Pain

Hendler (55) described four stages of psychological reaction to chronic pain, which are applicable and modifiable to chronic whiplash injuries. In the initial stage, lasting up to 2 months, the patient is generally calm and optimistic, confident that he or she will eventually recover. The second stage is marked by anxiety about outcome because of persistence of symptoms. Preoccupation with symptoms is not unusual. The third stage is characterized by depression, which generally starts within the first 6 months and may last for several years. This is a crucial point at which the patient realizes the pain and subsequent disability may persist indefinitely; at this stage the patient may view his or her situation as hopeless.

The final stage is the adjustment phase, which takes from 3 to 12 years after the onset of pain. During this stage depression resolves, but somatic complaints persist, resulting in psychological changes even in a previously well-adjusted individual (55). During this final stage the patient finally comes to terms with chronic pain and its subsequent disability and establishes a new equilibrium. Some patients never achieve this final stage, which represents a compromise between desired goals and previous activity levels.

Although these four stages are arbitrary and may not necessarily occur sequentially, they can be used empirically to explain the psychological reactions seen in many whiplash patients. Some patients never progress beyond the second or the third stages. Premorbid coping skills, ethnocultural behavior and attitudes, and marital or vocational stresses may contribute to the patient failing to reach the final stage of adjustment. Education of the patient and a supportive clini-

cian may help to reduce the psychological sequelae of these injuries.

## Premorbid Coping Skills

Patients bring to any stressful situation varying coping skills and strategies. Some patients cope better with persistent pain and disability than others. Poor copers generally are individuals with a history of premorbid psychological problems, poor self-esteem, or nonsupportive environments. Often their symptoms and subsequent disability are out of proportion to physical signs. These individuals are not hysterical or malingering but rather have dysfunctional coping styles that may augment their pain experience. They are often labeled histrionic or somatizers and are an important group since they account for a disproportionately large number of referrals to pain specialists and chronic pain clinics. Some characteristic features of poor copers are listed in Table 19.7.

## Social Consequences

Many whiplash patients have a difficult time dealing with the fact that they appear normal and their pain and disability are not immediately apparent to peers and relatives. Those around the patient find it difficult to recognize the impairment and subsequent disability; professionals also often find it difficult to recognize the disabilities as legitimate. The result is that the unwary observer may underestimate the injured individual's difficulties and overestimate his or her capabilities.

**Table 19.7.**
**Clues to Diagnosing Individuals with Poor Coping Skills**

Premorbid psychological problems (i.e., depression, suicide attempt)
Premorbid personality disorder
History of childhood abuse (physical, sexual, or psychological)
Coming from a broken home
Difficulty establishing interpersonal relationships
Marital problems
Dramatic presentation
Dependent and demanding behavior
History of alcohol and drug abuse
Females more likely than males
Immigrant with poor communication skills
Often limited education

There is a societal expectation that disabled individuals should have physical evidence of an impairment. So strong is this expectation that many patients who have not been given a proper diagnosis and explanation for their symptoms think they are "going crazy."

Whiplash victims who are experiencing continuous chronic pain often feel that they have little control over what happens to them. They complain that the pain rules their lives, determining when and where they can work, interfering with their social and leisure activities, and creating a cloud of uncertainty over their future. Once pain develops there is often little the individual can do to alleviate it. A sense of lack of control eventually leads to a state of "learned helplessness" and defeat, which in turn leads to chronic anxiety and depression. Personality changes are common in this setting. A kindly, well-adjusted individual may become irritable, argumentative, and depressed, with limited tolerance for children, friends, spouse, fellow employees, and others. These patients may go on to develop marital or employment difficulties and experience social isolation.

Many whiplash victims find it difficult to return to work after their injury, especially if their job involves working with their arms above the level of their shoulders, heavy lifting, repetitive arm work, prolonged sitting at a desk, and emotional tension. Where the individual is the principal breadwinner, financial and job security stresses may become overwhelming. As a result the individual often returns to work prematurely, causing an exacerbation of pain that leads the patient to again withdraw from work and further increases feelings of helplessness and hopelessness. Withholding or delaying financial compensation only contributes to anxiety about meeting financial obligations.

According to Ameis (47), role reversal by the family is the most "deadly" of the possible psychological consequences to recovery. When the dominant member is struck down by pain and impaired in daily function, some degree of sympathetic support is necessary and expected. However, when family members overprotect the injured individual, incentives to recover may be reduced. Family role reversal may occur out of genuine concern for the patient, through manipulation by the patient, or because the new dynamics of the family relationship develop maturity and independence in its other members. Unless such overcompensation is avoided, a state of dependency will be induced in the patient that may subsequently be difficult to reverse.

## Depression

In patients with persistent pain and disability, discouragement leads to despair and eventual depression. However, the relationship of pain to depression is an uncertain one. The prevalence of depressive disorders in patients with chronic pain is reported to be well over 30%, with significant variation depending on the target population (56), leading some to regard idiopathic chronic pain as a form of "masked depression." Chronic pain sufferers often deny feeling depressed and may instead complain of anxiety, focusing on their somatic complaints. The loss of control experienced by so many whiplash victims may play a central role in the development of depression. Depression may serve to heighten the pain experience, thereby intensifying the perception of pain, reducing motivation, and hindering therapeutic interventions.

## Posttraumatic Stress Syndrome

Posttraumatic stress syndrome is a form of anxiety neurosis that is seen in up to one third of accident victims. It is most prevalent in the first few weeks or months after the accident. The patient experiences panic attacks, often repetitively reliving the accident. The individual usually develops an unreasonable fear of riding in the car. This is considered to be a learned response and is closely related to the rape experience and other "assaults" of a deeply personal nature (47).

## MANAGEMENT OF WHIPLASH INJURIES

It is important to recognize that the symptoms associated with cervical soft tissue injuries may be prolonged, often with substantial disability. The successful clinician will develop a rational, progressive treatment program geared to the individual patient, taking into account not only the injury but the individual's peculiar reaction to the pain and disability and the impact it has on his or her family and vocational and avocational activities. The influence of outside environmental factors on the symptoms and subsequent disability must also be taken into account.

## NATURAL HISTORY OF WHIPLASH INJURIES

In the majority of cases, the natural history of soft tissue injuries following motor vehicle accidents is that of a slow, steady recovery. Only a minority of patients (10–15%) go on to develop chronic disabling pain. Recovery can be arbitrarily divided into three stages (47):

1. *Acute Posttrauma Phase:* During the acute stage the patient presents with pain, muscle spasm, and restriction of neck movement. The clinical picture generally develops over several hours after the accident and peaks the following morning or over the following few days. In more severe cases dysphagia may be present and the patient often complains of dizziness, tinnitus, or blurred vision. This acute phase usually lasts from one to several weeks.
2. *Postacute Phase:* Over time there is an easing of muscle spasm, allowing more neck movement to occur. This improvement may begin after the first week following the injury but generally takes longer. This phase may be delayed by injudicious collar use or excessive guarding on the part of the patient. Dizziness gradually disappears but associated new symptoms, in particular arm and low back pain, may appear at this stage. Patients often still have difficulty returning to work and experience pain every day, although they may begin to have pain-free periods, especially earlier in the day.
3. *Symptom Resolution/Persistence:* In this final phase most patients recover to almost full neck range of motion and strength, paralleled by the resumption of normal activities. At this point they are usually able to return to work. However, there are upper limits to the intensity and duration of activities they can perform without suffering from neck pain and headaches. Intolerance of prolonged positioning in one posture is very common and vigorous return to sport or heavy manual work often continues to be painful. Patient motivation and pain tolerance are important factors in determining the pace of recovery, especially during this last stage. This final stage is the longest and even the best motivated patient may fail to make a full "functional recovery."

### Functional Recovery

A functional recovery may be said to occur when a patient is able to carry out a full spectrum of normal activities, with a frequency and to a level of intensity and duration that are reasonable for his or her age, skills, and needs (47). What is often not appreciated is that whether a functional recovery is achieved varies significantly from individual to individual and is largely dependent on the external demands placed on him or her. For example,

Table 19.8.
**Factors Indicating a Poorer Prognosis following Cervical Whiplash Injury**

Rear-end collision
Wearing seat belt
Female sex
Increasing age
Preexisting cervical degenerative disc disease
Previous whiplash injury
Initial dysphagia, Horner's syndrome, or loss of consciousness
Arm numbness and pain
Persisting sleep disturbance
Prolonged collar use
Generalized pain syndrome (i.e., fibromyalgia)
Severe depression or anxiety
Vocation requiring manual labor
Lower socioeconomic group
Presence of litigation

an office worker or physician may achieve a functional recovery while a construction laborer doing heavy manual labor may not despite similar injuries.

Approximately 10–15% of patients suffering from cervical soft tissue injuries following motor vehicle accidents fail to achieve a functional recovery even after the passage of 2–3 years. This means that they are still left with pain and discomfort sufficient enough to seriously interfere with their ability to perform work or engage in leisure activities. It is these individuals who dominate chronic pain clinics and pain specialty practices. Many of these individuals have limited educational skills and are employed doing heavy manual labor or repetitive upper extremity work. The data suggest, therefore, that the patient with a cervical soft tissue injury following a motor vehicle accident has an 85–90% chance of achieving a functional recovery (47). Between 40 and 70% of these patients retain some degree of intermittent discomfort or "nuisance" symptoms (7, 57). These symptoms are distracting and may be occasionally intolerable, but do not detract from job performance and most leisure activities.

According to Macnab (9), if at the end of 6 weeks the patient has continuous pain, he or she can be expected to have intermittent symptoms for an additional 6–12 months. Similarly, Ameis (47) reported that the chance of achieving a functional recovery decreases with the duration of symptoms after injury. He indicated that 50% of patients will have made a functional recovery at the end of the first year; a further 25% may recover during the next 6 months. Patients still not able to return to full-time work or enjoy leisure activities after 18 months have a poor prognosis, with less than a 25% chance of recovery. Factors that indicate a poorer prognosis are listed in Table 19.8.

## THE TREATMENT PROGRAM

Treatment must take into consideration a variety of therapeutic interventions if the patient's recovery of function is to be maximized. Various treatment principles and options are listed below.

Ruling out treatable radiologic abnormalities (e.g., fractures of cervical spine, herniated disc).
Education of the patient as to the nature of injury and aggravating factors.
Avoidance of prolonged cervical collar use.
Use of graduated stretching exercises to be performed by the patient on a regular basis.
Attention to good posture.
Eventual strengthening of related musculature.
Promotion of general aerobic fitness.
Understanding the role of the patient's personality and emotional state in reaction to the injury.
Use of relaxation techniques and stress management.
Dealing with aggravating environmental factors.
Consideration of work modification and retraining.
Avoidance of surgery.
Emphasis on improved function and pain control as opposed to pain relief.

The idea that function takes precedence over pain relief is a difficult one for patients to grasp and accept. Patients hope and expect that treatment will result in a resolution of their pain. There are many treatment options available to the clinician treating whiplash victims (Table 19.9). Most available treatments have not been tested appropriately in proper clinical trials. The clinician must guide each patient through a pragmatic management program wherein the goals are pain control and a return to maximum functioning using whatever therapeutic intervention works for that individual. In this regard the doctor-patient relationship is vital, and it is important to understand conflicts that may endanger this relationship.

## PATIENT-PHYSICAN CONFLICTS

Patients with chronic whiplash injuries are among the most difficult to treat. Physicians are often ill-prepared to properly deal with these individuals because modern medicine emphasizes disease rather than illness. Traditional medical training focuses on physical pathology and demonstrable pathophysiology (i.e., disease) with little regard for the patient's perception of and response to his or her disease (i.e., the patient's illness). What often results is conflict between a difficult patient and an unprepared physician.

## The Difficult Chronic Whiplash Patient

Many chronic whiplash patients are the antithesis of the "ideal patient" (Table 19.10). The patient who comes to the physician for help may be threatened with loss of job, business, or home as well as marital discord and disintegration of relationships. Expectations of the medical system are often very high and as a result patients may continually (and often aggressively) seek different medical opinions and treatment. The result may be the development of an interaction style with physicians that can best be termed "hostile dependency."

These patients often express disillusionment with previous medical efforts to relieve their pain. Extensive testing, multiple medications, various therapies, and sometimes surgical operations fail to demonstrate an objective source of symptoms or provide a reliable relief of their pain. The pa-

**Table 19.9.**
**Elements of Treatment of Whiplash Injuries**

Therapeutic alliance
Reassurance
Education
Rest
Cervical collar
Early mobilization
Spray and stretch
Physical modalities
Transcutaneous electrical nerve stimulation
Posture—sleeping, sitting, standing
Traction
Manipulation
Acupuncture/acupressure
Massage
Injections
Medications
Psychology
Relaxation training
Biofeedback
Pacing of activities
Avoiding pain-aggravating activities
Vocational retraining

**Table 19.10.**
**Ideal Patient Versus Chronic Whiplash Patient**

| Ideal Patient | Chronic Whiplash Patient |
| --- | --- |
| Cooperative | Often hostile and resentful |
| Well motivated | Motivation in doubt |
| Optimistic | Depressed and frustrated |
| Compliant | Often poor compliance |
| Not demanding | Often demanding |
| Appreciative | Not always appreciative |
| High pain tolerance | At limits of pain tolerance |
| Confident in physician | Suspicious of physician |
| Never seeks second opinion | Seeks multiple opinions, including those of paramedical persons |
| Financially secure | Financial problems |
| Supportive family | Family does not understand |
| Flexible, nonmanual job | Inflexible manual labor |
| Good education/ skills | Limited education/skills |
| Not interested in litigation | Litigation pending |

tient naturally becomes suspicious of a medical system that he or she sees as impotent and often uncaring. Many drop out of the medical system entirely and enter a paramedical subculture populated by chiropractors, massage therapists, holistic healers, and the like, where easily understood explanations are given and the legitimacy of their symptoms is rarely questioned.

Dependency arises from a variety of factors. Patients often continue to see physicians to achieve adequate documentation for compensation purposes. Physicians therefore serve to legitimize the "sick role" in our society. In addition, physicians are the source of medications that may help to relieve pain. Patients often hold out the hope that the medical system can eventually resolve their pain.

## Medical Approach to Disease (Acute Medical Model)

With increasingly sophisticated technology and a better understanding of the pathophysiology of diseases, physicians are now able to effectively diagnose and treat a large number of medical conditions. This has resulted in better care for patients but it has brought with it marked changes in physician (and patient) attitudes. Medical training has emphasized teaching the "acute medical

model of disease." This is based on the premise that the patient's signs and symptoms can be reduced to a single disease state. The physician employs diagnostic tests to confirm clinical findings and then orders appropriate treatment based on the diagnosis. The goal is elimination of the disease state with amelioration of the patient's symptoms (Fig. 19.10). Deviation from this model is often considered unorthodox, and much of a physician's self-esteem as a clinician is related to his or her skill in effectively diagnosing and treating disease states.

## Physicians' Reactions to Chronic Whiplash Patients

Unfortunately, the chronic whiplash patient often presents with a plethora of complaints out of proportion to objective findings, refractoriness to standard medical therapy, psychosocial problems often as a consequence of symptoms, and complex litigation issues. The subjective complaints often fluctuate or are nonanatomic in nature. Therefore, chronic whiplash often fails to meet the criteria for a "disease state" as defined by traditional medical teaching. Furthermore, failure of the patient to respond to treatment may make the clinician feel inept and threatened.

When the patient's complaints fail to meet the

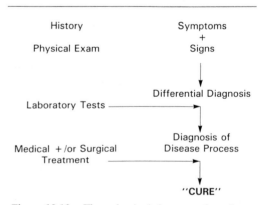

**REDUCTIONISTIC APPROACH TO DISEASE**
**(Acute Medical Model)**

**Figure 19.10.** The reductionistic approach to disease, better known as the acute medical model. The physician takes a history and examines the patient and then, with the help of diagnostic tests, is able to reduce signs and symptoms to a single disease diagnosis. He or she then applies appropriate medical and surgical treatments in an attempt to "cure" the disease process. Physicians often have difficulty applying this acute medical model to whiplash patients.

criteria of an acute disease state, many physicians quickly resort to a mind-body dualism that views problems as either physical or psychological. In truth the patient is held responsible for his or her continuing complaints. The chronic pain patient who has litigation pending or who is receiving compensation is particularly susceptible to this attitude, wherein symptoms may also be attributed to "secondary gain" or compensation neurosis. Diamond and Grauer (58), in their review of physicians' reactions to patients with chronic pain, stated, "The major reactions of physicians to patients with the chronic pain syndrome are frustration, disapproval, anger, uncertainty and rejection. The physician must understand that although these reactions are normal, they may interfere with optimal rapport and management. Understanding these reactions can help guide the physician in the management of patients with chronic pain."

## BASIC TREATMENT MEASURES

### Education

Education of the patient (and family) is very important in relieving anxiety and reducing the frustration that frequently accompanies chronic whiplash injuries. Knowledge brings with it a greater sense of control and confidence, which is so often lacking in these patients. Accurate information and reassurance should be provided as soon after the accident as possible. The mechanism of the injury should be explained to the patient and it should be emphasized that the symptoms experienced by the patient are common to this type of injury and entirely appropriate. The concept that properly educating patients regarding their injury causes prolongation of symptoms does not appear to be valid, and providing information appears to have only beneficial effects. Suggestions that the patient may be malingering or suffering from a "litigation neurosis" or that the symptoms are "in your head" are inappropriate and detract from optimal patient care. Finally, the patient must be aware of treatment goals (i.e., return of function versus complete relief of pain) and the likely prognosis. We provide our patients with a handout carefully outlining the above information.

After the acute stage is over, a very important concept for the patient to understand is that "hurt is not harm." Most patients believe that when they experience neck and shoulder pain they must be reinjuring the involved area. As a re-

sult they may limit their activities and movement of their neck in an attempt to limit the pain. This may result in subsequent loss of range of motion, which may result in further increases in pain. Advice against certain aggravating activities such as prolonged desk work, typing, lifting heavy loads, or reading with the neck in a prolonged flexed position may help to prevent significant exacerbations of pain. Symptomatic patients should avoid working overtime and working through their regular breaks. In many cases patients need to find a different job, especially if their work involves heavy lifting or working with the neck in a continuously flexed posture. Some patients must be temporarily withdrawn from work and in other cases the workload hours must be reduced substantially.

### Rest and the Cervical Collar

Patients with whiplash injuries are initially treated with rest to allow healing to occur and prevent excessive pain. Bed rest is sometimes recommended for the first 24 hr but is generally unnecessary. Resting the damaged neck for too long may itself have detrimental effects and may actually prolong subsequent disability. There is a growing trend toward early mobilization of these injuries to promote earlier recovery and reduce subsequent disability.

The initial use of a cervical collar is very common but remains controversial. A recent controlled, double-blind study demonstrated that patients mobilized early without a collar did better, with greater reduction of pain and improved cervical range of motion (59). The collar, if used, should splint the neck in slight flexion and should fit comfortably. A soft cervical collar splints but does not immobilize the neck. The duration of collar use in cervical soft tissues is controversial, but continuous use for more than 2 weeks should be discouraged. Prolonged collar use leads to a variety of complications, including:

Disuse atrophy of the neck muscles
Soft tissue contractures
Shortening of muscles
Thickening of the subcapsular tissues
Increased dependency and enhancement of feelings of disability

Collar use should not be abruptly withdrawn but rather weaned gradually. This is generally done by having the patient wear it 2 hr on and 1 hr off for several days, followed by 1 hr on and 2

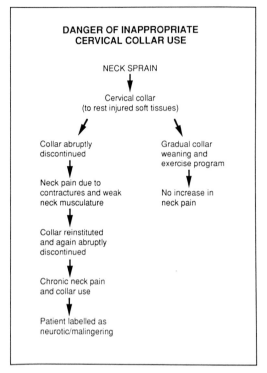

**Figure 19.11.** Excessive collar wearing in combination with lack of a collar weaning program may result in an iatrogenic dependency on the cervical collar.

hr off, with the collar then being discontinued. The collar weaning program should be performed in conjunction with a neck exercise program. Failure to use a collar weaning/exercise program may serve to perpetuate pain complaints during and after collar use (Fig. 19.11). The patient who abruptly stops wearing the collar may immediately experience an increase in pain as a result of cervical soft tissue contractures and weakened neck musculature. The patient may then be placed back in the collar for a further period, after which it is again abruptly discontinued. The cycle is continued and the end result is chronic collar use and perpetuation of chronic pain. At this point the patient may be considered either neurotic or a malingerer rather than suffering from an iatrogenic problem (19).

Examples of appropriate use of cervical collars include: (*a*) at night, especially if the patient has a tendency to sleep with the neck in prolonged forward flexion; (*b*) during long car rides; and (*c*) during periods of reading or studying. Cervical collars therefore remain a useful therapeutic tool, but their use must be carefully limited.

## Sleeping Posture

Poor sleeping postures can result in an intensification and prolongation of symptoms. In the ideal sleeping posture the patient is supine with adequate support of the cervical lordosis. Side lying is acceptable provided that the neck can be kept in a neutral position and not laterally flexed. Lying prone, or on the stomach, is contraindicated because it keeps the neck laterally rotated and under strain. Sleeping with no pillow causes the neck to go into lateral flexion or extension and should be avoided. Sleeping with one large pillow or several pillows causes lateral flexion (when sleeping on the side) or forward flexion (when sleeping supine) and is also best avoided. The patient should be encouraged to sleep with one small pillow or a special cervical pillow designed to support the cervical lordosis. The ideal cervical pillow is one that supports the neck in the neutral position while supine and prevents lateral flexion/rotation at the same time. A soft and sagging mattress or a motion waterbed makes proper positioning of the neck difficult and may also aggravate associated low back pain.

## Sitting and Standing Postures

Careful attention to posture is another important but often overlooked element of pain management. Prolonged sitting in one posture, particularly with the neck in a forward flexed position, generally results in an exacerbation of neck pain and headache. This is usually reported after long car rides, reading, or in clerical and typing/computer jobs, which whiplash patients find difficult. One way to limit the pain is to have the patient take a regular break every 30 or 40 min, moving the neck around and changing position during the break. Whiplash patients should be taught that the ideal posture when both sitting or standing is to keep the neck straight with the shoulders pulled back. Another difficult posture is working the arms above the level of the shoulders. Washing windows, painting, haircutting, filing, and reaching for things in a high cupboard all can result in an increase in neck and trapezius pain. Some special adaptations, such as using a drafting style of desk to allow it to be tilted up, thereby reducing neck forward flexion, are often quite helpful.

## PHYSICAL THERAPIES

Physical therapy should be directed along rational lines and its use should be time limited. Physical modalities such as local heat and cold, traction, manipulation, and massage therapy may provide temporary relief of pain but do not appear to provide long-term benefit. Therefore, use of these physical therapy techniques should not take away from time at work and must provide some improvement in terms of functional abilities. The emphasis of physical therapy should be on a graduated stretching routine designed to eventually restore full neck range of motion. In addition, some exercises should be designed to restore a measure of aerobic fitness.

## Physical Modalities

In the early acute phase of whiplash ice packs may be helpful to limit muscle swelling. After the acute phase (3–10 days after the accident) local hot packs, ultrasound, interferential or transcutaneous electrical nerve stimulation (TENS) may be helpful in temporarily reducing pain. Moist heat tends to be more effective than dry heat. Many patients find it useful to apply ice to involved areas for 3–5 min before stretching the involved muscles. Ice applied longer than 5 min tends to cool the muscles and may actually make the pain worse. Application of physical modalities seldom provides more than transient relief, and their use should not supplant time spent on postural education and exercises.

## Exercises

Exercises with the emphasis on stretching and increasing activity form the cornerstone of a successful treatment program. Exercises are initially best taught to the patient by a physiotherapist to ensure that they are being performed properly. After that emphasis is on a home exercise program with frequent monitoring by a therapist and/or clinician. This encourages the patient to take a more active role in his or her recovery. Early mobilization of the neck is to be encouraged even if it is uncomfortable. Early mobilization should be gentle and graduated to allow full healing of soft tissue damage and avoid excessive exacerbations of pain.

Between 1 and 2 days after the injury patients can be started on gentle, progressive stretching exercises. These exercises should not cause excessive pain and therefore need to be carefully monitored. The stretching of muscles to their normal length is necessary to restore normal function and minimize pain. Isometric strengthening exercises

of the cervical musculature should not be started until after the acute pain has subsided. Strong neck musculature helps to provide a strong, active physiologic splint. However, if exercises are done too aggressively, particularly in the early phase, exacerbations of pain often result.

## Traction

Traction has been advocated by some authors, but in our experience cervical traction often aggravates symptoms in both the acute and later stages. In the initial period traction is contraindicated because distractive forces may increase pain and further damage healing tissues. Manual traction provided by a physiotherapist may be useful in providing temporary relief of pain. Traction is no substitute for a proper stretching program.

## Manipulation

Of all therapeutic techniques available to treat whiplash victims, cervical manipulation is the most controversial. The aim of manipulation is to restore full range and quality of motion to affected muscles, ligaments, and joints. The best known form of manipulation is the "adjustment" or high-velocity, low-amplitude thrust. It begins with the patient positioned in such a way that muscles or joints are placed at maximum stretch so that the stretched muscle cannot effectively resist the manipulation thrust. At this point the manipulator applies additional stretch or "thrust," which results in the distraction of the joint or tissue being treated. There is a sudden yielding and an audible "crack" may be heard. Movement is now slightly increased beyond the physiologic limit into the paraphysiologic space. A second final barrier may then be met, formed by the stretched ligaments and joint capsule; this is the limit of anatomic integrity, and forcing movement beyond this point would damage ligaments and the joint capsule (Fig. 19.12). The additional abrupt stretch on the maximally extended muscles is said to stimulate muscle spindles and connective tissue proprioceptive organs, resulting in further sudden relaxation of the muscles and transient relief of pain.

We do not perform manipulation, but many of our patients report that although the "thrust" initially increases pain, after an hour they experience a marked lessening of the pain that can sometimes last for several days. This is followed by a gradual return of pain. It is still not known for certain how

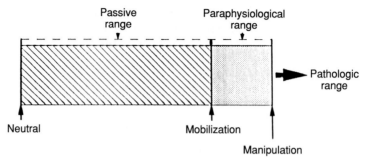

**Figure 19.12.** The stages of manipulation of a joint are shown. The apparent key to a successful manipulation is movement of the joint outside the passive range into the paraphysiologic range but not into the pathologic range.

manipulation works to relieve pain, but postulated mechanisms include alteration of sensory input from joints and soft tissues through mechanoreceptor stimulation, reflex effects upon increased muscle tone, restoration of extensibility to soft tissues, and the psychological effects of being carefully assessed and treated sympathetically. Manipulation may therefore disrupt, if only temporarily, the cycle of pain and muscle tension in some whiplash victims.

Forceful cervical manipulation procedures may result in rare but serious complications, such as vertebral artery dissection with stroke and cervical spinal cord injury. Disease processes and injuries that weaken bone and joint structures as well as other soft tissues, making them especially vulnerable to sudden stresses, are contraindications to forceful manipulation (Table 19.11). A transient worsening of pain and discomfort with no subsequent relief is not uncommon. The greatest difficulty with manipulation is that its effects are transient and generally need to be repeated. This may foster attitudes of passivity and dependency in patients. Practitioners of manipulation, in particular chiropractors, often use manipulation in isolation and not as a component of a more comprehensive pain management program.

## Massage

Massage therapy is a time-honored treatment for musculoskeletal problems, in particular myofascial pain and increased muscle tension. However, there is no evidence that it produces any long-lasting benefits. Massage, like manipulation, can play a role in keeping the patient functional by providing a temporary relief of pain. It is particularly effective in situations in which muscle tension and pain gradually build up (e.g., an office worker or a student studying for an exam) because it results

**Table 19.11.**
**Contraindications to Cervical Manipulation**

**Absolute contraindications**
  Malignant disease of the bone or soft tissues
  Osteomyelitis
  Osteoporosis of cervical vertebrae
  Spinal cord compression
  Recent fracture of cervical vertebrae
  Vertebrobasilar insufficiency
  Inflammatory arthritis, in particular rheumatoid arthritis
  Bony or ligamentous instability of cervical spine
  Severe nerve root irritation or compression
  *Acute* whiplash injury of the neck
  Anticoagulant therapy and current or recent steroid therapy
**Relative contraindications**
  Severe pain, made worse with manipulation
  Acute nerve root pain
  Worsening of signs and symptoms while being manipulated
  Developing psychological dependence on cervical manipulation

in muscle relaxation and a decrease in pain. Any massage therapy should be gentle; aggressive massage or deep friction techniques usually result in poorly tolerated increases in pain.

## MEDICATIONS

Medications have a limited role in the management of whiplash injuries and carry with them the potential for misuse and side effects. Many whiplash victims take substantial quantities of analgesics, often narcotics, even though they may provide limited benefit. The need for medication must be carefully assessed in chronic pain sufferers. Too often the side effects of the drug outweigh the benefits of pain reduction/control or improvement in function.

## Analgesics

Analgesic medications have their greatest application in the acute stage. Nonsteroidal anti-inflammatory drugs are more likely to benefit patients through their analgesic properties than through their anti-inflammatory properties. Narcotic analgesics may be needed in the first few weeks but their use must be carefully monitored and limited because of the risk of addiction. Their long-term use should be discouraged. More recently, there has been a trend toward more liberal use of narcotics in those individuals who remain functional with adequate analgesia and who are not considered likely to become psychologically dependent on narcotics. For patients who use large amounts of narcotic analgesics, the drugs are best given on a time-contingent basis rather than an "as-needed" basis. The total daily dose of analgesic should be determined and then divided into equal doses given at regular intervals such that the contingency of having pain is removed from the dosing schedule.

## Tricyclic Antidepressants

Tricyclic antidepressants such as amitriptyline, imipramine, trazodone, or doxepin, administered in small doses before bedtime, are often helpful in patients with a nonrestorative sleep pattern. It is important to avoid the trap of inducing artificial sleep with benzodiazepines, which themselves do not significantly affect stage 4 sleep. Tricyclic antidepressants such as amitriptyline or doxepin, administered in small doses at bedtime, may help ameliorate symptoms of pain in whiplash patients. The mechanism of action is not clear but may be related to the ability of tricyclic antidepressants to block the reuptake of serotonin in neurons of selected areas of the brain and spinal cord. These drugs therefore may enhance endogenous pain control pathways. Alternatively, they may act by reducing alpha wave intrusion into the normal delta wave pattern of non-REM stage 4 sleep, thereby reducing the prevalance of nonrestorative sleep so common in patients with this condition.

The major side effects of tricyclic antidepressants are dry mouth and morning drowsiness. We use amitriptyline and find that most patients who benefit from this medication need only 25–50 mg at bedtime; doses over 75 mg increase side effects

with little added therapeutic benefit. In our experience up to half of our patients taking amitriptyline obtain some or no benefit while the rest experience intolerable side effects, often at doses as low as 10 mg at bedtime, and must discontinue the medication.

## Cyclobenzaprine

Cyclobenzaprine (Flexeril) is similar to amitriptyline in its chemical structure. It is a tricyclic compound that has neurologic activity that results in reduced somatic motor tone (muscle relaxation). It is useful in some patients both in the acute and chronic stage. Cyclobenzaprine is prescribed in doses of 10 mg up to three times a day and may serve as an alternative drug for those patients intolerant to amitriptyline or other tricyclic antidepressant medications.

## SURGERY

Surgical intervention following cervical soft tissue injuries is rarely, if ever, indicated. Anterior cervical discectomy and fusion have been suggested (9) for those patients with intractable symptoms lasting over 2 years and localized to a single vertebral or intervertebral level (19). Even when computed tomography shows cervical disc herniation it is unlikely to be the sole source of pain in these complicated patients. Surgical intervention is therefore of little or no usefulness in most whiplash patients.

## PSYCHOLOGY

Psychological reactions to chronic pain and disability are common and may serve to intensify the experience or perception of pain. Patients differ in their coping strategies and many demonstrate poor coping abilities. The psychologist's role is to identify emotional problems common to chronic pain (i.e., anger, depression, and anxiety), poor coping strategies, and aggravating environmental factors. Assistance in developing better coping strategies, reducing muscle tension, proper pacing of activities, and family or marital problems may be used based on individual circumstances.

## Developing New Coping Strategies

A common maladaptive coping strategy is exhibited by individuals who attempt to work at preaccident levels too early in the recovery period. This usually results in a marked exacerbation of pain, and inactivity ensues. This cycle of overactivity/inactivity usually reflects a lack of acceptance of the injury. In this case the psychologist may be able to help the patient by using cognitive strategies to identify the maladaptive coping style, teaching proper pacing of activities and learning limits, and dealing with the inevitable frustration, anger, and depression resulting from the individual's inability to return to normal.

Alternatively some patients refuse to participate in any activity until the pain is "cured." This often reflects a common belief that pain indicates ongoing tissue damage. These patients avoid any activity that they believe will exacerbate their pain, fearing that this will cause further tissue damage. The psychologist may be able to reverse this style of coping by cognitive-behavioral methods, slowly encouraging the patient to become more active. A gradually increasing level of activity can be carefully planned and subsequently monitored.

## Reducing Muscular Tension

Another important goal of psychological intervention is muscle relaxation. While muscular tension can contribute to pain in any part of the body, the axial regions of the body, which include the neck, upper thorax, and lower back, appear to be the most susceptible. Muscle tension increases around the injured neck and upper thorax in response to pain. Anxiety, anger, and emotional stress can further increase muscle tension. The result is increased pain and discomfort, which may produce increased muscle tension, anxiety, and emotional stress. Eventually a self-perpetuating cycle develops (Fig. 19.13).

The goal of treatment is to reduce muscle tension before the pain reaches intolerable levels. Simply learning to rest or utilizing relaxation techniques may help prevent the perpetuation of severe pain. Electromyographic biofeedback techniques may help a patient learn to control muscle tension either through auditory or visual feedback. Self-hypnosis and imagery techniques are methods of mental manipulation of the experience of pain designed to reduce the pain. Pacing of activities and avoiding situations of emotional stress further aid in reducing muscle tension.

## VOCATIONAL ADJUSTMENTS AND RETRAINING

A key and often neglected aspect of the management of whiplash injuries is the patient's vocation

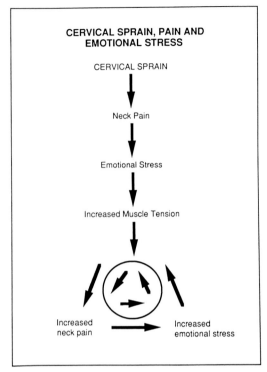

**Figure 9.13.** Emotional stress can influence pain from a cervical sprain by increasing muscle tension. The increase in pain further increases emotional stress and subsequent muscle tension. The result is a self-perpetuating cycle of pain → stress → muscle tension → increased pain, etc.

and its relationship to pain. Certain postures, heavy manual labor, and repetitive arm movements all aggravate symptoms. Often pain builds to the point at which the injured individual is no longer able to work. The inability to work often leads to loss of self-esteem, financial stresses, depression, and accusations of malingering or secondary gain. Type of employment is an important element in pain control. In our experience the most important prognostic factor in determining whether a patient will return to work is the type of work itself.

Heavy lifting tends to aggravate pain throughout the neck and upper thoracic regions. Workers such as manual laborers or nursing aides are particularly at risk. Repetitive arm work is also difficult, particularly when the arms are held above the level of the shoulders. Painting and hairdressing fall into this category of work. With both heavy lifting or repetitive arm work the volume and the intensity of work is important. If the work is not too intense, with frequent breaks, the patients may be able to cope; however, as the work increases in volume these individuals may no longer be able to continue without pain. Prolonged sitting and standing postures are well-known aggravators of neck, upper thoracic, and low back pain after whiplash injuries. Typists, secretaries, computer operators, truck drivers, file clerks, and students often find it difficult to sit or stand in one place for more than 20–30 min. This is further aggravated by having to keep the neck in a prolonged forward flexed position.

Many whiplash victims are housewives who have trouble with specific activities. The most difficult activities include vacuuming, washing walls, windows, or floors, and carrying children or groceries. Other pain-aggravating activities include washing dishes, doing laundry, making beds, ironing, and meal preparation. We recommend that housewives who have suffered a whiplash injury learn to pace their activities so that, for instance, instead of cleaning the whole house all at once they clean one room at a time, allowing adequate time to recover before proceeding to the next room; in some cases it may mean cleaning only one room a day. For heavier tasks like vacuuming, someone else should do the task, either the spouse or a hired housekeeper. It is important to stress to the patient that these measures will likely be only temporary and to encourage increased activity as the pain subsides.

Many individuals after a whiplash injury find they are unable to work and still maintain their pain within tolerable limits. A quick examination will show that they are able to actually perform the physical maneuvers required but will not reveal that with repeated or prolonged work the pain intensifies to intolerable levels. The jobs that are most likely to precipitate intolerable pain also tend to be boring and unfulfilling. For this reason the issue of secondary gain is often raised to account for the patient's continuing disabling pain and inability to work. These individuals are often in lower socioeconomic groups where there is a tendency to more pain-aggravating manual labor. Their work values are often questioned because it is thought they have the least to lose from not working. In contrast, professional and office workers generally do not engage in pain-aggravating activities and are able to modify their work and schedules to avoid exacerbations of pain and discomfort. These individuals generally complain of pain more after racquet sports, working in the yard or gardening, lifting weights, or sitting through long meetings or long car rides, or in times of stress.

## ROLE OF COMPENSATION

There are few issues in medicine as controversial as the role of compensation in prolonging chronic pain and disability after motor vehicle accidents. The growing tide of litigation after such accidents has had a significant socioeconomic impact, causing increased insurance rates, and in some states and provinces has led to "no-fault" legislation. Among many clinicians there has been a suspicion bordering on conviction that the availability of compensatory awards prejudices the outcome after injury. There is a widely held belief that litigants seeking compensation after such accidents improve and return to normal functioning within a short time of the finalization of the claim, irrespective of outcome. As a general principle, however, the role of litigation appears to be overrated by many clinicians, and the concept that patients rapidly recover following settlement of their compensation claim is not substantiated in the literature. There are a number of factors that contribute to the final level of chronic pain and disability and that must be considered when evaluating the prognosis for pain, disability, or return to work.

The term "compensation neurosis" has been used to describe symptoms following compensable accidents that fail to respond to treatment and rehabilitation. In 1946, Kennedy (60) wrote "compensation neurosis is a state of mind born out of fear, kept alive by avarice, stimulated by lawyers and cured by a verdict." The term was made popular by the influential writings of Henry Miller (61) in 1961 and has continued to persist to the present. Reasons for this mindset are complex and include the previously discussed patient-physician conflict as well as lack of objective evidence of continued anatomic injury, nonanatomic pain syndromes, poor understanding of musculoskeletal (referred) pain and the psychological sequelae of chronic pain, and apparent secondary gain in the form of litigation.

Secondary gain is the foundation upon which the concept of compensation neurosis is based. This assumes that the persistence of symptoms provides some financial, social, or psychological benefit to the patient. As a result the patient is thought to be practicing deception in order to achieve some personal gain. When the deception is unconscious it is labeled hysteria and when conscious it is called malingering. Both of these clinical entities are controversial and difficult to diagnose, and yet they are commonly used to explain continuing symptoms. Further discussion is beyond the scope of this chapter.

## Outcome Studies

Outcome studies of whiplash injuries suffer from a variety of problems, including lack of prospective design, selection bias in the group of patients reviewed, and a lack of measurable objective data. The literature that does exist, despite obvious deficiencies, provides some interesting insights into recovery after whiplash injuries. For clinicians who have been perplexed by persistent symptoms and the legitimacy of the whiplash syndrome in terms of the presence of a physiologic injury, some insights may be gained by reviewing these studies.

Gotten (57) surveyed 100 patients who were referred for neurosurgical consultation after cervical whiplash injury. After settlement of legal claims 12% were still sufficiently symptomatic to be wearing cervical collars, sleeping in traction, receiving physiotherapy, and periodically seeing their physicians for help. Another 34% suffered "minor" residual symptoms. Macnab (5, 7) reviewed 266 patients who had suffered cervical whiplash injuries and had court settlements 2 or more years previously and found at least 45% were still symptomatic. Notable in this study was the fact that the symptomatic group was comprised primarily of patients who had suffered hyperextension injuries. Most asymptomatic patients had lateral flexion or forward flexion injuries, pointing to the generally better prognosis in these types of injuries.

DePalma and Subin (62) found that, among 386 of their patients with cervical pain syndromes, only 25% were involved in litigation. Moreover, the outcome after therapy was the same in both litigation and nonlitigation groups, suggesting that litigation did not have a significant influence on outcome. Shutt and Dohan (10), in a study of 67 women, found that at 6 months 75% continued to experience neck pain. No difference was apparent between those patients who had pending litigation and those whose litigation had resolved.

Hohl (63) followed 146 patients with neck injuries following car accidents for 5 years. Within the first month following injury, virtually all patients experienced aching and stiffness in the neck, two thirds had headaches, and one third complained of shoulder pain. The duration of symptoms ranged from a few days to more than 5 years, with an average of about 24 months. At 5-year follow-up, 57% of these patients had made a "symptomatic recovery," defined as no residual problems related to the original injury; 43% were

still symptomatic. Interestingly, in those patients who had litigation pending, delays in court settlement were associated with worse outcome. Hohl also noted that of those patients who had no litigation pending only one half were asymptomatic at 5-year review.

Norris and Watt (64) reviewed 61 patients who were occupants of cars struck in rear-end collisions. They found residual neck pain at 6 months in 40% of patients with milder injuries and 90% of those with severe injuries. More recently **Deans** (23) reported the findings of a retrospective study of 137 individuals injured in motor vehicle accidents and seen in an emergency room over a 6-month period. Subjects were followed up by questionnaire over a further 2-year observation period. Sixty-two percent reported neck pain after their accident; of these, pain lasted 1 week in 17%, 6 months in 56%, and longer than 1 year in 42%. In this latter group, 36% had occasional pain while only 6% complained of continuous pain. Similarly, Wiley et al. (37) reviewed 320 cases of uncomplicated whiplash injuries referred for medical legal assessments. Of these, 156 were reviewed 1 year after initial assessment. A total of 142 of 156 cases had settled their litigation and of these 18% still had significant symptoms. The authors concluded that a "good" or "satisfactory" monetary settlement did not ensure the resolution of symptoms.

## SUMMARY

Whiplash or cervical flexion-extension injuries are a 20th-century phenomenon without natural parallel. The biomechanics of injury are relatively well understood but the pathophysiology of injury remains somewhat uncertain. Whiplash patients present with a consistent but often complex combination of pain, associated symptoms, and psychosocial consequences of chronic pain. Although a variety of treatments are available, none represents a cure.

Few issues generate as much controversy as the role of compensation in chronic pain and disability following motor vehicle accidents. Many of the patients are inappropriately labeled as suffering from a "compensation neurosis," and the belief that the presence of litigation prolongs symptoms is a persistent one. Lack of objective physiologic evidence of injury and poor therapeutic reponses appear to be the major concerns of many clinicians. However, the consistency of the clinical picture would suggest an organic basis for continuing complaints. Difficult patients, poorly informed physicians, and an adversarial system of seeking compensation have led to a suboptimal environment for recovery.

Recognizing that the problem is multifactorial and that there is no easy solution is a first step in improving the management of these unfortunate victims. Solutions involve helping patients develop better adaptive coping skills, training physicians to better recognize and treat chronic pain, and providing adequate and rapid fiscal rehabilitation.

## REFERENCES

1. Crowe ME: Injuries to the cervical spine. Presented at the meeting of the Western Orthopedic Association, San Francisco, 1928.
2. Erichsen JE: *Concussion of the Spine. Nervous Shock and Other Obscure Injuries to the Nervous System. Clinical and Medicolegal Aspects.* New York, William Wood & Company, 1886, p 57.
3. Croft AC: Biomechanics. In Forearm SM, Croft AC (eds): *Whiplash Injuries. The Cervical Acceleration Deceleration Syndrome.* Baltimore, Williams and Wilkins, pp 1–72, 1988.
4. National Safety Council: *Accident Facts.* Chicago, National Safety Council, p 47, 1971.
5. Macnab I: Acceleration injuries of the cervical spine. *J Bone Joint Surg [Am]* 46:1797–1799, 1964.
6. Macnab I: Acceleration extension injuries of the cervical spine. In: *AAOS Symposium of the Spine.* St. Louis, CV Mosby, 1969, pp 10–17.
7. Macnab I: The "whiplash syndrome." *Orthop Clin North Am* 2:389–403, 1971.
8. Macnab I: The whiplash syndrome. *Clin Neurosurg* 20:232–241, 1973.
9. Macnab I: Acceleration extension injuries of the cervical spine. In Rothman RH, Simeone FA (eds): *The Spine,* ed 2. Philadelphia, WB Saunders, 1982, pp 647–660.
10. Schutt CH, Dohan FCS: Neck injuries to women in auto accidents. A metropolitan plague. *JAMA* 206:2689–2692, 1968.
11. Bogduk N: The anatomy and pathophysiology of whiplash. *Clin Biomech* 1:92–101, 1986.
12. Commack KV: Whiplash injuries to the neck. *Am J Surg* 93:663–666, 1957.
13. Frankel VH: Pathomechanics of whiplash injuries to the neck. In Morley TP (ed): *Current Controversies in Neurosurgery.* Philadelphia, WB Saunders, 1976, pp 39–50.
14. LaRocca H: Acceleration injuries of the neck. *Clin Neurosurg* 25:205–217, 1978.
15. Severy DM, Mathewson JH, Bechtol CO: Controlled automobile rear-end collisions; an investigation of related engineering and medical phenomena. *Can Services Med J* 11:717–759, 1955.
16. McKenzie JA, Williams JF: The dynamic behavior of the head and cervical spine during "whiplash." *J Biomech* 4:474–490, 1971.
17. Wickstrom JK, Rodriguez RP, Martinez JL: Cervical spine syndrome: experimental production of acceleration injuries of the head and neck. In: *Proceedings, Prevention of Highway Injury.* Ann Arbor, MI, Highway Safety Research Institute, University of Michigan, Ann Arbor, pp 182–187, 1967.
18. Wickstrom JK, Martinez JL, Rodriguez R, et al: Hyperex-

tension and hyperflexion injuries to the head and neck of primates. In Gurdjian ES, Thomas LM (eds): *Neckache and Backache.* Springfield, IL, Charles C Thomas, 1970, pp 108–119.
19. Lieberman JS: Cervical soft tissue injuries and cervical disc disease. In: *Principles of Physical Medicine and Rehabilitations in the Musculoskeletal Diseases.* New York, Grune & Stratton, Inc, 1986, pp 263–286.
20. O'Neill BL, Haddon W Jr, Kelley AB, Sorenson WW: Automobile head restraints: frequency of neck injury claims in relation to the presence of head restraints. *Am J Public Health* 62:399, 1972.
21. States JD, Balcerak JC, Williams JS, et al: Injury frequency and head restraint effectiveness in rear-end impact accidents. In: *Proceedings of the 16th STAPP Car Crash Conference,* Detroit, Michigan, p 228, 1972.
22. Fox JC, Williams JF: Mathematical model for investigating combined seatback-head restraint during rear end impact. *Med Biol Eng* 14:263, 1976.
23. Deans GT: Incidence and duration of neck pain among patients injured in car accidents. *Br Med J* 292:94–95, 1986.
24. Hobbs CA: *The Effectiveness of Seat Belts in Reducing Injuries to Car Occupants.* Transport and Road Research Laboratory report No. 811, 1978.
25. Hobbs CA: *Car Occupant Injury Patterns and Mechanisms.* Transport and Road Research Laboratory supplementary report No. 648.
26. Rutherford WH, Greenfield AA, Hayes HRM, Nelson JK: *The medical effects of seat belt legislation in the United Kingdom.* Department of Health and Social Security Research Report No. 13. London, Her Majesty's Stationery Office, 1985.
27. Balla JI: The late whiplash syndrome. *Aust NZ J Surg* 50:610–614, 1980.
28. Hohl M: Soft tissue injuries of the neck. *Clin Orthop* 109:42–49, 1975.
29. Wickstrom J, LaRocca H: Management of patients with cervical spine and head injuries from acceleration forces. *Curr Pract Orthop Surg* 6:83, 1975.
30. Bland JH: *Disorders of the Cervical Spine.* Philadelphia, WB Saunders, 1987.
31. Croft AC: Developmental anatomy. In Foreman SM, Croft AC (eds): *Whiplash Injuries. The Cervical Acceleration Deceleration Syndrome.* Baltimore, Williams & Wilkins, pp 232–270, 1988.
32. Feinstein B, Langton JNK, Jameson RM, Schiller F: Experiments of pain referred from deep somatic tissues. *J Bone Joint Surg [Am]* 36:981–997, 1954.
33. Feinstein B: Referred pain from paravertebral structures. In Buerger AA, Tobis JS (eds): *Approaches to the Validation of Manipulation Therapy.* Springfield, IL, Charles C Thomas, 1977, pp 139–174.
34. Inman VH, Saunders JBdeCM: Referred pain from skeletal structures. *J Nerv Ment Dis* 99:660–667, 1944.
35. Speed WG: Psychiatric aspects of posttraumatic headaches. In Adler CS, et al (eds): *Psychiatric Aspects of Headache.* Baltimore, Williams & Wilkins, 1987, pp 210–206.
36. Balla JI, Moraitis S: Knights in armour. A follow-up study of injuries after legal settlement. *Med J Aust* 2:355–361, 1970.
37. Wiley AM, et al: Musculoskeletal sequelae of whiplash injuries. *Advocates Q* 7:65–73, 1986.
38. Raskin NH: *Headache,* ed 2. New York, Churchill Livingstone Inc, 1988.
39. Horwich H, Kasner D: The effect of whiplash injuries on ocular functions. *South Med J* 55:69–71, 1962.
40. deJong PTVM, deJong JMBV, Cohen B, Jongkees LBW:

Ataxia and nystagmus induced by injection of local anaesthetics in the neck. *Ann Neurol* 1:240–246, 1977.

41. Compere WE: Electronystagmographic finding in patients with "whiplash" injuries. *Laryngoscope* 78:1226–1232, 1968.

42. Pang LQ: The otological aspects of whiplash injuries. *Larynogoscope* 81:1381–1387, 1971.

43. Gay JR, Abbott KH: Common whiplash injuries of the neck. *JAMA* 152:1698–1704, 1953.

44. Travell J, Simons DG: *Myofascial Pain and Dysfunction: The Trigger Point Manual.* Baltimore, Williams & Wilkins, 1983.

45. Braaf MM, Rosner S: Symptomatology and treatment of injuries of the neck. *NY J Med* 55:237, 1955.

46. Croft AC, Foreman SM: Cited by Croft AC: Soft tissue injury: long-term and short-term effects. In Foreman SM, Croft AC (eds): *Whiplash Injuries. The Cervical Acceleration Deceleration Syndrome.* Baltimore, Williams & Wilkins, p 293, 1988.

47. Ameis A: Cervical whiplash: considerations in the rehabilitation of cervical myofascial injury. *Can Fam Physician* 32:1871–1876, 1986.

48. Torres F, Shapiro SK: Electroencephalograms in whiplash injury. *Arch Neurol* 5:28–35, 1961.

49. Ommaya AK, Faas F, Yarnell P: Whiplash and brain damage. *JAMA* 204:285–289, 1968.

50. Gibbs FA: Objective evidence of brain disorder in cases of whiplash injury. *Clin Electroencephalogr* 2(2):107–110, 1971.

51. Alves WM, Colohan ART, O'Leary TJ, Rimel RW, Jane JA: Understanding post-traumatic symptoms after minor head injury. *J Head Trauma Rehabil* 1(2):1–12, 1986.

52. Fisher CM: Whiplash amnesia. *Neurology* (NY) 32:667–668, 1982.

53. Frankel VH: Temporomandibular joint pain syndrome following deceleration injury to the cervical spine. *Bull Hosp Jt Dis* 26:47, 1969.

54. Wolfe F, Smythe MA, Yunus MB, Bennett RM, Bombardier C, Goldenberg DM, Tugwell P, and the Multicenter Fibromyalgia Criteria Committee: Criteria for fibromyalgia [abstract]. *Arthritis Rheum* 32(4)(Suppl):547, 1985.

55. Hendler N: Chronic pain patient versus the malingering patient. In Foly KM, Payne RM (eds): *Current Therapy of Pain.* Philadelphia, BC Decker Inc, 1985.

56. Romano JM, Turner JA: Chronic pain and depression: does the evidence support a relationship? *Psychol Bull* 97(1):18–34, 1985.

57. Gotten N: Survey of 100 cases of whiplash injury after settlement of litigation. *JAMA* 162:865–867, 1956.

58. Diamond EL, Grauer K: The physician's reactions to patients with chronic pain. *Am Fam Physician* 34(3):117–122, 1986.

59. Mealy K, Brennan H, Fenelon GCC: Early mobilization of acute whiplash injuries. *Br Med J* 292:656–657, 1986.

60. Kennedy F: The mind of the injured worker: its effect on disability periods. *Compens Med* 1:19–24, 1946.

61. Miller H: Accident neurosis—lecture II. *Br Med J* 1:992–998, 1961.

62. De Palma A, Subin D: Study of the cervical syndrome. *Clin Orthop* 38:135–142, 1965.

63. Hohl M: Soft tissue injuries of the neck in automobile accidents: factors influencing prognosis. *J Bone Joint Surg* [Am] 56:1675–1682, 1974.

64. Norris SH, Watt F: The prognosis of neck injuries resulting from rear-end vehicle collisions. *J Bone Joint Surg* [Br] 65:608–611, 1983.

## *20*

# FIBROMYALGIA AND CERVICAL PAIN

*Frederick Wolfe*

## FIBROSITIS, FIBROMYALGIA, AND MYOFASCIAL PAIN SYNDROMES: HISTORICAL AND CURRENT CONCEPTS

Within the last 15 years a very common syndrome of musculoskeletal pain has been reidentified and has become the subject of numerous research studies. The syndrome, fibromyalgia (previously known as fibrositis), is probably present in many individuals who have been classified as having other cervical and lumbar syndromes, including the various myofascial pain and regional pain syndromes.

Although fibromyalgia is very common, the recognition and understanding of the syndrome has been hampered by (a) a very confusing nomenclature, (b) changing concepts in the meaning of the sometimes synonymous syndrome of fibrositis, and (c) an impreciseness of definition in the older medical literature (1). A further contributing factor is the lack of communication between researchers and practitioners within the major medical specialties of general medicine, orthopaedics, pain, rheumatology, and physical medicine.

Until recently fibromyalgia was known as "fibrositis" (2–4), although the term "fibromyalgia" is probably now more common (5, 6). "Fibrositis" first appeared in the English literature in 1904 when Sir William Gowers used it to explain the presumed inflammation of fascia that he believed was the cause of "lumbago" or "muscular rheumatism" (7). Stockman (8), writing in 1920 from Edinburgh, found evidence of this inflammation on biopsy material from "fibrositis" patients. Thus in this early view there was a syndrome of

"muscular rheumatism" that had as its cause "inflammation." This was an attractive concept since it explained multiple medical problems for which there was, simply, no explanation. It is important to recognize that this "fibrositis" was actually ill defined and could apply to local, regional, and even generalized conditions, although it usually referred to the first two.

However, the concept of "muscular rheumatism," which included various local muscle and musculoskeletal disorders, dates well back into the 19th century (9–11). These disorders, most of which were local in nature, lacked an agreed upon pathophysiology, and often were similarly ill defined, gradually became known as fibrositis as well. The notion that "inflammation" was the cause of "muscular rheumatism" seemed incorrect clinically, and was later shown to be wrong (12, 13). Persistence of this notion of inflammation as the cause and the use of a name that implied inflammation impaired the credibility of the syndrome of fibrositis. However, the name had certain unifying properties, and attempts to repudiate it did not occur until recently (14).

Three other constructs of the fibrositis syndrome arose. In the first, the problems of poor definition (local, regional, generalized), the absence of criteria for diagnosis, and the suspicion that the term could be used to characterize almost any muscular problem found their culmination in a study by Halliday in 1941 in which the concept of fibrositis as a psychological rather than a physical disorder was promulgated (15). The second, a more traditional, better defined concept with emphasis on local and regional syndromes (2, 16–

319

18), in its most recent version emphasizes "trigger points" and referred pain. The major proponents of this concept are Travell and Simons, who have written about it in detail in their text (18). This construct has evolved into the "myofascial pain syndrome." In the third construct, Graham (19), followed by Smythe (3, 4), saw the fibrositis syndrome as a generalized disorder of pain associated with widespread local tenderness. This construct has evolved into the "fibromyalgia syndrome."

Thus by the mid-1970s "fibrositis" could have been (a) a term for any muscular or musculoskeletal syndrome, (b) a psychological disorder, (c) a local and regional disorder associated with trigger points, or (d) a generalized musculoskeletal pain syndrome. Clearly, the name had no specific meaning and little scientific validity. It added confusion wherever it was used.

During the last 15 years major changes have taken place that have largely ameliorated these problems. First, there has been a general trend toward the elimination of the term "fibrositis" in reference to local and regional muscular pain disorders and its replacement with "myofascial pain syndrome" (14). In addition, more precise definitions of these disorders have been developed (18). Even so, not all authors and clinicians understand the current nomenclature, and the waters not infrequently remain muddied.

The generalized musculoskeletal syndrome described by Graham and Smythe, with which this chapter is concerned, eschewed local and regional disorders and developed specific criteria for diagnosis (4–6). The term "fibromyalgia" (20) is gradually replacing "fibrositis" in this construct because it does not carry with it the "baggage" of all of the older constructs of fibrositis, and because it is different from those syndromes.

One may summarize the evolution of the nomenclature as follows (Table 20.1). Myofascial pain syndromes now refer to local and regional disorders; fibromyalgia refers to a generalized syndrome. The term "fibrositis" has too many connotations and imprecisions to be useful clinically or in research. Recent advances in fibromyalgia research have led to reliable criteria for diagnosis. Readers should carefully evaluate fibromyalgia studies for the use of appropriate criteria; those studies that refer to fibrositis should be similarly examined for the criteria that allow one to distinguish which syndrome is being reported. Finally, myofascial pain reports require scientific definition as well.

## THE FIBROMYALGIA SYNDROME

Briefly defined, fibromyalgia is a syndrome of generalized musculoskeletal pain *and* tenderness, and is associated with certain core features: stiffness, fatigue, and sleep disturbance (5, 21–26).

## WIDESPREAD PAIN

Widespread pain is an essential feature of fibromyalgia. Leavitt et al. (27) studied fibromyalgia patients using a pain localization sheet that scored 25 body regions. The mean number of sites reported as painful by fibromyalgia patients was 12.9 ($\pm 5.6$ SD). Of specific interest to this chapter is that shoulder/back pain was reported by 76% and neck pain was noted by 70% of patients. Other major sites of pain that were reported by more than 65% of patients were the lower back, thighs, legs, fingers, and knees.

Other studies have also reported high rates of pain (e.g., 26) (Fig. 20.1). The recent multicenter fibromyalgia criteria study (6) produced similar data on a larger sample. This study of 558 fibromyalgia patients and controls noted that 59.5% of fibromyalgia patients complained of pain in at least half of the 30 areas examined. Of interest, cervical region pain was a complaint in 85.3%! Thoracic and lumbar pain occurred in more than 70% of these patients. Thus pain is very widespread in this disorder, and axial skeletal pain and particularly cervical pain is invariably present.

**Table 20.1.**
**Evolution of Fibrositis Nomenclature**

| Current Terminology | | Constructs of Fibrositis |
| --- | --- | --- |
| | | 1. Generalized, local, regional syndrome (6) |
| | | 2. "Psychogenic rheumatism" |
| Myofascial pain syndrome | ⟵ | 3. Local, regional; trigger points |
| Fibromyalgia | ⟵ | 4. Generalized musculoskeletal pain disorder |

## Painful Regions

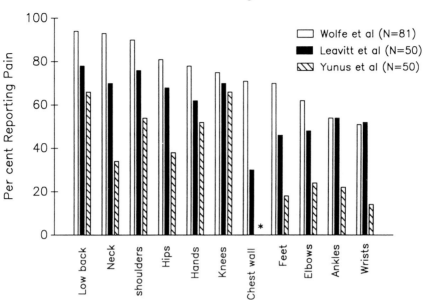

**Figure 20.1.**   Percentage of fibromyalgia patients reporting pain in various body regions in three studies (5, 22, 27). (From Wolfe F: Fibromyalgia: the clinical syndrome. *Rheum Dis Clin North Am* 15:1–18, 1989.)

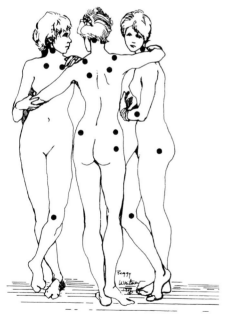

**Figure 20.2.**   Tender point locations for the 1990 classification criteria for fibromyalgia. (Drawing after *The Three Graces* by Baron Jean-Baptiste Regnault (1793), Louvre Museum, Paris.) See Table 20.3 for details. (From Wolfe F, Smythe HA, Yunus MB, et al: The American College of Rheumatology 1990 criteria for the classification of fibromyalgia: report of the Multicenter Criteria Committee. *Arthritis Rheum* 33:160–172, 1990. Copyright 1990. Used by permission of the American College of Rheumatology.)

## TENDERNESS

Along with pain, tenderness is a cardinal feature of fibromyalgia. Tenderness is most obvious in certain anatomic locations, known as tender point regions (Fig. 20.2), and the identification of tenderness in these areas is one of the criteria used in the diagnosis of fibromyalgia. Numerous studies have shown that subjects with fibromyalgia generally have tenderness at these locations, whereas

**Table 20.2.**
**Mean Scores of Pressure Required (kg/cm$^2$) to Elicit Intolerance in Fibromyalgia Patients Versus Controls[a]**

| Point No. | Anatomic Site | Patients | Controls | p< | Point No. | Anatomic Site | Patients | Controls | p< |
|---|---|---|---|---|---|---|---|---|---|
| 1 | Frontalis above orbit | 3.72 | 3.52 | 0.72 | 39[c] | Pectoralis muscle, upper clavicular section | 2.80 | 5.08 | 0.0001 |
| 2 | Temporalis above ear | 4.04 | 3.98 | 0.91 | 40[c] | Pectoralis muscle, lateral clavicular section | 2.62 | 4.91 | 0.0001 |
| 3 | Temporomandibular joint | 3.18 | 3.31 | 0.83 | 41 | Pectoralis muscle, upper sternal portion | 2.54 | 3.74 | 0.029 |
| 4 | Occipitalis above nuchal line | 4.53 | 4.12 | 0.55 | 42 | Pectoralis muscle, lower sternal portion | 2.44 | 3.86 | 0.01 |
| 5 | Upper sternocleidomastoid, below mastoid | 2.35 | 3.15 | 0.15 | 43 | Mid-serratus anterior | 2.69 | 4.38 | 0.0084 |
| 6[b] | Mid-sternocleidomastoid | 1.70 | 2.53 | 0.12 | 44[c] | Acromioclavicular joint | 3.26 | 5.23 | 0.0003 |
| 7 | Sternoclavicular joint | 3.39 | 4.46 | 0.10 | 45[c] | Tip of shoulder | 3.64 | 5.57 | 0.0008 |
| 8[b] | Low anterior neck, intertransverse C4–C6 | 2.74 | 3.36 | 0.26 | 46 | Mid-deltoid muscle, below shoulder tip | 4.13 | 5.26 | 0.069 |
| 9[b] | Mid-C1 | 3.44 | 4.25 | 0.23 | 47 | Supraspinatus tendon | 3.46 | 4.76 | 0.019 |
| 10[b] | Mid-C3 | 3.35 | 4.78 | 0.02 | 48[b] | Bicipital groove | 3.58 | 4.84 | 0.017 |
| 11[b] | Mid-C5 | 4.06 | 5.59 | 0.011 | 49 | Posterior upper triceps | 3.90 | 4.64 | 0.17 |
| 12[b] | Splenius capitis, just above mid-C1 | 2.47 | 3.96 | 0.018 | 50 | Posterior lower triceps | 4.83 | 5.41 | 0.15 |
| 13 | Splenius cervicis, T1 level | 2.84 | 4.59 | 0.003 | 51[c] | 2 cm distal medial epicondyle | 4.36 | 5.92 | 0.001 |
| 14[c] | Trapezius, at shoulder insertion | 3.82 | 5.85 | 0.0001 | 52[b] | 2 cm distal lateral epicondyle | 3.68 | 5.29 | 0.002 |
| 15[b] | Upper mid-trapezius | 3.67 | 4.87 | 0.018 | 53 | Fifth carpal bone | 4.49 | 5.06 | 0.22 |
| 16[c] | Trapezius, near vertebrae | 3.59 | 5.66 | 0.0005 | 54 | Mid-metacarpal area | 4.45 | 4.90 | 0.49 |
| 17[b] | Mid-T1 | 4.42 | 5.73 | 0.016 | | | | | |
| 18[b] | Mid-T3 | 4.61 | 5.79 | 0.003 | | | | | |

| | Site | | | |
|---|---|---|---|---|
| 19[b] | Mid-T5 | 5.00 | 5.34 | 0.51 |
| 20[b] | Mid-T7 | 5.56 | 5.60 | 0.91 |
| 21[b] | Mid-T9 | 5.34 | 5.82 | 0.084 |
| 22[b] | Mid-T11 | 5.10 | 5.60 | 0.11 |
| 23[b] | Supraspinatus origin | 3.29 | 5.04 | 0.002 |
| 24 | Mid-rhomboid at medial edge of scapula | 3.99 | 5.33 | 0.004 |
| 25[c] | Lower rhomboid at lower edge of scapula | 4.45 | 5.77 | 0.0005 |
| 26[c] | Mid-supraspinatus | 3.92 | 5.59 | 0.0005 |
| 27[c] | Mid-infraspinatus | 4.07 | 5.81 | 0.0001 |
| 28 | Mid-L2 | 4.87 | 5.64 | 0.044 |
| 29[b] | Mid-L4 | 5.43 | 5.81 | 0.25 |
| 30[b] | Mid-S1 | 4.63 | 5.64 | 0.028 |
| 31 | Over mid-coccyx | 5.52 | 5.91 | 0.12 |
| 32[b,c] | Top mid-outer iliac crest | 3.69 | 5.49 | 0.0002 |
| 33 | Multifidi, outer mid-iliac crest | 4.55 | 5.96 | 0.005 |
| 34[b] | Mid-buttocks, S1 joint | 5.53 | 6.00 | 0.019 |
| 35 | Ischial gluteal bursa | 5.49 | 5.60 | 0.82 |
| 36[b] | First costochondral junction | 2.57 | 3.38 | 0.17 |
| 37[c] | Third costochondral junction | 1.92 | 3.69 | 0.0004 |
| 38[c] | Over manubrial sternum | 2.25 | 4.08 | 0.0010 |
| 55 | Thumb metacarpophalangeal joint | 4.12 | 5.43 | 0.018 |
| 56 | Over lateral epicondyle | 4.35 | 5.42 | 0.036 |
| 57 | Mid-anterior forearm | 4.34 | 5.89 | 0.003 |
| 58[c] | Over wrist, anteriorly | 4.68 | 5.98 | 0.0004 |
| 59[b] | Greater trochanter | 5.23 | 5.89 | 0.041 |
| 60[c] | Mid-rectus femoris | 3.75 | 5.78 | 0.0001 |
| 61 | Mid-vastus lateralis | 4.55 | 5.64 | 0.031 |
| 62[b,c] | Medial fat pad proximal to knee | 3.80 | 5.89 | 0.0001 |
| 63 | Quadriceps tendon insertion at patella | 5.65 | 6.00 | 0.034 |
| 64[c] | Lateral joint line of knee | 5.32 | 6.00 | 0.005 |
| 65[c] | Medial joint line of knee | 4.56 | 6.00 | 0.0001 |
| 66[c] | Anserine bursa | 3.33 | 5.90 | 0.0001 |
| 67 | Mid-tibialis anterior | 4.68 | 6.00 | 0.004 |
| 68 | Mid-ankle joint | 5.44 | 6.00 | 0.133 |
| 69 | Mid-lateral tarsal area | 4.83 | 5.94 | 0.020 |
| 70 | First metatarsophalangeal joint | 4.57 | 5.66 | 0.023 |
| 71 | Mid-adductor magnus | 4.83 | 5.98 | 0.002 |
| 72[c] | Low posterior biceps femoris | 3.95 | 6.00 | 0.0001 |
| 73 | Mid-gastrocnemius | 5.37 | 6.00 | 0.02 |
| 74 | Upper achilles tendon insertion | 4.82 | 5.85 | 0.069 |
| 75 | Lower achilles tendon insertion | 6.00 | 6.00 | 1.00 |
| | Mean total pressure, all 75 sites | 295.80 | 387.00 | 0.0001 |

[a] From Simms RW, Goldenberg DL, Felson DT, Mason JH: Tenderness in 75 anatomic sites. Distinguishing fibromyalgia patients from controls. *Arthritis Rheum* 31:182–187, 1988. Copyright 1988. Used by permission of the American College of Rheumatology.

[b] Previously proposed tender points.

[c] Those tender points that best discriminated patients from controls ($p < 0.001$).

normal controls and even patients with other rheumatic conditions have less or no tenderness in these areas (28–32). A number of studies have identified the "best" tender point regions (those regions that best separate patients with the syndrome from controls) for use in the diagnostic examination. The studies of Simms and Goldenberg (33) and Yunus et al. (5) have provided useful data as to these sites.

Tenderness may be identified in two ways, by digital palpation or by dolorimetry. Dolorimetry is more precise but has little value in the clinic since it is time consuming to perform and requires the use of a special instrument. *Dolorimetry* is performed by advancing a spring (or electronic)-loaded instrument, which has a cork with an area of 1.54 cm$^2$ at its end, at a rate of about 1 kg/sec against the site to be examined. When the subject indicates that the site has become painful the amount of pressure that caused the pain is recorded. A pressure of 4 kg/1.54 cm$^2$ is often accepted as the level that separates patients from controls (28). When *digital palpation* is used the examiner should try to palpate with a similar force. When a patient states that the palpation is painful (not just "tender"), a tender point is recorded (6). Some scoring systems require a spontaneous verbal response, a grimace, or a movement for the tender point to be recorded as positive (5).

The study of Campbell and colleagues (28) provided data to support the concept of "control points," regions that were said to be no more tender in subjects with fibromyalgia than in controls. More recent studies (6, 29, 34), however, have suggested that fibromyalgia patients differ from controls at these sites as well, but that at the "control" sites the differences are quite slight and usually undetectable unless large samples are studied. Table 20.2 demonstrates the regions in which fibromyalgia patients and controls were most different in dolorimetry tenderness (29).

## CORE SYMPTOMS AND COMMON FEATURES OF FIBROMYALGIA

Three *core symptoms* predominate in fibromyalgia and give the characteristic features of the disorder: sleep disturbance, fatigue, and stiffness (Fig. 20.3). Although sleep disturbance was first defined on the basis of the sleep electroencephalogram (EEG) (4), in clinical practice this symptom has come to be associated with waking up tired or "nonrefreshed." As noted in Figure 20.3 this symptom and fatigue are the most common symptoms of the disorder. The recent multicenter study (6) defined sleep disturbance or fatigue to be present when patients noted it "often or usually or always," a method of definition that adds an objective dimension to such questions. Defined

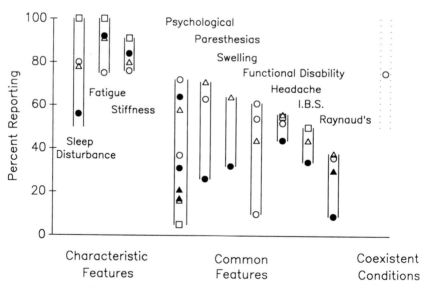

**Figure 20.3.** Percentage of fibromyalgia patients in clinical reports with characteristic and common features of the syndrome (I.B.S., irritable bowel syndrome). Symbols represent reports of different centers. (From Wolfe F: Fibromyalgia: the clinical syndrome. *Rheum Dis Clin North Am* 15:1–18, 1989.)

thus, more than 70% of the patients in that study had each of the three core symptoms of fibromyalgia.

Figure 20.3 also indicates the so-called *common features of fibromyalgia* (26). These features tend to differ in their prominence in the individual patient and are not specific for fibromyalgia, occurring in other medical conditions as well. However, the finding of such features integral to fibromyalgia may help to confirm the diagnostic impression, particularly in equivocal cases.

## EXACERBATING FACTORS AND ASSOCIATED CONDITIONS

Smythe first drew attention to factors that cause exacerbation of symptoms in fibromyalgia (3). Additional factors were later identified by Yunus and his colleagues (5). Fibromyalgia may be made worse by stress, weather changes, severe physical activity, anxiety, or tension; it may be improved by rest, heat, and vacation. Most of these symptoms are not effective in differentiating patients with fibromyalgia from those with other disorders (30). Even so, they are found frequently in fibromyalgia, and they constitute an important part of the syndrome.

Finally, fibromyalgia often occurs in concert with other rheumatic or nonrheumatic conditions. The presence of other conditions may influence the presentation of fibromyalgia or even may obscure its presence. Thus when fibromyalgia occurs in patients with low back pain or cervical pain syndromes, the underlying disorder becomes more prominent and appears more severe.

## DIAGNOSIS OF FIBROMYALGIA

The diagnosis of fibromyalgia is relatively straightforward and actually quite simple. However, it is useful first to consider potential modifiers to the diagnosis, the concepts of primary, secondary, and concomitant fibromyalgia. As originally proposed, fibromyalgia was thought of as a separate entity, a single diagnosis, but it was also clear that the signs and symptoms of the syndrome occurred frequently in those who had other rheumatic conditons. To distinguish the entities the term "primary" was applied to fibromyalgia that occurred in the absence of other conditions and the term "secondary" to fibromyalgia occurring with other, usually rheumatic conditions. However, both terms were problematic.

To identify primary fibromyalgia it was necessary to exclude all patients who had other disorders or who had abnormal laboratory or radiographic studies. The original diagnostic criteria of Smythe (4) and the later criteria of Yunus et al. (5) and others took this approach. However, radiographic abnormalities are common in the general population, as are isolated but unimportant laboratory abnormalities. In addition, excluding other medical conditions tended to limit patients to the young. Finally, occult disease might be present in those with the primary syndrome.

Secondary fibromyalgia was equally difficult to characterize. There was, for example, no way to determine when fibromyalgia was "secondary to" (read "caused by") another condition and when it was merely a concomitant disorder. Most investigators working in the field believed that actual secondary fibromyalgia was rare and the concomitant syndrome common. Also, there was no way of telling when "enough" secondary or concomitant disease was present for classification as concomitant fibromyalgia and when the associated disease might be "causative." An additional problem was that, although there were diagnostic criteria for primary fibromyalgia, none had been tested in secondary or concomitant disease, and it was uncertain if these criteria for the primary syndrome were appropriate.

The recent multicenter study of criteria for fibromyalgia (6) addressed these problems. This study tested (actually developed) criteria in patients labeled as "primary" as well as those labeled as "secondary or concomitant." It was found that the final criteria worked just as well in those labeled primary as in those in the other category. Therefore, to diagnose fibromyalgia one does not have to obtain radiographs or laboratory studies. Such tests should be obtained only when clinically indicated to identify or characterize another condition. With the radiographic, laboratory, and other disease exclusions eliminated, one can come up with a working definition of the fibromyalgia modifiers. Primary fibromyalgia is that condition in which the syndrome is recognized in the absence of another clinically important rheumatic disease. Concomitant fibromyalgia is fibromyalgia that occurs in the presence of another clinically important rheumatic condition. Practically, however, it is not usually important to make this distinction since fibromyalgia and any concomitant condition do not usually interact, and both should be addressed. For example, when fibromyalgia occurs in the presence of rheumatoid arthritis both conditions are treated, and our knowledge is not increased by labeling the fibromyalgia as "secondary." In fact, it is probably best to speak of the "fibromyalgia syndrome" without considering modifiers, much as one might address heart failure in an individual with psoriasis. At the level of diagnosis the newly proposed fibromyalgia classification criteria do not make any distinction between primary and secondary-concomitant fibromyalgia. The term "concomitant," quintessentially more precise, should replace "secondary."

A number of different diagnostic criteria have been proposed for fibromyalgia (35). Generally, all have been based on the identification of some combination of symptoms and a certain number of tender points. The newly proposed fibromyalgia criteria are based on the results of a 16-center study that enrolled 558 patients and controls (6, 36), and it is likely that they will be widely adopted as the *de facto* criteria for the syndrome. Only two criteria (Table 20.3) are required for diagnosis. First the patient must have "widespread pain." Widespread pain is defined as pain in the upper and lower body segments, pain on the left and right sides of the body, and pain in the axial skeleton. Second, a patient must have tenderness in at least 11 of 18 specified tender point sites (Fig. 20.2).

When fibromyalgia is sought in the clinic it is found to be quite prevalent. In a rheumatology clinic as many as 20% of new patients satisfied criteria for diagnosis (5). Using insensitive criteria about 5.5% of patients attending a general medical clinic were found to have the syndrome (28). The syndrome was reported to occur in about 2.3% of all patients seen in a family practice setting (37). Even so, the syndrome is not considered by or is unknown to many practitioners. As a consequence, many fibromyalgia patients have been misdiagnosed.

My experience and that of others is that misdiagnosis falls into two major categories. First, the syndrome may be erroneously identified as systemic lupus erythematosus or rheumatoid arthritis when fatigue and joint symptoms predominate. More frequently, however, fibromyalgia is mistaken for various forms of axial skeletal disease, including disc and entrapment syndromes. This is often the case when one symptom (e.g., neck and arm pain) predominates. The clue to the diagnosis of fibromyalgia lies in identifying the widespread nature of the pain even when the patient has one main complaint ("Yes, but do you have pain in your knees or legs?"). This should be followed up with the tender point examination. Stated simply,

---

**Table 20.3.**
**The American College of Rheumatology 1990 Criteria for the Classification of Fibromyalgia[a,b]**

---

1.  History of widespread pain.
    *Definition.* Pain is considered widespread when all of the following are present: pain in the left side of the body, pain in the right side of the body, pain above the waist, and pain below the waist. In addition, axial skeletal pain (cervical spine or anterior check or thoracic spine or low back) must be present. In this definition, shoulder and buttock pain is considered as pain for each involved side. "Low back" pain is considered lower segment pain.
2.  Pain in 11 of 18 tender point sites on digital palpation.
    *Definition.* Pain, on digital palpation, must be present in at least 11 of the following 18 tender point sites:
    *Occiput:* bilateral, at the suboccipital muscle insertions.
    *Low cervical:* bilateral, at the anterior aspects of the intertransverse spaces at C5–C7.
    *Trapezius:* bilateral, at the midpoint of the upper border.
    *Supraspinatus:* bilateral, at origins, above the scapula spine near the medial border.
    *Second rib:* bilateral, at the second costochondral junctions, just lateral to the junctions on upper surfaces.
    *Lateral epicondyle:* bilateral, 2 cm distal to the epicondyles.
    *Gluteal:* bilateral, in upper outer quadrants of buttocks in anterior fold of muscle.
    *Greater trochanter:* bilateral, posterior to the trochanteric prominence.
    *Knee:* bilateral, at the medial fat pad proximal to the joint line.
    Digital palpation should be performed with an approximate force of 4 kg.
    For a tender point to be considered "positive" the subject must state that the palpation was painful. "Tender" is not to be considered "painful."

---

[a]From Wolfe F, Smythe HA, Yunus MB, et al: The American College of Rehumatology 1990 criteria for the classification of fibromyalgia: report of the Multicenter Criteria Committee. *Arthritis Rheum* 33:160–172, 1990. Copyright 1990. Used by permission of the American College of Rheumatology.
[b]For classification purposes, patients will be said to have fibromyalgia if both criteria are satisfied. Widespread pain must have been present for at least 3 months. The presence of a second clinical disorder does not exclude the diagnosis of fibromyalgia.

in order to diagnose fibromyalgia, physicians must first consider it and then examine for it.

## DIFFERENTIAL DIAGNOSIS

Fibromyalgia is usually an easy diagnosis. The syndrome may, however, be confused with local and regional pain syndromes and with various axial skeletal syndromes in which some of the symptoms of fibromyalgia are also noted. Sleep disturbance, for example, is as common in low back pain as in fibromyalgia (30). It is also common in painful cervical syndromes. Headache, paresthesias, and psychological distress are also common in musculoskeletal pain syndrome. Thus it is hazardous to suspect fibromyalgia on the basis of behavioral patterns and symptoms without the performance of the tender point count. Tenderness is present on palpation in most regional syndromes, including the myofascial pain syndrome. The clue to these syndromes is that the tenderness is local or regional rather than generalized.

Cervical syndromes produce pain in the neck and shoulder girdles and associated tender points in these regions. Both cervical disease and lumbosacral disease are common, and they may frequently coexist. When this happens it may be difficult to separate this individual from one with fibromyalgia since most of the diagnostic features of fibromyalgia may also be present. A clue is that the pain may not be quite as widespread; it may be missing, for example, in the hands or feet or knees. Such patients may also have had a long history of pain in either the cervical or the lumbar area before the onset of pain in the other area. Finally, radiographic abnormalities may be severe. Even so it is sometimes impossible to separate the two syndromes.

In fibromyalgia, except for tender points, the physical examination is normal. The core and common symptoms, however, are usually present. When the count of tender points is below that needed for diagnosis one may think that the patient has early or mild fibromyalgia, but other diseases may present in this way as well. Both rheumatoid arthritis and systemic lupus erythematosus, in very early stages when joint swelling is absent or minimal, may present a rather similar picture. In such a setting one should be very cautious about diagnosis.

Similarly, it is important to recognize that joint pain and even tenderness may be present in those persons with fibromyalgia not on the basis of synovitis but on the basis of generalized hyperalgesia. A positive antinuclear antibody titer can lead the observer into the diagnosis of systemic lupus erythematosus when the real diagnosis is fibromyalgia. I and others interested in fibromyalgia have seen numerous patients erroneously diagnosed as having systemic lupus erythematosus or rheumatoid arthritis on the basis of spurious laboratory tests, joint pain that was hyperalgesia, and a failure to perform the fibromyalgia examination. It should be remembered that fibromyalgia and inflammatory disease can easily coexist.

## DEMOGRAPHICS

Most patients (>85%) with the syndrome are women (22, 26). The disorder appears at all ages, but seems to be most common between 30 and 60 years of age. One report describes 33 children with fibromyalgia (38), but in the absence of other reports insufficient data exist regarding estimates of prevalence among children. Most centers reporting on fibromyalgia have served middle-class, predominantly white populations, and few data are available regarding the proportion of nonwhite subjects with fibromyalgia.

## FIBROMYALGIA AND CERVICAL SPINE PAIN

The discussion above has emphasized that fibromyalgia is common, and that it frequently occurs together with other rheumatic syndromes. Thus fibromyalgia may be the cause of the patient's cervical pain, and fibromyalgia may occur together with another cause of cervical pain. In relation to cervical pain, it is useful to consider the symptoms of the disorder that suggest cervical spine involvement in the pain process.

A characteristic of fibromyalgia pain is radiation. Leavitt et al. noted that radiating pain was described by 48% of fibromyalgia patients as opposed to 12% of rheumatoid arthritis patients (27). As noted in Figure 20.3, paresthesias are a common feature of the syndrome as well. Among the common patterns of pain and pain radiation is cervical and shoulder girdle pain with aching and radiation of pain into the arms, hands, and fingers. Interestingly, fibromyalgia mimics lumbosacral disease in that "typical" sciatic and other characteristic forms of pain radiation may occur.

Seriousness and urgency are suggested by fibromyalgia complaints. Fibromyalgia is among the most painful of rheumatic conditions. Persons with the syndrome have greater pain levels and higher scores on visual analogue scales, for example, than do those with rheumatoid arthritis (39, 40). Clinicians react to pain severity and may initiate testing rather than continued observation.

## CERVICAL PAIN AND FIBROMYALGIA ETIOLOGY

A number of hypotheses have been suggested as to the etiology of fibromyalgia. One current hypothesis suggests that there are abnormalities in muscle, perhaps because of decreased oxygen uptake in muscle (41–45). Such a hypothesis, while it may explain the "muscle pain," fatigue, and weakness of the syndrome, does not explain the widespread nature of the pain, the nonmuscular complaints, and the abnormalities of autonomic hyperactivity that are frequently seen.

A hypothesis that more effectively explains fibromyalgia pain is the consideration of the syndrome as a central pain amplification syndrome or disorder of pain modulation (Table 20.2) (46). This concept is suggested by a number of observations. Tender point dolorimetry investigations indicate that fibromyalgia tenderness is widespread, existing even in the area of "control points" (29, 34). It seems likely that the "control regions" are intrinsically less sensitive, and that they respond to pressure with less pain. In this model the peripheral sites of tenderness are normal regardless of whether they are "control" sites or "tender point" sites.

Such a central model helps to explain the widespread pain reported by fibromyalgia patients: concomitant disease is uncovered or made worse. For example, Wolfe et al. noted in a study of fibromyalgia in patients with rheumatoid arthritis that, although fibromyalgia-positive and fibromyalgia-negative patients did not differ in their manifestations of rheumatoid arthritis, they had higher levels of pain, functional disability, and other global measures (40). I have suggested elsewhere that one might consider that all fibromyalgia is "secondary (concomitant)" (26) since in a pain amplification syndrome subclinical disease may become "amplified"just enough to be noted as pain. Finally, such a model explains the fact that pain is more severe in fibromyalgia patients than in those with a multitude of other rheumatic conditions. Within the context of more precise nomenclature, then, fibromyalgia would represent a conditon of *allodynia* and *hyperalgesia* (47).

It is of interest that a number of studies suggest that central mechanisms may operate in fibromyalgia. Vaeroy has found elevated levels of substance P in the cerebrospinal fluid of patients with the syndrome (48). Sleep studies have shown that deprivation of non–rapid eye movement (REM) sleep leads to intensification of musculoskeletal symptoms (49), and such sleep anomalies are characteristic of the syndrome (4). Reactive hyperemia as mediated through neurogenic inflammation is increased in fibromyalgia patients when compared with controls (50). A number of reports have demonstrated increased sympathetic activity in patients with the syndrome (50, 51), as well as a reduction in pain and tender points with sympathetic blockage (51). Sympathetic overactivity may be a part of the increased reports of Raynaud's phenomenon (52), "subjective swelling" and other neurologic-like symptoms (33).

At the clinical level, Smythe (3, 53, 54) has suggested that problems at the level of the lumbar and cervical spine may be causative or exacerbating factors in the syndrome. Within Smythe's concept structural abnormalities or abnormal stress on axial structures leads to increases in referred pain. Additional evidence for the role of the cervical spine comes from two sources. The first is the common experience that fibromyalgia develops in a number of individuals following trauma (22, 24). Most often the syndrome occurs after an event such as whiplash, a "back injury," or a "fall." The initial pain is usually unilateral, involving the neck, shoulder girdle and arm, but it soon spreads to involve the contralateral extremity and then the entire musculoskeletal system.

This type of pattern has been studied by Littlejohn (55, 56). He has reported in detail on the Australian epidemic experience with the "repetitive strain syndrome," a condition in which an extremity (and soon the shoulder girdle) becomes painful. This is often followed by involvement of the entire extremity. The extremity is often painful, with "local" "tender points" and evidence of sympathetic abnormality. A small number of these patients then develop contralateral symptoms and a full-blown fibromyalgia syndrome.

Although only a minority of patients develop fibromyalgia following (known) cervical or lumbar trauma (or other trauma), the pattern of development suggests that some "trigger" might exist that changes response at the level of the cord and leads to the development of fibromyalgia. Substance P and other neurotransmitters, and autonomic dysfunction, might be some of the effector mechanisms. To test the relationship between cervical trauma or injury and the subsequent development of fibromyalgia requires markers of cervical spine disease or injury that are more sensitive than those available today.

The presumed hyperalgesia of fibromyalgia suggests that (a) patients with fibromyalgia with various types of cervical spine disease will experience more pain and pain in a wider distribution than those without fibromyalgia, and (b) subclinical cervical spine disease may be unmasked in fibromyalgia. A third possibility is that fibromyalgia produces cervical pain in the absence of any disease or abnormality of the cervical spine. The study of Yunus et al. (5), which was restricted to relatively younger patients, found cervical pain in less than 40% of patients, as opposed to other studies in which 70% or more reported such pain (22, 27). Such data suggest that cervical pain is more common in older fibromyalgia patients who would be expected to have, intrinsically, more abnormalities of the cervical spine.

Although, the central nervous system likely plays a major role in fibromyalgia, the mechanism is certainly more complex than is suggested here. Psychological factors, infection, and other medical conditions may well lead to the development of the syndrome as well. As suggested by Graham in 1953 (19), fibromyalgia may be a final common pathway for a number of precipitating factors.

## PRACTICAL CONSIDERATIONS IN FIBROMYALGIA AND CERVICAL PAIN

It is extremely important to consider the diagnosis of fibromyalgia in any patients with neck and shoulder/arm pain. Failure to do this has led to unnecessary, expensive, and hazardous tests and treatments. Cathey and coworkers have documented high rates of hospitalization, diagnostic tests, and utilization of medical services prior to the diagnosis of fibromyalgia (57). These data have been confirmed anecdotally by other fibromyalgia investigators (5). Cathey et al. also noted 13 hospitalizations for surgery of the neck or back among their 81 patients. It is the sense of those involved in fibromyalgia research that almost all hospitalizations and surgical interventions in fibromyalgia patients have been unnecessary, the result of failing to consider the diagnosis.

## MANAGEMENT OF FIBROMYALGIA

Treatment of neck and shoulder/arm pain in fibromyalgia must consider fibromyalgia as well as the concomitant condition if one can be identi-

fied. It is almost certain that a treatment that aims at "anatomic" abnormalities and does not take fibromyalgia into consideration will fail. There are no prospective studies to support this assertion, but I have yet to see patients who have responded more than briefly to treatment for cervical pain with modalities such as cervical traction, ultrasound, trigger point injections, neck exercises, range-of-motion exercises, transcutaneous electrical nerve stimulation (TENS), and surgery in the absence of treatment for fibromyalgia as well. Indeed, axial skeletal surgery seems so universally unsuccessful that I believe that it should be undertaken in the fibromyalgia patient with great trepidation and only when there is strong evidence to support the belief that a specific anatomic lesion is present and is the cause of the pain.

Available data from Felson and Goldenberg (58) and Cathey et al. (57) suggest that fibromyalgia is a chronic disorder with few remissions. Thus the goal of treatment is not cure but reduction in symptoms and associated disability. Practically speaking, one wishes to reduce pain, psychological abnormality, functional disability, economic costs, side effects of treatment, and utilization of services and to make the patient more reliant on his or her own resources. The results of various treatment modalities are given in Table 20.4.

## PATIENT EDUCATION

Among the most important steps in fibromyalgia management is the explanation of the diagnosis to the patient. Patients must be taught that leg pain or arm pain is not a "pinched nerve," that knee or hand pain is not significant arthritis, that paresthesias are not neurologic disorders, and so forth, and that instead these symptoms are manifestations of the fibromyalgia syndrome and its hyperalgesia. If this can be accomplished there will be an immediate reduction in the demand for medical services, including hospitalizations and invasive and noninvasive investigations (57). Patients will be spared unnecessary expense and potential injury.

Explanation has other important benefits. Patients with fibromyalgia have usually seen multiple physicians without a certain diagnosis, and received multiple, and usually unsuccessful, treatments. Many tests have been performed, and were found to be normal. Patients frequently believe that physicians suspect their problems are psychological, and have been told that "nothing" could be found that was wrong. Patients are frequently

**Table 20.4.**
**Fibromyalgia Treatment**

| Treatment | Results | Reference |
|---|---|---|
| Amitriptyline | Effective | 61, 62 |
| Cyclobenzaprine | Effective | 63 |
| Exercise | Effective | 73 |
| Aprazolam | Possibly effective | (I.J. Russell, in press) |
| NSAIDS | Not effective | 62 |
| Corticosteroids | Not effective | 71 |
| Biofeedback | Possibly effective | |
| Local injections | Limited data, value dubious | |
| Physical therapy | No data, value dubious | |
| Analgesics | No data, probably effective | |
| Specific antianxiety and antidepressive therapy | No data | |

angry about the doctor shuffle and the unspoken insinuation of a psychological basis for their symptoms. If the physician who makes the diagnosis of fibromyalgia takes the patient through the usual findings in fibromyalgia—the sleep disturbance, fatigue, subjective swelling, paresthesias, and other symptoms—and then follows this with a description of the tender points, "which are not found in any other medical condition," several important benefits accrue. First, the patient is assured that what he or she has is a recognizable medical condition (syndrome), and one that is not primarily a psychological disorder. Second, there is an unspoken assurance that the physician understands the treatment of the disorder. Third, the anger that the patient may have brought with him or her is often dissipated, and a new physician-patient relationship can be established.

## PHARMACOTHERAPY

Pharmacotherapy has two principal aims: to address the presumed sleep abnormality that is present in fibromyalgia, and to reduce pain independently. Based on the work of Moldofsky and colleagues (49, 59, 60) related to the non-REM sleep anomaly (alpha-delta sleep) in the syndrome, a series of agents have been used that were presumed to improve sleep quality. Two agents, amitriptyline (61, 62) and cyclobenzaprine (63), have been shown to have benefit in well-controlled, blind clinical trials. In small doses (25–50 mg) amitriptyline reduces pain, sleep disturbance, and tenderness in fibromyalgia patients. Similar changes were found with cyclobenzaprine at doses of 10–30 mg/day. Although no studies have addressed this point, there appear to be certain patients who respond dramatically to such thera-

pies, whereas others respond in a limited fashion or not at all. Although these drugs reduce overall fibromyalgia severity, the overall improvement they bestow is small (perhaps 20%) and they are, alone, generally insufficient treatment for the syndrome. Although tricyclic drugs are frequently referred to as "antidepressants," they reduce pain in depressed as well as nondepressed individuals (64–69), and are effective at doses thought to be without antidepressant effect, doses commonly used in the treatment of fibromyalgia.

Two studies have examined the effect of nonsteroidal anti-inflammatory drugs in fibromyalgia. One study evaluated naproxen alone and in combination with amitriptyline; no benefit was found (62). A second study tried ibuprofen in fibromyalgia patients, but no benefit was noted (70). Although such studies confirm the clinical impression that nonsteroidal anti-inflammatory drugs have little value, it is important to recognize that patients with the disorder may have other musculoskeletal causes for pain (including cervical spine disease) that may benefit from treatment with these agents.

Analgesics are used frequently, but none has been studied scientifically. It is therefore a presumption, albeit a reasonable presumption, that they are effective in reducing the pain of fibromyalgia. There is almost no role for narcotic analgesics in this disorder, and there is a general consensus that they should not be used. Aspirin, acetaminophen, or propoxyphene (in small doses) are reasonable choices for therapy.

Although steroids have been suggested by some in the past, a controlled study has failed to suggest any benefit from this therapy (71), confirming the widely held view of experts that steroids should never be used in fibromyalgia.

The use of antidepressants and/or anxiolytic agents for treatment of psychological problems associated with fibromyalgia has not been addressed in controlled trials. It seems reasonable, however, to suggest that the indications for these agents are not different in fibromyalgia than in other medical conditions. A number of studies have reported that fibromyalgia patients have higher scores for anxiety and depression (as measured by a series of instruments) than do those with other rheumatic conditions (39, 40, 72). The issue as to whether such test abnormalities are intrinsic to the syndrome or instead represent a response to chronic severe pain has been raised. Regardless of the ultimate answer to that question, it seems clear that psychological stress can worsen the symptoms of fibromyalgia; therefore the physician should take into consideration the psychological status of the patient in the overall management plan.

## "TRIGGER POINT" INJECTIONS

Because of the relationship of the myofascial pain syndrome to fibromyalgia, it has been suggested that "trigger point" injections may be of benefit. Anecdotal evidence suggests that such therapies are frequently employed. On the face of it, however, there is little reason to suspect that such treatment would help fibromyalgia patients given the widespread nature of the pain and tenderness. It is not known whether trigger points (18) are increased in patients with fibromyalgia since no studies have specifically addressed that point. Bengstsson et al., using an idiosyncratic definition of trigger points, did find an increase in their fibromyalgia patients (24). A recent study (F. Wolfe, unpublished data) specifically addressing that point did not find that trigger points were prevalent in fibromyalgia patients.

Injection of trigger points should be accomplished when the treating physician believes that a second condition (myofascial pain syndrome) is coexistent with fibromyalgia and that that condition requires such therapy. The down side of injection therapy is that it makes the patient more rather than less dependent on the physician.

## PHYSICAL THERAPY AND EXERCISE

Physical therapy has been employed in the community for treatment of the syndrome. There are no data to suggest that it is of benefit, or to describe just what is meant by physical therapy. The strengthening of specific muscle groups and the use of range-of-motion exercises should not be expected to have any ameliorating effect on the signs and symptoms of the disorder, although H. Smythe has suggested (personal communication) that strengthening of abdominal musculature will be of benefit.

Exercise, however, has been shown to be of benefit in a carefully done, well-controlled trial that compared aerobic exercise (bicycle riding in a controlled setting) and stretching (in the same setting) (73). Patients in the aerobic group increased their aerobic capacity and had significant reduction in pain and the number of tender points. Since it has been shown that fibromyalgia patients are detrained (44, 74) and have lower muscular oxygen uptakes during exercise (44), there is reason to believe that aerobic exercise might benefit patients with the syndrome. The mechanism of such benefit is not known. It has been suggested, but not proven, that changes in neurotransmitters might occur following exercise. Other explanations are possible, including improvement in psychological status following physical conditioning. Whatever the mechanism, an attempt to get patients to exercise should be a part of any program of fibromyalgia management.

Selection of the best type of exercise is frequently a problem. Patients with significant low back pain may report intensification of pain following exercise, and the prescription of too vigorous an exercise will certainly lead to failure. It is good to attempt to get the patient to make exercise a part of his or her life. Therefore the exercise suggested ought to be more than a "chore." Bicycle riding (indoor or outdoor) is often an effective and acceptable exercise, although its availability as an outdoor activity depends on the community in which the patient lives and on weather considerations. "Fast walking" (fast enough to get the pulse to 140) may also be effective, but it may be harder to get patients to walk fast enough to achieve that goal. Swimming is difficult for most patients since it requires extra travel and may not be easily available. Exercise clubs and hospital "health centers" are uncertain entities since they tend to stress activities within their aerobic program that may increase pain in fibromyalgia patients.

## OTHER MODALITIES

Although modalities such as ultrasound, cervical traction, TENS, and similar devices are used in the community, they have little sound basis behind them. No studies have evaluated these expensive modalities in fibromyalgia patients. I believe that they are rarely indicated or required. Certainly chronic use of such treatments tends to enforce reliance on the health care system.

One study has investigated biofeedback in the syndrome in a small number of patients (75). Although benefit was reported, the study had a number of problems, and no firm conclusions can be drawn from it (76). Although biofeedback might help some patients, it remains an expensive treatment in this syndrome, and a treatment for which there exist no long-term data regarding efficacy.

Cervical collars have not been evaluated in fibromyalgia, but there is little reason to believe that they may be effective.

## CONCOMITANT CONDITIONS

Although the discussion thus far has addressed fibromyalgia as if it were primarily an isolated condition, it occurs frequently in combination with other medical disorders, including various neck pain syndromes. When possible, it is important to try to sort out manifestations of fibromyalgia from manifestations of the concomitant disorders. In concomitant conditions such as rheumatoid arthritis this is relatively easy to do. One looks for evidence of inflammatory disease and also for manifestations of the nonarticular condition (fibromyalgia). In cervical pain disorders this is a much more difficult problem since the manifestations of both syndromes may be the same. There are no guidelines as to how to apportion symptoms between the two conditions. When cervical pain is a prominent problem in fibromyalgia it is probably best to assume that some additional intrinsic disease of the cervical spine is present and to suggest therapy that may be helpful.

Therapy remains largely empiric since there are no studies that allow a choice between varying therapies or evaluation of their effects. Smythe, on the basis of his extensive experience in fibromyalgia and neck pain, suggests that neck pain and referred neck pain may be the result of "cervical strain" caused by stress to the "unsupported neck" during sleep (54). A reliable neck support specially designed to support the lower cervical spine may be of help. One may assume that such an inexpensive support can be helpful in the generalized syndrome of fibromyalgia, and it is reasonable to suggest that patients use such a device even in the absence of objective data concerning its benefit.

## ROLE OF THE WORKPLACE

It is beyond the scope of this chapter to discuss the role of the workplace (the home or the place of employment) in fibromyalgia. Nevertheless, it is worth noting that the patient's history may reveal that certain activities involving the neck include repeated movements and/or extremes of flexion, hypertension and rotation. It is probable that such motion in the patients with fibromyalgia neck pain can increase and continue the pain. Identification of such potential problems can lead to instruction regarding appropriate cervical joint protection.

## PROGNOSIS IN FIBROMYALGIA

The longest published study regarding fibromyalgia extended for only 2 years of follow-up (58). Studies of the therapeutic effect of tricyclics provide no data beyond 3 months. Data that are available, however, suggest chronicity of the syndrome. Hawley and her colleagues followed 75 fibromyalgia patients monthly during a 1-year period and assessed function, pain, global severity, and psychological variables using standardized questionnaire instruments (77). Scores for these variables did not change over the year in a repeated-measures analysis. Felson and Goldenberg interviewed 39 consecutive new patients during a 2-year period (58). At the final assessment, about 3.1 years after diagnosis, 92% of patients continued to have pain complaints. More than 60% of these 39 patients scored their symptoms as moderate or severe. Cathey et al. (57) studied 81 previously diagnosed fibromyalgia patients as to persistence of symptoms. Patients in this group had had fibromyalgia symptoms for a mean of more than 12 years. At interview all patients had symptoms. A past remission was noted by 23%, and the median duration of remission was 12 months. A remission lasting at least 12 months was noted by only 12.5% of patients.

These observations relating to chronicity and remission of symptoms represent the data of only two centers, both rheumatology centers. Whether such observations can be extrapolated to the community at large is uncertain. No data relating to fibromyalgia in the community are available. Longitudinal studies will be required to better describe the prognosis in the syndrome and to ascertain the long-term effects of therapy.

## MEDICOLEGAL ASPECTS OF FIBROMYALGIA

Fibromyalgia has been reported to follow trauma in approximately 22% of patients (22, 24), but no data have been collected as to the type of trauma. When such patients are seen in the clinic it is often in association with a compensation claim. The examining physician is usually asked if the trauma "caused" the fibromyalgia. Given the limited nature of our knowledge of the etiology of fibromyalgia, it is sometimes hardly more than a guess to answer such a question. The physician must try to decide if the patient is malingering or actually has the syndrome. One suggestion has been to test the "control point" regions as well as the "tender point" regions during the examination. Most often patients do not have significant tenderness in these regions. However, this is not always an effective means of differentiation since (a) some patients may be tender at all of the regions tested, (b) the worried and unsophisticated patient may be afraid to give a negative answer, and (c) even a patient who is clearly overreporting may also have fibromyalgia. A review of the symptoms of fibromyalgia may help here. The use of the dolorimeter may be another aid since the patient is less certain about where to place the level of pain than when asked if the examination is painful during the standard tender point palpation examination. Usually (perhaps 90% of the time) the examiner can establish the diagnosis accurately.

The diagnosis of fibromyalgia as an effect of trauma or injury is most secure when the following pattern is noted. An otherwise healthy person sustains some sort of trauma (injury) and then develops a local pain problem. The pain problem then becomes regional, then bilateral and finally generalized. This type of pattern is common and its identification offers a degree of security in an otherwise tenuous position.

Beyond the establishment of the diagnosis, and providing evidence regarding a causal pattern, the prognosis as to pain, medical expense, and work are important subsidiary questions. Since there are no data regarding what happens to patients whose fibromyalgia follows upon trauma, the only data that can be presented are the data relating to chronicity noted above. Clearly, fibromyalgia is not an expensive disorder unless unnecessary investigations and interventions occur.

Fibromyalgia is suspect as a source of disability since patients have no obvious anatomic abnormality and appear generally healthy. Fibromyalgia patients, however, score abnormally on standardized self-administered disability questionnaires. Our group administered the Stanford Health Assessment Questionnaire (HAQ) Functional Disability Index (78, 79) to fibromyalgia patients in a series of reports. Among 572 patients the mean HAQ score was 0.9 ($\pm$0.65 SD), indicating slightly less than moderate disability (80). By contrast, scores for 1285 rheumatoid arthritis patients were 1.1 ($\pm$0.68 SD), for 1068 low back pain patients 0.6 ($\pm$0.57 SD), for 744 knee osteoarthritis patients 0.7 ($\pm$0.57 SD), and for 493 hand osteoarthritis patients 0.5 ($\pm$0.54 SD). These data indicate that after the somewhat more impaired rheumatoid arthritis patients, patients with fibromyalgia describe more impairment than those with low back pain or osteoarthritis.

Results such as these might represent perceived rather than actual impairment. Cathey et al. used computerized simulated work testing in which the actual amount of work could be measured in inch-pound-degrees (Fig. 20.4) (81). In addition, they correlated work scores with pretest HAQ functional disability scores. Fibromyalgia patients and rheumatoid arthritis patients in that study were significantly impaired compared with normal controls, but performance scores for both disease groups were about equal. A moderately strong correlation ($r = .61$) was noted between HAQ scores and actual work impairment for the fibromyalgia patients, thus offering some additional validation to the functional status indicated on the HAQ disability assessments.

Further suggestions of impairment come from the data of Jacobsen and Danneskiold Samse (74), who tested fibromyalgia patients on a CYBEX machine and found evidence of muscle weakness, and from the data of Bennett and colleagues (44), who found patients poorly physically conditioned and with reduced exercise blood flow as measured by xenon-133 clearance.

Translation of these observations into actual work disability is precarious. Cathey and colleagues (57, 81) surveyed fibromyalgia patients on two occasions. In a study of 81 patients they found mean days lost from work during a 1-year period to be 9.8 days. Data from national statistics indicate that work loss for a similar period was 8.0, 7.4, and 5.2 days for patients with low back pain, rheumatoid arthritis, and osteoarthritis, respectively. In a study of 176 patients, 9.3% considered

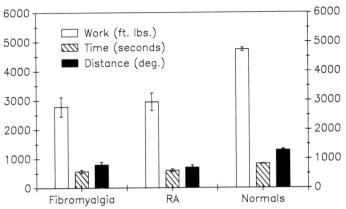

**Figure 20.4.** Total work, time, and distance score for fibromyalgia and rheumatoid arthritis (RA) patients and normal controls for five work tasks on a BTE work simulator (BTE Instruments, Baltimore, MD). The work tasks involved wrist twisting, pushing and pulling at the shoulder level, vacuum cleaning–like activity, working above the head, and lifting objects from the floor. Work is expressed in inch-pound-degrees $\times 10^3$. Distance represent total movement and is expressed as degrees $\times 10^3$. Time is the time used before stopping when completed (all of time used) or stopping prior to scheduled completion because of pain or lack of endurance. Error bars are SEM. (From Cathey MA, Wolfe F, Kleinheksel SM, Miller S, Pitetti KH: Functional ability and work status in patients with fibromyalgia. *Arthritis Care Res* 1:85–98, 1988. Copyright 1988 by Elsevier Science Publishing Co., Inc.)

themselves disabled but only 5.7% received disability payments from any source. Seventeen percent of patients reported that they stopped working because of fibromyalgia, and 30.4% stated that they changed jobs because of the syndrome (81). Similar data regarding work change and time lost from work have recently become available from Boston fibromyalgia researchers (83). In a different social setting, Bengstsson et al. reported that 22% of 55 Swedish patients were "disabled," and that 55% were unable to manage household tasks by themselves. Twenty-four percent were receiving pensions (24).

Even with data such as these the determination of work ability both within and outside of a compensation setting is extremely precarious, particularly since demographics, psychosocial factors, job satisfaction, and the actual type of work are important determinants of ability in chronic pain conditions. At a minimum, however, it seems possible to tell compensation and disability hearing officers that most patients can work provided they have jobs that do not impose physical hardships (i.e., do not cause or exacerbate pain), but that 15–20% of patients will stop working because of the syndrome. An important corollary of these observations is that most patients can work if they have the right job. Rather than making the patients "disabled" by encouraging the legal disability status, it is probably better therapeutically to

discourage the process and to aim the patient in the direction of improvement.

**REFERENCES**

1. Wolfe F: Methodologic and statistical problems in the epidemiology of fibromyalgia. In Ewad E, Fricton JR (eds): *Myofascial Pain and Fibromyalgia.* New York, Raven Press, 1989.
2. Kraft GH, Johnson EW, LaBan MM: The fibrositis syndrome. *Arch Phys Med Rehabil* 49:155–161, 1968.
3. Smythe HA: The fibrositis syndrome (non-articular rheumatism). In Hollander JL (ed): *Arthritis and Allied Conditions.* Philadelphia, Lea & Febiger, 1972, pp 965–968.
4. Smythe HA, Moldofsky H: Two contributions to understanding of the "fibrositis" syndrome. *Bull Rheum Dis* 28:928–931, 1977.
5. Yunus MB, Masi AT, Calabro JJ, Miller KA, Feigenbaum SL: Primary fibromyalgia (fibrositis): clinical study of 50 patients with matched normal controls. *Semin Arthritis Rheum* 11:151–171, 1981.
6. Wolfe F, Smythe HA, Yunus MB, Bennett RM, Bombardier C, Goldenberg DL, Tugwell P, Abeles M, Campbell SM, Clark P, Fam AG, Farber SJ, Fiechtner JJ, Franklin CM, Gatter RA, Hamaty D, Lessard J, Lichtbroun AS, Masi AT, McCain GA, Reynolds WJ, Romano TJ, Russell IJ, Sheon RP: The American College of Rheumatology 1990 Criteria for the classification of fibromyalgia: report of the Multicenter Criteria Committee. *Arthritis Rheum* 33:160–172, 1990.
7. Gowers WR: Lumbago: its lessons and analogues. *Br Med J* 1:117, 1904.
8. Stockman R: *Rheumatism and Arthritis.* Edinburgh, W Green & Son Ltd, 1920, pp 132.
9. Reynolds MD: The development of the concept of fibrositis. *J Hist Med Allied Sci* 38:5–35, 1983.

10. Simons DG: Muscle pain syndromes—part I. *Am J Phys Med* 54:289–311, 1975.

11. Simons DG: Muscle pain syndromes—part II. *Am J Phys Med* 55:15–42, 1976.

12. Glogoski G, Wallraff J: Ein beitrag zur klinic und histologie der muskelharten (myogelosen). *Z Orthop* 80:237–268, 1951.

13. Miehlke H, Schulze G, Eger W: Klinische und experimentelle untersuchungen zum fibrositissyndrom. *Z Rheumaforsch* 19:310–330, 1960.

14. Simons DG: Myofascial pain syndromes: where are we? Where are we going? *Arch Phys Med Rehabil* 69:207–212, 1988.

15. Halliday JL: The concept of psychosomatic rheumatism. *Ann Intern Med* 15:666–677, 1941.

16. Kelly M: The nature of fibrositis. *Ann Rheum Dis* 5:69–77, 1946.

17. Travell J, Rinzler SH: The myofascial genesis of pain. *Postgrad Med* 11:425–434, 1952.

18. Travell J, Simons DG: *Myofascial Pain and Dysfunction: The Trigger Point Manual.* Baltimore, Williams & Wilkins, 1983.

19. Graham W: The fibrositis syndrome. *Bull Rheum Dis* 3:33–34, 1953.

20. Hench PK: Nonarticular rheumatism (22nd rheumatism review of 1973–1976 literature). *Arthritis Rheum* 19:1088, 1976.

21. Bennett RM: Fibrositis: misnomer for a common rheumatic disorder. *West J Med* 134:405–413, 1981.

22. Wolfe F: The clinical syndrome of fibrositis. *Am J Med* 81:7–14, 1986.

23. Campbell SM, Bennett RM: Fibrositis. *DM* 32:653–722, 1986.

24. Bengtsson A, Henriksson KG, Jorfeldt L, Kagedal B, Lennmarken C, Lindstrom F: Primary fibromyalgia. A clinical and laboratory study of 55 patients. *Scand J Rheumatol* 15:340–347, 1986.

25. Goldenberg DL: Fibromyalgia syndrome. An emerging but controversial condition. *JAMA* 257:2782–2787, 1987.

26. Wolfe F: Fibromyalgia: the clinical syndrome. *Rheum Dis Clin North Am* 15:1–18, 1989.

27. Leavitt F, Katz RS, Golden HE, Glickman PB, Layfer LF: Comparison of pain properties in fibromyalgia patients and rheumatoid arthritis patients. *Arthritis Rheum* 29:775–781, 1986.

28. Campbell SM, Clark S, Tindall EA, Forehand ME, Bennett RM: Clinical characteristics of fibrositis. I. A "blinded," controlled study of symptoms and tender points. *Arthritis Rheum* 26:817–824, 1983.

29. Simms RW, Goldenberg DL, Felson DT, Mason JH: Tenderness in 75 anatomic sites. Distinguishing fibromyalgia patients from controls. *Arthritis Rheum* 31:182–187, 1988.

30. Wolfe F, Hawley DJ, Cathey MA, Caro X, Russell IJ: Fibrositis: symptom frequency and criteria for diagnosis. An evaluation of 291 rheumatic disease patients and 58 normal individuals. *J Rheumatol* 12:1159–1163, 1985.

31. Wolfe F, Cathey MA: The epidemiology of tender points: a prospective study of 1520 patients. *J Rheumatol* 12:1164–1168, 1985.

32. Wolfe F, Cathey MA: Prevalence of primary and secondary fibrositis. *J Rheumatol* 10:965–968, 1983.

33. Simms RW, Goldenberg DL: Symptoms mimicking neurologic disorders in fibromyalgia syndrome. *J Rheumatol* 15:1271–1273, 1988.

34. Tunks E, Crook J, Norman G, Kalaher S: Tender points in fibromyalgia. *Pain* 34:11–19, 1988.

35. Wolfe F: Development of criteria for the diagnosis of fibrositis. *Am J Med* 81:99–104, 1986.

36. Wolfe F: The design of a fibromyalgia criteria study. *J Rheumatol* 116(suppl 19):180–184, 1989.

37. Hartz A, Kirchdoerfer E: Undetected fibrositis in primary care practice. *J Fam Pract* 25:365–369, 1987.

38. Yunus MB, Masi AT: Juvenile primary fibromyalgia syndrome. A clinical study of thirty-three patients and matched normal controls. *Arthritis Rheum* 28:138–145, 1985.

39. Scudds RA, Rollman GB, Harth M, McCain GA: Pain perception and personality measures as discriminators in the classification of fibrositis. *J Rheumatol* 14:563–569, 1987.

40. Wolfe F, Cathey MA, Kleinheksel SM: Fibrositis (fibromyalgia) in rheumatoid arthritis. *J Rheumatol* 11:814–818, 1984.

41. Henriksson KG: Muscle pain in neuromuscular disorders and primary fibromyalgia. *Eur J Appl Physiol* 57:348–352, 1988.

42. Bengtsson A, Henriksson KG, Larsson J: Reduced high-energy phosphate levels in the painful muscles of patients with primary fibromyalgia. *Arthritis Rheum* 29:817–821, 1986.

43. Bengtsson A, Henriksson KG, Larsson J: Muscle biopsy in primary fibromyalgia. Light-microscopical and histochemical findings. *Scand J Rheumatol* 15:1–6, 1986.

44. Bennett RM, Clark SR, Goldberg L, et al: Aerobic fitness in patients with fibrositis: a controlled study of respiratory gas exchange and $^{133}$xenon clearance from exercising muscle. *Arthritis Rheum* 32:454–460, 1989.

45. Bennett RM: Muscle physiology and cold reactivity in the fibromyalgia syndrome. *Rheum Dis Clin North Am* 15:135–148, 1989.

46. Smythe HA: Fibrositis as a disorder of pain modulation. *Clin Rheum Dis* 5:823–832, 1979.

47. Merskey H, International Association for the Study of Pain: Classification of chronic pain: descriptions of chronic pain syndromes and definitions of pain terms. *Pain* S1–S226, 1986.

48. Vaeroy H, Helle R, Frre O, Kass E, Terenius L: Elevated CSF levels of substance P and high incidence of Raynaud phenomenon in patients with fibromyalgia: new features for diagnosis. *Pain* 32:21–26, 1988.

49. Moldofsky H, Scarisbrick P: Induction of neurasthenic musculoskeletal pain syndrome by selective sleep stage deprivation. *Psychosom Med* 38:35–44, 1976.

50. Littlejohn GO, Weinstein C, Helme RD: Increased neurogenic inflammation in fibrositis syndrome. *J Rheumatol* 14:1022–1025, 1987.

51. Bengtsson A, Bengtsson M: Regional sympathetic blockade in primary fibromyalgia. *Pain* 33:161–167, 1988.

52. Dinerman H, Goldenberg DL, Felson DT: A prospective evaluation of 118 patients with the fibromyalgia syndrome: prevalence of Raynaud's phenomenon, sicca symptoms, ANA, low complement, and Ig deposition at the dermal-epidermal junction. *J Rheumatol* 13:368–373, 1986.

53. Smythe HA: "Fibrositis" and other diffuse musculoskeletal syndromes. In Kelley WN, Harris Jr ED, Ruddy S, Sledge CB (eds): *Textbook of Rheumatology.* Philadelphia, WB Saunders, 1985, pp 481–489.

54. Smythe H: The "repetitive strain injury syndrome" is referred pain from the neck. *J Rheumatol* 15:1604–1608, 1988.

55. Littlejohn GE: Repetitive strain syndrome: an Australian experience [editorial]. *J Rheumatol* 13:1004–1006, 1986.

56. Littlejohn GO: Fibrositis/fibromyalgia in the workplace. *Rheum Dis Clin North Am* 15:45–60, 1989.

57. Cathey MA, Wolfe F, Kleinheksel SM, Hawley DJ: Socioeco-

nomic impact of fibrositis. A study of 81 patients with primary fibrositis. *Am J Med* 81:78–84, 1986.

58. Felson DT, Goldenberg DL: The natural history of fibromyalgia. *Arthritis Rheum* 29:1522–1526, 1986.

59. Moldofsky H, Scarisbrick P, England R, Smythe HA: Musculosketal symptoms and non-REM sleep disturbance in patients with "fibrositis syndrome" and healthy subjects. *Psychosom Med* 37:341–351, 1975.

60. Moldofsky H, Warsh JJ: Plasma tryptophan and musculoskeletal pain in non-articular rheumatism ("fibrositis syndrome"). *Pain* 5:65–71, 1978.

61. Carette S, McCain GA, Bell DA, Fam AG: Evaluation of amitriptyline in primary fibrositis. A double-blind, placebo-controlled study. *Arthritis Rheum* 29:655–659, 1986.

62. Goldenberg DL, Felson DT, Dinerman H: A randomized, controlled trial of amitriptyline and naproxen in the treatment of patients with fibromyalgia. *Arthritis Rheum* 29:1371–1377, 1986.

63. Bennett RM, Gatter RA, Campbell SM, Andrews RP, Clark SR, Scarola JA: A comparison of cyclobenzaprine and placebo in the management of fibrositis: a double-blind controlled study. *Arthritis Rheum* 31:1535–1542, 1988.

64. Leijon G, Boivie J: Central post-stroke pain—a controlled trial of amitriptyline and carbamazepine. *Pain* 36:27–36, 1989.

65. Ventafridda V, Caraceni A, Saita L, et al: Trazodone for deafferentation pain. Comparison with amitriptyline. *Psychopharmacology (Berlin)* 95:S44–S49, 1988.

66. Tollison CD, Kriegel ML: Selected tricyclic antidepressants in the management of chronic benign pain. *South Med J* 81:562–564, 1988.

67. Sharav Y, Singer E, Schmidt E, Dionne RA, Dubner R: The analgesic effect of amitriptyline on chronic facial pain. *Pain* 31:199–209, 1987.

68. Max MB, Culnane M, Schafer SC, et al: Amitriptyline relieves diabetic neuropathy pain in patients with normal or depressed mood. *Neurology* 37:589–596, 1987.

69. Butler SH, Weil Fugazza J, Godefroy F, Besson JM: Reduction of arthritis and pain behaviour following chronic administration of amitriptyline or imipramine in rats with adjuvant-induced arthritis. *Pain* 23:159–175, 1985.

70. Yunus MB, Masi AT, Aldag JC: Short term effects of ibuprofen in primary fibromyalgia syndrome: a double blind, placebo controlled trial. *J Rheumatol* 16:527–532, 1989.

71. Clark S, Tindall E, Bennett RM: A double blind crossover trial of prednisone versus placebo in the treatment of fibrositis. *J Rheumatol* 12:980–983, 1985.

72. Wolfe F, Cathey MA, Kleinheksel SM, et al: Psychological status in primary fibrositis and fibrositis associated with rheumatoid arthritis. *J Rheumatol* 11:500–506, 1984.

73. McCain GA, Bell DA, Mai FM, Halliday PD: A controlled study of the effects of a supervised cardiovascular fitness training program on the manifestations of fibromyalgia. *Arthritis Rheum* 31:1135–1141, 1988.

74. Jacobsen S, Danneskiold Samse B: Isometric and isokinetic muscle strength in patients with fibrositis syndrome. New characteristics for a difficult definable category of patients. *Scand J Rheumatol* 16:61–65, 1987.

75. Ferraccioli G, Ghirelli L, Scita F, et al: EMG-biofeedback training in fibromyalgia syndrome. *J Rheumatol* 14:820–825, 1987.

76. Wolfe F: Fibromyalgia: whither treatment. *J Rheumatol* 15:1047–1049, 1988.

77. Hawley DJ, Wolfe F, Cathey MA: Pain, functional disability, and psychological status: a 12 month study of severity in fibromyalgia. *J Rheumatol* 15:1551–1556, 1988.

78. Fries JF, Spitz PW, Kraines RG: Measurement of patient outcome in arthritis. *Arthritis Rheum* 23:137–145, 1980.

79. Wolfe F, Kleinheksel SM, Cathey MA, Hawley DJ, Spitz PW, Fries JF: The clinical value of the Stanford Health Assessment Questionnaire Functional Disability Index in patients with rheumatoid arthritis. *J Rheumatol* 15:1480–1488, 1988.

80. Wolfe F: A brief health status instrument: CLINHAQ [abstract]. *Arthritis Rheum* 32:S99, 1989.

81. Cathey MA, Wolfe F, Kleinheksel SM, Miller S, Pitetti KH: Functional ability and work status in patients with fibromyalgia. *Arthritis Care Res* 1:85–98, 1988.

82. Caro XJ: Immunofluorescent studies of skin in primary fibrositis syndrome. *Am J Med* 81:43–49, 1986.

83. Mason JH, Simms RW, Goldenberg DL, Meenan RF: The impact of fibromyalgia on work: a comparison with RA. [abstract]. *Arthritis Rheum* 32:S197, 1989.

## 21

# MANAGEMENT OF MYOFASCIAL PAIN

*Hans Kraus*

Most neck pain is muscular in origin. The overwhelming majority of complaints, varying from a simple "stiff neck" to a whiplash injury following trauma, can be traced to muscle problems. By comparison, mechanical injuries such as fractures and ligament tears, requiring surgical attention and immobilization, are relatively rare. In order to properly diagnose and treat the most frequent occurrences of neck pain, it is important to recognize and distinguish among four types of muscle pain: muscle deficiency, tension, spasm, and trigger points (1).

## MUSCLE DEFICIENCY

Muscle deficiency—itself a source of pain—is composed of two elements: weakness and stiffness. Weakness usually affects the anterior neck muscles and may occur after prolonged immobilization in a collar. To diagnose weakness, have the patient lie supine and raise his or her head against light resistance. Inability to do so indicates weakness of anterior neck muscles.

Muscle stiffness means that the muscle is shortened and unable to move within its normal range. It can result from chronic micro-trauma such as squeezing the telephone between the ear and shoulder, reading in bed, or typing at too high a keyboard. Stiffness often follows prolonged and repeated muscle tension or prolonged immobilization. Stiffness can be diagnosed by having the patient rotate and tilt the neck in the supine and sitting positions. Test flexion and extension in the sitting position. If range of motion is limited, the muscles are foreshortened and stiff.

## MUSCLE TENSION

Muscle tension is contraction of a muscle beyond physiologic need. When such contraction surpasses a certain threshold (depending on individual tolerance), pain ensues. Tension can result from emotional and/or postural stress. Combined causes (e.g., family problems coupled with poor working posture) increase tension manyfold. Conditions inherent in civilized societies, especially among city dwellers, prevent the release of the fight-or-flight response (Fig. 21.1) (2). That is, muscles are tightened in preparation for action that is subsequently not performed. This produces a tension syndrome that may cause a number of orthopaedic difficulties.

It has been demonstrated through electromyography (3) that tense muscles emit increased electrical discharge, which correlates with pain; as tension is released, electrical discharge and pain diminish (Fig. 21.2).

## MUSCLE SPASM

Spasm is the painful contraction of a muscle, both limiting and aggravated by movement (4). It can occur after acute trauma (e.g., whiplash), after major mechanical injury, following a sudden movement involving previously tense muscles, and as a result of temporomandibular joint problems. Several features contribute to a diagnosis of spasm: history, pain on motion that subsides when motion ceases, and palpation revealing tight, hard muscle. In the absence of major pathology, ethyl chloride spray and gentle motion

337

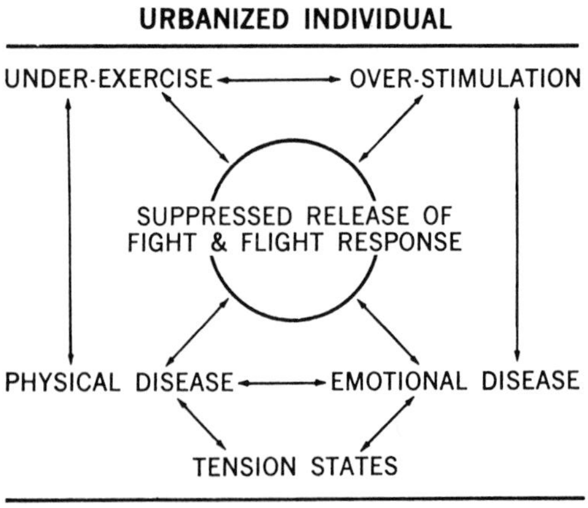

**Figure 21.1.** Tension syndrome produced by insufficient outlet for fight-or-flight response provides a basis for a large number of orthopedic difficulties, including stiff neck, painful shoulder, and painful back. Tension headaches belong in this group. (From Cannon WB: *Bodily Changes in Pain, Hunger, Fear, and Rage*, ed 2. College Park, MD, McGrath Publishing Co, 1970.)

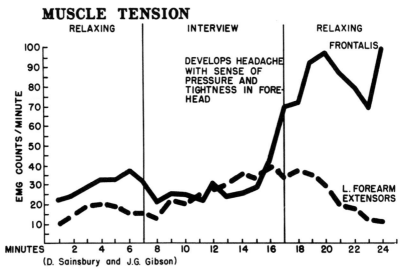

**Figure 21.2.** Electromyographic activity of tense muscle is highly increased, which goes hand in hand with increase of pain after irritating interview. (From Sainsbury P, Gibson JG: Symptoms of anxiety and tension and accompanying physiological changes in the muscular system. *J Neurol Neurosurg Psychiatry* 17:216–224, 1954.)

relieve pain and increase range of motion (5–9).

## TRIGGER POINTS

Trigger points are painful spots of degenerated muscle tissue that tend to develop after prolonged periods of unresolved spasm, tension, and/or stiffness. They usually occur near the insertion and origin of muscles because these areas are more vulnerable to tears when subjected to strain, as demonstrated by Malone and Garrett (10) in experiments with rabbit muscles.

The first person to discover and describe trigger points was a German orthopaedic surgeon,

Max Lange, in 1932 (11). Lange produced trigger points experimentally in dogs, biopsied the affected tissue, and noted the distribution of trigger points all over the body. He and his students Glogowski and Wallraff (12) also documented the pathohistology of trigger points in biopsied muscle (Figs. 21.3 and 21.4). Another German, a rheumatologist named Miehlke demonstrated through a series of biopsies that trigger points develop after a muscle has been in spasm or under tension for a prolonged period of time (13). Considerable literature on trigger points has accumulated in recent years (14–19).

Trigger points can be identified through palpation and measured with Fischer's pressure

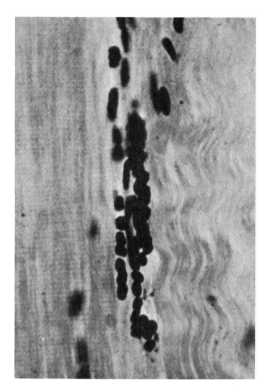

**Figure 21.3.** Clumps of nuclei between muscle fibers at a trigger point. Nuclei appear thickened and shrunken. (Formaldehyde, paraffin, hematoxylin-eosin; original magnification ×560.) (From Glogowsky G, Wallraff J: Ein Beitrag zur klinik und Histologie der Muskelharten (Myogelosen). *Z Orthop* 80:237–268, 1951.)

Since a healthy body does not respond with spasm to minor trauma, muscle tension can be diagnosed in such cases. Also how was the problem treated, if at all? For example, if the patient was immobilized in traction or with a collar, this kind of treatment can exacerbate the problem and set the stage for future occurrences.

Ascertain the time of day when discomfort is most severe. Morning pain is often the result of reading or watching television in bed the night before. Pain that increases during the course of the day and is most severe in the evening often results from a stressful day. Ask if the pain stops while the patient sleeps. If so, it is generally minor; severe pain prevents sleep. Is there numbness or paresthesia? This can indicate peripheral nerve entrapment or, less frequently, radiculitis. Does pain spread to the upper back and shoulders? If so, the trapezius is probably affected.

Since neck pain often arises from muscle ten-

threshold meter (20) (see below). They occur more frequently on the left side in right-handed people, in whom the left is the holding side and the right is the reaching side. In cases of occipital headache, they can be found in the suboccipital area.

## ETIOLOGY AND HISTORY

In order to make an accurate diagnosis, it is important to ask a variety of questions when taking the history of a patient with neck pain. For instance, what caused the first episode and when did it occur? It must be determined if pain originally appeared after trauma or during a time of stress. In the first instance the diagnosis would be muscle strain; in the second, muscle tension. It is also necessary to distinguish between major trauma, such as whiplash, and minor trauma, such as that caused by turning the neck suddenly in one direction or straining to raise a window that is stuck.

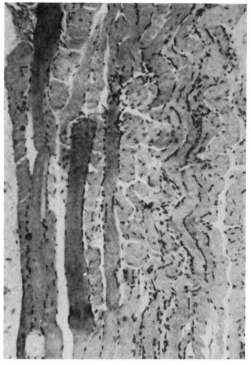

**Figure 21.4.** Biopsy specimen of a trigger point showing several darker, straightened out, club-shaped muscle fibers with a relative increase of nuclei. (Formaldehyde, paraffin, hematoxylin-eosin; original magnification × 80.) (From Glogowsky G, Wallraff J: Ein Beitrag zur Klinik und Histologie der Muskelharten (Myogelosen). *Z Orthop* 80:237–268, 1951.)

sion, it is important to ask about family history, tension in private life, and—most particularly—the type of work in which patient is engaged. Frequent sources of neck pain, resulting in constant tightening of neck and shoulder girdle muscles, are: squeezing the telephone between the ear and shoulder or using a computer (or typewriter) at a height that forces the patient to elevate his or her shoulders and arms to work the keyboard.

A necessary part of the interview includes questions relating to athletic activities. Weight-lifting or working out on weight machines, without relaxation and stretching, can cause neck pain. Any sport involving the upper extremities can result in neck and shoulder pain if the patient is not in shape. Tennis, squash, driving golf balls, or fencing may cause such problems, especially when the same motion is repeated frequently. This is true of any physical activity, ranging from gardening to working an automatic drill.

## EXAMINATION

Since each part of the body is related to the whole and cannot be considered separately, examination for neck problems should test strength and flexibility of all key postural muscles. I recommend using the Kraus-Weber tests for this purpose (Figs. 21.5 and 21.6). Weakness of abdominal muscles frequently correlates with neck problems, as does shoulder girdle stiffness. Weak abdominal muscles influence posture, force back muscles to carry the complete load of the body, and indirectly strain and tighten neck extensors. The floor-reach test is an excellent way to gauge muscle tension. If, because of tight back and hamstring muscles, the patient is unable to reach the floor, a second, more favorable result can be obtained by asking the patient to drop his or her head and relax the body first.

After an overall assessment, including a neurologic review, I examine the patient's neck movement in the supine position, noting degrees of flexion, extension, rotation, and tilt. To ascertain limitation of flexion and extension or to gauge weakness of anterior neck muscles, I have the patient elevate his or her head while I exert gentle pressure against the forehead.

Because a temporomandibular joint problem can be the cause of neck pain (21), I palpate for tenderness of masseter, temporal, and sternomastoid muscles and the pterygoids, with the patient supine. To assess tenderness of the temporoman-

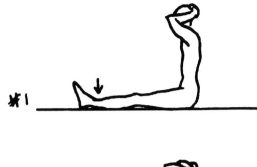

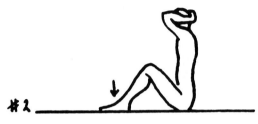

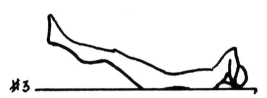

**Figure 21.5.**    The Kraus-Weber tests, tests 1, 2, and 3. These tests evaluate minimum muscular fitness. Test 1: Sit up from the prone position, hands behind head, legs straight, and ankles held down. Test 2: Repeat same position with knees flexed. Test 3: Raise both legs straight to a 30° angle and hold for 10 seconds. (*Arrows* indicate points at which the patient's body should be stabilized by another person.)

dibular joint, I insert my fingers into the patient's ears while having him or her move the jaw; I also consider his or her bite. I also check for postural vertigo; trigger points or spasm of neck muscles can produce dizziness (22).

To palpate shoulder muscles, I have the patient lie prone with a pillow under the hips and legs, resting the forehead on a plinth in order to relax. I then palpate the posterior neck muscles, suboccipital muscles, trapezii, interscapular muscles, infraspinati, and deltoids. Patients often make an evasive movement when a trigger point is pressed (23).

After identifying trigger points through palpation, they can be quantified with Fischer's pressure threshold meter (20). Fischer's gauge permits us to quantify the patient's pain perception and compare affected and nonaffected areas. The Fischer pressure threshold meter is a pressure gauge that measures the force needed to cause discomfort. A rod, tipped with a rubber cap whose surface is 1 cm², activates an indicator needle that registers the amount of pressure exerted (Fig. 21.7).

After thorough palpation has established the local tender spot, the gauge is applied and pressure gradually increased. The patient is instructed to call out "stop" as soon as he or she feels discomfort. After noting the amount of force needed to cause discomfort, the patient's contralateral side is tested using the same procedure. A difference in the force needed to cause discomfort quantifies the *localized tenderness*—the trigger

points. The values are expressed in newtons (N), measuring the force equal to 98 g exerted on 1 cm². Any difference greater than 20 (N) is significant. As a final measure the pressure threshold of a normal muscle, usually the deltoid, is gauged. Then the pain tolerance at this spot is tested. The patient is now requested to say "stop" only when pain becomes unbearable.

Besides identifying and quantifying trigger point pain, these pressure threshold measurements provide other valuable information:

Low pressure tolerance alerts us to the patient's low pain tolerance.

In persons with a very high pain threshold and tolerance we can identify trigger points that may go undetected by simple palpation.

The pressure threshold meter can establish and quantify improvement in localized tenderness. Immediately after injection or dry needling, pressure tenderness is greatly diminished; it increases the following day, but returns to normal after 7–10 days.

A generalized low pressure threshold often indicates systemic causes of muscle pain, endocrine imbalance being the most frequent (24). Hypothyroidism or lack of estrogen is usually responsible for general muscle tenderness and ache. In this event, the pressure threshold and tolerance—measured in the tibia—are higher than in normal muscle. The most frequent type of endocrine imbalance is hypothyroidism. Levels of thyroid-stimulating hormone, triiodothyronine, and thyroxine should be measured. Even if they are normal, in the presence of clinical signs and symptoms a therapeutic trial of thyroid medication may be worthwhile.

Although imaging should be part of the examination, it rarely correlates with pain. Computed tomography (CT) scans, magnetic resonance (MR) imaging, and bone scans may be necessary after severe trauma or when malignancy is suspected, but should be omitted, if possible, in other cases. I routinely use radiographs alone if the clinical picture points to a musculofascial syndrome.

I find in most cases that pain results from the muscles rather than from bone, ligaments, or nerve encroachment. Most whiplash injuries, for example, are muscle strains; bone and ligaments are seldom affected. Osteoarthritic changes in the neck are not necessarily the major cause of pain. Physiologic changes are often overstressed. The patient is told he or she has a "disc problem" when paresthesia in the hand or arm may be due to peripheral nerve entrapment. Anxious patients thus have an additional cause for concern, and

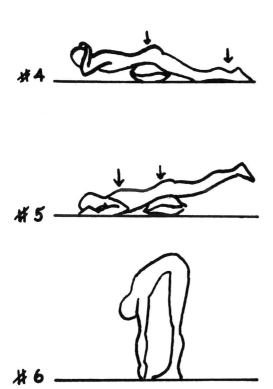

**Figure 21.6.** The Kraus-Weber tests, tests 4, 5, and 6. Test 4: Lie prone with pillow under hips, keep trunk raised, hands behind neck, and hold for 10 seconds. Test 5: Lying in the same position, raise both legs; hold for 10 seconds. Test 6: With knees straight, slowly reach toward the floor. (*Arrows* indicate points at which the patient's body should be stabilized by another person.)

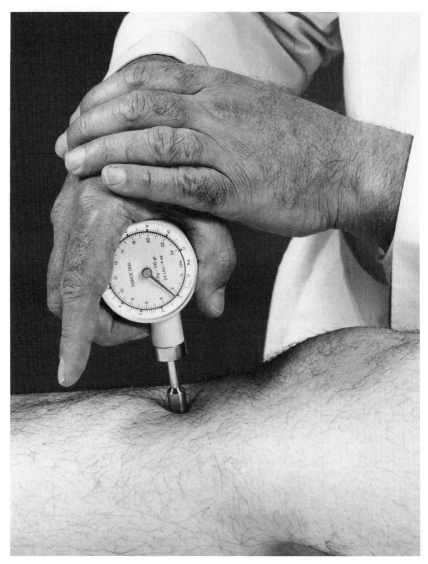

**Figure 21.7.** Fischer's pressure threshold meter. (From Fischer AA: Pressure threshold meter: its use for quantification of tender spots. *Arch Phys Med Rehabil* 67:836–838, 1986.)

their subsequent treatment becomes more difficult.

## TREATMENT

Treatment of muscle spasm consists of immediate controlled mobilization, relief of pain with ethyl chloride spray (5–7), and gentle manipulation (e.g., gentle rotation of head or slow shrugging of the shoulders). Before using ethyl chloride and gentle controlled motion, 10 min of tetanizing current followed by 10 min of sinusoidal current are applied to the affected area. The skin electrodes are usually applied bilaterally on the neck and trapezii.

In the absence of major pathology, response is generally satisfactory. A week or 10 days suffice to break the muscle spasm if its original cause, such as exaggerated tension or poor working posture, can be avoided. If the patient does not respond quickly to local therapy, the physician must suspect, and exclude, major pathology. A radiograph, CT scan, or MR image is then necessary. If there is no history of major trauma or malignancy, I prefer postponing these diagnostic measures until the spasm has been relieved.

The tests and examinations described under "Examination" are not feasible in the acute patient. The first step is to relieve pain, as described above. Once the acute phase is over, the patient should be reexamined for strength and flexibility of key posture muscles, degree of tension, and possible trigger points.

## REDUCTION OF TENSION

To avoid recurrences, one of the most frequent problems—*tension*—must be eliminated wherever possible. Sources of tension and irritation can be work stress, prolonged driving, reading in bed, squeezing the telephone (I advise earphones), and television viewing in bed. If emotional tension is a prime cause, a psychiatrist is recommended.

To reduce tension, relaxation exercises are instituted. As the patient lies supine with a pillow under the knees, he or she is asked to close the eyes, inhale and fully exhale, pull up the shoulders and let them go, let the head drop left and then right, and breathe deeply again. As the patient goes through this relaxation phase, he or she is told to pull up and relax the shoulders as often as possible during the day. Developing a habit of relaxing the neck and trapezius muscles, for example, whenever the telephone rings or someone enters the room or the patient stops for a red light can serve as a constant reminder to relax.

Another means of reducing tension is the use of tranquilizers in the acute phase. These should be gradually tapered off as soon as possible. Strenuous physical activities also have a great tension-relieving effect. It has been found that jogging to bring the heart rate up to 100–120 beats/min is more relaxing than meprobamate (25).

If a patient is hypnotizable it is worthwhile to have him or her learn self-hypnosis for frequent relaxation breaks in the course of the day. Spiegel and Spiegel's eye-roll test (26) can be used to determine if a patient is hypnotizable. The patient is asked to roll both eyes upward and focus on a point in the middle of the forehead; the more the eyes converge and the pupils disappear under the upper lid the greater is the patient's ability to be hypnotized. Hypnosis can also be used to control pain during trigger point injection. The use of posthypnotic suggestion can be helpful in inducing relaxation.

## IMMOBILIZATION

I do not recommend immobilization (e.g., collars) unless the patient is exposed to whiplash-type injuries in a bus, car, taxi, or subway, in which case a soft collar will prevent sudden movement. Hard collars should be reserved for truly mechanical injuries such as fractures, torn ligaments, or postsurgical repair of same. While a collar may give temporary relief, it freezes the muscles in one position, making neck stiffness and recurrence of acute episodes more likely. The same is true of cervical pillows.

## PHYSICAL CONDITIONING

Following treatment in the acute phase and reduction of tension, an exercise program is instituted to treat abdominal muscle weakness or back or shoulder girdle stiffness when necessary (see "Exercise," below). Long-range results can be expected only if the patient achieves good muscular conditioning and if the basic sources of his or her problem are contained. The patient's life-style in many instances has to be altered.

## TRIGGER POINT INJECTION

The objective of trigger point treatment is to destroy the painful nodules mechanically through needling. Injecting fluid is more effective than dry needling. I use lidocaine as a rule because of its analgesic effect. If a patient is sensitive to lidocaine, saline can be used; the results are the same.

To prepare for injection, two forceps, two syringes, and a set of 20- and 22-gauge needles, 1–3 inches long, are sterilized in an autoclave together with a sterilization indicator. When the latter changes color from tan to deep brown, this means that sufficient pressure has been reached (24 lbs pressure/cm$^2$ at a temperature of over 250°F). Although disposable needles can be used, I find them too sharp; furthermore, they make it more difficult to maintain sterile precautions. (Wear disposable gloves for injecting.)

After palpating and checking tenderness with the pressure gauge, mark the area to be injected with a needle scratch and clean it with alcohol. Inserting the needle near the scratch mark, probe in different directions for the trigger point (indi-

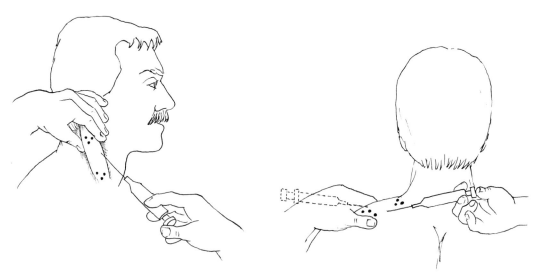

**Figure 21.8.** *Left,* Sternocleidomastoid muscle is grasped firmly with one hand and held firmly while the other hand directs the needle cranially, then caudally. *Right,* Upper trapezius os grasped between the thumb and index finger to avoid puncturing the apex of the lungs; the needle is directed medially and then laterally or vice versa. Dots indicate entry points of needle.

cated by the patient's flinching with pain) while injecting a small amount of lidocaine or saline solution (10 ml *in toto*). Making additional needle insertions, continue to needle in a full circle around the insertion and the origin of the muscle (Fig. 21.8). When each injection is completed, cover the needle puncture with a nonallergenic tape.

The patient is asked to return for treatment on three consecutive days following injection. Before treatment, sinusoidal current is applied for 15 min; this is followed by ethyl chloride spray and gentle movement to restore flexibility and relaxation to the injected area. The patient is never given injections in more than one area at a time or more than two areas in a week.

The areas most frequently requiring injection are the suboccipital muscles, the posterior neck muscles, the sternomastoid (often responsible for dizziness on change of position) (22), and the scaleni. Trigger points are also common in the trapezius and infraspinatus. Others can be found in the levator scapulae, rhomboids, and teres major. Sometimes trigger points exist at the medial or lateral epicondyle and adductor of the thumb.

Trigger point injections are painful. Patients who have low pain tolerance should be given an analgesic and a tranquilizer half an hour to an hour before injection. As a rule, we use Tylenol with Codeine 4 and Valium (5 mg).

If feasible, I prefer to inject trigger points as soon as they are detected on the first examination. However, I refrain from injecting trigger points when the patient is in spasm. Frequently, once muscle spasm is relieved completely no trigger-point is found. It is best to inject trigger points before beginning exercise and relaxation training because, for at least 4–5 days after injection, the patient is asked to avoid prolonged sitting, standing, or walking and to refrain from any strenuous activity, including driving. Patients should not sit for longer than 20–30 min at a time, walk more than two or three short blocks, or stand for more than 5 min at a time. Tension-creating work and postures should be avoided. It is especially important that they avoid driving, working on computers or typewriters, telephoning without using earphones, and reading or watching television in bed. If the patient lives further away than an hour's travel, injections should only be given if he or she can manage an easy and pain-free commute (e.g., being driven in a comfortable car).

## EXERCISE

It is seldom necessary to prescribe strengthening exercises for neck muscles. Neck weakness occurs primarily after injury and/or when the body is severely deconditioned and the abdominal muscles are weak. If strengthening exercises are deemed necessary, all patients should begin with relaxation exercises. Strengthening exercises begin with the patient in the supine position. The patient raises the head as far as possible, holds the position for a second, then rests. Next, the patient turns the head to one side, raises it, rests, turns the head to the other side, raises it, and rests again. Once these exercises have been performed three times each, gentle manual resistance can be added. After completing the strengthening phase, the patient should repeat the relaxation exercises.

To complete a program of neck rehabilitation, the patient who fails any of the six Kraus-Weber tests should be put on a program of exercise to strengthen key posture muscles and to stretch tight muscles. The exercises described here will correct the most common deficiencies—abdominal muscle weakness, back and hamstring stiffness, and tension. Without complete flexibility (floor touch) or adequate abdominal strength (sit-ups with knees flexed), persons suffering from back problems continue to experience pain when they resume normal activity.

Exercises should always begin and end with relaxation. New exercises are added one at a time, and no exercise is repeated more than two or three times in succession. Optimally, the patient should be trained and monitored by a therapist until he or she can do all the exercises slowly, in a relaxed fashion, with a second's rest between movements. The following exercises for the neck and back should be performed in the sequence given, proceeding from number 1 to the last exercise, as warm-up, and then performed in reverse as a cool-off.

## BACK EXERCISES

1. Lying supine, with hands resting at sides and with a pillow under the knees, slowly inhale through the nose. Exhale slowly through pursed lips. Repeat several times. Pull the shoulders up toward the ears; let go. Drop the head to one side, rest, then drop to the other side. Repeat the breathing exercise. Repeat all movements several times until relaxed.
2. In the supine position, with both knees flexed (*basic position*), bring one knee slowly to the chest, slide to full extension, return to basic position. Alternate with the other leg.
3. Perform the same leg movements as in exercise 2 while lying on the side. Alternate sides.
4. In the prone position, tighten buttocks. Relax.
5. In the supine position, bring both knees to the chest. Return to the basic position.

6. On hands and knees, arch back; then collapse to swayback ("catback").
7. In the basic position, lift head and shoulders; return to basic position.
8. Kneel with the forearms resting on a plinth; slowly slide the arms forward to stretch the pectoral muscles.
9. Sit on the edge of a plinth with the feet on the floor or a stool. Bend slowly, dropping the head between the legs.
10. In the basic position with the feet held down, curl up slowly to a sitting position. (Patients with weak abdominal muscles should keep their arms at their sides; later they can cross their arms over the stomach and chest, and finally clasp their hands behind the neck.)
11. Sit as in exercise 9; bend toward one side, then the other.
12. In the basic position, bring one knee toward the chest, straighten the leg with the foot toward the ceiling, then slowly lower the leg to full extension and return to basic position. Repeat once with the foot in dorsiflexion. Alternate with other leg.
13. In the basic position, straighten one leg, raise the leg while straight, lower the leg, and return to the basic position. Do once with foot pointing and once with foot in dorsiflexion. Alternate with other leg.
14. Standing with arms straight and hands joined behind back, slowly bend forward from waist.
15. Standing with knees straight, slowly reach toward floor.

## NECK EXERCISES

1. Perform relaxation and gentle neck movement as in exercise 1 in the back program.
2. While prone, bring the shoulder blades together; relax.
3. In the basic position, tilt the head to one side, then the other. Repeat exercise 1.
4. To do a pectoral stretch, sit with the hands joined behind the neck; bring the elbows backward.
5. In the supine basic position, bring the arm across the chest; alternate sides.

In acute cases, use only exercises 1 to 3 after applying ethyl chloride spray to the injured area. The number of exercises can be increased as the patient improves. In chronic cases, start with three or four exercises and add one, or at most two, as the patient improves.

## YMCA PROGRAM

The YMCA program, essentially the same as the one outlined above for back pain, is described in Melleby's book *The Y's Way to a Healthy Back* (27). More than 300,000 persons have completed this program—which includes sit-ups and floor reaches—without a single complication. This evidence proves that Nachemson's (28, 29) findings of high pressure in the L3–4 disc during these movements should not deter patients from their use. (Unfortunately a new National YMCA Director has changed the program, making its value questionable.)

## REMARKS

The most frequent mistakes in exercise programs are:

Neglecting relaxation.
Neglecting warm-up and cool-off.
Giving multirepetition exercises.
Giving too many exercises too soon, or giving exercises that are too demanding for patients. (It is a mistake to hand out written exercise sheets instead of demonstrating each exercise and working with the patient.)
Forgetting to use ethyl chloride for relieving discomfort, if indicated.

When the patient is completely free of pain and has normal strength and flexibility of key posture muscles, including full range of motion of neck muscles, he or she may gradually return to all previous activities. Before and after strenuous activity, the exercises learned should always be used as a warm-up and cool-off. If the patient's work is both strenuous and demanding, the patient will not be ready to resume work as soon as he or she is pain-free; such work must be returned to gradually.

## CASE HISTORIES

### SPASM THERAPY

G.B., a sedentary writer, came to the office in 1978, several months after her obstreperous dalmatian puppy pulled her down the steep back stairs in her house. Her neck muscles were in acute spasm. She had been treated by a local orthopedist with traction and advised to wear a collar at all times.

We treated her with electrotherapy, ethyl chloride spray, and gentle controlled exercise to relieve pain. Since the spasm was not prolonged, we were able to resolve the problem after three sessions.

### TENSION

G.R., an avid equestrian, was bucked off her horse in the summer of 1986. She suffered a broken nose and whiplash injury. Because G.R. was an old patient of ours, whom we had previously treated for several skiing and horse-related traumas, she was familiar with our procedures. Treating herself with ethyl chloride spray, relaxation exercises, and the gentle neck exercises she had learned in our office [recollection of which she reinforced by rereading the related chapter in our book (30)], G.R. was able to relieve the spasm without the need for traction or collar.

Whenever G.R. finds herself in tension-provoking situations, her neck muscles have a tendency to tighten up. At such times, relaxation and gentle exercise usually suffice to relieve pain. She carefully avoids reading or watching television in bed, types at a low keyboard, never holds the telephone between her neck and shoulder, and has bought a new horse.

## USE OF HYPNOSIS TO INDUCE RELAXATION

J.T., a traveling salesman, had suffered for several months from chronic pain in the right side of his neck and right shoulder. We relieved the acute spasm with electrotherapy, ethyl chloride spray, and gentle controlled movement (as outlined previously). We then injected several trigger points, following up with appropriate treatment.

Because his work required him to drive extensively, we could not ask J.T. to alter the work posture that had contributed to his previous pain. We did, however, note that he was readily hypnotizable. We therefore taught him self-hypnosis and recommended that he give himself a posthypnotic suggestion: "I will be relaxed when I drive, and my right shoulder will feel fine."

Some months later, J.T. returned to our office, complaining of pain in his left neck and shoulder. Since trigger points had not yet developed, we were able to relieve the painful spasm in short order. This time we told J.T. to change his posthypnotic suggestion to include both shoulders. He has been free of pain ever since.

## TRIGGER POINT TREATMENT

K.N., a 22-year-old female student, came in 2 years after a car collision in which she suffered whiplash, numbness of the left arm, and pain. After her injuries, K.N. had worn a collar and had been in traction for 2 weeks, after which she had received physical therapy (sine wave, hot packs, massage, and exercises) for 2 months. This treatment was followed by 2 months of manipulation—with no improvement. A year later the patient again had physical therapy (massage, exercise, traction), with no improvement.

Our examination yielded these findings:

Limitation of neck rotation to the right by about 30°.

Hypesthesia of the fourth and fifth fingers of the left hand and of the lateral aspect of the forearm.

Questionable weakness of the left finger flexors.

Trigger points in the left infraspinatus, trapezius, upper rhomboids, occipital muscles, and right posterior neck muscles.

K.N. had considerable tension. We found trigger points at C2, C3, and C4.

We injected the trigger points, with appropriate follow-up treatment. There was noticeable improvement after the third injection, and improvement continued with each injection. K.N. began an exercise routine. Two months later, upon discharge, she had full neck motion, full strength of the neck muscles, no tenderness, and improved relaxation.

This is an example of successful trigger point injection followed by strengthening exercises and relaxation training.

## CONCLUSION

Most neck pain is muscular in origin. Examination for muscle spasm, tension, muscle deficiency, and trigger points is essential to proper diagnosis. Treatment by controlled mobilization with the help of electrotherapy, ethyl chloride, relaxation exercises, strengthening, relaxing, and stretching of tight muscles, and trigger point injection where indicated is needed to obtain optimal results.

### REFERENCES

1. Kraus H (ed): *Diagnosis and Treatment of Muscle Pain*. Chicago, Quintessence Books, 1988.
2. Cannon WB: *Bodily Changes in Pain, Hunger, Fear, and Rage*, ed 2. College Park, MD, McGrath Publishing Co, 1970.
3. Sainsbury P, Gibson JG: Symptoms of anxiety and tension and accompanying physiological changes in the muscular system. *J Neurol Neurosurg Psychiatry* 17:216–224, 1954.
4. Kraus H: Muscle spasm. In Kraus H (ed): *Diagnosis and Treatment of Muscle Pain*. Chicago, Quintessence Books, 1988, p 11.
5. Kraus H: New treatment for injured joints [abstract]. *JAMA* 104:1261, 1935.
6. Kraus H: Use of surface anesthesia in the treatment of painful motion. *JAMA* 116:2582–2583, 1941.
7. Travell J: Ethyl chloride spray for painful muscle spasm. *Arch Phys Med* 33:291–298, 1952.
8. Kraus H: *Clinical Treatment of Back and Neck Pain*. New York, McGraw-Hill, 1970.
9. Travell J: Rapid relief of acute "stiff neck" by ethyl chloride spray. *J Am Med Wom Assoc* 4(3): 89–95, 1949.
10. Malone TR, Garrett W: Muscle strains: histology, cause and treatment. *Surg Rounds for Orthopedics* Jan, pp. 43–46, 1989.
11. Lange M: *Die Muskelharten (Myogelosen)*. Munich, JF Lehmann, 1931.
12. Glogowsky G, and Wallraff J: Ein Beitrag zur Klinik und Histologie der Muskelharten (Myogelosen). *Z Orthop* 80:237–268, 1951.
13. Miehlke K, Schultze G, Eger W: Clinical and experimental studies on the fibrositis syndrome [in German]. *Z Rheumaforsch* 19:310–330, 1960.
14. Travell J: Basis for the multiple uses of local block of somatic trigger areas. *Miss Valley Med J* 71(1):13–21, 1949.
15. Bonica JJ: Management of myofascial pain syndromes in general practice. *JAMA* 164(7):732–738, 1957.
16. Simmons DG: Myofascial trigger points: a need for understanding. *Arch Phys Med Rehabil* 62(3):97–99, 1981.
17. Travell J, and Simons D: *Myofascial Pain and Dysfunction: The Trigger Point Manual*. Baltimore, Williams & Wilkins, 1983.
18. Kraus H: Triggerpoints. *NY State J Med* 73:1310–1314, 1973.
19. Kraus H: "Pseudo-disc." *South Med J* 60:416–418, 1967.
20. Fischer AA: Pressure threshold meter: its use for quantification of tender spots. *Arch Phys Med Rehabil* 67:836–838, 1986.
21. Gelb H: In Kraus H. (ed): *Diagnosis and treatment of Muscle Pain*. Chicago, Quintessence Books, 1988, pp 67–84.
22. Weeks VD, Travell J: Postural vertigo due to trigger areas in the sternocleidomastoid muscle. *J Pediatr* 47:315–327, 1955.
23. Gillette HE: Office management of musculoskeletal pain. *Texas J Med* 62:47–53, 1966.
24. Sonkin L: In Kraus H (ed): *Diagnosis and Treatment of Muscle Pain*. Chicago, Quintessence Books, 1988, pp 91–95.
25. DeVries HA, Adams GM: Electromyographic comparison of single doses of exercises and meprobamate as to effects on muscular relaxation. *Am J Phys Med* 51:130–141, 1972.
26. Spiegel H, Spiegel D: *Trance and Treatment: Clinical Uses of Hypnosis*. New York, Basic Books, 1978.
27. Melleby A: *The Y's Way to a Healthy Back*. Piscataway, NJ, New Century Publishers, 1982.
28. Nachemson A: The lumbar spine: an orthopaedic challenge. *Spine* 1:59–71, 1976.
29. Nachemson A: The load on lumbar discs in different positions of the body. *Clin Orthop* 45:107–122, 1966.
30. Kraus H: *The Sports Injury Handbook*. Nick Lyons Books, 1981.

# 22

# INFLAMMATORY DISORDERS OF THE CERVICAL SPINE

*Frederick Wolfe*

Inflammatory involvement of the cervical spine by rheumatoid arthritis (RA) gives rise to a number of clinical manifestations, the most common of which appears to be pain; the least common is sudden death following compromise of the brainstem by the odontoid process. Understanding of the relationship of RA to cervical spine disease has been hampered by a number of factors (Table 22.1). First, there has been a systematic bias toward the identification and study of more severely afflicted RA patients, particularly within the orthopaedic and neurosurgical literature. In this instance the bias represents a referral bias, wherein patients with "worrisome," "important," or "severe" symptoms are referred for further study.

Second, cross-sectional studies from clinics with large RA populations tend to study patients with long duration of disease, usually 10 years or greater. Patients attending such clinics who are in the study sample are often those with worse RA since they attend the clinic more regularly. The consequence of such biases is to indicate that the incidence and prevalence of cervical spine disorders in RA is greater than it actually is, and that the cervical spine disease is more severe than it actually is.

The effect of this selection and identification bias is important in the evaluation of the various surgical and nonsurgical therapies that have been employed, since more severely afflicted persons will not respond as well as those with less severe disease (1).

Almost no studies of surgical outcome take into account covariates such as age, duration of disease, comorbidity, overall RA severity, and functional disability. Such factors might be important in the outcome—including mortality (1)—of patients undergoing surgery.

Most treatment studies involve small numbers of patients and lack any reasonable statistical power. Not a single report considered that the skill of the surgeon might be a factor in the outcome of the surgery. Different surgical procedures are performed in different centers, and, given the disagreement among surgeons, it is possible that some procedures are less effective than others. Very few outcome studies used blinded as-

**Table 22.1.**
**Bias in the Study of Rheumatoid Arthritis Involving the Cervical Spine**

Referral for study of more severely afflicted patients.
Study of patients with long duration of disease.
Severely afflicted RA patients cannot respond as well as those with less severe disease.
Most treatment series study only a few patients.
The skill of the surgeon is not considered.
Outcome of surgery may reflect a particular surgical technique.
Assessors in outcome studies were rarely blinded.
Criteria for neurologic abnormalities usually not well defined.
Indications for surgery differed among centers.

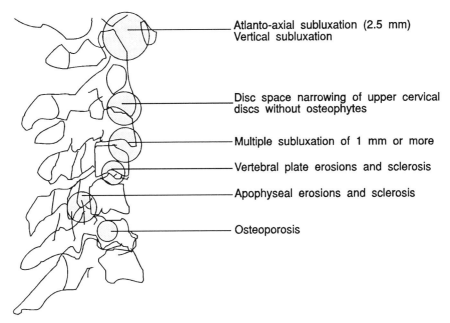

Atlanto-axial subluxation (2.5 mm)
Vertical subluxation

Disc space narrowing of upper cervical discs without osteophytes

Multiple subluxation of 1 mm or more

Vertebral plate erosions and sclerosis

Apophyseal erosions and sclerosis

Osteoporosis

**Figure 22.1.** Common sites of involvement in the rheumatoid cervical spine. [Adapted from Winfield et al. (7).]

sessors or observers, a fact that might have contributed to the greater success attributed to the surgical versus nonsurgical interventions. Only a few studies described in detail the "neurologic" abnormalities noted in their patients. It was often difficult to tell if those who benefited most from the surgery were different by virtue of severity, age, or duration of disease. Indications for surgical intervention differed from center to center. Finally, follow-up was usually of short duration. The net result of these problems is to make it extremely difficult to ascertain how effective surgery (and nonsurgical treatment) is in treating RA of the cervical spine. In this review the reader should be aware of these limitations, and I will try to stress them in the text.

## RHEUMATOID ARTHRITIS

### RADIOGRAPHIC ABNORMALITIES OF THE CERVICAL SPINE

The identification and diagnosis of RA changes in the cervical spine has traditionally been a function of the radiologic examination (Fig. 22.1) (Table 22.2). Although it may seem unusual or inappropriate to place the radiographic description of the disease before the clinical symptoms, most of what we know about the RA spine comes through radiographic assessment of the anatomic pathology,

**Table 22.2.**
**Radiologic Abnormalities in the Rheumatoid Arthritis Cervical Spine[a]**

Multiple subluxations of C2–3, C3–4, C4–5, C5–6
Narrow disc spaces with little or no osteoporosis
    Pathognomonic at C2–3 and C3–4
    Probable at C4–5 and C5–6
Erosions of vertebrae, especially verterbral plates
Odontoid small, pointed, eroded; loss of cortex
Basilar impression ("platybasia")
Apophyseal joint erosion; blurred facets
Osteoporosis generalized in cervical spine
Wide space (5 mm or more) between posterior arch of atlas and spinous process of axis (flexion to extension)
Osteosclerosis (secondary) in atlantoaxial-occipital complex
Atlantoaxial subluxation of 2.5 mm or more
Loss of subarachnoid space
Pannus in the region of the odontoid process

[a]Modified from Bland (3).

and it is easier to relate symptoms to underlying pathologic processes if the abnormalities are described first.

### Subluxations

**Atlantoaxial Subluxation.** Atlantoaxial subluxation (AAS) is generally diagnosed in adults when the shortest distance from the posterior surface of the anterior arch of the axis to anterior surface of the odontoid process is greater than 2.5 mm (2–7) [some authors suggest that the diagnosis be made when this distance is greater than 3.0 mm (8) or greater than 2.5 mm in women and 3.0 mm in men (4)]. In children, the atlantoaxial distance can normally be as great as 4 (9) or 5 mm (6). Atlantoaxial distances as great as 22 mm have been noted.

Identification of AAS requires several plain lateral films of the cervical spine with the head held in maximum flexion and in maximum extension. Inflammation and pannus invasion involving the synovial membranes anterior and posterior to the odontoid process (10–12) together with inflammation in the axial, alar, and transverse ligaments (13) lead to a weakening, stretching, or rupture of the involved ligaments (3, 4, 8, 14). AAS is usually reducible when the head returns to the neutral position (the reason that flexion views of the cervical spine are required), but occasionally fails to reduce, leading to the fixed irreducible form of AAS.

Interestingly, for mechanical reasons AAS may decrease over time as vertical subluxation (up-

ward migration of the dens) occurs. Winfield et al. noted two patients whose AAS decreased as vertical subluxation increased (7). One patient's AAS increased from 3 to 4 mm over a 5-year period, but then showed a decrease to 3 mm over the next 3 years as the vertical subluxation progressed. Santavirta et al. have demonstrated an inverse relationship between atlantoaxial displacement (AAS) and the degree of vertical subluxation (Fig. 22.2) (4). Similarly, Weissman et al. noted that AAS decreased over time in 19% of their patients (6). Within this group they noted that 57% developed atlantoaxial impaction. They suggested "improvement" in the remaining patients may have been related to "voluntary guarding, pain, or lack of flexion effort. . . ." Similarly, Winfield et al. cautioned that "it may be useful to remember that the full degree of atlanto-axial instability may not be seen radiographically if cervical spine flexion is markedly impaired" (7).

Clinically, then, absence of AAS does not, per se, mean absence of cervical abnormality. Moreover, the overall severity of cervical spine disease may not be correlated with the degree of AAS.

**Posterior Subluxation.** Posterior subluxation (PS) is an uncommon finding (less than 7% of

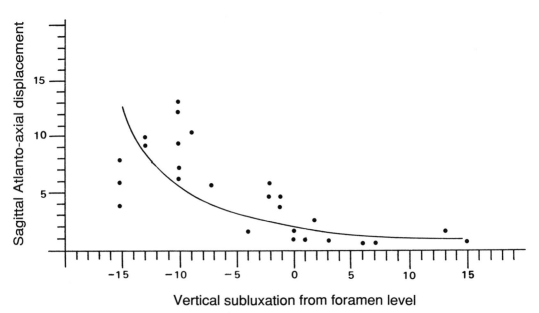

**Figure 22.2.**   The correlation of sagittal atlantoaxial displacement and vertical subluxation from the foramen level measured radiographically in 26 patients. The progress of vertical subluxation reduces the amplitude of anterior atlantoaxial subluxation. (From Santavirta S, Kankaanpaa U, Sandelin J, Laasonen E, Konttinen YT, Slatis P: Evaluation of patients with rheumatoid cervical spine. *Scand J Rheumatol* 16:9–16, 1987.)

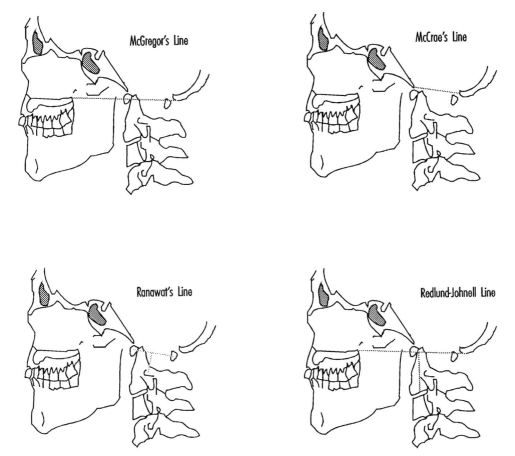

**Figure 22.3.** McGregor's line, McCrae's line, Ranawat's line, and the Redlund-Johnell line used in the determination of atlantoaxial impaction. [After Santavirta et al. (4); see text for details.]

cases) (6). It appears to be related to laxity of the supporting ligaments and erosion or fracture of the odontoid (4, 15–17).

**Atlantoaxial Impaction.** Atlantoaxial impaction (AAI) represents the condition wherein the odontoid process has migrated cephalad. It is also known as vertical subluxation, vertical settling, cranial settling, superior migration, basilar impression, and cranial subluxation.

A number of systems have been developed to measure AAI (Fig. 22.3). McGregor's line represents a line drawn "from the upper surface of the posterior edge of the hard palate to the most caudal part of the occipital curve in the true lateral X-ray" (18). Using McGregor's line, AAI is generally identified when the tip of the odontoid protrudes more than 4.5 mm above that line. McCrae's line (19) runs from the anterior to the posterior aspect of the foramen magnum. Extension of the odon-

toid process above this line is considered abnormal. Ranawat et al. (20) measured the length of a line drawn from the center of the pedicles of C2 to a line drawn from the anterior to the posterior arch of the atlas. In Ranawat's series a normal value of 15 or greater for men and 13 or greater for women was proposed. Redlund-Johnell et al. proposed a measurement for the distance between McGregor's line and the inferior margin of the body of the axis in lateral radiographs made in the neutral position (21, 22). A normal value of 34 mm for men and 29 mm for women was proposed.

Many of these measurements may be difficult to observe since erosion of the odontoid peg may occur or the landmarks of the Ranawat and Redlund-Johnell methods may be difficult to define (23). Kawaida et al. (22) and Morizono et al. (21) compared the Ranawat and Redlung-Johnell methods with McGregor's line (using an abnormal cutoff of 3 mm rather than the usual value of 4.5 mm), and studied the clinical manifestations associated with abnormalities of each. The Ranawat and/or Redlund-Johnell methods were thought to be superior since the McGregor line could not be identified in 18% of 209 patients. The percentage of patients found to be abnormal with the McGregor, Ranawat, and Redlund-Johnell methods were 15, 22, and 11, respectively. All patients found to be abnormal by the Redlund-Johnell method were also abnormal by the McGregor method. The correlation coefficient between the Ranawat and Redlund-Johnell values was .687, that between the Ranawat and McGregor values .592, and that between the Redlund-Johnell and McGregor values .772. Pain was noted more frequently in those with abnormal Redlund-Johnell values (95%) as opposed to those judged abnormal by the other methods (62–65%). Using magnetic resonance (MR) imaging, the authors found that all patients judged abnormal by the Redlund-Johnell method and from 74% to 89% of those judged abnormal by other methods had pathologic findings on the MR images.

The authors concluded that "[t]he Ranawat method, therefore, appeared to be more sensitive to mild VS [vertical settling], but abnormal Redlund-Johnell values indicated severe VS" (21, 22). It is possible that the Ranawat and Redlund-Johnell methods do not measure exactly the same process, since decreased Ranawat values reflect primarily decreased C1–C2 distance. Redlund-Johnell values also reflect occiput–C2 distance and may be influenced by destruction of the atlanto-occipital joints (21).

**Lateral and Rotary Subluxations and Lateral Mass Collapse.** For technical reasons lateral and rotary subluxations may be difficult to identify. They are brought about by synovitis leading to abnormalities in the atlantoaxial facet joints, including erosion, subchondral bone loss, and collapse of the lateral masses (4, 24–26). These abnormalities are best seen with open-mouth anteroposterior views if plain radiography is used. Weissman et al. defined lateral subluxation as being present when the lateral masses of C1 were positioned more than 2 mm lateral with relation to C2, provided the patient's head was not rotated (6). Lateral mass collapse is usually unilateral at the level of C1 and/or C2, related to erosive changes in the subchondral bone, and is associated clinically with painful, nonreducible rotational head tilt (Fig. 22.4) (24, 25).

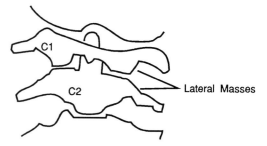

**Figure 22.4.** Collapse of the lateral masses of C1 and/ or C2 associated with nonreducible rotational head tilt (NRRHT). [After Santavirta et al. (4).]

**Subaxial Subluxations.** Subaxial subluxations, usually anterior, occur from C2 to C6 and are a characteristic feature of both early and late RA of the cervical spine (3, 7). They tend to occur in a staircase pattern (27) and are rarely seen at these levels in disorders other than RA. In the Winfield et al. study of early RA, of the 24 patients with such subluxation (defined as a subluxation of more than 1 mm or greater than 15% of the anteroposterior vertebral diameter), it was noted at C2–3 in 2, at C3–4 in 4, and at all levels from C2 through C5 in 8 patients.

## Subaxial Abnormalities

Bland (3) described additional abnormalities of the cervical spine, including disc space narrowing, vertebral erosions, apophyseal joint erosion, and osteoporosis (Table 22.2).

**Disc Space Narrowing and Erosions (Discitis).** Bland considered C2–3 and C3–4 narrowing with little or no osteophytosis as pathognomonic of RA of the cervical spine (3). Narrowing may be easily identified, but erosions are often not easily seen on plain radiography. It is believed that synovitis involving the uncovertebral joints (joints of Lushka) may play a role in this process (23, 28), but that mechanical trauma from associated instability is likely to be the most important factor (29, 30).

**Apophyseal Joint Abnormalities.** Apophyseal narrowing and sclerosis, reflecting the results of synovitis of these structures, is commonly identified. Such radiographic findings, however, are seen frequently in other, more common, conditions.

**Osteoporosis.** Commonly seen in RA, osteoporosis may reflect inflammation, disuse, and corticosteroid therapy. Like apophyseal joint abnormalities, it is commonly seen in other disorders.

**Bursitis.** Bursitis has been detailed by Bywaters, who noted bursae in between the spinous processes in four of nine RA necropsies (31). He posited that abnormal spinal mobility due to discal destruction and subluxation might be a factor in the aggravated bursal response. "In such cases the bursal synovial cavity may be the seat of rheumatoid disease, with resultant destruction of the spinous processes, visible radiologically" (31).

## SIGNS AND SYMPTOMS OF CERVICAL SPINE INVOLVEMENT

Pain is the most common symptom of cervical disease. Conlon et al. noted that 88% of 333 patients with RA were symptomatic (32). Wolfe et al., reporting on unselected patients seen in a longitudinal data bank (33), noted that of 675 patients "84 percent had evidence of cervical spine involvement (symptomatic or on physical examination) . . . at some time during follow-up." Such data should not be interpreted to indicate that all RA patients have clinically important neck pain, since the selection process and the method of follow-up favors identification of the symptom. In addition, most persons *without RA* will develop neck pain if followed longitudinally. Persistent and severe neck or occipital pain, however, is a characteristic feature and often the major reason for referral to surgical treatment centers (3, 4, 10, 34–37). Cervico-occipital pain is often precipitated or made worse by movement and has a deep, aching, and persistent quality (3). It is characteristically noted in the upper neck and occipital regions. Such pain is thought to arise from involvement of the first and second cervical nerves (3, 38–40), and rheumatoid involvement of the transverse and alar ligaments, the zygapophyseal joints, and similar structures. Involvement of levels below C2 leads to referral patterns in the lateral aspect of the neck, and to radicular pain (4).

Characteristic deformities may occur. Halla et al. have described in detail the nonreducible rotational head tilt (NRRHT) associated with unilateral collapse of C1 and/or C2 (24–26). NRRHT is defined clinical as a nonreducible lateral flexion deformity, usually with a rotational deformity as well. It presents a characteristic clinical picture, and is always associated with lateral mass collapse.

The head may also be held in the slightly flexed position because of tilting of the atlas on the axis

(3). Not uncommonly patients may lose the usual cervical lordosis and the head may be brought forward into a characteristic posture.

In the presence of C1–2 subluxation, bending of the head may demonstrate a bulge in the midline suboccipital region that represents the subluxing spinous process of C2 (3). Holding the spinous process posteriorly while carefully and slowly pressing backward on the forehead may produce severe pain in the presence of AAS (3).

With severe laxity at the C1–2 level the head may shift forward spontaneously, and patients may be aware of a shifting noise or clunk (3). Crepitus, stiffness, and pain are common with these movements of the cervical spine.

The major concern of cervical spine disease (along with the patient's pain) is neurologic abnormality (Table 22.3) (4). Such abnormalities can range from the transitory and trivial to sudden death if the brainstem is impaled upon the subluxing odontoid process. Ranawat has proposed a useful neurologic classification that has been widely accepted (Table 22.4) (20). However, the neurologic evaluation of rheumatoid patients may be very difficult because of inflammation, pain, muscle atrophy, and compression neuropathy. Stocking and glove paresthesias are an early symptom of rheumatoid myelopathy. Similarly, persistent occipital headache, dizziness, an electric shock–like sensation on moving the head (Lhermitte's sign), and spontaneous movement of the legs (including muscle spasm) should alert the examiner to the possibility of cervical myelopathy.

Cranial nerve abnormalities are usually associated with AAI, often in association with C1–2 nerve pain (4, 39). Reports of involvement of cranial nerves are common in the literature (3, 12, 39–43). Common symptoms are dysarthria, dysphagia (cranial nerve XII), diplopia (VI), and facial numbness and depressed corneal reflex (V) (4). AAS in itself does not usually involve cranial nerves, but is most often associated with pain in the C1–2 distribution. When subaxial subluxations occur they may be associated with other nerve root symptoms, including paresthesias, hyperalgesias, radicular pain, muscle weakness and atrophy, reduced tendon reflexes, and decreased sensations.

All forms of subluxations can be associated with long tract signs and symptoms in addition to those enumerated above. Weakness, spasticity, hyperreflexia, extensor plantar response, diminished bladder and bowel control, and Lhermitte's sign are among the signs and symptoms that may be noted (3, 4). Interference to blood supply by subluxing structures and by soft tissue masses may lead to syndromes of vascular insufficiency, such as vertebrobasilar artery insufficiency.

## PREVALENCE AND RATE OF PROGRESSION OF RADIOGRAPHIC ABNORMALITIES

Biases in patient selection, ascertainment, and follow-up have made it difficult to accurately assess the prevalence and clinical significance of the radiographic and clinical finding noted above, but several prospective studies allow reasonable estimates. As will be seen, the degree of radiographic abnormality found in the clinic when all patients with RA are assessed is far less than when those who are seen in surgical specialty clinics are assessed.

The best of the studies of cervical spine abnormality in RA is that of Winfield et al. (7), who followed 100 RA patients seen within the first years of illness for more than 7 years. Radiographs and clinical measurements of the 44 men and 56

women were obtained yearly. Twelve patients developed AAS, and 7 of 10 treated with aggressive penicillamine therapy increased their subluxation over 5 years of follow-up in spite of such therapy. Within 1 year of disease onset four patients already had AAS. Within 2 years 83% of those who would develop AAS already had that finding, suggesting that AAS develops relatively early in the course of RA.

Similar data regarding the proportion of patients with AAS were obtained by Wolfe et al. (33), who described the findings in 675 patients followed for more than 12 years in the Saskatoon data bank associated with the American Rheumatism Association Medical Information System (ARAMIS) (44, 45). They noted a 13% prevalence of AAS within the first decade of rheumatoid arthritis (33). Smith et al. noted AAS in 7.7% of 272 men and 10.1% of 383 women admitted to the hospital (5). Rasker and Cosh found AAS in 42% of 62 patients followed for 14 years (46). These patients, who have been reported elsewhere (47), appear to have had very severe RA and may not be typical of all RA patients. Taken as a whole, however, the data suggest that AAS develops early

**Table 22.3.**
**Some Common Correlations between Types of Rheumatoid Cervical Spine Change and Associated Neurologic Findings[a]**

| Rheumatoid Cervical Spine Lesions | Area Most Probably Affected | Common Clinical Symptoms/Signs |
|---|---|---|
| Vertical AAS | N. hypoglossus (XIII), n. vagus (XI), & n. glossopharyngeus (X) | Dysphagia, dysphonia |
| | N. abducens (IV) | Diplopia |
| | Spinal nucleus of trigeminal nerve (V) | Facial numbness, depressed corneal reflexes Palatal weakness |
| | Pons | |
| Anterior & posterior AAS | CI, CII roots | Occipito-cervical pain |
| Subaxial subluxation | Other cervical nerve roots | Radicular pain, paresthesias, hyperalgesias, & hyperaesthesias; muscular weakness & atrophy; diminished tendon reflexes; diminished cutaneous sensibility |
| All forms | Pyramidal tract | Uncontrolled jerks, weakness, spasticity, hemi or tetraparesis, Lhermitte sign, increased tendon reflexes, diminished abdominal reflexes, extensor plantar responses, incontinence |
| | Dorsal funiculus | Distal paresthesias, dissociated sensory loss |
| | Spinothalamic tract | Decreased pain sensation |

[a]From Santavirta S, Kankaanpaa U, Sandelin J, Laasonen E, Konttinen YT, Slatis P: Evaluation of patients with rheumatoid cervical spine. *Scand J Rheumatol* 16:9–16, 1987.

**Table 22.4.**
**Ranawat Classification of Neural Deficits**[a]

| Class | Deficit |
|---|---|
| Class I | No neural deficit |
| Class II | Subjective weakness with hyperreflexia and dysesthesia |
| Class III | Objective weakness and long tract signs |
| Class IIIA | Able to walk |
| Class IIIB | Quadraparetic and nonambulatory |

[a]From Ranawat CS, O'Leary P, Pellicci PM, Tsairis P, Marcchisello P, Dorr L: Cervical spine fusion in rheumatoid arthritis. *J Bone Joint Surg [Am]* 61:1003–1010, 1979.

within the course of RA, but that it is not particularly common within the first 10 years of disease.

Other estimates have placed the prevalence of AAS at 19–71% (48). At 20 years of disease, Wolfe et al. found AAS in 48% of patients (33), and Smith et al. noted that, among 153 patients admitted to the hospital for the treatment of RA with a duration of 15–30 years, 32% had AAS (5). Pellicci et al. followed a group of RA patients who had had radiographs of the cervical spine (49). At the onset of the survey of 106 patients, disease duration averaged 24 years. Most patients were in ARA Functional Class III and an equal number were in either Class II or IV. Thirty-seven percent had AAS. Five years later (disease duration about 29 years) that number rose to 58%.

Many of these studies were selective for more severely affected patients and for those with longer duration of disease. In addition, they were biased by left and right censoring, and these results are almost certainly not reliable estimates of the proportion of RA patients with AAS. Reporting utilizing unbiased samples of patients with early RA and life table methodology is the appropriate approach to the description of the subluxations of RA, but this has not been done in any study to date.

AAI was found in only 3 of the 100 patients studied by Winfield et al. during the first 8 years of disease (7), and in only 1 of the 675 patients studied by Wolfe et al. (33). Smith et al. reported 1% with this abnormality (5), and Henderson noted 4% (50). Pellicci et al. noted 3.7% at 24 years and 9.4% at approximately 29 years (49). By contrast, Rasker and Cosh found 32% of patients with AAI at 14 years (46).

It is difficult to obtain estimates of the proportion of RA patients with PS since the finding is relatively uncommon. Weissman et al. found it in 6.7% of 194 patients selected for the presence of AAS or AAI (6). It appears, therefore, to be an uncommon finding in RA. Lateral subluxation was found in 21% of this patient sample as well.

Subaxial subluxations were noted in 24% of the early RA patients followed by Winfield et al. for 7 years, and were present in 12% at the 2-year evaluation point (7). Subaxial subluxations were noted in 25% of patients with a disease duration of less than 10 years by the Saskatoon group (33). Other studies have found prevalence of 7–29% for this radiographic abnormality. Disc space narrowing has been reported in 18–25% of patients (26).

## RELATIONSHIP BETWEEN RADIOGRAPHIC ABNORMALITIES AND CLINICAL SYMPTOMS

As difficult as it is to obtain estimates of the prevalence of the various radiographic findings, it is equally difficult to obtain reliable and valid information regarding symptoms and physical findings in those patients with radiographic abnormalities. In studies reporting on such problems, very strong biases toward inclusion of symptomatic patients exist since it is within this group that radiographs are made. Patients with radiographic abnormalities but who were less symptomatic may have been excluded.

The study of Weissman et al. was a retrospective analysis of 194 RA patients seen in an arthritis specialty hospital during a 10-year period who had either AAI or AAS (6). Radiographic follow-up was for a mean of 4.9 years. Twenty patients (10.3%) had neurologic evidence of upper cervical cord compression. "Neurological findings consisted of objective motor weakness and Babinski reflexes in 16 patients and hyperreflexia with subjective weakness in four patients" (6). Forty percent of the 20 patients were men, but only 14.4% of the non–cord compression group were men. Posterior subluxation was found in 13 (6.7%) of the 194 patients, but in only one of the cord compression group. Atlantoaxial impaction was noted in 43 (22.2%). Forty-five percent of the cord compression group had this abnormality. The authors suggested that a patient with this abnormality had approximately a 20% chance of developing cord compression.

The data cited above are in contrast to those of Santavirta and Hopfner-Hallikainen, who evaluated 23 patients with long-standing, severe RA seen in a surgical hospital (51). Only 7 of 23 were in Ranawat class I. Ten patients had atlantoaxial impaction and all of those were in Ranawat class II or III. Twenty-two of 23 patients had chronic severe occipitocervical pain, and 14 had chronic dizziness.

Marks and Sharp evaluated 31 patients with rheumatoid cervical myelopathy (42). Sensory symptoms were the most common finding (23 of 31) and included paresthesias and numbness. Six patients were noted to have "spastic weakness." Their "typical complaint was 'my legs won't go.'" Flexor spasms, rarely reported by patients, were identified in five. One patient had Lhermitte's sign, and two had urinary urgency. AAS was noted in 25 of 31 patients, with a range of subluxaion from 4 to 18 mm. Subaxial subluxation was noted in 26 patients, and was most common at C3–4. No relationship was found between the degree of luxation and clinical symptoms.

Breedveld et al. used MR imaging techniques to evaluate 21 patients with cervical myelopathy (35). Pain, paresthesias, and numbness were found equally among those with increasing neurologic abnormality in a classification scheme similar to that of Ranawat et al. (20). Cord distortion was found in six of eight patients in class III, two of four in class II, and one of nine in class I.

Twelve patients with long-standing RA were studied by Semble et al. (10). Three patients with evidence of cord compression on MR imaging had neurologic signs of cervical myelopathy. Only 1 of the 12 patients with neck pain had no abnormalities on MR imaging examination.

A series of isolated disasters have been reported in association with RA of the cervical spine. These include bilateral hypoglossal nerve palsy (43), massive osteolysis (53), indrocephalus (54), spontaneous fracture of the atlas (55), laryngeal deviation (56), and sudden death following trauma (57).

## TREATMENT AND PROGNOSIS

Estimates of the prevalence of RA involving the cervical spine have exceeded 80% (3) and, given the crude methods we have to assess such disease, it is possible that involvement might approach 100%. However, since it is myelopathy that is of greatest concern, the various subluxations that are more directly linked to myelopathy should be assessed. At a rate of 20% for AAS and 5% for AAI (admittedly very hypothetical figures) we can use the data of Weissman et al. (6) to estimate the risk of neurologic abnormality (cervical cord com-

pression). This suggests that the risk of cord compression to a RA patient is about 2%. At one center 3.1% of RA patients registered at the arthritis unit underwent cervical spine surgery (58). One should also note that the mean duration of RA among those with cord compression in the Weissman et al. series was almost 16 years, and only four of their patients had disease duration of less than 10 years (6). This suggests that routine screening with cervical radiography is not cost effective or clinically effective.

Using the more severely afflicted sample of Pellicci et al. (49) (mean disease duration of 24 years), 9.5% of patients received surgery during the next 5 years of follow-up. This included 5 of the 40 patients with AAS (12.5%) and none of the four patients with AAI (0%).

A second measure regarding prognosis and treatment should be directed to the small proportion of patients who actually develop myelopathy. Patients with this problem require treatment since the clinical syndrome in and of itself is associated with significant pain and dysfunction. Second, progression of the myelopathy may lead to further worsening of signs and symptoms or even to death.

## Nonsurgical Treatment

Conservative treatment usually consists of various forms of splinting, with soft or hard collars or with surgical traction with skull tongs, a treatment (also used following some surgical interventions) associated with considerable "human suffering" (12). There are no controlled trials of this therapy and there is simply no way to judge if it is effective. A number of investigators suggest that it may be of no value, and that there is no reason to suppose that it can assist with AAI (59). Marks and Sharp (42) noted that of 15 patients treated with a collar alone 6 improved, 2 did not, and 7 died. In those receiving traction only all three died, and both of the two patients who received no treatment died. Meijers et al. reported that 9 of their 11 unoperated patients died within 1 year, 4 as a consequence of cord compression (60). Most patients appear to be intolerant of cervical collars, and they are frequently discarded although frequently prescribed.

## Surgical Treatment

Most studies that have compared surgical and nonsurgical outcomes have favored the surgical outcome, but the patients receiving nonsurgical treatment were usually more severely afflicted with RA or had other comorbid conditions that precluded surgical intervention. Symptomatic improvement and mortality were generally better in the operated groups.

It should be recognized that after 15–20 years of RA, almost all patients who receive surgical treatment are severely afflicted and generally dysfunctional. In this subset of patients almost any intervention will have a high failure rate. Various surgical procedures are employed, but I will not distinguish among them here. Santavirta et al. compared the operative ($n = 18$) and nonoperative treatment ($n = 16$) of 34 selected RA patients with AAS (61). Patients had a mean duration of disease of 19.4 years. Follow-up ranged from 6 months to 5 years (mean 2.2 years). Two who were not operated died of nonrelated causes and were excluded from the study! Patients undergoing surgery were more frequently in Ranawat class III, more frequently had cord compression, and had higher degrees of AAS. Occipital pain was releived in the nonsurgical group in only one of eight patients who had pain, but in 12 of the 15 operated patients who had pain. Deterioration in neurologic function was noted in the unoperated group, but neurologic function was unchanged or improved in those undergoing surgery.

Heywood et al. (58) reported high rates of success in 30 fusion operations performed in 26 patients (2 patients died postoperatively). Clark et al. (34) reported clinical improvement in 66% of 41 patients with a mean RA duration of 20 years. During a follow-up period of 40 months, no patients were reported to worsen clinically, pain relief was noted in 21 of 23 patients, and neurologic status was unchanged in 73% and improved in the rest. Crockard et al. reported excellent results in 23 patients with a mean RA duration of 17 years who underwent anterior decompression (12). All but one improved. There were no deaths. Similar data have been reported from numerous studies (20, 36, 40, 58, 61–63).

Not all reports have been so optimistic. Marks and Sharp noted that death occurred in three of eight operated patients (42). Meijers et al. noted 3 of 25 patients died following surgery (60). Zoma and coworkers performed 40 operations on 32 patients with RA for a duration of 18 years (37). They reported a success rate of 57%, a failure rate of 35%, and early postoperative mortality in 8%.

The exact role of cervical spine surgery is not clear. Some patients clearly benefit, some die because of it, and some die in spite of it. Mortality rates are hard to interpret because so little infor-mation is available about the overall status of the patients. Clearly, operating on more, rather than less, seriously afflicted RA patients will always lead to a higher mortality rate. A recent study by Saway and associates sheds light on this problem (1). They studied 26 patients who underwent cervical spine surgery. "The indications for surgery were either intractable pain ($n = 14$), neurological abnormalities ($n = 8$), or both ($n = 4$)." Six patients had evidence of myelopathy. Three control groups were identified: (a) a group matched for age, sex, disease duration, and rheumatoid factor positivity; (b) a group selected from a university clinic; and (c) a group selected from a private practice clinic where patients had been identified because of cervical symptoms and radiographic abnormalities in the cervical spine. Surgery patients had decreased survival compared with the matched RA patients, and the decreased survival was strongly associated with disease severity. Among the surgical group and one of the nonsurgical cervical disease control groups, those patients who died had much more severe features of RA, including interstitial lung disease, vasculitis, pericardial involvement, and ocular involvement. Interstitial lung disease was a particularly strong risk factor for mortality. Death was thought to be related to these extra-articular nonsurgical factors. The probabilities of survival at 1 and 5 years after surgery were 74% and 54%, respectively. The authors suggested, based on these analyses, that cervical spine disease per se is not a risk factor for surgery, but severity of RA is such a factor. These data are in accord with the observation of many reports that found high fatality rates in both operated and nonoperated RA patients with severe cervical spine disease.

Among the problems in evaluating this intervention (surgery) are some standard, basic ones. Objective and blinded methods of evaluation are rarely used. It is hard to know what "improved" means in the majority of cases. Patients with different types of cervical spine problems and surgery are lumped together in the various reports. Serious and important comorbidities are neither tabulated nor controlled for. There are no controls. Follow-up is brief. King has suggested that the major reasons for surgery on the cervical spine are cord compression, severe pain, and, in the absence of either of these two factors, a very severe degree of cervical subluxation (64). However, others have suggested, based on 5-year follow-up, that only progression of neurologic signs requires intervention (49). This is an important issue. It would be useful to know what the long-

term outcome of the apparently surgically improved RA patients reported in the above studies
has been. In the mean time, progression of neurologic signs appears to be the only absolute indication for surgical intervention.

## METHODS OF EVALUATING CERVICAL SPINE DISEASE

Plain radiography is the most common method of
assessing the cervical spine. Flexion, extension,
and neutral views can provide information regarding AAS, AAI, and subaxial subluxations;
open-mouth views can produce information regarding the lateral masses and the odontoid processes. A standard anteroposterior view offers
information regarding apophyseal joint involvement. Unfortunately, the correlation between
neurologic impairment and plain radiographs is
not good enough, and the exact indication for radiography remains unclear. We suggest that radiographs may be an appropriate screening tool
for use in patients with persistent cervical or occipital pain or those in whom neurologic symptoms are suspected. Although radiographs are less
expensive than MR imaging, they are by no means
inexpensive since the predictive value of both positive and negative results in an unselected RA population appears low.

Although multiplanar tomography and computed tomography (CT) provide much more information than plain radiographs, they are expensive techniques. It has been suggested that CT
scanning offers little benefit over conventional radiography, except perhaps in providing better definition. MR imaging appears to be a major tool in
the evaluation of the cervical spine. It provides excellent detail of soft tissues (although not of cortical bone), thus allowing direct visualization of
the spinal cord and nerve roots as well as RA pannus (10, 11, 26, 35, 65). Further studies are
required to define its exact role. The strong correlation between MR imaging results and neurologic signs suggests MRI imaging may play a more
important role in defining indications for surgery
(66).

## JUVENILE RHEUMATOID ARTHRITIS (JUVENILE ARTHRITIS)

Juvenile rheumatoid arthritis (JRA) characteristically affects the cervical spine. Several types of
JRA are distinguished, a pauciarticular type most
frequently encountered in girls in early child-

hood, a polyarticular type seen at any age, and a
systemic type seen at any age. In addition, spondyloarthropathies may present as peripheral arthritis in children. "Adult" seropositive RA may
develop, in the teenage years, although it is not
considered to be a form of JRA.

Seropositive JRA runs a course quite similar to
adult RA, including the cervical spine changes
noted above. Certain findings, however, appear to
be specific to JRA. Clinical involvement of the cervical spine occurs early in the course of JRA and,
unlike the adult disease, is frequently associated
with restriction in range of motion. The loss of
range often persists into adult life. Radiographic
abnormalities include AAS, but this is most common in children who are rheumatoid factor positive (67, 68). In children the upper limit of atlantoaxial separation is 4.5 mm (68), ranging from 4
(9) to 5 mm (6).

The most characteristic finding in JRA (> 50%
of cases) appears to be involvement of the apophyseal joint at C3–4 with subsequent ankylosis
(68). Perispinal calcifications were noted in 29%,
growth disturbances in 22%, AAS in 20%, and
odontoid erosion in 13% of the 120 JRA patients
described by Espada et al. (68). Hensigner et al.
studied 145 patients with JRA, however, and
found no evidence of cervical spine disease in 56
of 57 with pauciarticular onset disease (9). Cervical spine involvement was noted in almost all patients with polyarticular and systemic-onset disease. Neck pain was not a common complaint
among these patients. Hypoplasia of the vertebral
bodies (and associated discs) together with fusion
of the apophyseal joint may lead to the typical
clinical appearance associated with a fused cervical spine and micrognathia.

Although neurologic involvement can occur in
children with cervical spine disease (68), it appears not to be common. Fried et al. found only 2
children of 92 studied who had such impairment
(69). Of the 92, 31% had clinical evidence of cervical spine involvement. AAS was present in five
patients, two of whom had hyperreflexia and clo-
nus that subsequently resolved spontaneously.
With rare exceptions disease of the cervical spine
does not lead to neurologic complications in seronegative children.

## SERONEGATIVE SPONDYLOARTHROPATHIES

Seronegative spondyloarthropathies constitute
the third major class of inflammatory conditions

that affect the cervical spine. The signal condition is ankylosing spondylitis, a disorder that in its most characteristic manifestations is related almost entirely to the axial skeleton. Other disorders—Reiter's syndrome, psoriatic arthritis (70), the arthritis of inflammatory bowel disease, and less well-defined HLA-B27 arthropathies—can also affect the axial skeleton.

Ankylosing spondylitis (AS) almost always begins clinically in the sacroiliac joints, and may progress variably into other areas of the axial skeleton (as well as the large joints of the peripheral skeleton). Inflammatory involvement of the bone-ligament interface leads to the development of osseous erosion and sclerosis along the anterior vertebral surfaces. Better seen in the lower axial skeleton, these changes may give the vertebrae a square appearance with "shining corners." Ossification of the annulus fibrosus leads to the development of thin, vertical, radiodense lines known as syndesmophytes. A series of discovertebral erosive lesions has been described in detail (71). Within the cervical spine changes similar to those of RA may be seen. Erosions of the odontoid process, often with significant proliferative changes not seen in RA, may occur. Although AAS may occur, it is unusual compared with its incidence in RA, having been found in most large series in less than 2% of patients. The characteristic radiographic appearance in AS is associated with the extensive ligamentous calcification, which may lead to the appearance of a "bamboo spine." The major clinical manifestation of AS involving the cervical spine is pain associated with inflammation, marked limitation of motion, and fusion of the neck, often into a flexed "chin-on-chest" position.

## TRAUMA AND INFLAMMATORY DISEASE OF THE CERVICAL SPINE

Several factors predispose patients with inflammatory rheumatic disease to severe injury following trauma. First, the combination of inflammation, inactivity, and corticosteroid therapy renders the cervical spine, as well as the rest of the skeleton, osteoporotic, Next, the neural structures are vulnerable, particularly in the cases of the various subluxations where the bony structure may readily compress the cord, brainstem, nerve roots, or vascular structures such as the anterior spinal artery or the basilar arteries. Finally, in JRA and particularly in AS, the rigid spine is susceptible to fracture with associated severe cord dam-

age. Compounding these risk factors are the weakness and mechanical damage to joints as well as the sensory abnormalities inherent in the systemic inflammatory disorders that make falls more likely.

Fracture is the main hazard to the brittle and fragile cervical spine in AS (57, 72–85). Fractures may follow even minor trauma (74, 76, 79, 83–85). Chiropractic manipulation has caused fractures (75), as have other events such as falling from a bed or a chair (81–83), minor automobile accidents (57), or even riding a motorcycle over bumpy ground (81). Most fractures occur at lower cervical levels (C5–7), usually through a calcified intervertebral disc, but a hangman's fracture (C2) (85), fractures through the odontoid process (84), and fractures through the cervical body (74, 76) are known to occur. The usual injury in AS is transection of the cord (74, 83, 86), but extradural hematomas may follow trauma as well (87). Clearly, individuals with AS should be cautioned to avoid hazardous activities.

The spine is not brittle in RA as it is in AS, but it is subject to compression fracture related to osteoporosis, and spontaneous fractures of the atlas have been reported (55). Surgical intubation is a potential hazard in RA since the hypermobile upper segments of the cervical spine can, on flexion and other manipulation, produce cord compression. It has been suggested that all patients with RA who must undergo surgery should first have cervical spine films made, but this practice does not seem to be carried out routinely. Awareness of the fragile nature of the cervical spine in those patients with chronic inflammatory disorders and appropriate attention to safety seem to be the best protection. Awake intubation with the use of the fiberoptic bronchoscope (56, 88) and use of evoked potentials (88) to monitor neurologic status may be helpful in selected patients.

### REFERENCES

1. Saway PA, Blackburn WD, Halla JT, Alarcon GA: Clinical characteristics affecting survival in patients with rheumatoid arthritis undergoing cervical spine surgery: a controlled study. *J Rheumatol* 16:890–896, 1989.
2. Modic WT, Weinstein MA, Pavlicek W, Boumphrey F, Starnes D, Duchesneau PM: Magnetic resonance imaging of the cervical spine: technical and clinical observations. *AJR* 141:1129–1136, 1983.
3. Bland JH: Rheumatoid arthritis of the cervical spine. *J Rheumatol* 1:319–342, 1974.
4. Santavirta S, Kankaanpaa U, Sandelin J, Laasonen E, Konttinen YT, Slatis P: Evaluation of patients with rheumatoid cervica spine. *Scand J Rheumatol* 16:9–16, 1987.
5. Smith PH, Benn RT, Sharp J: Natural history of rheumatoid cervical luxations. *Ann Rheum Dis* 31:431–439, 1972.

6. Weissman BN, Aliabadi P, Weinfeld MS, Thomas WH, Sosman JL: Prognostic features of atlantoaxial subluxation in rheumatoid arthritis patients. *Radiology* 144:745–751, 1982.

7. Winfield J, Young A, Williams P, Corbett M: Prospective study of the radiological changes in hands, feet, and cervical spine in adult rheumatoid disease. *Ann Rheum Dis* 42:613–618, 1983.

8. Lipson SJ: Rheumatoid arthritis of the cervical spine. *Clin Orthop* 143–149, 1984.

9. Hensinger RN, DeVito PD, Ragsdale CG: Changes in the cervical spine in juvenile rheumatoid arthritis. *J Bone Joint Surg [Am]* 68:189–198, 1986.

10. Semble EL, Elster AD, Loeser RF, Laster DW, Challa VR, Pisko EJ: Magnetic resonance imaging of the cranioverte-bral junction in rheumatoid arthritis. *J Rheumatol* 15:1367–1375, 1988.

11. Reynolds H, Carter SW, Murtagh FR, Silbiger M, Rechtine GR: Cervical rheumatoid arthritis: value of flexion and extension views in imaging. *Radiology* 164:215–218, 1987. (Published erratum appears in *Radiology* 165:292, 1987.)

12. Crockard HA, Essigman WK, Stevens JM, Pozo JL, Ransford AO, Kendall BE: Surgical treatment of surgical cord compression in rheumatoid arthritis. *Ann Rheum Dis* 44:809–816, 1985.

13. Konttinen YT, Bergroth V, Santavirta S, Sandelin J: Inflammatory involvement of cervical spine ligaments in patients with rheumatoid arthritis and atlantoaxial subluxation. *J Rheumatol* 14:531–534, 1987.

14. Cabot A, Becker A: The cervical spine in rheumatoid arthritis. *Clin Orthop* 130–140, 1978.

15. Isdale IC, Corrigan AB: Backward luxation of the atlas. *Ann Rheum Dis* 29:6–9, 1970.

16. Crellin RQ, McCabe JJ, Hamilton EB: Severe subluxation of the cervical spine in rheumatoid arthritis. *J Bone Joint Surg [Br]* 52:244–251, 1970.

17. Weiner S, Bassett L, Spiegel T: Superior, posterior, and lateral displacement of C1 in rheumatoid arthritis. *Arthritis Rheum* 25:1378–1381, 1982.

18. McGregor M: The significance of certain measurements of the skull in the diagnosis of basilar impression. *Radiology* 76:572–584, 1961.

19. McCrae DL: Bony abnormalities in the region of the foramen magnum: correlation of anatomic and neurologic findings. *Acta Radiol [Diagn] (Stockh)* 40:335–354, 1953.

20. Ranawat CS, O'Leary P, Pellicci PM, Tsairis P, Marcchisello P, Dorr L: Cervical spine fusion in rheumatoid arthritis. *J Bone Joint Surg [Am]* 61:1003–1010, 1979.

21. Morizona Y, Sakou T, Kawaida H: Upper cervical involvement in rheumatoid arthritis. *Spine* 12:721–725, 1987.

22. Kawaida H, Sakou T, Morizono Y: Vertical settling in rheumatoid arthritis. Diagnostic value of the Ranawat and Redlund-Johnell methods. *Clin Orthop* 128–135, 1989.

23. Komusi T, Munro T, Harth M: Radiologic review: the rheumatoid cervical spine. *Semin Arthritis Rheum* 14:187–195, 1985.

24. Halla JT, Fallahi S, Hardin JG: Nonreducible rotational head tilt and lateral mass collapse. A prospective study of frequency, radiographic findings, and clinical features in patients with rheumatoid arthritis. *Arthritis Rheum* 25:1316–1324, 1982.

25. Halla JT, Fallahi S, Hardin JG: Nonreducible rotational head tilt and atlantoaxial lateral mass collapse. Clinical and roentgenographic features in patients with juvenile rheumatoid arthritis and ankylosing spondylitis. *Arch Intern Med* 143:471–474, 1983.

26. Halla JT, Hardin JG, Vitek J, Alarcón GS: Involvement of the cervical spine in rheumatoid arthritis. *Arthritis Rheum* 32:652–659, 1989.

27. Resnick D, Niwayama G: Rheumatoid arthritis. In Resnick D, Niwayama G (eds): *Diagnosis of Bone and Joint Disorders.* Philadelphia: WB Saunders, 1988, vol II, pp 954–1067.

28. Ball J, Sharp J: Rheumatoid arthritis of the cervical spine. In Hill AGS (ed): *Modern Trends in Rheumatology.* New York, Appleton-Century-Crofts, 1971, vol 2, pp 117–138.

29. Schils JP, Resnick D, Haghighi PN, Trudell D, Sartoris DJ: Pathogenesis of discovertebral and manubriosternal joint abnormalities in rheumatoid arthritis: a cadaveric study. *J Rheumatol* 16:291–297, 1989.

30. Martel W: The occipito-atlanto-axial joints in rheumatoid arthritis and ankylosing spondylitis. *AJR* 86:223–240, 1961.

31. Bywaters EGL: Rheumatoid and other diseases of the cervical interspinous bursae, and changes in the spinous processes. *Ann Rheum Dis* 41:360–370, 1982.

32. Conlon PW, Isdale IC, Rose BS: Rheumatoid arthritis of the cervical spine. *Ann Rheum Dis* 25:120–126, 1966.

33. Wolfe BK, Okeeffe D, Mitchel DM, Tchang SP: Rheumatoid arthritis of the cervical spine: early and progressive radiographic features. *Radiology* 165:145–148, 1987.

34. Clark CR, Goetz DD, Menezes AH: Arthrodesis of the cervical spine in rheumatoid arthritis. *J Bone Joint Surg [AM]* 71:381–392, 1989.

35. Breedveld FC, Algra PR, Vielvoye CJ, Cats A: Magnetic resonance imaging in the evaluation of patients with rheumatoid arthritis and subluxations of the cervical spine. *Arthritis Rheum* 30:624–629, 1987.

36. Fehring TK, Brooks AL: Upper cervical instability in rheumatoid arthritis. *Clin Orthop* 221:137–148, 1987.

37. Zoma A, Sturrock RD, Fisher WD, Freeman PA, Hamblen DL: Surgical stabilisation of the rheumatoid cervical spine. A review of indications and results. *J Bone Joint Surg [Br]* 69:8–12, 1987.

38. Santavirta S, Konttinen YT, Lindqvist C, Sandelin J: Occipital headache in rheumatoid cervical facet joint arthritis [letter]. *Lancet* 2:695, 1986.

39. Edmeads J: The cervical spine and headache. *Neurology* 38:1874–1878, 1988.

40. Slatis P, Santavirta S, Sandelin J, Konttinen YT: Cranial subluxation of the odontoid process in rheumatoid arthritis. *J Bone Joint Surg [Am]* 71:189–195, 1989.

41. Swinson DR, Hamilton EBD, Mathews JA, Yates DAH: Vertical subluxation of the axis in rheumatoid arthritis. *Ann Rheum Dis* 31:359–363, 1972.

42. Marks JS, Sharp J: Rheumatoid cervical myelopathy. *Q J Med* 50:307–319, 1981.

43. Macedo TF, Gow PJ, Heap SW, Wallis WE: Bilateral hypoglossal nerve palsy due to vertical subluxation of the odontoid process in rheumatoid arthritis. *Br J Rheumatol* 27:317–320, 1988.

44. Wolfe F, Fries JF: ARAMIS today: moving toward internationally distributed databank systems for follow-up studies. *Clin Rheumatol* 6:93–102, 1987.

45. Mitchell DM, Spitz PW, Young DY, Block DA, McShane DJ, Fries JF: Survival, prognosis and causes of death in rheumatoid arthritis. *Arthritis Rheum* 29:706–714, 1986.

46. Rasker J, Cosh JA: Radical study of cervical spine and hand in patients with rheumatoid arthritis of 15 years duration: an assessment of the effects of corticosteroid treatment. *Ann Rheum Dis* 37:529–535, 1978.

47. Rasker JJ, Cosh JA: The natural history of rheumatoid arthritis over 20 years. Clinical symptoms, radiological signs,

treatment, mortality and prognostic significance of early features. *Clin Rheumatol* 6:5–11, 1987.

48. Lipson SJ: Rheumatoid arthritis in the cervical spine. *Clin Orthop* 239:121–127, 1989.

49. Pellicci PM, Ranawat CS, Tsairis P, Bryan WJ: A prospective study of the progression of rheumatoid arthritis of the cervical spine. *J Bone Joint Surg [Am]* 63:342–350, 1981.

50. Henderson DRF: Vertical atlanto-axial subluxation in rheumatoid arthritis. *Rheumatol Rehabil* 14:31–38, 1975.

51. Santavirta S, Hopfner-Hallikainen D: Atlantoaxial facet joint arthritis in the rheumatoid cervical spine. A panoramic zonographic study. *J Rheumatol* 15:217–223, 1988.

52. Lachiewicz PF, Schoenfeldt R, Inglis A: Somatosensory-evoked potentials in the evaluation of the unstable rheumatoid cervical spine. A preliminary report. *Spine* 11:813–817, 1986.

53. Hardin CW, Manaster BJ: Case report 411: rheumatoid arthritis with massive osteolysis and deformity of cervical spine; consequent neuropathic arthropathy of the shoulders. *Skeletal Radiol* 16:232–235, 1987.

54. Rillo OL, Rabadán A, Houssay R, Schillaci R, Pardal E: Atlantoaxial subluxation and indrocephalus in rheumatoid arthritis. *J Rheumatol* 16:121–125, 1989.

55. Sandelin J, Santavirta S, Laasonen E, Slatis P: Spontaneous fracture of atlas of cervical spine affected by rheumatoid arthritis. *Scand J Rheumatol* 14:167–170, 1985.

56. Keenan MA, Stiles CM, Kaufman RL: Acquired laryngeal deviation associated with cervical spine disease in erosive polyarticular arthritis. Use of the fiberoptic bronchoscope in rheumatoid disease. *Anesthesiology* 58:441–449, 1983.

57. Skold G: Injuries to pathologically changed cervical vertebrae. *Am J Forensic Med Pathol* 6:163–166, 1985.

58. Heywood AW, Learmonth ID, Thomas M: Cervical spine instability in rheumatoid arthritis. *J Bone Joint Surg [Br]* 70:702–707, 1988.

59. Konttinen YT, Santavirta S, Slatis P, et al: Pathogenesis of the rheumatoid cervical spine. *Scand J Rheumatol [Suppl]* 67:50–55, 1987.

60. Meijers KA, Cats A, Kremer HP, Luyendijk W, Onvlee GJ, Thomeer RT: Cervical myelopathy in rheumatoid arthritis. *Clin Exp Rheumatol* 2:239–245, 1984.

61. Santavirta S, Slatis P, Kankaanpaa U, Sandelin J, Laasonen E: Treatment of the cervical spine in rheumatoid arthritis. *J Bone Joint Surg [Am]* 70:658–667, 1988.

62. Santavirta S, Sandelin J, Slatis P: Posterior atlanto-axial subluxation in rheumatoid arthritis. *Acta Orthop Scand* 56:298–301, 1985.

63. Glynn MK, Sheehan JM: Fusion of the cervical spine for instability. *Clin Orthop* 179:97–101, 1983.

64. King TT: Rheumatoid subluxations of the cervical spine [editorial]. *Ann Rheum Dis* 44:807–808, 1985.

65. Aisen AM, Martel W, Ellis JH, McCune WJ: Cervical spine involvement in rheumatoid arthritis: MR imaging. *Radiology* 165:159–163, 1987.

66. Stevens JM, Kendall BE, Crockard HA: The spinal cord in rheumatoid arthritis with clinical myelopathy: a computed myelographic study. *J Neurol Neurosurg Psychiatry* 49:140–151, 1986.

67. Ansell B, Kent PA: Radiological changes in juvenile chronic polyarthritis. *Skeletal Radiol* 1:129–144, 1977.

68. Espada G, Babini JC, Maldonado Cocco JA, Garcia Morteo O: Radiologic review: the cervical spine in juvenile rheumatoid arthritis. *Semin Arthritis Rheum* 17:185–195, 1988.

69. Fried JA, Athreya B, Gregg JR, Das M, Doughty R: The cervical spine in juvenile rheumatoid arthritis. *Clin Orthop* 179:102–106, 1983.

70. Blau RH, Kaufman RL: Erosive and subluxing cervical spine disease in patients with psoriatic arthritis. *J Rheumatol* 14:111–117, 1987.

71. Resnick D, Niwayama G. Ankylosing spondylitis. In Resnick D, Niwayama G (eds): *Diagnosis of Bone and Joint Disorders.* Philadelphia, WB Saunders, 1988, vol II, pp 1103–1170.

72. Hunter R, Dubo H: Spinal fractures complicating ankylosing spondylitis. *Arthritis Rheum* 26:751–759, 1983.

73. Hunter T, Dubo H: Spinal fractures complicating ankylosing spondylitis. *Ann Intern Med* 88:546–549, 1978.

74. Murry GC, Persellin RH: Cervical fractures complicating ankylosing spondylitis. *Am J Med* 70:1033–1041, 1981.

75. Rinsky LA, Reynols GG, Jameson RM, Hamilton RD: A cervical spinal cord injury following chiropractic manipulation. *Paraplegia* 13:223–227, 1976.

76. Harding JR, McCall IW, Park WM, Jones BF: Fracture of the cervical spine in ankylosing spondylitis. *Br J Radiol* 58:3–7, 1985.

77. Hollin SA, Gross SW, Lewin P: Fracture of the cervical spine in patients with rheumatoid spondylitis. *Am Surg* 31:532–536, 1965.

78. Salathe M, Johr M: Unsuspected cervical fractures: a common problem in ankylosing spondylitis. *Anesthesiology* 70:869–870, 1989.

79. Foo D, Sarkarati M, Marcelino V: Cervical spinal cord injury complicating ankylosing spondylitis. *Paraplegia* 23:358–363, 1985.

80. Guttmann L: Traumatic paraplegia and tetraplegia in ankylosing spondylitis. *Paraplegia* 4:188–201, 1966.

81. Lemmen LJ, Laing PG: Fracture of the cervical spine in patients with rheumatoid spondylitis. *J Neurosurg* 16:242–250, 1959.

82. Raine GE: Fractures of the cervical spine in ankylosing spondylitis. *Proc R Soc Med.* 63:657–658, 1970.

83. Kiwerski J, Wieclawek H, Garwacka I: Fractures of the cervical spine in ankylosing spondylitis. *Int Orthop* 8:243–246, 1985.

84. Govender S, Charles RW: Fracture of the dens in ankylosing spondylitis. *Injury* 18:213–214, 1987.

85. McCall I, el Masri W, Jaffray D: Hangman's fracture in ankylosing spondylitis. *Injury* 16:483–484, 1985.

86. Braunstein EM, Weissman BN, Seltzer SE, Sosman JL, Wang AM, Zamani A: Computed tomography and conventional radiographs of the craniocervical region in rheumatoid arthritis. A comparison. *Arthritis Rheum* 27:26–31, 1984.

87. Garza Mercado R: Traumatic extradural hematoma of the cervical spine. *Neurosurgery* 24:410–414, 1989.

88. Ovassapian A, Land P, Schafer MF, Cerullo L, Zalkind MS: Anesthetic management for surgical corrections of severe flexion deformity of the cervical spine. *Anesthesiology* 58:370–372, 1983.

## 23

# DEGENERATIVE DISC AND OTHER NEURAL LESIONS

*William I. Smulyan*

The management of neck pain in the office and the operating room setting is a challenging and pitfall-laden problem that demands of the physician in general, and the orthopaedic surgeon in particular, a constant awareness of anatomy and the need to correlate it to the many differential diagnostic considerations that can cause or be associated with neck pain. The patient with acute neck pain and torticollis is as uncomfortable as any patient in all of orthopaedics. The patient with chronic neck pain that has been refractory to any modality of treatment is difficult to manage and often chronically depressed as a result of the ongoing pain problem. Discussion of the embryology, anatomy, and examination of the cervical spine is helpful in facilitating an understanding of the manifestations of the disease entities that can afflict this region.

## EMBRYOLOGY

Embryologically, the bony cervical spine arises from the mesoderm. This layer develops between the endoderm and ectoderm during the third week of embryonic life. The mesoderm develops into an axial rod called the notochord as the ectoderm forms the neural tube on the dorsal surface of the embryo directly above or posterior to the notochord. Segmentation then occurs in the fourth week. Cellular quantities increase as mesodermal cells differentiate into myotome, dermatome, and sclerotome. Resegmentation of these primitive segments occurs at 5–6 weeks of embryonic life. These segments, or somites, are now called vertebrae.

During this time, the cells that give rise to the intervertebral disc differentiate around a cleft called the fissure of Von Edner. Cells migrate dorsally over the neural tube from the vertebral body to form the vertebral arches dorsally. Ventrally, these cells form the costal processes or ribs.

During the fetal phase of development the mesenchymal predecessors or anlage of the vertebrae undergo the processes of chondrogenesis and subsequently osteogenesis without change in their shape or fundamental structure. Obviously, however, they acquire a different tissue matrix as they increase in size. Chondrification, which begins in two centers on each side of the midline, ultimately forces notochordal tissue out of the vertebral body into the intervertebral disc space to remain there as the nucleus pulposus. At the same time, chondrification continues in the neural arch and in each costal process.

These steps in the development process are typical for most of the vertebrae except in the area of the occipitoatlantoaxial articulation. This area arises from the first four somites in the embryo. The intervertebral disc between the atlas and the axis is represented by the apical and alar ligaments. The vertebral body of C1 results from the fusion of the caudal part of the C1 somite and the cranial part of the C2 somite. The odontoid process and the body of C2 also arise from this cellular mass.

Ossification begins in the vertebrae from three ossific nuclei, one in the vertebral body and one in each of the two neural arches. This process continues from birth through late childhood, with lit-

362

tle potential for longitudinal growth in the cervical spine.

## ANATOMY

Anatomically, the cervical spine consists of the first seven vertebrae in the spinal column and may be thought of in two halves, the upper and the lower. There is a typical lower cervical vertebra (C3–7) in which there is a small vertebral body, concave superiorly and convex inferiorly. Transverse processes are noted in the inferior four vertebrae. Posteriorly there are the spinous processes, which are usually bifid in C3, C4, and C5 and more prominent in C6 and C7. The spinous process of C7 is called the vertebra prominens.

In the upper cervical spine, the atlas, or C1, is the most unique of the vertebrae because it has no centrum or body. That portion has been absorbed into the body of the axis, or C2, to form the odontoid process. C1 therefore has a thick anterior arch with bulky lateral masses for the articulation with the occiput superiorly. The transverse process of C2 contains a forament for the vertebral artery called the foramen transversarium. All of the cervical vertebrae protect this vessel except for C1.

The bony elements of the cervical spine and skull are linked together with ligaments and discs that provide the neck with a stable but flexible framework. The major stabilizers are the anterior and posterior longitudinal ligaments extending over the entire length of the spine. The anterior ligament is closely attached to the intervertebral discs and thickens over the concave part of the vertebral body, whereas the posterior ligament is widest in the upper spine and narrows caudally. It is waisted over the vertebral bodies and fans out over the intervertebral discs.

The intervertebral disc consists of the nucleus pulposus at its center, two cartilaginous endplates that are adjacent to the facing vertebral surfaces, and the annulus fibrosus or outer ring. The area of closest contact between the superior surface of a given vertebra and the inferior surface of the next higher vertebra is at the point of origin of the pedicle from the vertebral body. This articulation is called the uncovertebral joint or the joint of Luschka. The articulations between the vertebral arches are maintained by the ligamentum nuchae, the interspinous ligament, the ligamentum flavum, and the facet joints. These joints are diarthrodial, with typical synovial membranes and fibrous capsules.

The articulation of the occiput with C1 and C2 is different from that of the joints of the lower spine. Stability is more reliant on ligaments than in the lower portion of the spine. The anterior and posterior longitudinal ligaments are present. The posterior extends upward to be called the tectorial membrane at the level of the occiput and overlies the body of the axis. The transverse ligament forms from the axis to the base of the occiput. At the apex of the dens is an apical ligament that attaches to the anterior rim of the foramen magnum and is flanked by two alar ligaments. Additionally, the joints between the dens and the atlas, the occiput and the axis, and the atlas and axis are synovial joints.

Motion occurs with the use of muscle groups interacting in a complex way to move the rigid osseous framework supported by its ligamentous system. These muscles work the neck in flexion, extension, rotation, and lateral bending. These various muscular groups are layered and interwoven to provide supportive and complimentary function. The muscles are arranged in triangles in which muscular groups are enclosed within other muscular groups. These muscular triangles protect the important visceral, vascular, and neural structures, including the larynx, trachea, esophagus, carotid sheath, and cervical sympathetic chain.

The cervical spine houses the cervical portion of the spinal cord. The vertebral arteries run parallel with each side of the spinal column to provide a blood supply to the cervical cord and brainstem. With the cervical spine are the two layers of the mater, dura and pia, and the system of dentate ligaments of the pia mater, which also serve to protect the spinal cord. The cervical nerve roots pass almost directly lateral to the cord at each level to exit from the spinal canal at the neural foramen of that level.

## DIFFERENTIAL DIAGNOSIS OF NECK PAIN

Neck pain may be caused by degenerative disorders of the spine, including variations of cervical discogenic disease such as disc rupture and cervical spondylosis. Additionally, noninfectious, inflammatory disorders such as rheumatoid arthritis and other variations of collagen vascular diseases, infections, tumor, and acute trauma all contribute to the development of neck pain and necessitate its management in the adult patient.

In the consideration of the problem of neck pain from its clinical aspects, it is important again to emphasize that the five lower cervical vertebrae are connected in five areas—the intervertebral disc, the two facet joints, and the neurocentral or uncovertebral joints bilaterally. Cervical disc degeneration, the destruction of the mechanical integrity of the disc, seems to be the initiating factor in the development of cervical spondylosis.

## CERVICAL SPONDYLOSIS

One of the major causes of pain in the neck is cervical spondylosis, a condition of progressive degeneration of the cervical spine associated with the aging process. It begins in the cervical intervertebral disc with a loss of mechanical integrity of the disc. This degeneration leads to changes secondarily in the surrounding bones and soft tissues of the cervical spine. Osteophytes develop as hypertrophy occurs in the facets and the laminae. While this is very much a part of the aging process, disc rupture or protrusion is a specifc manifestation of this condition. Symptoms are produced because of tension on the dura or the nerve root. Symptomatic difficulty ultimately develops because of resultant changes in the mechanical function of the spine. Early in the stages of disc degeneration, there is mechanical evidence of instability at a single level of the cervical spine. That segment develops a predisposition to be injured, and symptoms may therefore arise because of injury to the ligaments or the joints.

In addition to neck pain, the patient may also describe some phenomenon of referred pain in the shoulder, headache particularly about the occipital portion of the skull, interscapular pain, pain in the arm, or even pain in the chest. In the late stages of cervical disc degeneration, when spondylosis or the development of bony outgrowths about the area of the uncovertebral joint has developed, symptoms may be associated with nerve root compression or irritation. During degeneration, there is loss of intervertebral disc space height as osteophytes develop in the neurocentral (uncovertebral) joints.

Radiographic studies at this time might show encroachment on the intervertebral foramen by osteophytes. These changes, when observed in the joints of Luschka, are most visible on anteroposterior views. Osteophytes in this location may be implicated as a cause of vertebral artery compression. Disc degeneration occurs most commonly in the midcervical region, causing a decrease in extension in the spine and the normal cervical lordosis. This produces a loss of motion in that segment or segments and subsequent hyperextension of the head.

Patients who have chronic headache associated with cervical spondylosis have a pain in the distribution of the greater occipital nerve. This pain typically originates in the suboccipital region. It may be associated with neck muscle fatigue, recurrent motion of the spine, and emotional tension. Additionally, some investigators believe that there is a vascular component as well. There may be nausea and vomiting in association with other migraine-like complaints. Etiologically, this is thought to be due to compression or irritation of the greater occipital nerve. Relief may be achieved with attempts at nerve blocks. Successful use of this technique would also confirm the diagnosis. Biofeedback techniques, in addition to the standard forms of nonsurgical management, may be very beneficial in such cases.

In the case of advanced spondylosis, the patient may continue to have significant long-term symptoms. Complaints may consist of neck pain with associated grinding and cracking sounds and sensations. The patient may describe aching in the shoulders and upper arms and radiation of pain into the hands as well as into the upper back and interscapular region. Physical examination may be expected to reveal diminished mobility in the neck and possibly in the shoulders as well. This latter problem may demand separate diagnosis and treatment of its own. Patients with this symptom complex may have already had previous surgery directed at management of cervical spondylosis or cervical disc rupture.

In the management of such patients, it is imperative that a satisfactory evaluation be carried out in order that no evidence of any other systemic problem—specifically, neoplasms of the apex of the lung and metastatic disease to the cervical spine—is missed. These entities may frequently masquerade as problems associated with "advanced cervical spondylosis." Nonsurgical treatment modalities remain the treatment of choice in these situations. Patients with long-term chronic complaints must always be considered in terms of various psychiatric, psychosocial and vocational factors that may be complicating, or in actuality causing, the complaints the patient is experiencing.

## TRAUMATIC CERVICAL NEURITIS

Traumatic cervical neuritis as a result of disc herniation, osteophytic compression, or trauma—

both surgical and nonsurgical—may be quite disabling. Pain of this nature is radicular in character, following the course of the nerve root that is injured. The pain may be burning and constant. In addition, it may be refractory to the use of analgesics. Neurologic examination may indicate loss of sensory and/or motor function. Standard history and physical examination will probably provide the diagnosis. However, the use of diagnostic techniques such as plain radiography, magnetic resonance (MR) imaging, computed tomographic (CT) scanning, and myelography may be of benefit. Nonsurgical treatment should be initiated. It should fail before any surgical intervention is considered.

## REFLEX SYMPATHETIC DYSTROPHY

Reflex sympathetic dystrophy may occur when there has been an injury to the cervical nerve root, possibly of a surgical nature. This type of injury may also occur when a fusion collapses or if infection has developed. In addition to the complaint of pain, there is evidence of autonomic instability—complaints of coldness or sweating in the affected limb, loss of muscular strength, and stiffness. Neurologic examination will not be consistent with the diagnosis of radiculopathy. Radiographically, there may be loss of mineral from the bones of the limb about which the patient is complaining. Diagnostically, electrical studies are nonspecific and thermography may, at best, be of some benefit. Treatment is largely symptomatic and is directed at encouraging the patient to be able to live with the symptoms. Biofeedback techniques can be helpful. Surgically, upper thoracic and cervical sympathectomy can provide some relief. This should be considered only if sympathetic nerve blocks have provided symptomatic relief.

## AMPLIFIED PAIN SYNDROME

Another entity in the differential diagnosis of neck pain is an amplified pain syndrome. A patient with this problem will often exaggerate or overemphasize symptomatic difficulty. There is little evidence of age or sex predilection, and etiologic trauma is often trivial. Secondary gain motivations are frequently seen in these situations. Evaluation of patients of this nature must be thorough and directed at both systemic and local diagnoses. Plain radiography, myelography, CT

scanning, MR imaging, and appropriate electrical studies, as always, must be done to initiate this evaluation. Psychological evaluation is important in order to determine whether or not sociopathy or some other form of character disorder may be contributing to the patient's difficulties. Therapy is obviously arduous. Surgery is of little benefit, and nonsurgical management, particularly behavioral therapy, should be the primary goal in treatment.

## TRAUMATIC LESIONS

Traumatic lesions also are a part of the differential diagnosis of neck pain. The first recorded reference to paraplegia following injury to the cervical spine is found in the Edwin Smith Papyrus (1). In 1838, Key provided the first modern account of a spondylotic bar producing compression of the cervical cord (2). In 1911, this compression was reported to be a sequela of osteoarthritis of the spine (3). By 1926, radicular symptoms due to narrowing of the intervertebral foramen were recognized (4), and by 1932 Schmorl had developed an understanding of the anatomic and abnormal aspects of intervertebral disc protrusion (5). By 1940, three clinical manifestations of cervical disc rupture were described by Stukey—bilateral anterior pressure on the spinal cord, unilateral anterior pressure with a Brown-Séquard–type syndrome, and nerve root compression (6).

In 1948, the importance of the neurocentral joints of Luschka was emphasized by Bull (7). Osteophytic changes and their significance in nerve root compression were also emphasized. Brain (8) emphasized the importance of vascular changes. He believed that acute cervical disc protrusion, more typically traumatic in origin, was more likely to produce nerve root compression, whereas chronic changes associated with osteophytic compression were more likely to cause cord compression. In 1957, studies by Payne and Spillane demonstrated narrowing in the cervical canal in patients with myelopathy-associated cervical spondylosis (9).

Radiographically, cervical spondylosis has all variations. Initially, there is no evidence of any radiographic abnormalities. By the end of the course of the disease, specific studies such as MR imaging and CT become necessary to localize an involved level. Disc space narrowing is expected to be a constant feature of late-stage changes in cervical spondylosis. These are noted most commonly at C5–6 and next most commonly at C6–7.

The vertebral bodies undergo secondary changes of remodeling, characterized by sclerosis in the cortex as well as osteophytic changes, either anteriorly or posteriorly. Oblique radiographic studies of the cervical spine are necessary to demonstrate posterolateral osteophytic change as well as changes in the neurocentral joints.

Brain's studies indicated that there is no satisfactory correlation between abnormal radiographic appearances and symptomatology (8). It is well known that patients with many of the radiographic stigmata of cervical spondylosis may be without symptoms. Some of this discrepancy may be explained by the premorbid size of the diameter of the cervical canal. Cord compression may therefore be expected if the sagittal diameter at any level is less than or equal to 10 mm.

## CERVICAL RADICULOPATHY AND MYELOPATHY

There are two main clinical syndromes associated with cervical spondylosis—cervical radiculopathy and myelopathy. Radiculopathy, particularly in spondylosis, may be single or multiple, and it may be unilateral or bilateral, as well as symmetrical or asymmetrical.

Radiculopathy may be acute or subacute to chronic. The acute type is associated with a tear of the annulus fibrosus and prolapse or extrusion of a free fragment of nucleus pulposus. Frequently there is no evidence of osteophytic change or spondylosis. Vigorous trauma ranging from a pure soft tissue injury to fracture-dislocation is usually necessary to produce this type of change. Lesions are frequently intraforaminal. They are associated with pain in the neck and shoulder radiating in a dermatomal distribution. Sensory symptoms, including paresthesia, hypesthesia, and hyperalgesia, are far more common than motor or reflex changes. Radicular pain is also accentuated by activities such as the Valsalva maneuver that place the involved nerve root under increased stretch. The patient will typically complain of pain in the neck, top of the shoulder, and scapula. Some of the sensory symptoms are thought to be due to stimulation of the sinuvertebral nerve fibers in the annulus fibrosus, and the anterior and posterior longitudinal ligaments.

Nontraumatic radiculopathies may be considered to be more subacute. Overusage with or without a combined inflammatory process may be responsible for initiating this sequence of events. Symptoms occur as the result of direct mechanical compression of individual nerve roots within the foramen as well as stretching of the nerve roots due to abnormal angulation of the vertebral bodies around degenerated disc fragments. It would then seem clear that a patient with preexisting foraminal osteophytic encroachment is more prone to develop discogenic signs than one who does not have this difficulty. This occurs most commonly at C5 and C6.

Cervical myelopathy seems to be associated with the development of transverse bars in cervical spondylosis. Other anatomic changes seen in this situation include facet hypertrophy and canal stenosis. This latter finding may be a preexisting but previously unrecognized condition. The clinical picture seen is typically that of an incomplete lesion—dysesthesias of the hands, paresthesias in the fingertips, weakness and clumsiness of the hands, and weakness of the lower limbs. There is a decrease in the appreciation of light touch and tactile discrimination. Muscular atrophy may be noted. If there is corticospinal tract involvement, deep tendon reflexes will be exaggerated distal to the lesion. Also seen is the inverted radial reflex: percussion of the lower end of the radius will produce reflex flexion of the digits. Sphincter impairment, as well as the jaw jerk reflex, may also be seen, occurring most commonly at C5. Symptoms typically are insidious in onset. Acute trauma, particularly hyperextension, is the most common cause of acute symptoms.

## CERVICAL DISC LESION

Obviously, the most common cause of neck pain is some manifestation of a lesion of the cervical disc. Entrapment of the cervical cord may be caused by tumors of the cervical cord, most typically the neurofibroma. Typically, a patient with this problem will be in the middle decades of life and will complain of stiffness in the neck as well as pain in the shoulder. The patient may also describe pain about the arm and forearm in addition to paresthesias in the digits. Pain in the thumb and index finger indicates an involvement of the sixth cervical root at C5–6. This is the most common site of this lesion. When there is involvement of the seventh root, the middle fingers are involved in the complaint. Fifth finger involvement indicates a lesion at the C7–T1 interspace.

## ARTHRITIS

Neck pain is also caused by arthritis and the various arthritic disorders such as rheumatoid arthritis. This polyarthritic disorder is a lesion of the synovium and eventually involves all elements of the musculoskeletal system. Sixty percent of the patients with this disorder will manifest some involvement of the cervical spine. When the atlantoaxial articulation is affected, subluxation of C1 and C2 will occur in 25%. Anatomically, the joint surfaces in this area or in the facets will become eroded and irregular. Only infrequently will neurologic symptoms occur. If surgical treatment is necessary, it should be justified on the basis of radiographically demonstrable instability as well as pain. The halo is a valuable adjunct to the postoperative management. When upper cervical spine subluxations are neurologically significant, myelopathy is evident and the prognosis is guarded. The natural history of this disorder is poor. In addition to the diagnostic studies already discussed, discography may be employed by certain physicians.

## EVALUATION OF THE PATIENT WITH NECK PAIN

In discussing neck pain, the basic approach to the patient is still the traditional form of complete history taking and physical examination. Accurate information about pain patterns is very important. Pain radiating into the shoulder or down the arm may be a primary cervical spine problem and/or a primary extremity problem. It may also represent retrograde radiation of pain in the upper limb as a result of carpal tunnel syndrome or some other form of peripheral nerve entrapment in the distal aspect of the upper limb.

Neck problems alone tend to be associated with chronic types of pain, whereas shoulder problems, such as acute calcific tendinitis or an injury to the rotator cuff, are usually a more acute type of pain causing sleep disturbance. Questioning the patient about the effect of neck motion on pain is significant because patients with cervical discogenic complaints will experience an exacerbation of pain with motion in the neck. Patient occupation and typical neck posture also influence development of neck pain. Questioning the patient with regard to the possibility of sleep disturbance in association with change of position should also be considered. If trauma has occurred, then the mechanism of injury must be ascertained. Recreational and occupational factors producing repeated wear and tear on increasingly brittle elastic tissues should be sought because they contribute to these symptoms quite frequently.

Examination of the neck begins with observation of the patient with regard to overall appearance, facial expression, and posture of the neck. Palpation of the cervical spine is extremely important to assess for tenderness, deformity, or palpable masses. A lesion of the spinal accessory nerve may be detected by observing for the presence or absence of atrophy in the sternocleidomastoid and trapezius. It is important to observe for evidence of muscular cramping or spasm. Palpation for points of tenderness is extremely important. Observe the neck for range of motion. A patient with a normal examination should be expected to demonstrate the ability to flex the neck to bring the chin to the chest and extend the neck to 90°. Lateral bending should be at 45° bilaterally. Rotation is next, with normal being 60° bilaterally. Finally, of all of the muscular structures, particularly anteriorly and superiorly over the apices of the lungs, should be palpated for adenopathy. Differential diagnosis of neck pain must certainly include any lesion found in this area.

Evaluation of the cervical spine is next done radiographically. A basic series of neck radiographs consists of anteroposterior and lateral views, an open-mouth view for the odontoid, and oblique views. Additionally, a set of basic studies may also include flexion and extension views to assess the stability of the cervical axis. In the anteroposterior view, overall alignment of the vertebral bodies can be assessed. Rotational variations can be determined by attempting to draw a straight line through the spinous processes. Cervical ribs may be detected in this study. The lateral view is helpful in the diagnosis of a fracture of the vertebral body and in looking for changes in bony density. The oblique view facilitates the assessment of the alignment of the facet joints as well as the patency of the neural foramina.

Myelography is the traditional form of diagnostic radiographic study beyond plain films in the imaging of degenerative disorders of the spine. Although it has largely been supplanted by CT and MR imaging, this procedure, now performed with water-soluble contrast material, remains a valuable adjunct in the armamentarium of evaluative procedures. Even after a positive MR image has been obtained, it has been the policy of this author to continue to require myelography before contemplating any surgical intervention.

In addition to the traditional methods of imaging the spine, CT scanning and MR imaging have now become sufficiently reliable that they are regarded as excellent screening studies to be employed before any types of invasive studies are performed. In the diagnostic imaging of the cervical spine MR imaging resonance studies are becoming more repeatedly reliable, and are rapidly becoming the second-choice study after the plain radiograph. There are those who believed that it may now be an appropriate first study for the evaluation of the cervical spine in a patient in whom symptoms of degenerative disease or other problems such as tumor or infection are suspected. $T_1$-weighted sagittal images with 3-mm slice thicknesses provide excellent contrast for evaluation of the marrow of the vertebral body, disc space height, neural canal, and spinal cord and fluid. Oblique views through the neural foramen can be obtained. All of the anatomic structures, including the cerebrospinal fluid–dural interface, can be studied in a single modality without any invasive methods. Imaging of this type makes it possible to diagnose disc herniation, canal stenosis, subluxation, malalignment, and neoplasm. Only if studies of this nature then fail to provide a specific diagnosis should the use of contract CT be considered.

Other diagnostic testing to be considered for conditions of the cervical spine should include nuclear medicine studies such as the bone scan and possibly a gallium scan. Additionally, if nerve compression is thought to be a diagnostic possibility, then electromyography and nerve conduction studies are important to help in the localization of a lesion. The ability to do this aids in planning precise surgical treatment of the properly diagnosed problem.

## MANAGEMENT

Nonsurgical treatment for these conditions of the neck is directed at decreasing pressure on the affected nerve root. Various modalities may be utilized. Traction, either dynamic or static, is frequently the method of choice. Static traction may be provided in the hospital setting, maintaining the patient in the supine position and achieving the maximum benefits of bed rest and inactivity at the height of the severity of a patient's symptoms.

This basic method may be employed in the outpatient setting with various types of home devices. Theoretically, foraminal spaces are being opened to permit enlargement of the neural pathway. Medication to be used would consist of anti-inflammatory and analgesic drugs. Occasionally muscle relaxants are of some benefit, probably because of their sedative properties.

A detailed technical discussion of the surgical treatment for painful disorders of the cervical spine is beyond the scope of this particular chapter. However, a brief review is helpful in completing a general consideration of the problem. In the case of the patient with a discogenic or spondylotic lesion that is being considered for surgery, it has been the policy of this author to manage the problem nonsurgically coincident with the performance of diagnostic studies. Surgery is offered if nonsurgical treatment has failed. Failure of nonsurgical treatment means that the patient's symptoms have not been relieved and there may be progression of neurologic findings in the form of increased weakness, reflex loss, or increased numbness in the appropriate radicular distribution.

Invasive therapy is directed at both decompression of the involved neural tissue and preserving or regaining stability of the spine. In cervical disc rupture, discectomy may be performed either posteriorly or anteriorly. If the posterior approach is employed, then typically no fusion or prolonged postoperative bracing is necessary. however, these is a tendency for the disc space to collapse secondarily, potentially creating the need for a second procedure anteriorly in the form of a fusion. The primary use of anterior interbody fusion for disc rupture, osteophytic foraminal encroachment, or a combination of the two has, in the hands of this author, been a reliable method for the decompression of the affected nerve root and for stabilization of the cervical spine. To be sure, the postoperative course is more prolonged. However, if the surgery is confined to one level, the fusion rate is greater than 90–95% with generally satisfactory results.

Finally, it should be emphasized that the use of any surgical treatment for the cervical spine is reserved in virtually all cases for those lesions that appear to be specifically identifiable by history, physical examination, and diagnostic studies. Particularly in the case of a degenerative discogenic lesion, when the diagnosis is accurately established preoperatively and nonsurgical treatment has failed, a favorable surgical outcome may be predicted.

## REFERENCES

1.
2. Key, 1838.
3.
4.
5. Schmorl, 1932.
6. Stukey, 1940.
7. Bull, 1948.
8. Brain
9. Payne, Spillane, 1957.

## SUGGESTED READINGS

Bateman JE: *The Shoulder and Neck.* Philadelphia, WB Saunders, 1972.

Cervical Spine Research Society: *The Cervical Spine.* Philadelphia, JB Lippincott, 1983.

Lestini WF, Weisel SW: The pathogenesis of cervical spondylotic radiculopathy and myelopathy. *Clin Orthop Rel Res* 239:69–93, 1989.

Rothman H (Ed): Symposium on the disease of the intervertebral disc. *Orthop Clin North Am* 2:2, 1971.

Rothman RH, Simeone FA: *The Spine.* Philadelphia, WB Saunders, 1975.

# 24

# RADIATING TEMPOROMANDIBULAR DYSFUNCTION AND FASCIAL TRAUMA PAIN

*Jerome D. Buxbaum, Steven G. Ashman, and Alan S. Exler*

It is well established in the literature (1, 2) that a profound interrelationship exists between orofacial and cervical structures. Most patients who present with traumatic injury in these areas really are afflicted with pathologies of multifactorial origin that affect both orofacial and cervical structures. The problem is compounded because most physicians are unaware and poorly trained in the diagnosis and triage of temporomandibular dysfunctions (TMD), and most dentists are unappreciative of the cervical implications that often logically are associated with TMD symptoms.

Temporomandibular dysfunction syndrome was first described by Costens, and through the years a number of different terms have been used to describe temporomandibular joint pathology and/or neuromuscular nociception in the orofacial area. Some of these terms are temporomandibular joint (TMJ) disease, myofacial pain dysfunction (MPD), and myo-oral facial pain (MOFP). All of these terms have proven to be inappropriate. The term "TMD" is simply a description of a set of symptoms analogous to the term "heart disease." Neither term describes a specific pathology. At present over 100 pathologic and psychological entities produce one or more symptoms and findings that fall under the umbrella term of TMD.

The result of this lack of integrated information is that the patient is referred from one specialist to another without benefit. It is imperative that an accurate diagnosis of both orofacial and cervical disease be obtained prior to the initiation of any definitive therapy. It is also imperative that treatment of both areas be conducted simultaneously.

Two of the major causative categories of TMD are musculoskeletal and traumatic. The musculoskeletal category includes not only mandibular position but craniocervical posture as well. Traumatic injuries to the cranium, jaw, neck, or shoulders will produce effects in all of these structures. Therefore, any pathology that hinders normal physiologic activity in the stomatognathic system may produce pain involving the head, neck, throat, and ears.

## ANATOMY AND PHYSIOLOGY

The stomatognathic system in general and the mandible in particular do not exist in isolation. Rather, these structures are designed to function in harmony with the upper vertebral column, cranium, hyoid bone, and shoulder area coupled with all of the involved musculature. The masticatory system is balanced and supported posteriorly by the vertebral column, anteriorly by the hyoid complex, inferiorly by the clavicle and shoulder girdle, and superiorly by the cranium.

Cinefluorographs made by Schemen and others clearly demonstrate the interaction between mastication and cranial movement. These films demonstrate that as incision of foodstuffs occurs the head moves quickly backward, helping to tear the bite from the portion.

Simplistically, the muscles in this area can be divided into four groups:

1. The muscles of mastication
    a. Masseter
    b. Temporalis
    c. Medial pterygoid
    d. Lateral pterygoid
2. The suprahyoid muscle group
3. The infrahyoid muscle group
4. Associated neck musculature

The anatomic details of these muscles are summarized in Table 24.1.

Of major significance is the neuromuscular interrelationship between the cervical and stomatognathic areas. Kirveskari (3) has shown that the physiologic status of the stomatognathic system was significantly associated with both mobility of the cervical area and neck-shoulder muscle tenderness. During clenching of the mandible there is significantly increased activity in the trapezius, sternocleidomastoid, and other muscles of the neck and cervical areas (4). These studies have been well substantiated in both the medical and dental literature. The result of this physiologic fact is that many patients with TMD have an associated craniocervical dysfunction. This statement has equal validity if the pathologies are juxtapositioned (5).

The articular capsule of the TMJ is especially susceptible to extension-flexion–type trauma to the neck area. The capsule is composed of dense fibrous tissue in its posterior, superior, inferior, medial, and lateral aspects. However, its anterior component is simply loose connective tissue. Therefore, there is no resistive structure to forces that tend to displace the joint structures in an anterior dimension. Approximately 80% of patients who have been subjected to flexion-extension trauma of the neck also develop internal derangements of the TMJ (6). If myogenous pathologies are added to the number of internal derangements, the number of patients having TMD complications following extension-flexion trauma exceeds 90%.

## THE TMD WORKUP

As a result of the numerous pathologies that may produce symptoms in the orofacial area, the diagnostic procedures involved in a thorough TMD workup are numerous. Some are simple and can readily be performed by a knowledgeable physician or dentist. Others are complex and should be referred to an appropriate specialist for implementation.

The basic evaluation should include a thorough systems review and history, an examination of the oral and perioral hard and soft tissues, measurement of the mandibular range of motion, determination of patterns of mandibular movement, auscultation of the TMJ, palpation of the masticatory and adnexal musculature of the TMJ and a complete hematologic study, including thyroid function, arthritic profile, and erythrocyte sedimentation rate. The more esoteric studies include appropriate radiographs and magnetic resonance (MR) imaging, deprogrammed occlusal analysis, a study of occlusal relationships, and electromyographic studies. For additional information the reader is referred to any one of a number of texts devoted to the diagnosis and treatment of temporomandibular pathologies (7, 8). However, it is appropriate to elaborate on several of these items.

The mandibular range of motion can easily be measured by any clinician. The amount of vertical movement is determined by first measuring the number of millimeters an upper central incisor overlaps its lower counterpart. The patient is then asked to open as far as possible without pain and the distance between the incisal edges of the upper and lower central incisors is recorded. The opening range of motion is the sum of the interincisal distance plus the amount of overlap. The patient is then asked to open as far as possible even though pain is present. This maximum opening is again added to the amount of overlap to obtain a maximal opening range of motion. Lateral excursion is the number of millimeters that the lower central incisors move either left or right from their normal central position. Protrusive excursion is the number of millimeters that the lower central incisors can move forward from their normal closure position. The currently accepted values for these movements are: left and right lateral, at least 9.1 mm; protrusive, at least 6.1 mm; and vertical, 50.3 $\pm$ 6.9 mm (9).

Joint auscultation is accomplished by placement of a stethoscope over the preauricular areas bilaterally. As each side of the TMJ is examined the patient is asked to open, close, move left, move right, and protrude the mandible. Note should be made of the presence of any ''clicks'' or crepitus and at which location in the opening and/or clos-

**Table 24.1.**
**Muscles of Masticatory System and Surrounding Structures**[a]

| Muscle | Origin | Insertion | Vascularization | Innervation | Function |
|--------|--------|-----------|-----------------|-------------|----------|
| | | | **A. Muscles of Mastication** | | |
| Masseter | *Superficial:* tendinous aponeurosis from zygomatic process of maxilla and anterior two thirds of inferior border of zygomatic arch<br><br>*Deep:* medial aspect and inferior border of posterior one third of zygomatic arch | Lateral aspect of ramus and angle of mandible as far anteriorly as last molar tooth, as far superiorly as base of coronoid process | Masseteric branch from maxillary artery | Masseteric branch from mandibular division of trigeminal nerve | Powerful elevator of jaw; deep fibers aid in retracting mandible |
| Temporalis | Inferior temporal line and bones of temporal fossa | As a tendon on coronoid process and anterior border of ramus of mandible as far inferiorly and anteriorly as third molar | Anterior and posterior deep temporal arteries from maxillary artery (these anastomose with middle temporal from superficial temporal artery) | Anterior and posterior deep temporal nerves of the mandibular division of trigeminal nerve | Primarily an elevator of mandible; some fibers (posterior and middle) act as retractor |
| Medial (internal) pterygoid | Pterygoid fossa and medial surface of lateral pterygoid plate; one slip from lateral portion of pyramidal process of palatine bone and adjacent maxillary tuberosity | Medial surface of mandibular ramus as far superiorly as sphenomandibular ligament, inferiorly to mylohyoid groove | Branch from maxillary artery | Medial pterygoid nerve from trunk of mandibular division of trigeminal nerve | Primarily elevator of mandible |
| Lateral (external) pterygoid | *Superior head:* greater wing of sphenoid and infratemporal crest<br><br>*Inferior head:* lateral surface of lateral pterygoid plate | *Superior head:* articular capsule of TMJ—disc and superior portion of mandibular neck<br><br>*Inferior head:* anterior surface of mandibular neck | Branch from maxillary artery | Lateral pterygoid nerve from mandibular division of trigeminal nerve | *Superior head:* disc stabilizer<br><br>*Inferior head:* jaw depressor and protruder, initiates jaw opening; the two heads operate antagonistically |

**B. Infrahyoid Muscles**

| Muscle | Location | Origin | Insertion | Innervation | Action |
|---|---|---|---|---|---|
| Sternohyoid | Anterolateral aspect of neck | Posterior aspect of sternoclavicular joint area | Inferior border of hyoid bone | Ansa cervicalis | Depresses and fixes hyoid bone |
| Sternothyroid | Deep to sternohyoid | Manubrium | Oblique line of thyroid cartilage | Ansa cervicalis | Depresses larynx |
| Thyrohyoid | Deep to sternohyoid | Oblique line of thyroid cartilage | Greater cornu and body of hyoid bone | C1, via hypoglossal nerve | Depresses and fixes hyoid bone |
| Omohyoid | Posterior and anterior triangles of neck | Superior border of scapula just medial to scapular notch | Inferior border of body of hyoid bone | Ansa cervicalis | Depresses and fixes hyoid bone |

**C. Muscles of Back of Neck Supporting Neck Musculature**

| Muscle | Location | Origin | Insertion | Innervation | Action |
|---|---|---|---|---|---|
| Sternocleidomastoid | Bisects lateral aspect of the neck | *Lateral head:* medial one third of clavicle *Medial head:* manubrium | Mastoid process of temporal bone and lateral half of superior nuchal line | Spinal accessory and C2, C3 (for proprioception) | Unilaterally, approximates ear of the same side to shoulder; in unison with its counterpart, tips head back, raising chin |
| Trapezius | Most superficial layer covering back of neck and upper back | External occipital protuberance, superior nuchal line, ligamentum nuchae, and spinous process of C7–T12 | Lateral one third of the clavicle; acromion, spine, and tubercle of spine of scapula | Accessory nerve and ventral primary rami of C3, C4 (for proprioception) | Most of its action is on shoulder in suspending, squaring, shrugging, and pulling it in; it is also a rotator of scapula. Fixing shoulder, it assists in pulling head posteriorly and laterally |
| Splenius capitis | Immediately deep to trapezius | Ligamentum nuchae, spinous processes of vertebrae C7–T4 | Mastoid process of temporal bone and lateral one third of superior nuchal line of occipital bone | Dorsal primary rami of middle cervical nerves | Pulls head back and rotates |
| Splenius cervicis | Lateral and inferior to splenius capitis | Spines of vertebrae T3–T6 | Transverse processes of vertebrae C1–3 | Dorsal primary rami of lower cervical nerves | Pulls head back and rotates |
| Iliocostalis cervicis | Back of neck to angle of upper few ribs | Angles of ribs 3, 4, 5, and 6 | Transverse processes of vertebrae C4–6 | Dorsal primary rami of lower cervical nerves | Extends and rotates cervical spine |

**Table 24.1.**
**Muscles of Masticatory System and Surrounding Structures[a]—Continued**

| Muscle | Origin | Insertion | Vascularization | Innervation | Function |
|---|---|---|---|---|---|
| Longissimus cervicis | Medial to iliocostalis cervicis | Transverse processes of vertebrae T1–5 | Transverse processes of vertebrae C2–6 | Dorsal primary rami of cervical nerves | Extends and inclines cervical spine laterally |
| Longissimus capitis | Medial to longissimus cervicis | Transverse processes of vertebrae T1–5 and articular processes of vertebrae C4–7 | Posterior aspect of mastoid process of temporal bone | Dorsal primary rami of cervical nerves | Extends and inclines head laterally |
| Spinalis cervicis | Inconstant | Inferior portion of ligamentum nuchae; spine of vertebrae C7, T1, and T2 | Spine of vertebrae C2–4 | Dorsal primary rami of cervical nerves | Extends cervical vertebral column |
| Spinalis capitis | Usually fused with medial part of semispinalis capitis | Transverse processes of vertebrae T5 and T6 | Lateral to external occipital crest, between superior and inferior nuchal lines | Dorsal primary rami of cervical nerves | Extends head |
| Semispinalis capitis | Deep to splenius capitis | Transverse processes of vertebrae C7–T6 and articular processes of vertebrae C4–6 | Occipital bone between superior and inferior nuchal lines | Branches of dorsal primary rami of cervical nerves | Extends head and, acting unilaterally, tilts it to one side |
| Semispinalis cervicis | Deep to semispinalis capitis | Transverse processes of vertebrae T1–6 | Spinous processes of vertebrae C2–5 | Branches of dorsal primary rami of upper thoracic and cervical nerves | Extends cervical vertebral column and, acting unilaterally, tilts it to one side |
| Multifidus (cervical portion) | On either side of spinous process of each cervical vertebra | Articular processes of vertebrae C4–7 | Spine of vertebrae C2–7 | Branches of dorsal primary rami of upper thoracic nerves | Extends cervical vertebral column and, acting unilaterally, tilts it to one side |
| Rotatores longus and brevis spinae (cervical portion) | Dorsal aspect of vertebrae | Transverse processes of C3–7 | Base of spinous processes of vertebrae above | Branches of dorsal primary rami of cervical nerves | Pull back spinal column and rotate neck to opposite side |
| Interspinalis (cervical portion) | Between spines of cervical vertebrae | Spine of each cervical vertebra, except C2 | Spine of cervical vertebra immediately above, except C1 | Branches of dorsal primary rami of cervical nerves, except C1 | Extends the cervical spinal column |

| Muscle | Origin | Insertion | Arterial Supply | Nerve | Action |
|---|---|---|---|---|---|
| Intertransversarii anterior (cervical portion) | Anterior tubercles of transverse processes C2–T1 | Between transverse processes of cervical vertebrae, placed anteriorly | Anterior tubercles of transverse processes of vertebrae C2–T1 | Ventral primary ramus of nerves C2–T1 | Unilaterally, tilts cervical spinal column to one side; in unison with its counterpart, fixes cervical spinal column |
| Intertransverarii posterior (cervical portion) | Posterior tubercles of transverse processes C2–T1 | Behind intertransversarii anterior | Posterior tubercles of transverse processes of vertebrae C2–T1 | Ventral primary rami of nerves C2–T1 | Unilaterally, cervical spinal column to one side; in unison with its counterpart, fixes cervical spinal column |
| Obliquus capitis superior | Transverse process of atlas | Deep to semispinalis capitis | Inferior to superior nuchal line of occipital bone | Dorsal primary ramus of suboccipital nerve (C1) | Pulls head back and, acting unilaterally, tilts it to one side |
| Obliquus capitis inferior | Spinous process of axis | Deep to semispinalis capitis and inferior to obliquus capitis superior | Transverse process of atlas | Dorsal primary ramus of suboccipital nerve (C1) | Rotates altantoaxial joint to turn face laterally |
| Rectus capitis posterior major | Spine of axis | Medial to obliquus capitis superior | Below and on inferior nuchal line of occipital bone | Dorsal primary ramus of suboccipital nerve (C1) | Draws head back and turns face laterally |
| Rectus capitis posterior minor | Tubercle of posterior arch of atlas | Medial to rectus capitis posterior major | Above superior lip of foramen magnum to inferior nuchal line | Dorsal primary ramus of suboccipital nerve (C1) | Pulls head directly posteriorly |
| **D. Suprahyoid Muscles** | | | | | |
| Digastric | *Anterior belly:* mandibular arch *Posterior belly:* develops in hyoid arch | Intermediate tendon looping around body and greater cornu of hyoid bone | Posterior auricular artery–anterior-submental branch of the artery | *Posterior belly:* facial nerve *Anterior belly:* trigeminal nerve | *Combined:* elevates hyoid bone, assists in opening mandible *Anterior:* draws hyoid bone anteriorly *Posterior:* draws hyoid bone posteriorly |
| Stylohyoid | Posterior and lateral surfaces of styloid process of temporal bone | Body of hyoid bone | Posterior auricular and occipital branches of external carotid artery | Branch of facial nerve that enters its midbelly as the nerve approaches its inferolateral border | Draws hyoid bone superiorly and posteriorly, in addition to assisting in fixing it |
| Mylohyoid | Entire length of mylohyoid line of mandible from symphysis menti to region opposite last molar tooth | *Anterior:* insert into a median raphe *Posterior:* insert into body of hyoid bone | Anastomoses from submental branch of facial artery and sublingual branch of lingual artery | Mylohyoid nerve of trigeminal | Assists in depressing mandible when hyoid bone is fixed |

**Table 24.1.**
**Muscles of Masticatory System and Surrounding Structures**[a]—*Continued*

| Muscle | Origin | Insertion | Vascularization | Innervation | Function |
|---|---|---|---|---|---|
| Geniohyoid | Inferior mental spine of mandible before descending to anterior surface of body of hyoid bone | Muscle is in contact with its counterpart from opposite side of mandible | Sublingual branch of lingual artery | Fibers of first cervical nerve | Draws hyoid bone anteriorly and, in so doing, draws tongue as well |
| **E. Tongue Muscles** | | | | | |
| Genioglossus | Superior mental spine | *Anterior:* into tip of tongue *Posterior:* pass to base of tongue | Deep lingual artery | Hypoglossal nerve | Protrudes tongue; anterior fibers depress tongue tip |
| Hyoglossus | From side of body and greater cornu of hyoid bone | Styloglossus muscle | Deep lingual artery | Hypoglossal nerve | Major depressor of tongue |
| Styloglossus | From anterior surface process of temporal bone and stylomandibular ligament | Enter styloid aspect of tongue | Deep lingual artery | Hypoglossal nerve | Retracts tongue, while more anterior fibers elevate tongue tip |

[a]Adapted from Hiatt JL, Gartner LP: *Textbook of Head and Neck Anatomy.* New York, Appleton-Century-Crofts, 1982.

ing stroke the sound occurs. During these opening and closing maneuvers the mandible should be observed for the presence of any deviations or deflections from the midline. Normal subjects should be capable of depressing and elevating the mandible without deviation or deflection.

Palpation of the TMJ and its associated musculature is essential. If the reader is not familiar with this technique the authors urge that this skill be obtained. Although a number of texts describe the process, the better way of learning palpation is by "hands-on" practice with the assistance of a trained clinician.

If TMD is suspected from the examination, the patient should be referred to an appropriate specialist. Muscle relaxants, tranquilizers, and narcotics are of little benefit in support of these patients. Symptoms can temporarily best be handled medically by use of nonsteroidal anti-inflammatory drugs and tricyclic antidepressants (10).

## PAIN OF TMJ ORIGIN (11–15)

When the clinician evaluates the patient complaining of pain in the head and neck region following a traumatic episode, he or she must be able to differentiate between pain that is associated with TMJ pathology and pain that may be associated with cervical pathology. The pain referral patterns can and do overlap.

## MASTICATORY ARTHRALGIA

Pain originating from within the TMJ is called masticatory arthralgia. Masticatory arthralgia can emanate only from structures within the joint that have nociceptors. These structures are (*a*) the ligamentous attachments to the condyle, (*b*) the posterior attachment, (*c*) the capsule, and (*d*) the articulating surfaces.

### Ligamentous Attachments to the Condyle

The articular disc (meniscus) is a fibrocartilagenous structure within the temporomandibular joint space that has a specialized shape and function. It is divided into four zones: (*a*) the thickened anterior band, which is primarily loose connective tissue; (*b*) the thin intermediate band, which is the functional part of the disc; (*c*) the thickened posterior band, the purpose of which is to prevent the anterior displacement of the disc; and (*d*) the posterior attachment. The posterior band is usually thicker than the anterior band. It functions to adapt to the shape of the glenoid fossa and articular eminence above and the mandibular condyle below. The disc is firmly attached to the condyle by ligamentous attachments on the medial and lateral poles. Although the functional areas of the disc are avascular and not innervated, the ligamentous attachments and the anterior and posterior attachments contain nerve endings that respond to stretching. Thus when the joint is inflamed or traumatized or when the disc is obstructed, the patient will experience pain originating from the attachment of the disc to the condyle.

### Posterior Attachment

Posterior to the articular disc is a two-zone tissue attachment connecting the posterior surface of the disc to the tympanic plate of the temporal bone and the neck of the condyle. This tissue, the posterior attachment (which has historically been called the bilaminar zone), consists of fibroelastic tissue and collagen fibers. It is highly vascular and innervated. In pathologic states wherein the disc is anteriorly displaced, this posterior attachment becomes the intermediate tissue between the condyle and the articular eminence. Compression of this tissue between the articulating structures of the joint therefore results in pain. The main purpose of the posterior attachment is to prevent negative pressure from developing as the disc translates forward with the condyle. It does this by means of elastic fibers and arteriovenous shunts. It does not place any posterior traction on the disc.

### Capsule

The capsule of the TMJ is the thin, loose fibrous connective tissue enveloping the joint. The capsule attaches to the rim of the temporal articular surface and extends inferiorly to the periosteum of the neck of the condyle. The lateral portion of the capsule is thickened and is called the lateral capsular ligament or temporomandibular ligament. The inner lining of the articular surface of the capsule is covered by a synovial membrane that lubricates the joint. Trauma, both macrotrauma and microtrauma, results in synovitis or capsulitis and results in pain during translatory movements of the joint (protrusion, lateral excursion, and wide opening).

## Articulating Surfaces

The articulating surfaces of the TMJ are covered by an avascular, noninnervated fibrocartilage rather than by hyaline cartilage. Devoid of blood vessels and nerve endings, these surfaces are insensitive of painful stimuli under normal circumstances. Inflammatory processes that occur in the joint alter this situation. In patients with rheumatoid arthritis that affects the TMJ, the inflamed synovial membrane proliferates onto the articular surfaces. Patients with joints undergoing degenerative arthritic changes have erosion of the articular surface, which exposes the innervated and vascular underlying osseous tissue. Thus, pain can originate from these inflamed articular surfaces of the joints.

## PAIN OF PREAURICULAR AND JAW AREAS

Pain of the preauricular and jaw areas can be myalgic or arthralgic in origin. The muscles that refer pain into these areas include the sternocleidomastoid, masseter, medial (internal) pterygoid, lateral (external) pterygoid, suboccipital, splenius cervicis, trapezius, temporalis, digastric, platysma, orbicularis oculi, and zygomaticus major (16). Pain of muscle origin is usually diffuse and not well localized. Jaw function may or may not cause or exacerbate the pain. Refrigerant sprays such as ethyl chloride or fluorimethane will frequently temporarily reduce the pain. The pain is frequently responsive to muscle relaxants and physical therapy.

Intermittent pain originating from the joint will usually localize itself to the joint region. It is usually responsive to palpation and to functional movements such as protrusion, excursion, and wide opening. Diagnostic local anesthetic injection into the joint and capsule will frequently eliminate symptoms. When there is an acute episode of pain that originates from the joint, muscle splinting will sometimes exist. If the splinting becomes chronic myospasm may occur, thus masking the etiology of the pain and making the diagnosis more difficult.

## CAUSES OF INJURY TO TMJ

The temporomandibular apparatus is subject to trauma from various sources. Microtrauma represents those subclinical traumatic episodes that cumulatively result in symptoms of TMD. It is the chronicity of the microtraumatic episodes that results in the damage to the joint and adnexal structures. A slight blow can exacerbate a preexisting degenerative arthritic condition or internal derangement, resulting in a patient presenting with symptoms out of proportion to the degree of trauma. Macrotrauma can result in lasting TMD symptoms, usually proportional to the degree of injury to the joint. The injury may present as a condylar fracture, a hemarthrosis, or just muscle contusion.

## RADIOGRAPHIC DIAGNOSIS

An aid in the diagnosis of TMJ pathology is radiographic and diagnostic imaging. The hard and soft tissues of the TMJ can be studied by several imaging techniques now available.

## CONVENTIONAL RADIOGRAPHY

Conventional radiography is useful as a screening study to rule out fracture and gross bony abnormalities but is unable to diagnose soft tissue structures. A TMJ series (open and closed) may give some information as to range of condylar movement. Transcranial and transorbital views allow visualization of the condyle and fossa, but give less than an adequate assessment of the joint space.

## TOMOGRAPHY

Tomography may be used to study the bony structures of the joint. It is useful to rule out fractures and degenerative arthritis and identify osteophytes. Lateral and anteroposterior views allow visualization of the condyle in both mediolateral and anteroposterior slices. The relatively high radiation dose and lack of soft tissue in the image make these radiographs valuable only when some pathology is suspected.

## ARTHROGRAPHY

Arthrography is the injection of a contrast medium into the inferior and/or superior joint space under fluoroscopic control. This may also be performed utilizing tomography with a view of the joint under function. It allows the diagnostician to dynamically evaluate the moving, functioning joint. It is presently the only study that will show a perforation of the disc. Test results may be video recorded for future reference. The invasive and sometimes painful nature of this test has led to less frequent use. This procedure is contraindicated in patients who are allergic to contrast dye.

## COMPUTED TOMOGRAPHY SCAN

Computed tomography scanning is a good technique for evaluation of the bony structures of the joint. It can be used to diagnose fractures and tumors, but it does not give dependable information about the soft tissue structures of the joint. The views are static and give little information about the joint under function.

## MAGNETIC RESONANCE IMAGING

MR imaging is very useful to study both the hard and soft tissue of the joint, especially the disc. It is used to determine the position of the disc relative to the condyle. It cannot determine the presence of a perforation of the disc (17). Cine MR imaging allows a semi-dynamic view of motion. Recent advances in equipment and diagnostic ability have made this the single most valuable imaging technique. MR imaging is contraindicated in patients with cerebral vascular lips or ocular metallic foreign bodies.

## BONE SCANNING

Single photon emission computed tomography (SPECT) and planar imaging techniques are useful for diagnosing organic TMJ disease (degenerative joint disease, acute injury, hyperplasia, and tumors) (18).

## TREATMENT

### TEMPOROMANDIBULAR DYSFUNCTION

Obviously, the treatment of patients with the symptoms that have been described is dependent upon an accurate diagnosis. Pathologies that are diagnosed in the TMJ and/or its associated musculature may be treated by the following methods.

### Nonsurgical Treatment

The treatment for patients with TMD is aimed at relieving pain and improving function. Most patients who present with symptoms of TMD will respond positively to nonsurgical treatment. This treatment usually consists of a combination of intraoral orthopaedic devices, physical therapy, drugs, and counseling. One of the most common types of orthopaedic devices are deprogramming splints, which eliminate the effects of bruxism and grinding and allow the masticatory muscles to relax. Another type of splint is the anterior repositioning splint, used to position the mandible anteriorly in attempt to recapture a displaced disc when this pathology has been diagnosed. Physical therapy includes the use of ultrasound, heat, transcutaneous electrical nerve stimulation, exercise, and massage. Muscle relaxant, nonsteroidal anti-inflammatory, and antidepressant drugs are sometimes used in conjunction with splints and physical therapy. Drug therapy in the absence of adequate diagnosis and other supportive therapy is of little benefit.

### Arthroscopy

The small percentage of patients who do not respond to nonsurgical treatment may be surgical candidates. These usually are the patients who exhibit frank pathology within the joint on imaging and in whom the symptoms are usually localized to the joint itself. TMJ arthroscopy has been looked at as a possible therapeutic approach to TMJ pathology since 1975, when it was first described by Ohnishi (19). Within the past few years this procedure has been found to be especially helpful for patients who exhibit a displaced disc that does not move relative to the condyle when it translates. The arthroscope is used to lyse adhesions and lavage the superior joint space at the same time. When accompanied with splinting and physical therapy, this procedure has been found to be very effective in improving the mobility of the joint and reducing pain (20).

### Arthroplasty

Patients who are not candidates for arthroscopy and patients for whom arthroscopy has not eliminated symptoms and improved function may undergo arthroplasty. This is an open joint surgery wherein the displaced disc can be repaired (meniscoplasty or meniscal plication) or removed (meniscectomy). The diseased articular surfaces can be recontoured and the obstructions to normal condylar movement can be removed. Certain cases will require autogenous or alloplastic grafting within the joint to reestablish function. Patient response to both arthroscopy and arthroplasty is quite good, with greater than 80% of patients reporting improvement of symptoms postoperatively (20, 21). Total joint replacement is reserved for the most intractable cases in which these other procedures have not allowed the patient to resume adequate function.

## FRACTURES

Most condylar fractures are treated with closed reduction and immobilization of the mandible via intermaxillary fixation. This is the only time immobilization of the joint is indicated. Following a period of about 3–6 weeks, the jaw is mobilized and active physical therapy is begun to overcome the propensity to adhesions and scarring. Severe fracture trauma and poor physical therapy can lead to ankylosis of the joint. Open reduction is generally reserved for severely displaced condylar fractures or bilateral fractures with loss of vertical dimension of the mandible. In this latter case, one may chose to perform an open reduction on one side to restore the vertical length of the jaw. Early mobilization and less time of immobilization may be accomplished by use of internal rigid plates and screws. The goal of any of these treatments remains to achieve a stable bite and satisfactory range of motion (i.e., interincisal opening, protrusion, and lateral excursions).

## HEMARTHROSIS

Hemarthrosis and joint effusion are seen in the TMJ as in other acutely injured joints. Typically, no fractures are diagnosed on radiographs but the patient presents with pain and swelling directly over the joint. A hallmark finding is an ipsilateral open bite. Heat, anti-inflammatory analgesics, and occasionally arthrocentesis are useful in resolving this problem. Untreated, the patient with this type of pathology may progress to TMD and ankylosis.

## CONCLUSION

The authors have attempted to explain the intimate interrelationship and interdependence that exists between the stomatognathic and cervical systems. These anatomic and physiologic facts require that both areas be considered in the diagnosis and management of patients presenting with symptoms in either site.

### REFERENCES

1. Davis PL: Electromyographic study of superficial neck muscles in Mandibular Function. *Dent Res* 58:537, 1979.
2. Travell J: Temporomandibular joint pain referred from muscles of the head and neck. *Prosthet Dent* 10:745, 1960.
3. Kirveskari P, Alanen P, Karskela V, Kaitanierrú P, Holtari M, Virtanen T, Laine M: Association of functional state of stomatognathic system with mobility of cervical spine and neck muscle tenderness. *Acta Odontol Scand* 46:281–286, 1988.
4. Hagberg C: EMG versus force relationship in painful masseter muscles before and after intramuscular anesthetic and saline injections. *Scand J Dent Res* 95:259–265, 1987.
5. Clark GT, et al: Craniocervical dysfunction levels in a patient sample from a temporomandibular joint clinic. *Am Dent Assoc* 115:251–256, 1987.
6. Weinberg S, LaPointe H: Cervical extension-flexion injury (whiplash) and internal derangements of the temporomandibular joint. *J Oral Maxillofac Surg* 45:653–656, 1987.
7. Buxbaum J, Myers D, Myslinski M: *The Physiology, Pathophysiology, Diagnosis and Treatment of Temporomandibular Dysfunction and Related Facial Pain.* Baltimore, University of Maryland Dental School, Department of Physiology, 1986.
8. Morgan DH, House LR, Hall WP, Vamvas SJ: *Diseases of the Temporomandibular Apparatus,* ed 2. St. Louis, CV Mosby Company, 1982.
9. Clark GT, Lynn P: Horizontal plane movements in controls and clinic patients with TMD. *J Prosthet Dent* 155:730–735, 1986.
10. Buxbaum J, Myers D, Myslinski N: Dental management of orofacial pain. In Tollison CD (ed): *Handbook of Chronic Pain Management.* Baltimore, Williams & Wilkins, 1988, pp 305–310.
11. Bell WE: *Orofacial Pains,* ed 4. Chicago, Year Book Medical Publishers, Inc, 1989, pp 285–331.
12. Morgan DH, House LR, Hall WP, Vamvas SJ: *Diseases of the Temporomandibular Apparatus,* ed 2. St. Louis, CV Mosby Company, 1982, pp 8–25.
13. Dolwick MF, Sanders B: *TMJ Internal Derangement & Arthrosis.* St. Louis, CV Mosby Company, 1985, pp 1–26.
14. Helms CA, Katzberg RW, Dolwick MF: *Internal Derangements of the Temporomandibular Joint.* San Francisco, Radiology Research and Education Foundation, 1983, pp 1–14.
15. Rees LA: The structure and function of the mandibular joint. *Br Dent J* 96:125, 1954.
16. Travell JG, Simons DG: *Myofascial Pain and Dysfunction: The Trigger Point Manual.* Baltimore, Williams & Wilkins, 1983, pp 165–282.
17. Katzberg RW, et al: Temporomandibular joint: MR assessment of rotational and sideways disk displacements. *Radiology* 169:741, 1988.
18. Kircos LT, et al: Emission imaging of patients with craniomandibular disorders. *Oral Surg* 65:249, 1988.
19. Ohnishi M: Arthroscopy of the temporomandibular joint. *J Jpn Stomatol Assoc* 42:207, 1975.
20. Moses JJ, et al: The effect of arthroscopic surgical lysis and lavage of the superior joint space of TMJ disc position and mobility. *J Oral Maxillofac Surg* 47:674–687, 1989.
21. Benson B, Keith D: Patient response to surgical and nonsurgical treatment for internal derangement of the temporomandibular joint. *J Oral Maxillofac Surg* 43:770, 1985.

## 25

# HEADACHE FOLLOWING CERVICAL TRAUMA

*Seymour Diamond and Frederick G. Freitag*

Trauma to the cervical spine may result from several different mechanisms. The most common form of trauma to the neck results from acceleration-extension injuries that accompany motor vehicle accidents (1). Other forms of trauma may occur to the cervical spine, such as direct or blunt trauma (2) and trauma resulting from manipulation of the neck (3).

## PHYSIOLOGIC MECHANISMS

Cervical trauma may induce injury-related headache through several mechanisms, such as direct injury to the musculoskeletal tissues (4). The injury may occur to the cervical nerves or nerve roots, and sympathetic nerve fibers passing through the neck. Injury to the vertebral artery may also be involved (5), as well as brain injury occurring without direct head trauma.

Janecki and Lipke (4) reviewed the cervical tissue changes associated with acceleration-extension injuries of the cervical spine. There is a wide variation in the injuries sustained. Minor tears were found within the sternocleidomastoid muscles with minimal trauma. Disruption of the longus colli occurred if the trauma was of sufficient severity to cause disruption of the anterior longitudinal ligament with injury to the intervertebral disc (4). The researchers cited the force of a 15 mile/h accident producing an accleration of $10G$ on the cervical spine.

Injury to the nerve roots and fibers may occur, and could involve the brachial plexus. The development of thoracic outlet syndrome (6) associated with headache and upper extremity symptoms is typical of this disorder. Bogduk (7) discussed traumatic injuries to the second cervical nerve and the development of occipital neuralgia. Extremes of rotation and extension could lead to injury of C2 between the posterior arch of the atlas and the superior articular facet of the axis. Another possible injury could occur at the site at which the greater occipital nerve penetrates the semispinalis capitis muscle. However, this injury would not typically result in headache. A reduction of blood flow through the vertebral artery may result from either acceleration-extension injuries to the cervical spine (4) or manipulation of the cervical spine (5). Mueller and Sahs (3) indicated that normal motion of the neck may result in decreased blood flow through the vertebral arteries. Rotation of the neck with extension can completely occlude the flow of the vertebral artery through the contralateral artery. Injury to the artery may produce thrombus formation and its ramifications, such as stroke.

The cervical sympathetic plexus could sustain injury associated with tears of the longus colli (4). Vijayan (8) proposed, in his series of cases, that the syndrome of posttraumatic dysautonomic cephalgia resulted from injury to cervical sympathetic fibers. This injury occurs beyond the emergence of these fibers from the first thoracic segment and before their separation into the internal and external carotid sympathetic plexuses.

Concussive-type injuries may occur without direct head impact in acceleration-extension injuries. Ommaya and his colleagues demonstrated alterations in the level of consciousness in Rhesus monkeys (9). Evidence of contusions and hemorrhage associated with the concussive injuries was found in various sites throughout the brain. No correlation was determined between the loss of consciousness and the occurrence of cerebral contusions or hemorrage. These results were confirmed by magnetic resonance (MR) imaging. The study by Jenkins and his group assessed brain trauma associated with closed head injury (10). On MR imaging four patients who had not lost consciousness and four patients who experienced only a brief alteration in their level of consciousness demonstrated evidence of contusion or intracerebral bleeding. The MR images were performed shortly after the injury. In cases of severe head trauma, prolonged decreases in regional and global cerebral blood flow were also reported (11).

Psychological or psychiatric factors may also contribute to posttraumatic headaches, and are discussed later in the chapter. The resulting headaches are classified broadly as muscle contraction, vascular, or neurologic in nature. Considerable overlap between the various forms of headache may occur in certain patients. Exacerbation of preexisting headaches may also occur.

## MUSCLE CONTRACTION HEADACHES

Muscle contraction headaches are the most common form of headache that result from trauma to the cervical spine. Following the injury, the headache occurs on a daily basis. It also occurs as an exacerbation of an underlying tendency to experience episodic muscle contraction headache. The headache develops from the actual time of the injury in about 11% of reported cases. Within the first week following the injury, an additional 75% of the patients develop headaches (12).

The pain intensity of muscle contraction headache may vary widely between individuals, or in a given patient, at different times. Although most patients with these headaches complain of mild to moderate pain, some patients will experience severe and incapacitating pain (13).

## CLINICAL FEATURES

Most patients with muscle contraction headaches describe the pain as located in a generalized pattern over the entire head. The pain may occur in other distributions such as frontal, occipital, or over the vertex, and it may localize at the temporoparietal areas. At times the headache may be unilateral; pain may radiate from these regions into the facial area, over the temporomandibular joint, and into the mandible. The muscle contraction headache with a traumatic origin can be associated with neck pain. It can localize to specific areas of the neck, such as the suboccipital areas and the region of the cervicothoracic junction. In some patients the pain may be unilateral if rotation of the cervical spine occurred at the time of the injury. Extension of the pain into the arms may sometimes occur. Other patients report radiation of suboccipital pain to the eyes and forehead.

The pain of muscle contraction headaches is usually described as a steady, nonpulsatile ache. However, patients use a variety of other descriptions, including drawing, cramping, squeezing, soreness, tightness, a vise-like sensation, and a band-like sensation as if a hatband had shrunk while placed on the head. Patients also describe the pain as shooting or stabbing, and may identify other sensations as being unpleasant, although vague and indistinct.

In some patients, pain of muscle contraction headaches may be both exacerbated and relieved by application of heat and cold, as well as movement of the neck. In about 55% of patients reported by Balla and Karnaghan (12), any activity could exacerbate muscle contraction–type headaches, and heat provided comfort while cold exacerbated the headaches. These results may occur because of the increased muscle spasm that occurs with shivering.

In order to obtain relief, patients may also assume certain postures that restrict the degree of motion of affected joints. Examination of the patient with muscle contraction headaches rarely reveals distinct neurologic signs unless significant brain injury has occurred with direct cranial trauma. However, signs of peripheral neurologic dysfunction may be present. Involvement of the upper extremities may be present if damage has occurred directly to the nerve roots as they exit the foramina, or if there is nerve impingement from marked spasm of the muscles through which the nerve fibers pass.

Observation of the patient with muscle contraction headache will reveal abnormalities. In order to minimize resting pain, postural changes of the back and neck will occur. The patient will fail to open the jaw fully when talking. Also the patient will not fully open the oropharynx. Palpation of the sites of the headache or neck pain may reveal spasm in the involved muscle, with associated tenderness. In some patients, localized painful nodules can be demonstrated in the involved musculature. Palpation of these nodules may increase headache pain and, in certain areas, may elicit tinnitus, vertigo, and lacrimation.

Following trauma to the spine, limitation of the range of motion of the cervical spine occurs. Early in the interval following the injury, spasm of the neck muscles occurs. Spondyloarthritic changes may occur in some patients after a long period following the trauma that may also serve to limit the motion of the neck. In patients with limitation of jaw motion, examination may reveal dysfunction of the temporomandibular joint (14), with localized pain over the joint proper. If internal derangement of the joint has occurred, auscultation over the joint may reveal audible noise, such as crepitus.

A variety of psychological symptoms may occur in the posttraumatic headache patient, including symptoms of depression (15), anxiety, irritability, aggression, and apathy. These emotional factors may be significant in causing muscle contraction headache. Martin and his associates reviewed the psychiatric evaluations of 25 patients with muscle contraction headache (16). No single psychological factor was found to be a provocateur of these headaches. Most patients demonstrated multiple conflicts, such as repressed hostility, sexual conflicts, and unresolved dependency needs. This study suggests that, in cases of muscle contraction headaches, somatization of anxiety in the form of either increased skeletal muscle tension or psychophysiologic expression is occurring.

## CHRONIC MUSCLE CONTRACTION HEADACHES AND DEPRESSION

Chronic muscle contraction headaches may conceal a serious emotional disorder such as depression (17, 18). The patient will present with a persistent and vague headache, without organic cause. For the patient, the physical symptoms are more socially acceptable than the anxiety or depressive symptoms. Many patients insist that there is a somatic basis for their pain. The physican must be cognizant of other signs of depression, such as insomnia, irritability, loss of energy or spontaneity, lack of interest, and early morning fatigue or awakening (19).

Physicians readily recognize depression in its classical presentation with disturbances of mood and affect. Many patients, however, present with vague, chronically recurrent symptoms that may be physical, emotional, or psychic in nature. A headache occurring secondary to depression is usually classified as a muscle contraction headache. There are several distinctive features that may help distinguish the headache related to depression. The patient with depression describes the headache as occurring on a daily basis, with a history of headaches lasting for many years. A diurnal variation is demonstrated when the headaches are associated with depression: The periods between 4:00 and 8:00 in the morning and again in the evening are the periods during which the depressive headache is most conspicuous to the patient.

Several other factors may be present in those patients with chronic muscle contraction in whom depression is a potential etiology. During the patient interview, determining a family history of depression or a prior history of depression in the patient is important. In these patients, eliciting a history of recurrent symptoms of depression may be possible. Also, onset of depression-related headache may be attributed to a specific event. The nature of the event may have been traumatic to the patient or may have been associated with personal loss. Frequently the impact of the event may appear to be disproportionate to the subsequent severity of the headache.

## MECHANISMS OF MUSCLE CONTRACTION HEADACHE

Several mechanisms are involved in the genesis of muscle contraction headache. This headache may result from a postconcussion injury of the brain or a whiplash-type injury (7). The headache may be caused by direct traumatic effects on the muscles and ligaments of the cervical spine and scalp muscles that result from rapid stretching and tearing that evolves from acceleration-extension injuries. This process is normally short lived, and will resolve over several weeks with the healing of the tissues. The chronic muscle spasm is maintained by local pathologic processes related to the injury and their central influences.

The development of chronic muscle contraction headaches (20) following trauma involves three independent reflex arcs and four consecutive steps. A multisynaptic reflex of withdrawal initiates this muscle spasm. Local pathologic processes cause stimulation of nerve fibers, and the impulses are transmitted directly to the spinal cord and then to the ventral roots. The stimulus then passes over the efferent nerves to the neuromuscular junction, which eventually causes the muscle to contract acutely and spread the painful stimulus. Second, stimulation of the polysynaptic spinal pathways and the lemniscal system occurs. The initial impulse travels up the spinal cord to the thalamus and central levels. At these areas, the stimulus is recognized as being painful. From these centers, the brain then transmits impulses through the reticulospinal system, activating the γ-efferent neurons that contract the muscle spindle. This contraction yields a monosynaptic stimulus that travels directly to the ventral horn, augmenting the discharge in the peripheral nerve and thereby augmenting the muscle contraction. The contraction of the muscle spindle itself is a monosynaptic stimulus and relates to the tendon stretch reflex. In the normal state, the contracting muscle fibers inhibit firing of the muscle spindle and terminate the third reflex arc stretch, leading to muscle relaxation.

The muscle spindle remains tight as the state of activity of γ-efferent nerves determines muscle tone and cortical or local processes activate it. The muscle continually contracts until it becomes painful, thereby leading to a cycle of spasm, anxiety, and pain associated with a chronic muscle contraction headache.

Olesen and Langemark (21) have suggested four different forms of muscle contraction–type headache based on the state of the muscle, afferent nociceptive impulses, spinal cord gating of these impulses, and the brain. The relative states of these systems determine the occurrence of muscle contraction headache and muscle tenderness.

The "myogenic headache" results from activation of the muscle fibers with strong afferent nociceptive impulses passing through an open spinal cord gate, thus leading to headache with muscle tenderness. If the spinal cord gate is closed and the other factors remain constant, the patient experiences muscle tenderness without headache. In patients without significant muscle fiber activation but with an open spinal cord gate, any amount of nociception will be amplified thus leading to a hypersensitized state of brain activation from these impulses and a "dysnociceptive headache." "Psychogenic headache" is produced despite normal muscle fiber activation. The normal afferent nociceptive information processed through the spinal cord may be gating in a normal fashion, although the patient experiences headache pain without nociception.

## ROLE OF NEUROTRANSMITTER DYSFUNCTION

Neurotransmitter dysfunction may play an important role in the development of muscle contraction headache following trauma. Nappi and his colleagues (22) have suggested that β-endorphin may play a role in nociception: a defect in the secretion of this compound may lead to a hyperalgesic state. They found that the patients with "chronic daily headaches" had depressed blood levels of β-endorphin. (Their term "chronic daily headache" is synonymous with muscle contraction headache.) However, in patients with posttraumatic headache, Nappi et al. found β-endorphin levels comparable to those of healthy controls without headache, and responses of both groups to traditional Chinese acupuncture were similar. Sicuteri (23) also advanced the concept of impairment of opioid receptors playing a role in the genesis of pain disorders, such as chronic muscle contraction headache.

In two reports, Rolf and coworkers (24) and Skulka and his colleagues (25) demonstrated that platelets of patients with muscle contraction headaches had basal levels of serotonin similar to those of migraine headache patients and controls. However, these platelets demonstrated significantly greater uptake of serotonin in patients with tension headache as compared to patients with migraine or control subjects. This finding suggests an alteration in central mechanisms of serotonin release as well as in the platelets of patients with muscle contraction headache as compared to migraine patients. In another study by Nappi and his associates (26), the relationship between the biochemical states of chronic muscle contraction headache and depression were studied. They were unable to demonstrate a change in β-endorphins in the cerebrospinal fluid (CSF) of patients with depression absent of headache, and of control patients. However, in patients with chronic muscle contraction headache, CSF values were about 50% of those of controls and depressed patients without headache. In depressed patients, there is an alteration in platelet serotonin function and plasma serotonin (27). The levels of serotonin are 30–60% less than those of control patients. Treatment of the depression with antidepressants did not normalize plasma serotonin but the platelet serotonin levels dropped to 8% of pretreatment levels.

The focus of most research into depression and pain, including headache, has centered on the role of norepinephrine and serotonin (17, 28). The brain's analgesia system involves a serotonergic-mediated pathway descending in the dorsal horn of the spinal cord. It originates in the raphe nucleus and interlaces with norepinephrine- and opioid-containing neurons in the locus ceruleus.

The biochemical basis of depression remains under investigation. However, most of our knowledge of depression evolves from work performed in the mid-1950s (29). At that time, one of the drugs used to treat *Mycobacterium tuberculosis* was isoniazid, a monoamine oxidase inhibitor (MAOI). Patients treated with this drug developed euphoric states resulting from the increased norepinephrine and serotonin concentrations in the brain caused by this agent. Treatment of hypertension with rauwolfian alkaloids such as reserpine caused severe depression in a small percentage of patients. The rauwolfian alkaloids result in depletion of both of these biogenic amines from the brain.

Siever and Uhde (30) investigated the relationship between the noradrenergic system and depression during clonidine treatment. This $\alpha_2$-adrenergic agonist produced more variance in measures of basal noradrenergic secretion in depressed patients as compared to controls. The parameters that were measured included heart rate, plasma norepinephrine, and plasma 3-methoxy-4-hydroxyphenylglycol (MHPG). Additionally, Siever and Uhde found that clonidine reduced plasma cortisol to levels comparable to those of controls. This finding suggests that depression is similar to hypercortisolemia secondary to noradrenergic dysfunction.

Fawcett (31) suggested that other neurotransmitters, including dopamine and the endorphins, also play a role in the genesis of depression. Over the years, several tests were developed to evaluate depression and assist in the selection of the appropriate therapeutic agent. One of these, the dexamethasone suppression test (DST) (31) involves administering a small amount of dexamethasone to the patient at midnight and measuring serum cortisol levels on the following day. It demonstrates that a subgroup of patients with endogenous depression also exhibit nonsuppression. Most of these patients have a normal suppression in the morning and nonsuppression later in the day.

About 45% of endogenously depressed individuals have an abnormal DST. Because the test is 96% specific for endogenous depression, an abnormal DST will occur in only 4–7% of patients with other psychiatric disorders. These include schizophrenia, mania, personality disorders, and minor or neurotic depression. If a patient has an abnormal response to the test, the physician must rule out organic illnesses that can also cause an abnormal result, including Cushing's syndrome, pregnancy, and uncontrolled diabetes mellitus. The physican must also review the patient's current medications because a variety of drugs may alter the results. Currently DST is the most valuable method of monitoring the patient's response to therapy. Normalization of the DST seems to correlate with an improved clinical picture. Patients with an abnormal DST appear more likely to suffer from recurrent depression than those patients who exhibit normal suppressions.

Another diagnostic test is the thyroid-stimulating hormone (TSH) response to thyrotropin-releasing hormone (TRH). A large percentage of endogenously depressed patients have a blunt TSH response to the administration of TRH. The mechanism for this blunted response is unknown, and the clinical value of this test remains uncertain.

The MHPG urine test is useful for evaluating the main metabolite of norepinephrine in the central nervous system (urinary levels of MHPG may reflect the degree of norepinephrine metabolism) (29, 32). Some groups of depressed patients have decreased MHPG in the urine and other groups have normal or increased levels of MHPG. This finding suggests that two groups of depression may exist. One group would be characterized by disruption of norepinephrine metabolism with serotonin and dopamine systems that are normal. The second group would have a disorder of serotonin metabolism but not norepinephrine or dopamine metabolism.

Studies have revealed that depressed patients with low MHPG levels have a higher response to imipramine and desipramine as opposed to amitriptyline and nortriptyline. Maas (29) argued that patients with low MHPG levels had low norepinephrine levels but normal serotonin levels. The patients with high MHPG levels had converse results. This finding suggests the possibility of three distinct subgroups of depressive disorders, which can be distinguished based on their MHPG levels (33).

Sandler and various colleagues (34) have studied the relationship between urinary excretion of tyramine and its metabolites after ingestion of an oral loading dose of tyramine and lifelong predilection to the development of depression. They also demonstrated an inverse correlation between the amount of tyramine and its metabolites excreted in the urine of depressed patients and their likelihood of response to antidepressant therapy. Patients with the lowest tyramine excretion were most likely to have a favorable outcome with antidepressant therapy (35). Reynolds and his associates (36) suggested a link between depression and a deficiency in folate-altering metabolism of homocysteine to methionine. Based on their findings, S-adenosylmethionine was considered useful in the relief of depression.

## MIGRAINE HEADACHE

Since the 1946 report of Simons and Wolff (37) regarding the mechanisms of chronic posttraumatic headache, a number of reports have been presented on the occurrence of migraine following trauma. The majority of these reports have focused on direct head trauma causing migraine attacks. Whiplash injury is also a possible mechanism for this form of posttraumatic headache (38).

Simons and Wolff described three forms of posttraumatic headache. In their report, the type 3 headache resembled migraine and occurred in 4 of their 63 cases. Of interest, this headache occurred with type 1 headache, a muscle contraction–type headache, in their series of patients. Since their patients obtained relief of the headaches by using ergotamine, they determined that these headaches were caused by distention of extracranial arteries.

Reports by Bonham-Carter's group (39) and Diamond (17) have suggested a link between depression and migraine headache. Alterations in tyramine metabolism and in neurotransmitter function were identified as possible links between the two disorders. Raskin (40) suggested that dysfunction of the neurotransmitter receptor system may occur in posttraumatic migraine and migraine occurring without head trauma. Jacome reported on four cases of basilar artery migraine following uncomplicated whiplash injuries with apparent cranial insult (38). He believed that several mechanisms could, in this situation, contribute to the development of migraine. He suggested five theories to explain his findings: direct concussion of the brain, rotational shearing of the brain, dysfunction of the spinal afferent system, injury to the cervical sympathetic chain, and vascular damage to the vertebral artery.

## OTHER HEADACHES OF POSSIBLE VASCULAR ORIGIN RELATED TO CERVICAL TRAUMA

### POSTTRAUMATIC DYSAUTONOMIC HEADACHE

Vijayan (8) described a syndrome, posttraumatic dysautonomic cephalgia, that is associated with trauma to the anterior neck region. His series included seven cases presenting with headache subsequent to various forms of trauma to the anterior neck. The reported forms of trauma were direct or blunt injury, whiplash, and acceleration-extension injuries. The patients had periodic headaches occurring from two to 12 times per month. The headache attacks occurred in association with pupillary dilatation and facial sweating. Additionally, the lead case of this series described pain that was throbbing, localized to the frontotemporal region, and 8–12 hr in duration. Other associated symptoms were identified, including photophobia, nausea, and vomiting. In these cases, the patients were headache-free between attacks. However, between attacks, four patients experienced meiosis and ptosis on the affected side. One patient complained of a decreased sweating response in the interim period between attacks.

### CERVICAL MIGRAINE

Initially, Bärtschi-Rochaix (41) described the syndrome of cervical migraine as related to cervical trauma. He later added other pathologic causes related to the neck as additional contibuting factors to the development of the syndrome. Cervical migraine is characterized by headaches that resemble migraine and, if triggered by trauma, are unilateral. The headaches may be bilateral or may switch sides if the syndrome results from arthritis or atherosclerotic disease. The pain typically occurs in the frontotemporoparietal regions but may radiate to the neck. In some patients paroxysms of pain can occur, and certain head postures may precipitate these paroxysms. The pain has been described as either dull and migrainous or neurologic and, less often, throbbing. A variety of other symptoms may accompany the migraine, including giddiness, auditory symptoms including "auditory scotomata," visual symptoms typical of migraine, cervicobrachial radicular symptoms, and psychiatric manifestations. Nuchal symptoms were rarely absent in association with these headaches.

A variety of forms of this disorder were described under the term "posterior cervical sympathetic syndrome of Barré-Liéou," as reviewed by Gayral and Neuwirth (42). They identified facial, vertiginous, ocular, asthenic, and psychoneurotic forms of the syndrome. Although trauma may be the precipitating factor, cervical arthritis is the most common cause of this syndrome. In addition to the spinal articulation disorders, this syndrome could be extended by the skin that overlies the involved vertebral segment.

Objective findings are relatively rare in this syndrome. Neck stiffness and tenderness of the spinous processes from C3 to C5 may accompany paravertebral spasm and tenderness, and often involve the trapezius.

Diagnostic studies, including radiologic examination, were considered important in the diagnosis of this syndrome. Degenerative changes in the zygapophyseal joints at one or more cervical segments were identified as responsible for producing distortion of the vertebral nerve as it passed over this segment. Also, irritation of this nerve was considered as a factor in cervical migraine. Additionally, concomitant stretching of the vessel could thereby lead to constriction of the artery related to various motions of the cervical spine. Bogduk et al. (43) however, demonstrated electrical stimulation of the vertebral nerve as having no effect on vertebral blood flow, and stimulation of the sympathetic system produced marked effects on carotid artery flow and resistance. Anthony has further distinguished the problem of migraine with occipital pain from that of greater occipital neuralgia (44). Pain localization and increasing patterns of occipital pain may define a greater occipital neuralgia component as distinct from the underlying migraine.

Carotidynia may occur following cervical trauma. This self-limiting condition may only last for several weeks. It is characterized by a dilated carotid artery with distinct pulsatile blood flow and tenderness on palpitation, especially when pressed against the cervical transverse processes. Carotidynia usually occurs in those who experience other vascular headaches, such as migraine. Simple analgesics usually will relieve the accompanying pain. Other treatments usually used for migraine are rarely needed to obtain relief.

## CERVICOGENIC HEADACHE

Sjaastad and Dale (45) have described chronic paroxysmal hemicrania (CPH). Characteristically, attacks are of short duration, and certain movements of the neck precipitate the attacks in some patients. Eventually, Sjaastad and his colleagues recognized a group of patients similar to those with CPH who experienced attacks of headache triggered by neck movement (46). As compared to CPH, this syndrome did not consistantly affect females (9); only two thirds of the cases occurred in women. The pain was strictly unilateral and occurred in the frontotemporoocular areas, with or without facial pain. In contrast to classical, nonclassical, or cervical migraine, the attacks do not switch sides.

Attacks of cervicogenic headache are accompanied by ipsilateral symptoms of lacrimation, rhinorrhea, tinnitus, erythema, conjunctival injection, or flushing of the forehead. Symptoms that are often associated with migraine, such as gastrointestinal and neurologic complaints, may accompany severe attacks. Some patients report pain radiating to the ipsilateral shoulder and arm. A distinguishing hallmark of this disorder is difficulty swallowing. Between attacks, neck stiffness, crepitus, and painful neck movement have been reported. The attacks may be triggered by neck movement or maintaining the head in a specific position for a prolonged period. The duration of the attacks are variable, and could range from minutes to days. Examination of the neck may reveal areas of tenderness of the C2 root, along the greater occipital nerve, or over the transverse processes of C4 and C5. Six of 11 cases reported by Fredriksen's group involved trauma to the cervical spine (47).

Relief of the headache by lateral blocks to C2 suggested a cervical origin for these headaches. Surgical intervention to the cervical spine, in the form of uncoforaminectomy, may be useful in this disorder.

As compared to cervical migraine, cervicogenic headache occurs in younger patients. It is strictly unilateral and does not switch sides. The visual symptoms of cervicogenic headache are not typical of any type of migraine, including cervical. The occurrence of nausea, a typical migraine symptom, is more frequent in cervicogenic headache than in cervical migraine.

Sjaastad et al. (48) have further suggested that a relationship between migraine, cervicogenic headache, and occipital neuralgia via the second cervical nerve may exist. They base their theory on the response of cervicogenic headache and occipital neuralgia to nerve blocks of C2. They also contend that many patients diagnosed with common migraine who fail to respond to conventional migraine therapy may in fact be suffering from cervicogenic headache instead of migraine. A similar scenario may occur in patients with muscle contraction headache.

## OCCIPITAL NEURALGIA AND THIRD OCCIPITAL HEADACHE

### OCCIPITAL NEURALGIA

The term "occipital neuralgia" may refer to all types of pain involving the posterior portion of the head. This term is most appropriately restricted to those pain disorders that have neurologic characteristics that only involve the greater occipital nerve. The greater occipital nerve arises primarily from the C2 root but it also has contributions from both the C1 and C3 roots. Its sensory boundaries extend to the vertex, the region immediately posterior to the auricle, and into the neck itself to the level of the third cervical vertebra. Sigwald and Jamet described two major forms of occipital neuralgia, paroxysmal and continuous (49).

Paroxysmal occipital neuralgia describes superficial pain occurring only in the distribution of the greater occipital nerve. The attacks are unilateral, the pain onset is sudden, and the pain is severe from the outset. The patient may describe the pain as sharp, twisting, a dagger thrust, or an electric shock. It rarely demonstrates a burning characteristic. Although single flashes of pain may occur, a volley of attacks presents more frequently. The attacks may occur spontaneously. Specific maneuvers applied to the back of the scalp or neck regions, such as brushing the hair or moving the neck, provoke attacks.

In the second form of occipital neuralgia, the pain is continuous instead of intermittent and has two forms, acute and chronic. In contrast to the paroxysmal form of occipital neuralgia, the continuous form often has an underlying etiology. Its attacks last for many hours and are typically devoid of any trigger zones. In the acute form, the entire bout of neuralgia will continue up to 2 weeks before remission. Exposure to cold is a common trigger. The greater occipital nerve may be tender but palpation will not elicit attacks.

In chronic, continuous occipital neuralgia, the patient may experience painful attacks lasting for days or longer, which are accompanied by localized muscle spasm. The most common etiologies for this form include cervical arthritis, cranial cervical malformations (50) syringomyelia, medullary tumors, or Pott's disease of the suboccipital region. In a series by Hammond and Danta (2) 12 of 19 patients suffered trauma of the cervical spine as a factor in the development of occipital neuralgia. Four patients were injured in motor vehicle accidents that induced whiplash. Another patient received a similar injury as a result of an attempted strangulation. Two patients incurred direct trauma to the cervical spine from motor vehicle accidents, and another two patients had direct injuries due to other events. Three patients suffered injuries of an unspecified nature that involved the cervical spine.

Although the cases in this series were older (average age of 42 years), this disease may also present in young patients. Both Dugan and his colleagues (51) and Rothner (personal communciation) studied series of adolescent or young adult patients with occipital neuralgia. Rothner failed to find any radiologic evidence of underlying pathology. Dugan's group, however, found a variety of objective findings, including platybasia with basilar impression and malformation of the first two cervical vertebrae, fusion of the second and third cervical segments, and subluxation of cervical vertebrae. In both series of cases, strenuous exercise or minimal neck trauma served to initiate occipital neuralgia.

### THIRD NERVE HEADACHE

Bogduk and Marsland (52) described a series of 10 patients who experienced headache arising from the occipital and suboccipital regions with radiation, in many cases, to the vertex or orbits. The pain was usually constant and was frequently described as an aching sensation. As with some cases of occipital neuralgia, various neck movements could aggravate third nerve headache attacks. Restricted neck movements associated with this form of headache were reported by four patients. Five of the cases complained of tenderness of the C2–3 region. In 4 of these 10 cases, industrial accidents or motor vehicle trauma played a role in developing the headache.

## TREATMENT OF HEADACHE FOLLOWING CERVICAL TRAUMA

Because a considerable overlap may exist between types of posttraumatic headaches, treatment strategies must be developed for the patient with multiple headaches. Most patients with posttraumatic headaches will respond to medical regimens. Other therapeutic modalities, such as injection techniques, physical therapy including manipulation, and surgical intervention, may be considered for these various forms of headache.

## MEDICAL THERAPIES

Two major divisions of medications are utilized in the treatment of posttraumatic headache—drugs for the relief of acute headache and drugs to reduce the frequency and severity of the headaches. These divisions are respectively known as abortive and prophylactic therapies.

### Abortive and Acute Therapies

The choice of agents for acute headaches is partially dependent on the type of headache the patient is experiencing and the patient's ability to distinguish types. The role of trauma in the genesis of headache does not influence the selection of treatment.

In selecting an appropriate abortive agent for an acute migraine attack, ergotamine preparations are usually the drugs of choice. These medications are taken at the earliest sign of the migraine attack, or during the aura phase of classical migraine. A variety of dosage forms of ergotamine are available, including oral, rectal, sublingual, parenteral, and inhalation. The ergotamine preparations are used for the treatment of posttraumatic migraine, migraine and muscle contraction headaches, posttraumatic dysautonomic cephalgia, cervical migraine, cervicogenic headache, and type 2 posttraumatic headache as described by Simons and Wolff (37).

The patient must be instructed to avoid frequent use of the ergotamine preparations because daily use may lead to the development of ergotamine-dependent headaches or ergotism. It is essential that the patient realize that a 4-day hiatus between uses must be strictly followed. The risk of complications associated with the ergot agents is significantly reduced if these instructions are followed.

For patients in whom the ergotamine preparations fail to abort the acute migraine or in whom the ergotamine preparations are contraindicated, alternative therapies are available. A combination compound containing isometheptene mucate may prove useful and well tolerated. Another agent, GR43175 (Sumatriptan), has serotonergic agonist actions similar to the ergotamine preparations. Since this agent is devoid of the adrenergic effects found in the ergotamines, it may be free of the potential for rebound headache. Preliminary reports have been promising (53).

The use of nonsteroidal anti-inflammatory drugs (NSAIDs) may be beneficial in the treatment of a variety of posttraumatic headache syndromes, and they have been demonstrated to be successful for aborting the migraine attack (54). Also, the NSAIDs have direct analgesic actions. This effect proved successful in double-blind placebo-controlled trials (55, 56). These results have an impact on the patient with both common migraine and muscle contraction headaches. Difficulties arise for the patient in differentiating, early in an attack, which type of headache is occurring. The NSAIDs may relieve the pain of acute muscle contraction headache or may abort the acute migraine. In selecting an NSAID, the patient's previous response to these drugs must be considered.

A variety of muscle relaxant agents are available alone or in combination with analgesics. These drugs may also prove beneficial in the treatment of posttraumatic headaches, especially those with a muscle tension component (57). These agents and their use are discussed elsewhere in this book.

The patient with posttraumatic headache may at times require a narcotic analgesic or an analgesic agent combined with a barbiturate in order to control the pain or anxiety associated with severe headaches. Using these agents on a regular basis is best avoided. Curtailing daily use of these drugs for extended periods helps prevent dependency problems.

### Prophylactic Therapies

Many patients who experience headache following cervical trauma have a pattern of either daily headaches or headaches occurring with sufficient frequency to warrant prophylactic therapy. A useful guide in considering prophylactic therapy is determining if the patient experiences more than two severe or incapacitating headaches per month. In addition, prophylactic therapy should be considered for those patients unable to achieve prompt and consistent relief with abortive agents, or in whom abortive agents are contraindicated.

In treating patients with migraine headaches following cervical trauma, many agents can be considered, including $\beta$-adrenergic blocking agents, calcium channel antagonists, NSAIDs, and various antidepressant agents. $\beta$-Adrenergic blocking agents are useful in treating posttraumatic dysautonomic cephalgia. Muscle contraction headaches occurring on a chronic basis, which may or may not be associated with depression, may respond to daily use of antidepressant agents. These agents may be very effective in the treatment of patients with both migraine and muscle contraction headaches. The antidepressants may be used alone or in combination with other agents specific for migraine headache treatment. The NSAIDs may also be useful in providing generalized analgesic effects in both abortive and prophylactic use. Inflammation associated with the occurrence of degenerative changes in cervical or temporomandibular joints as a result of trauma may be reduced by the NSAIDs. These agents are also useful, with limited success, in patients with cervicogenic headache. In occipital neuralgia, agents used in trigeminal neuralgia, such as carbamazipine, may provide benefit.

Of the $\beta$-adrenergic blocking agents available, only those agents without partial agonist activity have provided substantial benefit in the treatment of headache. Propranolol is the only $\beta$ blocker approved by the Food and Drug Administration (FDA) for migraine treatment. Diamond and Medina (58) demonstrated the effectiveness of propranolol in the prophylaxis of migraine. A long-acting preparation has also proven effective (59). A decrease in the frequency and severity of headaches usually occurs after starting propranolol. Progressive remission occurs over several months. In a long-term controlled trial by Diamond and his associates (60), approximately 50% of patients who had experienced a remission of their migraine for at least 6 months continued to maintain this remission after discontinuing therapy. Other $\beta$ blockers, including atenolol (61), metoprolol (62), nadolol (63), and timolol (64), have also proven beneficial in controlled clinical trials in the prophylaxis of migraine. Metoprolol has demonstrated effectiveness in preventing the headache associated with posttraumatic dysautonomic cephalalgia (8). Although several calcium channel blockers are currently available in the United States, only two have been used in the treatment of migraine. The use of verapamil for the treat-

ment of migraine was started following a successful clinical trial (65). Nimodopine, recently released by the FDA for the treatment of subarachnoid hemorrhage, also proved useful in clinical trials for migraine prevention (66). Ongoing research with another calcium channel antagonist, flunarizine, is underway, although the drug is only available in countries other than the United States. In clinical research with this drug, significant reduction in migraine frequency occurred (67).

The NSAIDs have demonstrated excellent results in the prophylactic treatment of migraine. A variety of NSAIDs have been studied in both placebo-controlled trials and other comparative trials with propranolol and pizotifen. These studies are the gold standards of migraine research. Fenoprofen calcium (68), indomethacin (69), ketoprofen (70; S. Diamond, F. G. Freitag, R. M. Gallagher, and D. Feinberg, unpublished results) mefenamic acid (71), naproxyn and its sodium salt (72–74), and tolfenamic acid (75) were previously studied. Significant reduction in headache parameters occurred in these clinical trials, producing results similar to the standards of migraine comparative studies. In cervicogenic headache, limited success was demonstrated with piroxicam and aspirin (47) but little benefit was noted from other NSAIDs. Degenerative changes may occur following cervical trauma. Neck trauma may exacerbate these changes, which are present on radiologic examination in some patients with headaches arising from the cervical spine. In these patients, a trial of NSAIDs may be useful.

The antidepressant drugs have broad application in the treatment of headache following cervical trauma. The method by which antidepressant agents relieve headache and other pain states is not fully understood. Two major mechanisms of action may account for their effectiveness: relief of depression presenting as pain and direct analgesic effects (76). Their actions may affect neurotransmitter concentrations, neurotransmitter receptor sensitivity, blocking receptor uptake, or altering neuronal firing rates. However, since these agents also relieve pain in nondepressed patients, direct analgesic actions have been suggested. Other antidepressants have demonstrated effects on the endorphin-modulated pain system.

Both the tricyclic antidepressants and MAOIs have proven useful in the treatment of migraine and muscle contraction headaches. Following work by Diamond (77) on depressive headaches, Lance and Curran (78) demonstrated the effectiveness of amitriptyline in the treatment of tension headache in a placebo-controlled crossover study. In a study of patients who developed headaches following trauma, over 90% of these cases showed good or excellent recovery (79). Solitary use of amitriptyline has also proven useful in patients with both migraine and muscle contraction headaches, or as an addition to combination therapy with propranolol. In another study, combination therapy was more effective than using amitriptyline alone (80). Another tricyclic, doxepin, proved to have comparable efficacy in similar cases (81). The presence or absence of a sleep disorder is the basis for selection of an antidepressant. In general, patients who experience insomnia tolerate and benefit from the more sedating types of antidepressants. In contrast, the patient who is hypersomnolent demonstrates better results with one of the nonsedating tricyclics.

The patient's prior experience with antidepressants may also enhance the selection process. The occurrence of adverse effects, which are frequent with the antidepressants, may also be considered. Slow upward titration of antidepressant doses may minimize the side effects experienced by patients during therapy with these agents.

In patients failing to achieve a satisfactory response with the tricyclic agents, use of nontricyclic antidepressants may be attempted. In an unpublished study, the majority of patients who had failed on various tricyclics and MAOIs achieved improvement with fluoxetine in an open trial over several months (S. Diamond and F. G. Freitag, unpublished results). Alternatively, the MAOIs may be of significant benefit in recidivist patients. Anthony and Lance (82) found a greater than 50% reduction in the frequency of migraine in 20 of 25 patients involved in their study of the late 1960s. Their patients had been unresponsive to both cyproheptadine and methysergide prior to treatment with the MAOI phenelzine. Freitag and his associates (83) studied patients with failed response to multiple drug therapies, including β blockers, calcium antagonists, NSAIDs, and various tricyclic antidepressants. They found that 8 of 19 patients with migraine, 12 of 16 patients with mixed headache syndrome, and 2 of 4 patients with pure muscle contraction headache had at least a 50% reduction in their headaches following treatment with phenelzine or isocarboxazid. Although the use of combination therapy with the MAOIs and tricyclic agents has not been in widespread use, this type of treatment has been successful for patients who were nonresponsive to

singular MAOI therapy. Six of their eight patients with mixed headaches and two patients with muscle contraction headaches achieved at least a 50% decrease in their headaches. In the study, the MAOIs used were isocarboxazid and phenelzine, and the tricyclics used were amitriptyline, doxepin, trazadone, and trimipramine. The use of amitriptyline in combination with MAOIs may prevent the occurrence of hypertensive reactions related to consumption of tyramine-containing foods by patients on MAOIs (84). Patients using these agents must adhere to the restricted tyramine-free diet and avoid the use of concomitant therapy with contraindicated medications, such as the sympathomimetics.

Patients with occipital neuralgia may be given a trial of therapy with agents usually used in the treatment of trigeminal neuralgia. Carbamazepine, phenytoin, maolate, and lioresal given alone or in combination should be considered for patients with trigeminal neuralgia who are refractory to single-drug therapy. Muscle relaxants and other conservative therapies may be beneficial in cases of occipital neuralgia.

## OTHER THERAPIES FOR TREATMENT OF POSTTRAUMATIC HEADACHES

Three major categories of alternative therapies have been recommended for the treatment of posttraumatic headaches: physical modalities, injection therapy, and surgical intervention.

### Physical Modalities

The use of heat, cold, rest, and exercises, with attention to acute areas of muscle spasm, may sometimes benefit patients who experience headache following cervical trauma. The use of cranial electrotherapy has also proven beneficial in the acute treatment of muscle contraction headache (85). Physical therapies such as massage and traction administered alone (41) or with manipulations of the neck (40) may help some patients with tension headache. However, these manipulative techniques (86) may cause life-threatening complications, related to vertebrobasilar stroke, in a number of patients (3, 87).

### Injection Therapy

Some authors advocate local anesthetic blocking techniques for treating a variety of headaches related to neck trauma. Primarily, the techniques involve nerve blocks of the second cervical ganglion (88) for a variety of headache types within the cervical or occipital regions. The greater and lesser occipital nerves are also blocked in treatment of occipital neuralgia (2). In cervicogenic headache a block of the second cervical root may be useful, and the same situation may exist in cervical migraine (48). Blocking of the third cervical nerve root is a recommended treatment in third occipital nerve headache (52). Injection of the C1–2 arthrosis may be useful for occipital neuralgia (88).

The use of percutaneous denervation nerve blocks has been suggested for treating cervical and other headaches (89). In Hildebrandt's group, 13 of 35 patients experienced significant reduction in their pain or became pain-free. Blume et al. (90) have advocated similar techniques for the treatment of occipital neuralgia and cervicogenic headaches.

## Surgical Intervention

In some patients who obtain benefit from local anesthetic injections, surgical intervention may be indicated. Occipital neurectomy has been successful in some cases of occipital neuralgia (2). Uncoforaminectomy performed for cervicogenic headache was successful in 15 of 26 patients (46). In a case of posttraumatic occipital neuralgia with subsequent development of cervical arthritis, decompression of the C2 and C3 nerve roots was successful (91). Jamieson and Merskey (6) described surgery for thoracic outlet syndrome associated with posttraumatic headache, with favorable outcome in three cases.

### REFERENCES

1. Macnab I: Acceleration injuries of the cervical spine. *J Bone Joint Surg [Am]* 46:1797–1799, 1964.
2. Hammond SR, Danta G: Occipital neuralgia. *Clin Exp Neurol* 15:258–270, 1978.
3. Mueller S, Sahs AL: Brainstem dysfunction related to cervical manipulation. *Neurology* 26:547–550, 1976.
4. Janecki OJ, Lipke JM: The whiplash syndrome. *Am Fam Physician* 17:144–151, 1978.
5. Coburn DF: Vertebral artery involvement in cervical trauma. *Clin Orthop* 24:61, 1962.
6. Jamieson WG, Merskey H: Representation of the thoracic outlet syndrome as a problem of chronic pain and psychiatric management. *Pain* 22:195–200, 1985.
7. Bogduk N: The anatomy of occipital neuralgia. *Clin Exp Neurol* 17:167–184, 1981.
8. Vijayan N: A new post-traumatic headache syndrome, clinical and therapeutic observations. *Headache* 17:19–25, 1977.
9. Ommaya AK, Fass F, Yarnell P: Whiplash and the rain. *JAMA* 204:285–289, 1968.
10. Jenkins A, Hadley MDM, Teasdale G, Macphearson P,

Rowan JO: Brain lesions detected by magnetic resonance imaging in mild and severe head injuries. *Lancet* 2:445–446, 1986.
11. Barclay L, Zemcov A, Reichert W, Blass JP: Cerebral blood flow decrements in chronic head injury syndrome. *Biol Psychiatry* 20:146–157, 1985.
12. Balla J, Karnaghan J: Whiplash headache. *Clin Exp Neurol* 23:179–182, 1987.
13. Oleson J: Clinical characterization of tension headache. In Oleson J, Edvinsson L (eds): *Basic Mechanisms of Headache*. New York, Elsevier, 1988, pp 9–14.
14. Forresell H, Kangasniemi P: Mandibular dysfunction in patients with muscle contraction headache. *Proc Finn Dent Soc* 80:211–216, 1984.
15. Kwentus JA, et al: Psychiatric complications of closed head trauma. *Psychosomatics* 26:8–17, 1985.
16. Martin MJ, Rome HP, Swenson WM: Muscle contraction headache, a psychiatric review. *Res Clin Stud Headache* 1:184, 1967.
17. Diamond S: Depression and headache. *Headache* 23:123–126, 1983.
18. Magni G: On the relationship between chronic pain and depression when there is no organic lesion. *Pain* 31:1–21, 1987.
19. Barolin GS: Headache and (concomitant) depression. *Psychopathology* 19(suppl 2):165–171, 1986.
20. Diamond S: Muscle contraction headache. In Dalissio DJ (ed): *Wolff's Headache and Other Head Pain*, ed 5. New York, Oxford University Press, 1987, pp 173–174.
21. Oleson J, Langemark M: Mechanisms of tension headache, a speculative hypothesis. In Oleson J, Edvinsson L (eds): *Basic Mechanisms of Headache*. New York, Elsevier, 1988, pp 457–461.
22. Nappi G, Faccinetti F, Bono G, Micieli G, et al: Plasma opioid levels in post-traumatic chronic headache and trigeminal neuralgia; maintained response to acupuncture. *Headache* 22:276–279, 1982.
23. Sicuteri F: Opioid receptor impairment: underlying mechanism in pain diseases. *Cephalalgia* 1:77–82, 1981.
24. Rolf LJ, Wiele G, Brune GG: 5-hydroxytryptamine in platelets of patients with muscle contraction headache. *Headache* 21:10–11, 1981.
25. Shukla R, Shanker K, Nag D, Verma M, Bhargava KP: Serotonin in tension headache. *J Neurol Neurosurg Psychiatry* 50:1682–1684, 1987.
26. Nappi G, Faccinetti F, Martignoni E, Petraglia F, et al: CSF beta-EP in headache and depression. *Cephalalgia* 5:99–101, 1985.
27. Sarrias MJ, Artigas F, Martinez E, Gelpi E, et al: Decreased plasma serotonin in melancholic patients: a study with clomipramine. *Biol Psychiatry* 22:1429–1438, 1987.
28. Feighner JP: Pharmacologic management of depression. *Fam Pract Recert* 4(suppl 1):13–24, 1982.
29. Maas J: The biology of depression: where we stand. *Psychiatry* 5:67–69, 1973.
30. Siever LJ, Uhde TW: New studies and perspectives on the noradrenergic receptor system in depression: effects of the alpha 2-adrenergic agonist clonidine. *Biol Psychiatry* 19:131–156, 1984.
31. Fawcett J: Depression at the biochemical level. *Psychiatry Annu* 109(suppl):362–368, 1980.
32. Cobbin D, Requin-Blow B, Williams RL, et al: Urinary MHPG and tricyclic antidepressant drug selection. *Arch Gen Psychiatry* 36:1111–1115, 1979.
33. Schatzberg AF, Orsulak PJ, Rosenbaum AH, et al: Toward a biochemical classification of depressive disorders V: Het-

erogeneity of unipolar depressions. *Am J Psychiatry* 139:471–475, 1982.

34. Bonham-Carter SM, Reveley MA, Sandler M, Dewhurst J, et al: Decreased urinary output of conjugated tyramine is associated with lifetime vulnerability to depressive illness. *Psychiatr Res* 3:13–21, 1980.

35. Hale AS, Hannah P, Sandler M, Bridges PK: Tyramine conjugation test for prediction of treatment response in depressed patients. *Lancet* 1:234–236, 1989.

36. Reynolds EH, Carney MWP, Toone BK: Methylation and mood. *Lancet* 2:196–198, 1984.

37. Simons DJ, Wolff HG: Studies on headache: mechanisms of chronic post-traumatic headache. *Psychol Med* 8:227–242, 1946.

38. Jacome DE: Basilar artery migraine after uncomplicated whiplash injuries. *Headache* 6:515–516, 1986.

39. Bonham-Carter S, Sandler M, Goodwin BL, Sepping P, Bridges PK: Decreased urinary output of tyramine and its metabolities in depression. *Br J Psychiatry* 132:125–132, 1978.

40. Raskin NH: *Headache,* ed 2. New York, Churchill Livingstone, 1988, p 272.

41. Bärtschi-Rochaix W: Headaches of cervical origin. In Vinken PJ, Bruyn GW (eds): *Handbook of Clinical Neurology.* Amsterdam, North Holland, 1970, pp 192–203.

42. Gayral L, Neuwirth E: Oto-neuro-ophthalmologic manifestations of cervical origin: posterior cervical sympathetic syndrome of Barre-Lieou. *NY State Med* 1:1920–1926, 1954.

43. Bogduk N, Lambert GA, Duckworth JW: The anatomy and physiology of the vertebral nerve in relation to cervical migraine. *Cephalalgia* 1:11–24, 1981.

44. Anthony M: Unilateral migraine or occipital neuralgia? In Rose FC (ed): *New Advances in Headache Research.* London, Smith-Gordon, 1989, pp 39–43.

45. Sjaastad O, Dale I: A new (?) clinical headache entity: chronic paroxysmal hemicrania. *Acta Neurol Scand* 54:140–159, 1976.

46. Sjaastad O, Saute C, Hovdahl H, Breivik H, Gröbæ KE: "Cervicogenic" headache. An hypothesis. *Cephalalgia* 3:249–256, 1983.

47. Fredriksen TA, Hovdahl H, Sjaastad O: Cervicogenic headache: clinical manifestations. *Cephalalgia* 7:147–160, 1987.

48. Sjaastad O, Fredriksen T, Stolt-Nielsen A: Cervicogenic headache, C$_2$ rhizopathy and occipital neuralgia: a connection? *Cephalalgia* 6:189–195, 1986.

49. Sigwald J, Jamet F: Occipital neuralgias. In Vinken PJ, Bruyn GW (eds): *Handbook of Clinical Neurology.* New York, Elsevier Publishing, 1968, pp 368–374.

50. Scott M: Occipital neuralgia. *Pennsylvania Med* 71:85–88, 1968.

51. Dugan MC, Locke S, Gallagher JR: Occipital neuralgia in adolescents and young adults. *N Engl J Med* 267:1166–1172, 1962.

52. Bogduk N, Marsland A: On the concept of third occipital headache. *Neurol Neurosurg Psychiatry* 49:775–780, 1986.

53. Doenicke A, Brand J, Perrin VL: Possible benefit of GR 43175, a novel 5-HTL-like receptor agonist, for the acute treatment of severe migraine. *Lancet* 1:1309–1311, 1988.

54. Diamond S, Freitag FG: Do non-steroidal anti-inflammatory agents have a role in the treatment of migraine headaches? *Drugs* 37:755–760, 1989.

55. Diamond S: Ibuprofen versus aspirin and placebo in the treatment of muscle contraction headache. *Headache* 23:206–210, 1983.

56. Diamond S, Medina JL: A double blind study of zomepirac

sodium and placebo in the treatment of muscle contraction headache. *Headache* 21:45–48, 1981.

57. Bakris G, Mulopulos GP, Tiwari S, Franklin C: An effective alternative for muscle contraction headache: orphenadrine citrate. *Ill Med J* 161(2):106–108, 1982.

58. Diamond S, Medina JL: Double blind study of propranolol for migraine prophylaxis. *Headache* 16:238–245, 1976.

59. Diamond S, Solomon GD, Freitag FG, Mehta ND: Long-acting propranolol in the prophylaxis of migraine. *Headache* 27:70–72, 1987.

60. Diamond S, Kudrow L, Stevens J, Shapiro DB: Long term study of propranolol in the treatment of migraine. *Headache* 22:268–271, 1982.

61. Stensrud P, Sjaastad O: Comparative trial of Tenormin (atenolol) and Inderal (propranolol) in migraine. *Headache* 20:204–207, 1980.

62. Vilming S, Standnes B, Hedman C: Metoprolol and pizotifen in the prophylactic treatment of classical and common migraine, a double blind investigation. *Cephalalgia* 5:17–23, 1985.

63. Freitag FG, Diamond S: Nadolol and placebo comparison study in the treatment of migraine. *J Am Osteopath Assoc* 84:343–347, 1984.

64. Tfelt-Hansen P, Standnes B, Kangasniemi P, Hakkarainen H, Olesen J: Timolol versus propranolol versus placebo in common migraine prophylaxis: a double-blind multicenter trial. *Acta Neurol Scand* 69:1–8, 1984.

65. Solomon GD, Steel JG, Spaccavento LJ: Verapamil prophylaxis of migraine: a double-blind placebo-controlled study. *JAMA* 250:2500–2502, 1983.

66. Meyer JS, Hardenberg J: Clinical effectiveness of calcium entry blockers in the prophylactic treatment of migraine and cluster headaches. *Headache* 23:266–277, 1983.

67. Diamond S, Schenbaum H: Flunarizine, a calcium channel blocker in the prophylactic treatment of migraine. *Headache* 23:39–42, 1983.

68. Diamond S, Solomon GD, Freitag FG, Mehta N: Fenoprofen in the prophylaxis of migraine: a double-blind placebo-controlled study. *Headache* 27:246–249, 1987.

69. Anthony M, Lance JW: Indomethacin in migraine. *Med J Aust* 1:56–57, 1968.

70. Stensrud P, Sjaastad O: Clinical trial of a new anti-bradykinin, anti-inflammatory drug, ketoprofen, in migraine prophylaxis. *Headache* 14:96–100, 1974.

71. Johnson RH, Hornabrook RW, Lambie DG: Comparison of mefenamic acid and propranolol with placebo in migraine prophylaxis. *Acta Neurol Scand* 76:490–492, 1986.

72. Lindegaard KF, Ovrelio L, Sjaastad O: Naproxyn in the prevention of migraine attacks. A double blind placebo controlled cross-over study. *Headache* 20:96–98, 1980.

73. Ziegler DK, Ellis DJ: Naproxyn in the prophylaxis of migraine. *Arch Neurol* 42:582–584, 1985.

74. Behan PO, Connelly K: Prophylaxis of migraine: a comparison between naproxyn sodium and pizotifen. *Headache* 26:237–239, 1986.

75. Mikkelsen BM, Falk JV: Prophylactic treatment of migraine and tolfenamic acid. *Acta Neurol Scand* 66:105–111, 1982.

76. France RD: The future for antidepressants: treatment of pain. *Psychopathology* 20(suppl 1):99–113, 1987.

77. Diamond S: Depressive headaches. *Headache* 4:255–259, 1964.

78. Lance JW, Curran DA: Treatment of chronic tension headache. *Lancet* 1:1236–1239, 1964.

79. Tyler GS, McNelly HE, Dick ML: Treatment of post-traumatic headache with amitriptyline. *Headache* 20:213–216, 1980.

80. Mathew NT: Prophylaxis of migraine and mixed headache. A randomized controlled study. *Headache* 21:105–109, 1981.

81. Mørland TJ, Storli OV, Mogstad TE: Doxepin in the treatment of mixed "vascular" headaches and tension headache. *Headache* 19:382–383, 1979.

82. Anthony M, Lance JW: Monoamine oxidase inhibition in the treatment of migraine. *Arch Neurol* 21:263–268, 1969.

83. Freitag FG, Diamond S, Solomon GD: Antidepressants in the treatment of mixed headache: MAOIs and combined use of MAOIs and tricyclic antidepressants in the recidivist headache patient. In Rose FC (ed): *Advances in Headache Research.* London, Libbey, 1987, pp 271–275.

84. Pare CMB, Hallstrom C, Kline N, Cooper TB: Will amitriptyline prevent the "cheese" reaction of monoamine oxidase inhibitors? *Lancet* 2:183–186, 1982.

85. Solomon S, Elkind A, Freitag FG, Gallagher RM, et al: Safety and effectiveness of cranial electrotherapy in the treatment of tension headache. *Headache* 29:445–450, 1989.

86. Hoyt WH, Shaffer F, Bard DA, Benesler JS, et al: Osteopathic manipulation in the treatment of muscle contraction headache. *J Am Osteopath Assoc* 78:322–325, 1979.

87. Laughlin TM: Complications of spinal manipulation. *Osteopathic Ann* 14(1):21–23, 1985.

88. Ehni G, Benner B: Occipital neuralgia and $C_1$-$C_2$ arthrosis. *N Engl J Med* 310:127, 1984.

89. Hildebrandt J, Argyrakis A: Percutaneous nerve block of the cervical facets—a relatively new method in the treatment of chronic headache and neck pain. *Manual Med* 2:48–52, 1986.

90. Blume H, Atac M, Golnick J: Neurosurgical treatment of persistent occipital myalgia-neuralgia syndrome. In Pfaffenrath V, Lundberg PO, Sjaastad, O (eds): *Headache.* Berlin, Springer-Verlag, 1985, pp 24–34.

91. Poletti CE: Proposed operation for occipital neuralgia: $C_2$ and $C_3$ root decompression. *Neurosurgery* 12:221–223, 1983.

## 26

# COGNITIVE DEFICITS FOLLOWING CERVICAL TRAUMA

*Donald W. Hinnant and H. Dennis Kade*

Mild brain injury and cognitive deficits are commonly yet frequently unrecognized concomitants of traumatic spinal cord injury. In cervical trauma or whiplash injury, there can be mild cerebral damage that may go undetected because of a lack of evidence of a direct blow to the head. Following cervical trauma, some individuals may exhibit cognitive symptoms that may be more readily identified as psychological symptoms, emotional overlay, or litigious behavior. Current pathologic, epidemiologic, and neuropsychological data are merging to suggest that minor head injury and whiplash injuries are capable of producing cognitive deficits and neurobehavioral symptoms due to neural damage to axons (1, 2). A shear-strain model has been proposed to explain how the damage occurs in acceleration-deceleration injury resulting in axonal tearing and microscopic degeneration (3).

In the unfortunate event of cervical trauma that also includes a serious impact to the cranium, a clear delineation of procedures for medical evaluation and treatment is often indicated. A continuum of care exists between patients who experience minor trauma and those who suffer severe traumatic head injury. In whiplash, mild head injury, and injuries in which there is a diagnosis of concussion, the extent of diagnostic evaluation and expectations about recovery are not as clear. The following case report may help to illustrate this.

A 27-year-old female was referred to the Pain Center for evaluation and treatment of persistent headaches,

insomnia, and vague somatic complaints. The patient had been involved in a rear-end collision 2 months prior to referral and suffered a severe whiplash injury. Medical records indicated that she had been evaluated in the emergency room and there were no objective neurologic findings. There was also no indication in the record of concussion, unconsciousness, or amnesia. Following routine radiographs and a 4-hr period of observation, the patient was discharged home with a prescription for muscle relaxants, cervical collar and analgesics. After approximately 1 week, the patient sought treatment from her family practitioner because of persistent headaches and difficulty in performing her job as a computer programmer. The patient was considered to have diminished coping skills and her headaches led to a neurologic consultation, which again produced negative findings. Problems developed between the patient and her employer as a result of missed time from work and her decreased performance. At the time of referral to our clinic, the patient had hired an attorney. The referral report from the neurologist provided additional diagnoses of depression, hysterical personality, and a probable "supratentorial component."

Evaluation at the Pain Center revealed a young woman with possible embellishment of symptoms, as if she was attempting desperately to convince us of the severity of her problems. A psychological evaluation was performed in order to get a better understanding of her headache complaints as well as psychological factors affecting her condition. The initial evaluation produced evidence of problems with concentration and attention, irritability, and reactive depression. The patient's Minnesota Multiphasic Personality Inventory (MMPI) profile suggested somatic preoccupation, depression, and hysterical features. The profile also suggested severe hostility and pervasive anxiety. Because of the patient's problems with attention and concentration as well as her difficulty in performing her job, a neuropsychological screening was conducted. Test results found the patient to have symptoms of mild diffuse cognitive impairment, including decreased concentration and processing speed, distractibility, and consistent memory deficits. The patient's emotional problems were considered to be a behavioral manifestation of her frustration and reaction to her inability to perform as she was accustomed in her job. She also was having considerable difficulty in maintaining her relationship with her employer because of her irritability and reduced productivity. The patient was particularly frustrated with reports of negative findings from her doctors and the fact that she was never provided valid explanations for her problems.

It became more apparent that the patient was exhibiting classical symptoms of "postconcussive" or "posttraumatic syndrome," although there was no objective evidence of the patient ever having received a concussion or a direct blow to the head. The patient's employer was contacted, and work-related problems were discussed along with suggestions for establishment of a structured plan for gradual resumption of her responsibilities. She received medications and physical and behavioral therapy for her headaches in addition to supportive psychotherapy.

## DEFINITIONS

### COGNITION

The term "cognitive function" is often used interchangeably with "intelligence." Lezak (4) described four major classes of cognitive functions:

(1) Receptive functions, which involve the abilities to acquire, process, classify, and integrate information; (2) memory and learning, by means of which information is stored and recalled; (3) thinking, which concerns the mental organization and reorganization of information; and (4) expressive functions, through which information is communicated or acted upon. Each functional class comprises many discrete activities—such as immediate memory for spoken words, or color recognition. Although each function constitutes a distinct class of behavior, normally they work in close interdependent concert.

In an assessment of cognitive impairment following whiplash or closed head injury, intellectual dysfunction is more accessible to evaluation than are associated psychological factors and behavior. The functions of the intellect can be measured and correlated with well-identified neurobehavioral and anatomic systems, whereas the behavioral and emotional components following an in-jury are more easily considered to be reactive to the injury itself or possibly preexisting factors. Because of the typically diffuse nature of brain trauma associated with mild head injury, as opposed to focal injury and severe head trauma, the tissue damage—no matter how slight—may affect intellectual, emotional, and behavioral expression to some degree (4).

Intellectual or cognitive behavior is a very complex characterization of behavior that includes higher level processes of abstract thought, verbal reasoning, and arithmetic calculation. These high-level processes are dependent upon the individual's intact capacity for perception, memory, and adequate language development. These three basic functions allow the individual to develop behavior and control within the environment through highly sophisticated systems of cortical and subcortical relationships. Emotional behavior and intellectual processes depend upon a state of awareness within the individual of both the environmental stimuli and the individual's thought processes. This complex system of interrelationships between the arousal system, the limbic system, and the cortex in conjunction with the frontal lobes provides the basis for intellect and personality. Although the higher cortical regions and the limbic system serve to provide the basis for the intellect, the frontal lobes serve as a modulator between emotion and behavior. The prefrontal cortical lobe structures are the most recent phylogenetic development in the human nervous system (5).

Cognitive impairment may therefore be defined as a deficiency in intellectual functions that are dependent upon basic attention, information processing ability, language, and memory. Neuropsychological evaluation of cognitive function may include assessment of the individual's ability to manipulate well-learned material and demonstration of abstract reasoning, problem solving, and calculation ability. Particular attention is also paid to subtle deficits in any of the perceptual and sensory functions as well as evaluation of perceptual-sensorimotor systems.

### CLOSED HEAD INJURY, MILD HEAD INJURY, AND CONCUSSION

The term "closed head injury" is commonly used to describe an impact to the head that does not create a skull fracture or involve penetration through the skull into the interior of the cranium. The term "mild head injury," however, is used much more loosely to describe a minor injury to the head. Mild head injury could include superficial lacerations or any other associated minor injuries to the head that may or may not involve injury to brain tissue. As Rutherford (6) has proposed, the term "minor brain injury" would be less open to confusion.

The term "concussion" has often been described as one of the most complicated concepts to define in the fields of neurology and neuropsychology. Although no definition can accurately describe all of the possible manifestations of a concussion, the Ad Hoc Committee of the Congress of Neurological Surgeons has described two consistent features: (a) concussion results from a mechanical impact to the head, and (b) there is an immediate impairment of neurologic function. Loss of consciousness has often been described as a required symptom for diagnosis of concussion, as well as a period of brief amnesia, eventual resumption of full orientation, and lack of prolonged neurologic deficits. Strub and Black (5) reported that definitions of concussion often propose that neurologic deficits must return to complete normal function without residual impairment. We agree with Strub and Black that this definition is too restrictive and that patients often have undetermined and/or subtle neuropathologic injury to nerve tissue. It is important to note that definitions of concussion usually do not provide any limit in terms of severity, and various authors have described concussion in degrees ranging from very mild to extremely severe. An in-depth discussion of postconcussion syndrome follows because of the widespread use of this description of symptoms that may follow head injury.

Traditionally concussion has been considered to be primarily a psychological group of symptoms. However, a mounting body of more recent research has demonstrated that even in mild concussion there are microscopic injuries to neural tissue. In concussion the neurologic examination is typically normal. Cognitive, psychological, and somatic sequelae combine to form the postconcussion syndrome. Long and Novack (7) cited reports suggesting that the severity of postconcussion symptoms increases with the severity of head injury, with headache and memory problems being most prevalent. However, they also reported evidence suggesting a higher incidence of postconcussion symptoms among mildly injured patients as compared to those severely injured. They provided several suggestions for this contradiction: "Minor problems labelled as post concussion symptoms in patients less severely injured may be overshadowed by significant cognitive and physical problems in those severely injured. In addition, severely injured patients often are not fully aware of their deficits and they respond inconsistently to questions concerning problems in recovery." The authors suggest that there is a curvilinear relationship to explain that the incidence of postconcussion symptoms increases from mild to moderate head injury and then drops with severe injuries (7).

In the ninth *International Classification of Disease* (ICD) (8) postconcussional syndrome (ICD-9-CM310.2) is defined as:

> . . . states occurring after generalized contusion of the brain in which the symptom picture may resemble that of the frontal lobe syndrome (310.0) or that of any of the neurotic disorders (300.0–300.9), but in which in addition headache, giddiness, fatigue, insomnia, and a subjective feeling of impaired intellectual ability are usually prominent. Mood may fluctuate, and quite ordinary stress may produce exaggerated fear and apprehension. There may be marked preoccupation. The symptoms are more common in persons who have previously suffered from neurotic or personality disorders, or when there is a possibility of compensation. This syndrome is particularly associated with the closed head type of head injury when signs of localized brain damage are slight or absent, but may also occur in other conditions (ICD-9-CM).

The National Head Injury Foundation and Lishman (9) have provided information on the postconcussion syndrome that suggests that this syndrome involves a variety of temporary somatic and cognitive dysfunctions experienced from several weeks to 1 year after head injury. The postconcussion syndrome may be comprised of the following complaints:

Headache
Transient diplopia
Drowsiness
Positional vertigo
Depression
Fatigue
Anxiety
Hyperacusis
Loss of concentration ability
Loss of abstract thinking
Loss of inhibitions
Loss of judgment
Loss of libido
Avoidance of crowds
Loss of recent memory
Insomnia

Emotional lability
Irritability
Photophobia
Need to dwell on major life events

In this chapter, the terms "closed head injury" (CHI), "mild head injury" (MHI), and "concussion" are used interchangeably. "Posttraumatic syndrome" is another description of symptoms following head injury that is often used interchangeably with "postconcussion syndrome." These terms are also used synonymously in this chapter. The term "organic brain syndrome" has been used consistently by the American Psychiatric Association to describe two categories, organic mental disorders and organic brain syndromes. For a review of the organic brain syndrome classification, please refer to the *Diagnostic and Statistical Manual* published by the American Psychiatric Association (10).

## INCIDENCE

Estimates of head trauma vary considerably from source to source. Estimates have ranged from 3 million to 10 million in the United States (11, 12). Statistical evidence of head injury remains highly uncertain because of the multitude of variables utilized in data collection. Symptoms of head injury range from the obvious in severe trauma to highly subtle and often undetectable symptoms following mild injury and concussion. Statistics of occurrence depend upon the researcher's selection of symptoms, time since injury, severity of the injury, and the probably unreliable recording of the length of unconsciousness and the period of posttraumatic amnesia. Of the 10 million estimated head injuries in the United States, approximately 90% have been described as mild to moderate in severity (8).

It becomes obvious that in the case of flexion-extension injuries and deceleration injuries in which there is no recorded injury to the cranium, statistical evidence of cognitive impairment becomes very elusive.

## INCIDENCE OF COGNITIVE DEFICITS ASSOCIATED WITH SPINAL CORD INJURY

A significant proportion of victims of spinal cord injury have been found to have a concomitant CHI that is often undiagnosed because primary attention was paid to the stabilization of spinal-orthopaedic and other physical injuries. Recent studies by Davidoff et al. (13, 14), Wilmot et al. (15), and Morris et al. (16) have highlighted the incidence of CHI with associated spinal cord injury. Davidoff's group reported that 57% of spinal cord–injured patients were found to have cognitive deficits 8–12 weeks following injury. Wilmot et al. found that 64% of their sample had mild to profound cognitive dysfunction, with 70% falling in the mildly impaired category. Interestingly, only 23% of those patients with cognitive impairment were noted to have head injury or cognitive problems by their treating physicians, even though the physicians were aware of the ongoing neuropsychological investigations of their patients (15)! These studies point toward the prevalence of cognitive deficits in the spinal cord injury population and, more importantly, to the impact these deficits may have on the rehabilitation process. For example, cognitive impairment may impede the rehabilitation process through deficits in attention, response to medications, memory problems, and difficulty in learning new skills as well as psychological behavior such as irritability, lack of motivation, confusion, and depression.

Morris et al. (16) suggested that more attention be paid to evaluation of cognitive deficits in spinal cord–injured patients. They provided an excellent review of the incidence of head injury in patients with spinal cord injury (Table 26.1). Most cases of brain pathology in spinal cord–injured patients are found to be associated with upper cervical lesions, although other studies have found as many as 50% of patients evaluated had lower spinal cord injuries (15).

In Wilmot et al.'s investigation, 87% of subjects who had a premorbid history of academic problems were found to have significant impairment on neuropsychological testing. This is not surprising since patients with prior intellectual and academic problems more typically show cognitive deficits on testing. However, 56% of patients *without* prior academic or intellectual problems were found to have impaired cognitive function associated with spinal cord injuries. This body of research suggests there is a higher correlation between spinal injuries and neuropsychological deficits than is commonly reported in the literature (15).

## VALIDITY OF PATIENT COMPLAINTS

Minor CHI and whiplash injuries do not produce cognitive deficits that can readily be detected in the usual neurologic examination, mental status

**Table 26.1.**
**Reported Incidence of Head Injury in Patients with SCI[a,b]**

| Reference | $n$ | % with Head Injury | Criteria for Head Injury | Head Injuries at Each SCI Level | Comments |
|---|---|---|---|---|---|
| Guttmann, 1967 | 396 | 2 | Death from head injury | * | Only deaths from head injury were noted. |
| Harris, 1966 | 114 | 27 | * | 27% of cervical | All subjects in the study had cervical injuries. |
| Meinecke, 1968 | 595 | 25 | Concussion/contusion = 74%; skull wounds = 26% | * | Sports injuries were the most common etiology. |
| Harris, 1965 | 150 | 33 | "Minor" (LOC × min or PTA × 12 hrs) = 60% "Major" = 40% | 45% of cervical 24% of thoracolumbar | |
| Maynard et al., 1979 | 123 | 10 | "Cognitive impairment" persisting at 72 hrs | 10% of cervical | All subjects in study had cervical injuries. "Cognitive impairment" was not defined. |
| Silver et al., 1980 | 100 | 50 | "Minor" (head abrasions with "short" LOC) = 82%; "Serious" (long PTA with contusion) = 18% | 33% of cervical 67% of thoracolumbar | |
| Rimel, 1981; Young et al., 1982 | 253 1615 | 47 16 | Cerebral concussion (60% skull fracture) = 20%; major brain injury = 20% | 14% of cervical 18% of thoracolumbar | |
| Schueneman and Morris, 1982 | 35 | 51 | History of LOC or PTA associated with SCI | | |
| Wagner et al., 1983 | 167 | 25 | "Mild" (Glasgow Coma Score of 13–15) = 63%; "Moderate/ Severe" (Glasgow Coma Score of ≤ 12) = 37% | 27% of cervical 20% of thoracolumbar | |
| Dubo and Delaney, 1984 | 101 | 58 | * | * | All subjects in study were involved in motor vehicle accidents. |
| Davidoff et al., 1985 | 101 | 42 | History of LOC or PTA associated with SCI | Of assessed upper cord injuries, 41% had LOC. Of assessed upper cord injuries, 88% had PTA. Of assessed lower cord injuries, 20% had LOC. All of assessed lower cord injuries had PTA. | Of total sample, 87% were assessed for LOC; of total sample, 22% were assessed for PTA. Gunshot wounds were the least common etiology. |

[a]From Morris J, Roth E, Davidoff G: Mild closed head injury and cognitive deficits in spinal cord injured patients: incidence and impact. *J Head Trauma Rehabil* 1(2):31–42, 1986.
[b]CHI, closed head injury; LOC, loss of consciousness; PTA, posttraumatic amnesia; SCI, spinal cord injury.
*Not specified.

examination, or IQ test. A physician might be tempted to (mis)diagnose malingering in a patient who has unsuccessfully attempted to return to work following a minor injury but shows no apparent neurologic damage.

Although opinions about the influence of litigation upon persistence of complaints continue to be divided, the literature suggests that litigation is not as significant a factor as was believed in the past. There is evidence that patients seeking compensation do not actually differ in the number of symptoms or deficits, but rather complain more about the deficits that they have. Rimel et al. (17) found no difference in adjustment associated with the patient's being involved in litigation. Rutherford's most recent data (6) on patients in litigation reveal that 57% of minor CHI patients had symptoms at the time that their medical reports were written (mean 12.9 months after accident), 39% at the time of settlement (mean 22.1 months after accident), and 34% at 1 year after settlement (mean 34.1 months after accident). It is notable how many patients were symptom free before their medical reports were written and how many improved over the next 10 months leading up to the settlement. Yet the long-term symptom rate is double that generally reported for mild CHI. Two interpretations have been proposed: (a) involvement in litigation reduces the recovery rate or (b) those patients with injuries likely to produce resistant symptoms (such as falls) and/or positive neurologic findings (which also correlate with more resistant symptoms) are more likely to be involved in litigation. Note that the receipt of financial reward in litigation (which is usually emphasized in discussing such cases) did little to reduce symptoms (less than or equal to 4%)! Also, there is a small group of patients who report continued symptoms for many years (perhaps lifelong) regardless of litigation status. Russell (18) has questioned whether MHI patients ever recover completely even if clinical symptoms are no longer apparent.

The physician who may be suspicious of a MHI will find the usual interview with the patient to be of little or no help since the chief complaint is usually not related to the patient's decrements in cognitive function. If the patient has noticed any cognitive changes they are usually difficulties with attention and concentration, which the patient will often attribute to the effects of medication, headache, or his or her own problems in coping. A standard psychological evaluation will have difficulty determining whether these complaints are indeed organic or are psychogenic. All of these complaints may be attributable to both organic and psychological factors, which obviously can complicate interpretation of any test result.

It is helpful for the physician to be thorough in evaluating the quality and depth of complaints. Answers to questions about the patient's current situation and coping style are usually quite informative. Complaints of forgetfulness, misplacement of objects, or forgetting information more frequently may obviously impair productivity at work, but also may create difficulty with the patient's family. Patients may begin to make notes and attempt to hide their problems from others. Decrements in job performance may be related more to an inability to cope adequately with distractions than to an inability to perform routine, customary tasks. Neuro-otologic evaluation of CHI patients reveals a high incidence of vestibular dysfunction and asymmetrical hearing loss consistent with the frequent complaints of dizziness and hyperacusis. A very thorough history helps to attribute symptoms to the current injury and/or prior causes such as previous injury or psychological-intellectual factors (19). An evaluation by a competent neuropsychologist, behavioral neurologist, or psychologist with training and experience in evaluation and treatment of postconcussive patients may provide evidence of mild brain dysfunction.

## BRIEF OVERVIEW OF BRAIN FUNCTION AND BEHAVIORAL MANIFESTATIONS OF CHI

When one area of the brain suffers greater injury than other regions, the symptoms observed may reflect the specific areas of trauma. In diffuse injury, common in cases of MHI, the individual may experience a variety of symptoms reflecting several areas of contusion. Coup (direct area of impact) and contrecoup (contusion opposite the area of impact) injuries are common in concussion (4).

The brain may be damaged both directly and indirectly in trauma. During acceleration-deceleration injuries the brain experiences rapid movement as it sits on the brainstem inside the vault of the skull. During cervical trauma and in concussion, the frontal and temporal areas are more likely to sustain damage caused by the bony protrusions on the interior surfaces of the skull. Ommaya and Gennarelli (20) identified evidence for the effects of diffuse injury caused by shear-strain that is especially apparent in the areas in which the skull's bony protrusions and uneven surfaces in the area of the temporal and frontal lobes cause minute lesions and lacerations. When there is a great deal of momentum on impact, as seen commonly in automobile accidents, focal defects are not as evident and there is typically a pattern of multifocal, bilateral, diffuse injury (4). However, in most cases this diffuse injury is more likely to occur in the frontal and temporal lobes.

The distribution of lesions and behavioral manifestations of damage are correlated with the severity of impact and the extent of damage from superficial to deeper brain structures. The depth of parenchymal lesions as shown on magnetic resonance (MR) imaging is highly correlated with the duration of amnesia and the quality of recovery (21). There is evidence that during acceleration-deceleration injury extreme stress is placed on the reticular formation and the brainstem (3, 17). Obviously, potentially dangerous effects on the lower brainstem structures may result from swelling and the deleterious effects on vital functions (19). A common cause of death in more severe CHIs is increased intracranial pressure (4). The contusions and strains caused by the impact are considered to be the direct effects of the trauma to the brain, while the complications involving hematoma and edema are secondary effects that lead to clinical manifestations that require closely supervised observation and medical management (4, 17, 19).

## LEFT AND RIGHT HEMISPHERIC FUNCTION

In the cortex, it is well known that the two cerebral hemispheres serve different functions. The left hemisphere is commonly associated with learning fine motor movements in 90% of right-handed individuals (4, 5). The left hemisphere is also considered the dominant hemisphere for development of language. The auditory cortex of the left hemisphere is greater in size and is responsible for language development and verbal processes. Left-handed individuals, however, have less left hemisphere dominance for language (approximately 60% with the other 40% having some right hemisphere dominance for language). It has been estimated that approximately 80% of left-handed individuals have some degree of language function in both cerebral hemispheres. The left hemisphere also mediates the numerical symbol system and the ability to perform abstract calculations. In summary, the left cerebral hemisphere is involved in reading and writing, speech, verbal memory, and complex logical analysis of information processing (4, 5).

The right hemisphere, often referred to as the nondominant hemisphere in right-handed people, is more commonly associated with processing and storage of nonverbal information, including visual information, shapes and forms, and perception of spatial orientation and perspective. The right hemisphere functions in calculations involving a characteristic spatial organization as opposed to the left hemisphere's linear format for computation. Damage to the right hemisphere may result in defects in visual-motor ability, construction of form in manual tasks, and perception. The right hemisphere therefore has a superior capacity for spatial concepts and synthesizing information in a holistic manner (4, 5).

Emotional differences in the left and right hemispheres have been shown to be characteristic of patients suffering lateralized brain injury. Damage to the left hemisphere is often associated with intense anxiety and catastrophic reaction with recognition of loss of normal function. Depression is also often associated with injury to the left hemisphere. Damage to the right hemisphere is often associated with an apathetic response and a seeming inability to appreciate subtle emotional responses considered to be normal for particular situations. Right hemisphere injury is therefore correlated with an inability to synthesize limbic control and appropriate emotional response to environmental demands (4, 5, 19).

## TEMPORAL-LIMBIC REGIONS

During injury to the side of the head, the temporal lobes are often concussed against the rigid encasement of the middle fossa. When this occurs, the hippocampal functions are disturbed, creating difficulty for retrieval of memory through the limbic system. Consolidation of stimuli into memory is often disturbed. If the damage is not permanent, the memory process returns to normal over a period of time. These effects are often evidenced by the period of retrograde and anterograde amnesia common in concussion. Memory is mediated by the cortex, which catalogs and stores visual, verbal, and tactile memory, in association with the limbic system, which is responsible for registering, storing, and retrieving information for the complete memory process. Memory function is commonly referred to in evaluation as immediate memory, recent memory, and remote or long-term memory (4, 5).

## FRONTAL-LIMBIC REGIONS

Frontal lobe injury presents with or without intact intelligence. Frontal injury often results in an inability to plan ahead or judge the consequences of one's actions, affective lability, lack of insight, and a loss of social inhibitions or spontaneity. The process of concentration requires a voluntary conscious effort in order to sustain attention. This process originates in the frontal area of the cortex and is mediated through the limbic system. This region is involved in an individual's ability to screen out extraneous stimuli in the environment. The process of attention and concentration requires an intact limbic system, intact ascending activating tracts from the reticular formation into the cortex, and intact frontal lobes. Damage in any of these three areas results in impaired attention and concentration. Such impairment obviously would affect memory and ability to function in a logical and efficient manner when a high degree of concentration and attention is required for performance (4, 5, 19, 22).

## FRONTAL LOBES

Much has been written about the frontal lobe syndrome (which is described later in this chapter). The frontal lobes are responsible for a variety of emotional and interpretive functions. Emotional lability and irritability reflect frontal lobe injury. A patient may demonstrate apathy, euphoria, and social inappropriateness. The frontal lobes serve as mediators between the limbic system and the cortex for balancing emotional expression. The prefrontal regions are responsible for aspects of the personality as well as judgment, decision-making ability, and abstract thinking and analysis. Injury to the frontal lobes may manifest in the individual's difficulty in distinguishing right from wrong, formulating proper business and work functions, or analyzing abstract concepts. Some patients with frontal lobe injury may develop phobic-type reactions in public, resort to isolation, or dwell obsessively on prior life experiences (22).

## VISUAL-EXTRAOCULAR REGIONS

Following cervical trauma and often in CHI, patients may complain of diplopia, which usually results from abnormal eye movements. The trochlear, oculomotor, and abducens cranial nerves may be affected. The oculomotor nerve is often injured in head trauma either at the nucleus in the midbrain or peripherally. Transient diplopia probably reflects extraocular incoordination secondary to traction on the muscles during the trauma. Photophobia is also a very common complaint following head injury, and probably results from autonomic disruption to the pupil causing it to have abnormal dilation and a hypersensitivity to bright light (23).

## ACOUSTIC NERVE AND INNER EAR

The complaint of dizziness is very common in the first week following head injury. Electronystagmographic, caloric, and audiographic findings have been reported in patients complaining of postconcussion dizziness. An intact acoustic nerve and labyrinth system are required in the normal process of hearing and equilibrium. Patients also complain of increased sensitivity to loud noises. This may be due to stretching of the stapedius muscle, which is attached to the vestibule and the stapes. The tensor tympani extends from the eustachian tube and attaches to the malleus. These muscles may suffer from the effects of traction forces on them during the injury, resulting in patient complaints of difficulty in hearing, tinnitus, and disequilibrium (24).

## NEUROPATHOLOGY OF MHI AND CONCUSSION

Brain injury is followed by the succession of three major physiologic events: (*a*) a period of shock or diaschisis, (*b*) a period of recovery, and (*c*) a chronic impairment that reflects a locus in the tissue damaged. In severe trauma, considerable torsional and shearing forces create damage at the level of the deep white matter of the cerebral hemispheres and at the level of the upper brainstem, primarily the midbrain. The brainstem reticular formation is often disturbed in these injuries, resulting in deep coma and symptoms of severe neurologic abnormality (25).

This chapter will focus on the neuropathology of MHI and the available (minimal) literature indicating physiologic damage found to occur in whiplash injuries. In milder head injuries, investigations have found small capillary hemorrhages, surface shearing, contusion, and injured nerve fiber tracts to be the basic causes of neuronal dysfunction and distortion of synaptic connections (1).

The current evidence supports the use of the model referred to as shear-strain for explaining the microscopic lesions in the brainstem and in the area of the rostral pyramids (3). Experimental studies of shear-strain injury caused by acceleration-deceleration and rotational forces have led to confirmation of various physiologic and morphologic explanations for the effects seen in MHI and concussion (20).

Because the majority of damage in milder injuries occurs at a microscopic level following concussion, computed tomography (CT) scans and MR images may appear normal. Some studies of autopsied patients who died from multiple injuries and were considered to have mild head trauma have produced evidence of numerous "retraction balls" representing axonal damage in addition to small clusters of hypertrophied microglia. Fiber tracts have also been detected showing specific damage along the fiber tract path associated with the shear force occurring during the trauma (26). Various theories and degrees of cerebral disconnection in the central nervous system have been proposed as explanations for the long-term neuropsychological and postconcussive symptoms seen following milder trauma (1, 20, 26).

Secondary effects dependent upon the degree of injury are commonly observed following trauma. Intracranial hypertension may occur and create distortion and displacement of the hemispheres and enlargement of the cerebral ventricles. Undue pressure may be applied in a downward direction on the brainstem formation. Ischemic changes may affect circulation in the brain, including that in the occipital cortex and hippocampus and anteriorly between the middle and anterior cerebral arteries. Fat embolism and subarachnoid hemorrhage may develop, contributing to further secondary changes that can create a neurosurgical emergency (19). A lengthy discussion of the secondary changes is beyond the scope of this chapter, but the topic can be reviewed in other sources (19).

## EXPERIMENTAL MODELS OF NEUROPATHOLOGY FOLLOWING MILD HEAD INJURY

Because mild concussion is not typically associated with mortality, there are few morphopathologic and histopathologic studies available for investigation of neurologic substrates involved in minor head injury. Experimental models utilizing animals—in particular monkeys—have attempted to simulate acceleration-deceleration injuries typical of human accidents, such as automobile accidents and other forms of concussion. Extensive experimental studies in the cat using a fluid-percussion model of experimental brain injury have been done in recent years in order to assess the microscopic damage to neural tissue. In these studies, the degree of impact in concussion can be accurately controlled by the researchers, who can create a range of injury from mild to severe (27).

These experimental studies show, unfortunately, that even minor injury causes immediate and irrevocable axonal damage following CHI. Research by Povlishock and Coburn (27) has shown that, following minor injury, damaged axons react with swelling although surrounding parenchyma and vessels may not necessarily be altered. The researchers speculated that diffuse axonal damage contributes to the disconnection in the central nervous system pathways that underlies neurobehavioral abnormalities seen in these MHI subjects. These studies are quite significant in that they suggest that axons are possibly more vulnerable to the effects of shear-strain forces than other tissues and that the direct tearing of focal axons is not required for evidence of injury. It appears that axonal damage may occur without evidence of proximal abnormalities in parenchymal tissue, intraparenchymal tissue, or nearby vasculature. Thus trauma may cause disruption of axonal function without actually tearing the membrane. Disruption of function may trigger deafferentation, leading to neurobiologic consequences that may disrupt communication of nerve fibers and neurotransmission. This disruption and disconnection of the central nervous system pathways has been considered the major underlying morphologic substrate that leads to the behavioral and clinical abnormalities described following minor CHI.

Traditionally, neurophysiology researchers have proposed that a regenerative effort would not occur following injury in the brain because of axonal disruption and probable cell death. Povlishock and Coburn found that some of the injured axons did degenerate and die, although others were found to show a regenerative effort through sprouting (27). The authors have proposed that the recovery seen following MHI may indeed be due to the sustained sprouting and growth cone formation similar to regeneration seen in the peripheral nerves. In milder injuries with known axonal damage but without injury to related microtissue, this regeneration may explain the recovery phase following mild head injury, which, as Levin et al. (28) have shown, averages approximately 3 months.

## NEUROCHEMICAL STUDIES

Neurochemical studies in MHI have indicated that loss of consciousness following concussion may be attributable to binding of acetylcholine to muscarinic receptors. The rostral pons has been found to be the brain region associated with the components of behavioral suppression seen in unconsciousness following concussion. The research of Hayes and coworkers (29) provides extensive support for the role of the cholinergic systems in the symptoms following concussion. In their research, they have attempted pharmacologic blockade of cholinergic systems to study the effects on coma. It appears that anticholinergic antagonists can affect the level of behavioral suppression seen in concussion. Their use of scopolamine 15 min prior to trauma significantly reduced mortality and the duration of unconsciousness. They cite evidence that mechanical brain injury and injury to the spinal cord can result in increased levels of acetylcholine in both the cerebrospinal fluid and the brain. The increased levels of acetylcholine are considered to be injurious to tissue, thereby effecting higher degrees of injury and increased likelihood of poor clinical outcome.

In summary, this research suggests that the temporary unconsciousness and resultant syndrome common to concussion is due to increases in activity within the inhibitory neural systems in the brain. Long-term behavioral deficits may result from widespread excitation of neurons produced by excessive release of acetylcholine and other excitatory neurotransmitters following CHI (29).

## NEUROPATHOLOGY IN WHIPLASH INJURY WITHOUT KNOWN IMPACT TO THE HEAD

Objective scientific evidence has documented that whiplash injuries can create diffuse damage in brainstem tissue. Early research by Unterharnscheidt and Higgins (30) showed, in precisely controlled studies with monkeys, that graded acceleration-deceleration injuries could produce damage throughout the central nervous system. Their investigations of rotational acceleration forces produced lesions in the brain as well as throughout the entire length of the spinal cord, including the cauda equina. Trauma was applied in a controlled manner that produced nondeforming tensile forces on the skull that were thought to be similar to the trauma produced in cervical whiplash injuries. Cortical layers were found to have subdural and subarachnoid hemorrhages, with tearing and avulsion of veins and arteries. Rhectic hemorrhages in cranial nerves were observed in addition to small hemorrhages throughout the entire length of the spine. Differences in the degree of injury were found to be associated with angular acceleration as compared to cortical contusions found in translational trauma. It was concluded that rotational acceleration of the head produced lesions in the brain and throughout the length of the spinal cord, providing support for more recent research by Wilmot et al. (15) and Davidoff et al. (14) in which concomitant CHI was found to occur in association with spinal cord injuries.

Electroencephalography (EEG) has been used extensively in the clinical evaluation of cervical trauma patients and victims of CHI. Common postconcussional complaints that also are frequently seen following whiplash injuries (headaches, dizziness, nausea, and vomiting) have been associated with mild EEG abnormalities. Some authors have recommended EEG as a serial follow-up evaluation to monitor mild brain abnormalities (31). Specific abnormalities include depressive, irritative, or epileptic changes. Torres and Shapiro (32) compared EEG studies of patients suffering from whiplash injuries with EEGs of patients with CHI. The possible mechanisms for these abnormalities were summarized as "1) direct influence on the brain tissue by acceleration and deceleration; 2) injury to the brain as the head and neck move rapidly backward and forward, occurring as the brain hits the inner table of the skull; [and] 3) acute and chronic vascular insufficiency produced by constriction or occlusion of one or both vertebral arteries as they traverse the vertebral foramina in the cervical region." Arterial occlusion and compression of vertebral arteries have been reported as a complication of acceleration-deceleration injuries by many authors (30–32). It has been proposed that this compression may lead to insufficiency in the territories of the basilar and posterior cerebral arteries (32).

Experiments utilizing implanted subcortical electrodes in addition to surface EEG electrodes demonstrated that the "whiplash syndrome" is in part due to electrophysiologic changes, and that at the time of subcortical onset of EEG abnormalities (6–8 weeks) surface EEG recordings were normal. Hippocampal spiking was proposed in these studies as a subclinical form of posttraumatic epilepsy (33). Schoenhuber and Gentilini (34) cautioned that even in moderate or severe head injuries there is no strong correlation between persistent EEG abnormalities and patients' subjective complaints. Abnormal EEG readings do not necessarily demonstrate evidence for an organic basis for symptoms. Auditory brainstem responses have been used in recent years as a means for evaluating symptoms following concussion, yet there is insufficient literature available to describe the utility of these responses in support of damage following whiplash injury (34).

The effects of rapid acceleration-deceleration injury on blood vessel permeability have been attributed to distortion of vessels in the brainstem and upper cervical spinal cord. There is also evidence that cerebrospinal fluid may be forced into the cisterna magna and subarachnoid space. Some researchers believe that practically all head injuries involve some degree of hyperextension-hyperflexion to the cervical spine at the time of impact. Therefore, it is possible that the whiplash component could play a major part in the symptoms found following head trauma, such as coma (35).

As evidence continues to accumulate in support of the shear-strain model as the basis for explanation of symptoms common in MHI, perhaps more attention will also be paid to the combined effects of cervical trauma and minor brain injury. It is the opinion of the authors that continued conceptualization of whiplash injury and MHI as two separate and distinct entities by the medical profession will only perpetuate the confusing clinical symptoms and management problem characteristic of these patients.

## ASSESSMENT OF OCCULT HEAD INJURY

### ESTIMATING DEGREE OF SEVERITY FOLLOWING ACUTE CHI

Evaluation of the severity of acute CHI is a difficult task. Duration of unconsciousness and depth of coma are used as indicators of severity. Prolonged unconsciousness lasting over 6 hr typically leads to a progression of complicating symptoms. Rate of recovery and prognosis is related to various clinical symptoms, including oculovestibular defect, pupillary abnormalities, abnormal motor response, EEG slowing and paradoxical arousal, and CT abnormalities suggesting hematoma, in-

creased intracranial pressure, or other conditions (5, 19, 28).

According to reports by Levin et al. (28), early neurobehavioral symptoms may represent diffuse axonal injury, alteration of neurotransmitters, and occult intracerebral lesions undetected typically by CT scanning. Their reports indicate that MR imaging may visualize acute intracranial lesions that are not present on CT scan. Vestibular disturbance involving the labyrinth and temporary changes in the superficial cranial vessels may contribute to the manifestation of postconcussion symptoms.

## ASSESSING LEVEL OF CONSCIOUSNESS

Traditionally the severity of a CHI was estimated by the presence and duration of coma. The Glasgow Coma Scale, developed by Teasdale and Jennett (36), is a systematic and reliable tool for assessing the degree of impairment in consciousness based on observations of eye movements, motor response, and verbal response (Table 26.2). A score of 7 or less defines coma, 9 or more is not comatose, and 53% of those with a score of 8 are comatose (19). An initial score of 13 to 15 defines mild brain injury.

## DURATION OF LOSS OF CONSCIOUSNESS

Duration of loss of consciousness (LOC) has long been used as an index of severity of brain injury. Lewin (37) documented the poor outcome of pa-

**Table 26.2.**
**Glasgow Coma Scale[a]**

| Dimension | | Score |
|---|---|---|
| Eyes open | Spontaneously | 4 |
| | To speech | 3 |
| | To pain | 2 |
| | Not at all | 1 |
| Best verbal response | Oriented | 5 |
| | Confused | 4 |
| | Inappropriate | 3 |
| | Incomprehensible | 2 |
| | None | 1 |
| Best motor response | Obeys commands | 4 |
| | Localizes pain | 3 |
| | Flexion to pain | 2 |
| | None | 1 |

[a]From Teasdale G, Jennett B: Assessment of coma and impaired consciousness: a practical scale. *Lancet* 2:81–84, 1974.

tients unconscious for more than a month. A MHI is usually indicated by a LOC of less than 20 min.

It has been suggested by Jennett and Teasdale (19) that a severity digit for head injury be added to several ICD codes. Duration of LOC could be used to index severity for code 850 (concussion), 800 (Fracture of Vault of Skull), 851 (Cerebral Laceration and Contusion), 852 (Subarachnoid, Subdural, and Extradural Hemorrhage), 853 (Other and Unspecified Intracranial Hemorrhage), and 854 (Intracranial Injury of Other and Unspecified Nature).

## POSTTRAUMATIC AMNESIA

The period of posttraumatic amnesia (PTA) is not always easy to assess and it is certainly not always absolute. Following injury, patients have dramatic fluctuations in memory for the traumatic event, along with confused behavior and lucid periods that may leave partial memories for the accident. This "spotty" memory for the injury does create difficulty in assessment, yet PTA is the most useful clinical measure of severity of injury following trauma. Russell (18) has shown the clinical usefulness of assessing PTA as an index of the existence and severity of CHI in spinal cord–injured patients. It was observed that the last obvious step in regaining full consciousness was restoration of ongoing (anterograde) memory. The interval between the CHI and the return of speech is about one fourth of the interval between the CHI and the end of PTA; the latter correlates with the end of spatial disorientation (19). The duration of PTA is directly related to objective neurologic findings (19, 38), personality changes and psychiatric disability (9, 39), and the time it takes to return a patient to work (39).

The duration of PTA is defined as the time from the injury until the patient is able to recall events on a day-to-day basis. The following expanded scale by Jennett and Teasdale (19) is useful for classifying the severity of a patient's injury according to the span of time the patient requires to recall the injury:

Less than 5 min—very mild
5–60 min—mild
1–24 hr—moderate
1–7 days—severe
1–4 weeks—very severe
More than 4 weeks—extremely severe

Logically, any LOC creates at least an equal PTA. However, a patient may show PTA without LOC, suggesting the former is potentially more sensitive. Research evidence verifies the sensitivity of PTA. Davidoff and associates (14) found that 35% of spinal cord injury patients were falsely negative for CHI when assessed by duration of LOC but were positive when assessed by duration of PTA. As Jennett and Teasdale (19) pointed out:

Amnesia for even a few minutes after a blow to the head is evidence of diffuse brain damage. The duration of this PTA normally exceeds by a considerable margin the length of time for which the patient was regarded as unconscious, because it includes the time during which he was awake but confused. Football players are familiar with the phenomenon of the player who resumes the game after a brief concussion, who responds to situations appropriately and may even play confidently, but who subsequently has no memory at all of that part of the game. A period of PTA is not infrequently discovered on close questioning of patients whom reliable witnesses report never to have been unconscious at all after the injury. . . . there are many instances of patients recorded by doctors as having been fully conscious, who have no subsequent memory of this encounter at all.

Lishman (9, 40) has used PTA as a predictor of cognitive loss and capability of return to work. His studies of psychiatric sequelae following CHI led to the following time frame for return to work:

1. PTA less than one hour = return to work in one month
2. PTA less than one day = return to work in two months
3. PTA less than one week = return to work in four months
4. PTA greater than one week = loss of work for one year or more

Davidoff et al. (14) have shown PTA to be superior to LOC as an index of CHI in patients with acute spinal cord injury. Yet PTA is assessed in only 14–22% of cases, and radiographic workup of the head is not performed consistently. This is difficult to understand since PTA is easily evaluated. A standard protocol for assessing PTA is the Galveston Orientation and Amnesia Test (GOAT) developed by Levin et al. (41). It can be administered within 10 min by nursing staff, and, if administered on admission and daily until the patient achieves a score of 90 or above, it will give a reliable index of the severity of CHI. A score of 66 or less indicates that the patient is not encoding new memory for daily events and thus continues to experience ongoing PTA.

Duration of LOC is useful as a supplement to

the GOAT because it can be obtained from witnesses to the injury, emergency medical service personnel, and police reports. It should correlate with the PTA assessment obtained from the patient. Since multiple etiologies are possible for PTA (e.g., hypoxia, alcohol ingestion, medication effects), these should be considered when PTA is present without LOC.

## DEFICITS IN HIGHER COGNITIVE FUNCTIONING

### INTELLECTUAL DEFICITS

Tests of intelligence are easily obtained for patients but are limited in their usefulness and potentially misleading. Since part of what is measured by an intelligence test is overlearned verbal information (skills often spared by mild CHI), a patient's performance in this area is often a better indication of premorbid functioning than of current deficit. Focal damage to the dominant hemisphere (possibly unrelated to the CHI), as well as cultural and educational limitations, can lower the patient's performance on the verbal portion of the test.

Nonverbal tests depend heavily on visuospatial abilities and manual manipulation of materials. Performance on these tests is much more independent of educational and cultural background, but significantly declines in the elderly, leaving a restricted range of possible values to assess deficits in the older patient. More importantly, performance on these tests can be impaired by any one or more of the following: perceptual deficits in the nondominant hemisphere, central or peripheral impairment in the use of the upper extremities, and general cognitive or psychomotor slowing (since most are timed). If academic records or previous ability test scores (from high school, college, armed forces, etc.) are available, they can help to clarify the interpretation of the patient's present scores. Still, intelligence tests tap skills that are largely in the posterior cortex, and some CHI patients will do surprisingly well.

The research setting allows some clarification of these multiple influences on IQ scores to reveal general trends in intellectual deficits and recovery. Verbal abilities are more resistant to decline and recover more rapidly, with maximum improvement 3–6 months following injury. Nonverbal intellectual performance continues to improve for 12 months or more (19). A minor CHI may not produce changes in IQ that can be clearly

attributed to the CHI in an individual case because of the multiple influences on performance discussed above and the fact that a test of intelligence is simply not designed to detect acquired deficits in specific cognitive functions. The commercial neuropsychological test battery standardized on general neurology patients tends to emphasize functions that may underestimate the subtle cognitive deficits of a minor CHI (4). Detection of acquired deficits in these patients is most sensitively done by an experienced neuropsychologist.

### DEFICITS IN JUDGMENT, REASONING, AND COMPLEX PROBLEM SOLVING

In reviewing deficits in specific cognitive functions, it must be remembered that CHI deficits in specific functions are seen as points of emphasis against a background of diffuse dysfunction. Also, defects in high-level concept formation and reasoning can result from diffuse damage, but are associated with more severe injuries and thus less likely in the mild CHI cervical patient (4). Still, Rimel and associates (17) examined 424 mild CHI patients at 3 months after injury and found deficits in higher level cognitive functioning, novel problem solving, and attention and concentration in spite of the fact that only 2% had positive neurologic exams.

Deficits are apparent on tests requiring the patient to concentrate, rapidly shift attention, quickly notice stimulus changes, solve novel problems, and formulate abstract concepts (1, 2, 4, 19). Arithmetic reasoning may be affected, but this may simply appear poor as a result of difficulty in mentally tracking the sequential steps needed to arrive at a correct solution. Patients show confusion with elements of orally presented questions and feel uncertain about the correctness of their answers (4). It has been suggested that in mild CHI these higher cortical functions actually remain intact but are difficult to utilize efficiently in novel or distracting settings (42).

### MEMORY DEFICITS

The temporal lobes are in an anatomic position of high risk in a CHI. It is not surprising that patients frequently complain of memory difficulty even after the period of PTA. Since the degree of temporal lobe damage correlates with the severity of the CHI, the mild CHI cervical patient can be expected to show mild symptoms (4). It should also be considered that a patient with deficits in attention, concentration, and/or perception may have faulty initial registration and consolidation of the information to be remembered. Inertia, impaired learning ability, and/or retrieval problems can present as a complaint of poor memory. Careful assessment will determine the underlying problem (4). Retrieval problems tend to relate to specific verbal or visuospatial deficits (rare in mild CHI patients).

It is useful to distinguish between short-term and long-term memory when assessing a patient. Jennett and Teasdale (19) offered the following neurophysiological explanation:

> It is believed that short-term memory depends on neurophysiological (electrical) processes, while the finite time required for imprinting a permanent image indicates a chemical event, probably involving protein synthesis. Failure of recall may be because the "memory" was never imprinted, or has decayed, or cannot be retrieved. Sometimes cueing can release a memory that was temporarily inaccessible, suggesting that it was loss of the address to an intact imprint that was the explanation of the memory difficulty in such cases. In patients with prolonged retrograde amnesia, the usual recovery of much of the memory of events that happened prior to the injury indicates that this was a retrieval defect. By contrast there is always a permanent loss of memory for a short period immediately prior to impact, the trace of those happenings presumably never having been imprinted. This is certainly the case with post-traumatic amnesia.

In spite of memory complaints, simple tests of immediate memory may be performed within normal limits by the CHI patient (similar to the demented patient) because it involves only immediate recall. It is an interesting parallel that demented patients also have generalized cortical deficits, but the chief complaint is usually memory. It may be that, as an end behavior, functional memory is so complex and demands so much from so many areas of both cortex and subcortex that generalized brain deficits are most apparent as memory dysfunction. Moving to an unfamiliar setting and lack of structure make the deficit more apparent. The patient and family should be told to keep the home environment unchanged at least until the maximum recovery period has passed. Having the patient keep a notebook in which to record a daily schedule and list of things to do will greatly reduce the effect on day-to-day life. Most mild CHI patients will be sufficiently intact to maintain their own notebook or daily schedule for activities.

## DEFICITS IN ATTENTION, CONCENTRATION, PROCESSING SPEED, AND MENTAL TRACKING

The mild CHI patient's attention span may be impaired. Often this deficit can be demonstrated by poor ability to repeat a series of digits. This function recovers quickly, reaching a plateau within the first 6–12 months after injury. The ability to learn new information recovers more slowly (4). Other studies have used a variety of tests or batteries of tests, but found similar results: only mild deficits in sustained attention and memory by 1–3 months following injury (43). It is important to remember that attention and concentration may also be impaired by severe pain and analgesic medication. These factors must be considered in the patient who is showing a prolonged period of recovery.

Diffuse damage is readily apparent on tests requiring the patient to mentally keep track of information over a period of time. Examples include a timed, nonpictorial, connect-the-dots task or orally administered arithmetic problems that must be computed without the aid of pencil and paper. These tasks involve both maintaining information from a previous step in the sequence to the next and at the same time maintaining the problem-solving strategy (4).

## PROCESSING SPEED

Slowed thinking and reaction times are apparent when the patient is given a test demanding accuracy within a time limit. These deficits may put the patient at risk of injury when operating dangerous machinery (such as driving a car) and at risk for poor productivity if returned to work too soon. A test commonly used to assess processing speed and tracking ability is the Paced Auditory Serial Addition Test (PASAT).

The PASAT is a neuropsychological technique of sufficient difficulty that it is particularly useful for documenting the frequent complaints of loss of concentration in mild CHI patients. Of patients with mild concussion, half are normal on this test within 2 weeks and 90% by 35 days, and the rest are complicated by complaints of post-concussional syndrome (19). More recent research suggests that the direct effect of mild CHI on concentration dissipates by 3 months after injury even in postconcussional syndrome. Yet a mild physiologic stress (hypoxia associated with being at a high altitude) has been found to reproduce the neuropsychological deficits even as long as 1 year following injury (4, 19). These findings suggest that, although there may be an apparent remission of symptoms, a degree of fragility remains. The deficits may reappear as a result of a broad range of physiologic stressors (e.g., medication, alcohol, insomnia, and nutritional factors) that should be considered by the clinician faced with a patient showing slow recovery or a return of symptoms.

## EMOTIONAL, PSYCHOSOCIAL, AND PERSONALITY CHANGES

It is a very difficult task to attempt to evaluate and compare a cervical trauma victim's premorbid personality and psychological makeup to the patient's psychological reactions and characteristics following trauma. Measurement of psychological variables is fraught with controversy even among clinical psychologists and psychiatrists.

Rutherford (6) has proposed a model of viewing the postconcussion syndrome in terms of early and late symptoms. Early symptoms have been identified as those complaints immediately following trauma, including headache, dizziness, vomiting, nausea, drowsiness, and blurred vision. Late symptoms are those that are reported weeks following trauma. Late symptoms may include headache, dizziness, irritability, anxiety, depression, memory complaints, concentration problems, insomnia, fatigue, and other symptoms that imply psychological disorder. It is suggested that late symptoms are caused by interaction between organic and neurotic factors.

Depression is one of the more frequent psychological reactions to mild CHI and cervical trauma. The depression may be reactive to the loss of functioning, pain, and even the stress of litigation. Some patients may develop an endogenous depression with a biologic etiology. Symptoms of depression may alternate with periods of agitation and anxiety. Frontal and temporal brain damage have been most often associated with posttraumatic depression. Damage to norepinephrine neurotransmission in the locus ceruleus has been proposed as a mechanism for depression associated with frontal lesions, and a few studies have suggested decreased serotonin. Some patients may have an abnormal sleep pattern that may be detected by a sleep-deprived EEG. Sleep fragmentation, interruption of rapid-eye-movement (REM) sleep, and nonrestorative sleep patterns have been reported following CHI (44).

Fatigue has been proposed as one of the more problematic symptoms that greatly affects the patient's ability to return to work and to function in a normal manner. Wrightson and Gronwall (45) have elaborated on the significance of fatigue and its relation to the patient's ability to work within limits. If the fatigue exceeds a critical level and the patient pushes beyond that level, functional capacity deteriorates, stress accumulates, and other symptoms such as dizziness and headache reappear.

## PERSONALITY CHANGES

Personality changes have been traditionally associated with a frontal lobe syndrome that may follow CHI. [There are numerous other sources for a detailed review, such as Kolb and Whishaw (25), Luria (22), and Strub and Black (5).] Since the degree of frontal lobe damage correlates with the severity of the injury, the symptoms described in this section may be *mild or nonexistent* in the mild CHI cervical patient.

Injury to the convex lateral surface of the frontal lobe affects intellectual and motor function. Personality changes associated with damage to this area include apathy, lack of drive, and a tendency to approach problems with a stereotypical strategy rather than assessing the situation and selecting an optimum strategy (i.e., lack of restraining oneself from acting on the first obvious strategy in order to evaluate alternatives). It should be remembered that the apathetic patient may report that he or she is doing fine, just as demented patients are usually unaware of any cognitive deficits. Occasionally a patient who was aggressive or overanxious will show personality changes actually seen as a positive "calming down" by the family (4).

Damage to the orbital portion of the frontal lobe produces a personality change involving a different sort of self-restraint problem. This patient shows euphoria, irritability, disinhibition, attention deficits, hyperactivity, sexual indiscretion, and aggression. Usually these changes are simply a nuisance to others, but they can occasionally be so extreme as to lead to criminal acts. The changes can be summarized under the rubric of defects in social restraint and judgment and are usually childish (typical of an 8–10-year-old) in character (19).

Temporal lobe damage may also be associated with change in personality. Some patients develop complex partial seizures associated with personality changes including talkativeness and a tendency toward tedious, detailed speech often described as circumstantiality. Aggressive discontrol may also occur with temporal lobe damage (44).

Personality changes combine with the cognitive sequelae to produce adjustment problems following trauma. In moderate to severe CHI the personality changes are more common and often more disabling than the cognitive changes, although they can be more difficult to objectively measure.

Other personality changes following CHI and the postconcussion syndrome can be attributed to hypersensitivity to alcohol and medications. Patients may exhibit only vague changes in personality but often family members may report unusual behavior and atypical reactions to ingestion of alcohol, resulting in violent outbursts, mood fluctuations, and manifestations of depression. These changes may be brought on by smaller amounts of consumption than that previously required to create the state of intoxication.

In general, a broad range of psychological reactions may occur following cervical trauma. Goldstein (46) made a distinction between symptoms due to direct loss of neurons (i.e., cognitive deficits) and symptoms due to the patient's attempts to compensate for the residuals from the injury (i.e., anxiety, agitation, irritability, social withdrawal, possible embarrassment, depression, etc.). In some cases, CHI may result in traditional psychiatric syndromes such as posttraumatic stress disorder, organic personality disorder, and affective disorders. Patients may also develop a dependency on pain medications or tranquilizers, or meet the criteria for a somatization disorder. The reader is encouraged to review Chapters 6 and 29 for information regarding psychological issues common to victims of cervical trauma and CHI.

## PSYCHOSOCIAL ISSUES

The patient may initially be in a state of emotional upheaval. If there was no PTA to obscure the memory of the accident or if the patient denies the acquired cognitive impairment, then the later development of neurotic symptoms is common (46). Most patients worry about potential for recovery, return to work, and resumption of a normal life-style. The patient's whole identity may be tied to an occupation for which he or she is no longer suited. The cognitive, emotional, and personality changes associated with CHI seriously complicate the patient's ability to deal with these issues. If there are deficits in problem solving, these complex life issues seem even more overwhelming. Conversely, a patient with significant damage to the frontal lobes may have little awareness or concern that a problem even exists.

## FAMILY PROBLEMS

The concerns, conflicts, and emotional upheaval of the patient are often experienced by family members (16). Just as family members are often the first to notice the subtle changes at the onset of a degenerative dementia, they may be more acutely aware of the effects of mild CHI in the patient than are the health care professionals involved. This is particularly true in the patient who has had a brief stay in the hospital before being discharged to the care of the family. The clinician must be prepared to discuss the effects of CHI with concerned family members. A volatile family may need family counseling to adapt to the changes. Conversely, the patient who has a longer hospital stay with less intense family contact may be discharged to a family that is completely unaware of the cognitive changes that have taken place. This family will need education about the effects of CHI and any adjustments they need to make in life-style (who drives the car, balances the checkbook, etc.). A great service can be performed if the patient can be spared the failure experienced in returning to cognitively demanding tasks too soon (e.g., the patient who returns to work, performs below acceptable levels, and is fired). Such a failure can produce a blow to self-esteem that lasts even longer than the effects of the brain injury.

The irritability that is a concomitant of mild CHI tends to keep a degree of friction in the patient's relationships as a backdrop to the above issues. Sensitivity to noise can make the usual din of a house with playful children unbearable to an irritable and hostile patient who finds himself or herself in a constant struggle to keep family members quiet. The family's adjustment is influenced by several factors: the premorbid psychodynamics of the family, the patient's current emotional state (ranging from apathy or lack of awareness to frustration and anger or depression), and the role changes that may have taken place as a result of the injury (e.g., a wife who is now the sole breadwinner, sole parent, and master of the house). The mild CHI patient with no visible symptoms may be treated with suspicion by outsiders (particularly if litigation is involved) while the family closes ranks in total support of the patient's complaints. Once the situation becomes chronic, the change of roles and the emotional support that is contingent on complaint both persist via the law of inertia. They can create a perpetual identity of patienthood for the injured party without psychological intervention.

## WORK

Rimel and associates (17) studied patients with spinal cord injury and minor CHI (LOC of 20 min or less). At 3 months following injury 59% of the patients complained of memory disturbance and 34% of those previously employed had failed to return to work. A significant number also complained of fatigue, headache, vertigo, and an inability to drive an automobile. Since Davidoff et al. (14) have shown that the level of spinal cord injury has no relationship to CHI, fingings should be similar for cervical patients with mild CHI. A potential complication to returning the patient to work is the fact that 5% of CHI patients will develop epilepsy, the second leading cause of occupational difficulty (36). The most common type in these patients is temporal lobe epilepsy, and its presence is likely to further complicate the patient's emotional adjustment (10).

At the very least, the common irritability and difficulties in memory and concentration will interfere with performance on the typical job. Indeed, if the patient has lived a sheltered life from the time of injury until returning to work these difficulties may not be apparent until work becomes demanding. Thus, the patient may not attribute job difficulties directly to the effects of the CHI, but instead may attribute them to time away from the job or the like. The more mentally demanding the patient's job (such as the computer programmer discussed above) the more likely work performance will be impaired. Thus, the higher the premorbid function the greater the occupational disability when returning to the same occupation. A similar observation has been made by Kolb and Whishaw (25) in that bright patients are acutely aware of the loss of cognitive function that is preventing a return to a premorbid level of competence.

## RECOVERY

Following cervical trauma associated with mild cognitive impairment, the course of recovery may be difficult and is often unpredictable. Although the patient may have physical symptoms associated with cervical injury, cognitive deficits may not be apparent to friends, family members, coworkers, or supervisors. The patient's expectations of recovery, in addition to the expectations of family members, may be confused and this may set the stage for conflict. Cervical trauma victims may not have initial explanations for their cognitive deficits unless there is an associated head injury. In the case in which there is not direct impact to the head, cognitive deficits may lead to feelings of insecurity and the full expression of the postconcussion syndrome may develop and continue to complicate rehabilitation. The postconcussion symptoms may occur whenever environmental demands exceed cognitive capacities for dealing effectively with the demands.

Research by Dikmen and associates (43) presents evidence that suggests that many mild CHI patients continue to have major life disruption 1 month following the injury. Fortunately, most cases of MHI have shown recovery in approximately 3 months (28). Dikmen et al. identified the tendency for these patients to have postconcussional complaints that exceed symptoms expected based upon the degree of neuropsychological impairment found upon evaluation. Although patients in their group were considered to be mildly impaired, at 1 month they continued to report a high degree of posttraumatic symptoms.

A return to work and resumption of leisure activities is also hampered by the combined effects of the cervical trauma and the MHI. Data collected on patients following MHI also failed, as one might expect, to show a return to work within 1 month following injury. Most patients in this group resumed leisure and recreational activities but with limitations. The majority of patients returned to work and had completely resumed social activities within a 1-year period (Table 26.3).

It is often helpful to caution patients that postconcussion symptoms are expected and will often occur if they attempt to push too hard or are under stress. Symptoms of headache and dizziness should be anticipated as a natural consequence of the injury. The stress and fatigue cycle should be explained thoroughly. When an exacerbation of postconcussion symptoms does occur, it is important to caution the patient that cognitive capabilities as well as the ability to cope with the sequelae of the injury are being overwhelmed by expectations and external demands. In other words, attempts to recover too rapidly and return to com-

**Table 26.3.**
**Resumption of Major and Other Activities**[a]

| Modified Function Status Index | One Month | One Year |
|---|---|---|
| *Return to major activity* | | |
| With no limitations | 4 | 15 |
| With limitations | 4 | 2 |
| No return | 9 | 2[b] |
| Could not determine—summer | 2 | 0 |
| *Resumption of leisure/recreational activity* | | |
| With no limitations | 3 | 12 |
| With limitations | 15 | 6 |
| No resumption | 1 | 0 |
| No resumption, not injury related | 0 | 1 |

[a]From Dikmen SS, McClean A, Tempkin N: Neuropsychological and psychosocial consequences of minor head injury. *J Neurol Neurosurg Psychiatry* 49:1227–1232, 1986.
[b]One of the two head injury patients who had not returned at one year had problems that were not head injury related.

plete premorbid functioning might encourage an increase in symptoms and result in frustration for both the physician and the patient.

When symptoms of the acute stage of concussion and the cervical trauma have subsided considerably and the patient is amenable to further evaluation, it is often helpful to pursue a complete neuropsychological evaluation. The neuropsychological assessment should provide useful information regarding the patient's deficits and the effects the deficits will have on recovery. The purpose of the evaluation should be explained to the patient as well as the family. The information contained in the evaluation should provide insight into the patient's combined emotional and neuropsychological condition. Reevaluation of the patient's cognitive status at subsequent intervals allows for predictions in recovery as well as provision of a time frame for resumption of vocational and other activities. In more severe cases, the evaluation may provide recommendations for an individually tailored program such as cognitive retraining. Specific recommendations in the report should address adjustment counseling and the need for referral to a psychologist or psychiatrist. Often the patient can benefit from psychopharmacologic treatment directed toward control of many disturbing symptoms such as depression, anxiety, headache, and insomnia. Some patients may benefit by referral to a concussion clinic or to other community resources associated with various hospitals and universities. Information on re-

sources available in the patient's area may be obtained from the National Head Injury Foundation, Inc., Framingham, MA 01701 (617/879-7473).

## CONCLUSION

When a patient suffers both cervical trauma and associated impairment of brain function, multidisciplinary evaluation and treatment is indicated. One can imagine the problems encountered when the cervical trauma patient develops the chronic pain syndrome. This problem is only compounded when the cervical patient also has minor brain dysfunction. The problems encountered by the mild head injury patient are practically identical to those of the chronic pain patient. Both usually have continued complaints beyond the time expected by the treating physicians. Because of the magnitude of problems and complications common in the recovery process with the combined cervical trauma and head injured patient, an interdisciplinary approach to treatment is encouraged (47).

### REFERENCES

1. Barth JT, Macciocci SN, Giordani B, Rimel R, Jane JA, Boll TJ: Neuropsychological sequelae of minor head injury. *Neurosurgery* 13:529–533, 1983.
2. Rimel RW, Giordani B, Barth JT, Boll TJ, Jane JA: Disability caused by mild head injury. *Neurosurgery* 9:221–228, 1981.
3. Holburn AHS: Mechanics of head injuries. *Lancet* 2:438–441, 1943.
4. Lezak M: *Neuropsychological Assessment.* New York, Oxford University Press, 1983.
5. Strub RL, Black FW: *Organic Brain Syndromes: An Introduction to Neurobehavioral Disorders.* Philadelphia, FA Davis Company, 1982.
6. Rutherford WH: Post concussion symptoms: relationship to acute neurological indices, individual differences, and circumstances of injury. In Levin HS, Eisenberg HM, Benton AL (eds): *Mild Head Injury.* New York, Oxford University Press, 1989.
7. Long CJ, Novack TA: Post concussion symptoms after head trauma: interpretation and treatment. *South Med J* 79:728–732, 1986.
8. *International Classification of Disease—9.* Ann Arbor, MI, Edwards Bros, Inc, 1978.
9. Lishman WA: The psychiatric sequelae of head injury: a review. *Psychol Med* 3:304–318, 1973.
10. American Psychiatric Association: *Diagnostic and Statistical Manual of Mental Disorders,* Washington, DC, APA, 1987.
11. Irving J: Impact of insurance coverage on convalescence and rehabilitation of head injured patients. *Conn Med* 36:385–391, 1972.
12. Kasbeek W, McLaurin R, Harris B, et al: The National Head and Spinal Cord Injury Survey: major findings. *J Neurosurg* 53:519–531, 1980.
13. Davidoff G, Morris J, Roth E, Bleiberg J: Cognitive dysfunction and mild closed head injury in traumatic spinal cord injury. *Arch Phys Med Rehabil* 66:489–491, 1985.

14. Davidoff G, Morris J, Elliott R, Bleiberg J: Closed head injury in spinal cord injured patients: retrospective study of loss of consciousness and post traumatic amnesia. *Arch Phys Med Rehabil* 66:41–42, 1985.

15. Wilmot CB, Cope N, Hall KM, Acker M: Occult head injury: its incidence in spinal cord injury. *Arch Phys Med Rehabil* 66:227–231, 1985.

16. Morris J, Roth E, Davidoff G: Mild closed head injury and cognitive deficits in spinal cord injured patients: incidence and impact. *J Head Trauma Rehabil* 1(2):31–42, 1986.

17. Rimel RW, Jiordani B, Barth JT, Boll TJ, Jane JA: Disability caused by mild head injury. *Neurosurgery* 9:221–228, 1981.

18. Russell WR: Recovery after minor head injury. *Lancet* 2:13–15, 1974.

19. Jennett B, Teasdale G: *Management of Head Injuries.* Philadelphia, FA Davis, 1981.

20. Ommaya AK, Gennarelli TA: Cerebral concussion and traumatic unconsciousness: correlation of experimental and clinical observations on blunt head injuries. *Brain* 97:633–654, 1974.

21. Levin HS, Eisenberg HM, Amparo EG, Williams DH, High WM, Crofford MJ: Depth of parenchymal lesions visualized by magnetic resonance imaging in relation to level of consciousness after closed head injury. Paper presented at the American Association of Neurological Surgeons Meeting, April, 1988, Canada.

22. Luria AR: *The Working Brain.* New York, Basic Books, 1973.

23. Bannister R: *Brain's Clinical Neurology,* ed 5. London, Oxford University Press, 1977.

24. Toglia JU, Rosenberg E, Ronis M: Post traumatic dizziness. *Arch Otolaryngol* 92:485–492, 1970.

25. Kolb B, Whishaw IQ: *Fundamentals of Human Neuropsychology,* ed 2. New York, WH Freeman and Co, 1985.

26. Oppenheimer DR: Microscopic lesions in the brain following head injury. *J Neurol Neurosurg Psychiatry* 31:299–306, 1968.

27. Povlishock JT, Coburn TH: Morphopathological change associated with mild head injury. In Nevin HS, Eiseberg HM, Benton AL (eds): *Mild Head Injury.* New York, Oxford University Press, 1989.

28. Levin HS, Mattis S, Ruff RM, Eisenberg HM, Marshall LT, Tabaddor K, High WM, Frankowski RF: Neurobehavioral outcome following minor head injury: a center study. *J Neurosurg* 66:234–243, 1987.

29. Hayes RL, Lyeth BG, Jenkins LW: Neurochemical mechanisms of mild and moderate head injury: implications for treatment. In Levin HS, Eisenberg HM, Benton AL (eds): *Mild Head Injury.* New York, Oxford University Press, 1989.

30. Unterharnscheidt F, Higgins LS: Traumatic lesions of the brain and spinal cord due to non-deforming angular acceleration of the head. *Texas Rep Biol Med* 27:1, 1969.

31. Gibbs FA: Objective evidence of brain disorder in cases of whiplash injury. *Clin Electroencephalogr* 2(2):107–110, 1971.

32. Torres F, Shapiro S: EEG in whiplash injury. *Arch Neurol* 5:28–35, 1961.

33. Liu YK, Chandran KD, Heath RG, Unterharnscheidt F: Subcortical EEG changes in rhesus monkeys following experimental hyperextension-hyperflexion (whiplash). *Spine* 9:329–338, 1984.

34. Schoenhuber R, Gentilini M: Neurophysiological assessment of mild head injury. In Nevin HS, Eisenberg HM, Benton AL (eds): *Mild Head Injury.* New York, Oxford University Press, 1989.

35. Domer FR, Liu YK, Chandran KB, Krieger KW: Effects of hyperextension-hyperflexion (whiplash) on the function of the blood-brain barrier of rhesus monkeys. *Exp Neurol* 63:304–310, 1979.

36. Teasdale G, Jennett B: Assessment of coma and impaired consciousness. *Lancet* 2:81–84, 1974.

37. Lewin W: The management of prolonged unconsciousness after head injury. *Proc R Soc Med* 52:880–884, 1959.

38. Smith A: Duration of impaired consciousness as an index of severity in closed head injuries: a review. *Dis Nerv System* 22:69–74, 1961.

39. Steadman JH, Graham JG: Head injuries: an analysis and follow up study. *Proc R Soc Med* 633:23–28, 1970.

40. Lishman WA: Brain damage in relation to psychiatric disability after head injury. *Br J Psychiatry* 114:373–410, 1968.

41. Levin HS, O'Donnell VW, Grossman RG: Galveston Orientation and Amnesia Test: practical scale to assess cognition after head injury. *J Nerv Ment Dis* 167:675–684, 1979.

42. Schwartz DP, Barth JT, Dane JR, Drennan SE, DeGood DE, Rowlingson JC: Cognitive deficits in chronic pain patients with and without history of head/neck injury: development of a brief screening battery. *Clin J Pain* 3:94–101, 1987.

43. Dikmen SS, Temkin N, Armsden G: Neuropsychological recovery: relationship to psychosocial functioning and post concussional complaints. In Levin HS, Eisenberg HM, Benton AL (eds): *Mild Head Injury.* New York, Oxford University Press, 1989.

44. Kwentus JA, Hart RP, Heck ET, Cornstein S: Psychiatric complications of closed head trauma. *Psychosomatics* 26:8–17, 1985.

45. Wrightson P, Gronwall D: Time off work and symptoms after minor head injury. *Injury* 12:445–454, 1981.

46. Goldstein K: The effect of brain damage on the personality. *Psychiatry* 15:245–260, 1952.

47. Golden CJ, Moses JA Jr, Coffman JA, Miller WR, Strider FD: *Clinical Neuropsychology: Interface with Neurologic and Psychiatric Disorders.* Orlando, FL, Grune & Stratton, 1983.

# MEDICAL-LEGAL ISSUES

## 27

# PSYCHOSOCIOECONOMIC IMPACT OF CHRONIC CERVICAL PAIN

*Paul Leung*

The title of this chapter suggests a subject straightforward enough and relatively easy to present, yet the chapter was a struggle to put together because a litany of potential such impacts would be numbing for the reader. This chapter reflects much of the difficulty associated with the state of clinical work related to chronic pain. It would be difficult to say that the impact of pain is not important, and few would deny the potential negative effects of any type of chronic pain on the person as well as on others close to that person. At the same time, much of what is known about the psychosocioeconomic impact of chronic cervical pain comes from common sense, clinical experience, anecdotes, and extrapolations from work related to chronic illness. There has not been much research with regard to the impact of chronic cervical pain. With relationships between all of the elements of pain and their impact on the person and family being exceedingly complex, it is difficult to decipher or dismantle for study these various aspects resulting from chronic pain.

On a societal level, the psychosocioeconomic impact of chronic pain, and of chronic cervical pain in particular, is enormous, but even this statement must be tempered with some caution. Much of the available information, although staggering, is about chronic disease and disability rather than pain itself. An Institute of Medicine report (1) estimated that total disability expenditures from all sources for members of the U.S. population between 18 and 64 years of age more

than doubled between 1970 and 1982, from \$60.2 billion to \$121.5 billion in 1982 dollars. Epidemiologic surveys indicate that back pain was the most prevalent diagnosis, with few data available as to what portion was cervical or neck pain. Estimates from 1984 are that \$14 billion was spent that year in the United States for treatment or compensation of low back pain alone (2). Bonica suggested that 700 million work days are lost each year because of pain (3). While the number of persons and the amount of dollars involved for cervical pain is unknown, it is probably not inconsiderable. One study involving a comprehensive pain center found that the primary location of pain for 17% of its patients was in the cervical area (4).

Given the complexity of the anatomy of the neck and its vulnerability (5), the number of persons with chronic cervical pain is probably significant and the toll that it takes worth considering. For example, a recent book on chronic illness cites a composite history of a woman suffering from pain in the neck and the impact of that pain on her life (6):

> It controls me. It's limiting. I can only go so far and then the pain stops me. Whenever I have to do something really physical or deal with a stressful situation, the pain increases terrifically. I've had to stop thinking about decisions I need to make in my marriage and relax and get the pain under control. Can't deal with my financial and career needs when the pain is back.

It is very difficult for me to be independent and not give in. Financially because I am not secure, it makes the whole process more difficult. I don't have the sense I can be completely independent. Also, the guilt I feel at breaking up the family. Other side is to be free, in charge of my own life. Right now things are in the balance. I'm feeling somewhat depressed.

You know what I think? The stiff neck is a kind of symbol, an icon of what I need to become; tough, stiff necked. The weak, vulnerable neck—it's the opposite. That is what I am, or fear I am. Stiff-necked or weak-necked? Is it the result of the pain or is the pain merely the vehicle to express this tension at the center of my life? I don't mean the pain is unreal. But being there, it comes to carry, to express this meaning. I would go on with the metaphor. Have you seen the great Renaissance and medieval paintings of Christ hanging there limp on the cross? Head down, neck under such stress, arms out. That's the position, when I stop to look at what I've done in my painting, that places the pressure on my neck and brings out the pain the worst. (p. 91)

There is perhaps no better descriptor of the impact of chronic cervical pain than the old adage "pain in the neck." Next to pain in the posterior, it is probably difficult to think of something worse. While the term may mean different things to different people, few would not have a conception of its meaning. "Pain in the neck" refers to something so persisting and so all encompassing that it affects all that happens to a person. A person's entire perspective on self, others, and environment is affected by the pain.

Fortunately, the incidence of chronic cervical or neck pain is much less than that of chronic low back pain, and most cervical or neck pain is generally not chronic (7). However, for the person with the pain the impact is no less important. Everything that occurs to the person and to persons close to him or her is affected by the pain. Neck mobility "is essential for the full appreciation of the world around us" (7). Communicating "yes" and "no" is probably the most common nonverbal expression used and involves the cervical region. Interference with the most basic mode of communication is sure to have an impact on a person's life.

Much of the literature concerned with chronic pain has dealt with the impact of psychological and social factors on pain and the role of these factors in either increasing or decreasing pain (8–10). The focus for this particular chapter is a bit different. It is not about how pain is influenced by factors and processes around an individual, but rather about the consequence of "any and all outputs of the individual that a reasonable observer would characterize as suggesting pain, such as (but not limited to) posture, facial expression, verbalizing, lying down, taking medicines, seeking medical assistance, and receiving compensation" (11, p. 334). Another definition that helps in understanding how pain can have an impact on a person involves five specific aspects: (a) autonomically mediated pain indicators, (b) visible and audible nonverbal signals that pain is experienced, (c) verbal reports of pain (d) requests for ministrations or assistance because of pain, and (e) functional limitation or restricted movement because of pain (12). Obviously, this definition involves the entire continuum of what pain is all about. This definition suggests that it may be necessary, in explaining the impact of pain, to be specific about the area to which one is referring. The schematic in Figure 27.1 illustrates another approach to the various components of pain.

Little is found in the literature on how chronic pain has an impact on the psychological, social, and economic aspects of the life of the person with pain (13). While knowing what factors may either decrease or increase the perception of pain is important, knowing what aspects of a person's life are affected is also important. Understanding the impact or consequences of the pain on the person and his or her environment can be particularly useful in designing appropriate intervention. For example, knowing that there may be certain psychological costs to the individual as a result of a loss of function because of pain may suggest the need for specific psychological supports to augment that individual. Knowing that there are economic impacts or changes that are documentable may suggest intervention of a different nature.

The emphasis of this chapter is on the impact of chronic cervical pain on the various psychological, social, and economic elements of the pain patient's life. Little has been written on the psychosocioeconomic impact of pain, and even less on cervical pain, so many of the references cited in this chapter relate to chronic pain in general and to chronic illness rather than to cervical pain specifically. It is assumed that the same dynamics of chronic disease apply to the person with chronic cervical pain. Chronic pain is like chronic illness in that it is something that a person will have to learn to live with and that will not go away. The presence of a chronic condition such as chronic pain will have an impact on a person socially, psychologically, and economically (14). This impact is often manifested in a cyclic manner. The chronic

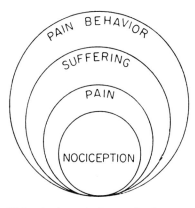

**Figure 27.1.** A schematic diagram for the components of pain. Only pain behavior is measurable and observable. (From History and Organization of the University of Washington Multidisciplinary Pain Center. In Loeser JD, Egan KJ (eds): *Managing the Chronic Pain Patient.* New York, Raven Press, 1989, p 6.)

condition can change the psychological situation, which in turn can affect the economic status, which then affects the family and a host of other interrelationships (15).

## ASSESSMENT/MEASUREMENT

A particular problem in exploring the impact of chronic pain on the person and his or her situation is the accurate assessment or measurement of that impact. While there is no totally satisfactory method, a number of relatively recent developments have systematized the gathering of data and information about the impact of chronic disease and specifically pain on the person. The development of the West Haven–Yale Multidimensional Pain Inventory (WHYMPI) (13) was a good first step. The WHYMPI was designed as an instrument to specifically inventory the impact of pain on the patient's life. The first part of the inventory was designed to evaluate perceived pain and the impact of that pain. Specifically, six areas are covered: (*a*) pain severity and suffering; (*b*) pain-related life interference, including interference with family and marital functioning, work and work-related activities, and social-recreational activities; (*c*) dissatisfaction with present level of functioning in each of the areas listed in *b* above; (*d*) appraisal of support received from spouse, family, and significant others; (*e*) perceived life control, incorporating the perceived ability to solve problems and feelings of personal mastery and competence; and (*f*) affective distress, including mood, irritability, and tension (16).

Another instrument of some utility in measuring the impact of pain is the Millon Behavioral Health Inventory (MBHI) (17). Unlike the WHYMPI, the MBHI was designed to assess a variety of behavioral health factors related to medical conditions. The individual is required to answer "true" or "false" to statements such as "Lots of people would care about me if I became very rich," "I really hate to have my work pile up," and "I get so touchy that I can't talk about certain things." The basic premise is that pain can affect these areas of a person's life.

## CAUTIONS

Each person who experiences pain is different. Part of the difficulty in understanding how pain has an impact on a person is understanding the individualized response. Physicians and health professionals must recognize the individual nature of pain and its impact and not expect that similar reactions will always occur. One person with an occupational background and age similar to those of another individual may have a totally different family structure that may affect the impact of the pain on that individual. There is some evidence that a person's reaction may be related to premorbid experience and accumulated strengths and weaknesses (14). One concept helpful in understanding the cause of chronic pain is the notion of trajectory. A trajectory is a psychosocial concept of thinking about the cause of illness or disease. Inherent in the concept of trajectory is the idea that there is more to an illness than the physiologic aspects and that there is a need to focus on differences in perception of the source of the disease as well as its impact by the professional, the patient, and the family (14). Using the concept of a pain trajectory, it may be possible to analytically order a variety of events and thus understand a bit more about what perspective the person with pain may have (14).

While the discussion in this chapter appears to categorize specific aspects of the person on which chronic cervical pain has an impact, these categories should not be considered as separate entities within themselves but rather as interrelated, each affecting the other (14). For example, the economic impact of pain is particularly obvious, involving the loss of earnings that comes from not being employed, but the loss of employment has many other ramifications. The loss of earnings is related to inability to function in a specific role as a productive employee. This role change, in turn, is related to changes in self-perception, which may have a specific psychological impact on the individual, such as heightened anxiety or depression.

There must also be caution in interpreting the meaning of the psychosocioeconomic impact of chronic cervical pain on the person and family. There is an enormous range of what can be considered a "normal" response. It is all too easy to not spend time in analyzing carefully what has occurred and instead make the easy diagnosis that pain has had a pathologic impact on the person and family. While dysfunction from pain can be pathologic, dysfunction does not suggest only pathology. This is tremendously important in working with persons with chronic cervical pain and their families. Persons in pain and their families may have a need to believe that what is happening to them is "normal" and not necessarily pathologic. At the same time, the impact of the pain can be of such severity that the reactions of both the individual and the family can be pathologic and require intensive intervention. Flexibility of response rather than a "canned approach" on the part of the health care professional is necessary.

## IMPACT ON THE PERSON

The impact of chronic pain on the psychology of the person is at once complex, profound, and subtle. Particularly difficult is deciding what role the pain has in interfering with the functioning of the individual. The impact of the pain has been described as the result of interaction with a particular set of circumstances in a way that has been termed an "unfortunate juxtaposition" (18). The manifestation of the pain's impact may be due to long-standing personality patterns or it may be circumstantial and nothing more than the "luck of the draw." It is extremely difficult to be definitive in this regard, and this often adds to the negative impact of chronic pain.

While it may be possible to read more into the equation than what is apparent, there may be some psychological meaning that patients place on the location of the pain that is important in understanding the impact of the pain on that individual. In other words, what a person believes to be important may be symbolic and idiosyncratic to that person. Because chronic pain in the cervical region may mean limited function in basic communication associated with anatomic structure, chronic cervical pain may come to mean limitation both in a symbolic and in an anatomic sense to the individual affected, and the person would behave accordingly. For example, not being able to nod becomes symbolic to the individual of limitations on the ability to communicate. With this perspective, the psychological impact is greater than one would perhaps expect.

## LOSS

The notion of loss is an important psychological impact resulting from chronic pain. Chronic pain results in affected persons being able to do less than they were before the onset of the pain. They feel that they are less as persons and no longer whole. The change of perception of who they are and what they can or cannot do involves dealing with the loss. As will be noted later, roles become twisted and identity can become confused as a result of chronic persistent pain. Even something that is as ingrained as sexual identity may be affected when sexual behavior is limited by the pain.

## CHRONIC DISABILITY SYNDROME

A major impact of chronic pain is often the development of the "chronic disability syndrome" (19). The decreased ability to function depends not only on injury or etiology of the pain but on what has been described as "illness or pain" behaviors (12). Specifically, one psychological impact of the pain is the development or learning of a set of behaviors that in effect bring about disability or further decreased function (Fig. 27.2). The concept of the chronic disability syndrome has been used to describe persons capable of working but who choose not to work. However, the concept may be useful in defining all areas of activity and not only employment. Also, use of the term "chronic disability syndrome" in the context that persons "choose" not to work may be a matter of interpretation. It appears that these persons in reality may not be able to work as a result of both physiologic and psychological factors. Five elements of the syndrome provide a framework for conceptualizing the result of a chronic pain situation. Strang (19) listed these factors as:

1. Being out of work for at least 6 consecutive months, claiming disability and entitlement of financial compensation
2. Having subjective complaints that are disproportionate to objective findings
3. Having psychological findings underlying subjective complaints and perception of disabled status
4. Having decreased or absent motivation to recover and a negative attitude about return to work
5. Duration of the above features for at least 6 months,

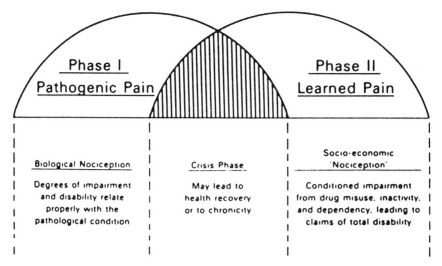

**Figure 27.2**    The nociceptive spectrum. (From McAlary PW, Aronoff GM: disability syndrome: contributing factors, detection, prevention and treatment. In Aronoff GM (ed): *Pain Centers: A Revolution in Health Care.* New York, Raven Press, 1988, p 216.)

not secondary to any other medical or psychiatric condition

A related way of thinking about the impact of chronic pain on the individual has been termed the "five Ds" (20), in which the following occur: (*a*) dramatization involving vague, diffuse, non-anatomic pain; (*b*) drug abuse involving various habit-forming pain medications; (*c*) dysfunction or impairments related to various physical and emotional factors; (*d*) dependency with accompanying passivity, depression, and helplessness; and (*e*) disability with pain contingent on financial compensation.

The development of the chronic disability syndrome is important when there is a "lack of physical findings and difficulties with defining a specific diagnosis" for the person with chronic cervical pain (21). A diagnosis of chronic intractable benign pain is sometimes used to describe a variety of difficulties of a psychosocioeconomic nature, which indicate that intervention should begin as soon as the person demonstrates that he or she is adapting poorly, with the pain becoming the focus of life (18). The primary emphasis of intervention is upon changing behavior rather than the elimination of pain.

## DISTRACTION

Another psychological impact of chronic pain is distraction, involving a lack of attention to or concentration on the world or environment around the person. Others may describe the person as being very selfish in that he or she seems to think only about the self. The individual's life is almost totally consumed by the pain itself. Energy is focused within, and the person becomes difficult to live with and to work with. Not only does the individual with pain think only of the self, but other persons and things become irritants rather than a source of satisfaction or pleasure.

## SELF-WORTH

Another critical area in which pain has an impact on the person is self-esteem or self-worth. While not always easy to define, self-worth refers in this context to what a person believes about who he or she is in relationship to what he or she was prior to injury and the person's perception of societal norms and how he or she measures up to those norms. Not being able to do what he or she was able to do before, the person believes that he or she is less of a person. The consequences of this include being easily frustrated, irritable, and especially hard on oneself, not being able to see progress, and having difficulty setting goals. Self-concept undoubtedly is related to behavior. This is especially true in American society, where so much of life is tied to what one does.

## AFFECT

Chronic pain can also have an impact on the emotional or affective responses of the person. The literature on the emotional aspects of chronic pain is difficult to assess because many of these studies were done in pain clinics with selective populations (9). "Those individuals with chronic pain who do not seek medical attention and continue to function despite their pain constitute an important group rarely subject to psychological studies" (9). Very little is known of persons who function with their pain because most of the available data are biased toward individuals who do not function well and who not only voice complaints but are more likely to enter pain programs. Thus, there is a need to be careful in interpreting the available information. It is probably safe to say that many persons do experience affective changes as a result of their chronic pain or perception of pain. Very often there is much anxiety related to what the pain means and the changes that have occurred in their lives. Notwithstanding that anxiety may lead to more pain, the impact on the individual is that he or she has a sense of living on edge. Feeling uncertain about oneself and what one is able to do is energy consuming and leaves the person feeling drained and unable to cope.

## DEPRESSION

Another aspect of the affective realm often associated with chronic pain is depression (22). "It seems logical that chronic pain would cause depression; however, the task of determining the incidence, severity, and quality of the depressive symptoms caused by chronic pain is complicated by the fact that primary depressive illness is so common" (9). Although not well understood, there may well be an intimate link between depression and pain. On the one hand depression can serve to heighten awareness of pain; on the other hand pain can produce depressive symptoms directly (9). Elevated Minnesota Multiphasic Personality Inventory (MMPI) scores on the Depression scale are not uncommon in persons with pain complaints (19).

## IMPACT ON RELATIONSHIPS

Chronic cervical pain disrupts relationships and roles, and can literally turn life into chaos. Not only may the individual turn inward and withdraw, but previous roles and relationships and all of the learned expectations associated with those relationships may be changed. Chronic pain has been noted to affect four social aspects of the person's life: the patient's family, ethnic/cultural

community, work site, and health care organization (23). Of particular significance is the change that often takes place within the family unit. The pain patient lives in a context of others, and it is extremely rare for pain not to affect those others. The impact is perhaps the greatest on those persons closest to the person in pain. Chronic pain and the changes that occur create an uncertainty in relationships that can be very difficult to live with (24). As with individuals, the impact on families is very idiosyncratic, and can be negative as well as positive.

A typology useful for understanding the effect of chronic disease or pain on the family unit is one proposed by Rolland (25). Rolland's typology utilizes a phase approach, characterizing chronic illness as having a crisis phase, a chronic phase, and a terminal phase. Within each phase are specific tasks that the family unit must accomplish. The first phase involves the initial sensing by the family that something is wrong. The tasks that must be dealt with in the crisis phase include creating a meaning for the illness event that maximizes the family's sense of mastery over their lives, grieving for the loss of the preillness family identity, moving toward an acceptance of the change but maintaining continuity with their past, pulling together for short-term reorganization, and developing a way to move toward the future. After the initial crisis comes a chronic phase in which the family must dig in for the "long haul." The primary task of the family during this phase is to maintain maximum autonomy of all family members. The final phase involving the terminal nature of many chronic diseases is generally not one of major concern in chronic cervical pain. This typology helps the practitioner to identify what families must do in order to deal with a family member who becomes ill or, in the context of this chapter, experiences chronic pain. The ultimate impact of the pain is to create a situation in which the family is stressed.

Examining the effects of chronic pain on the family is a relatively recent phenomenon, and there are few scientific data that describe the impact of chronic pain in a family context (25, 26), although family theorists have attempted to conceptualize the effect of stress for whatever reason for some time (27).

## EMPLOYMENT

One of the immediate effects of pain is often the loss of employment or of the ability to do work that was done prior to the onset of pain. This may be either inability to perform the work itself, inability to work full time, or the need to do a different type of work. Regardless of the particular configuration, the change itself, however minor, can be stressful and disrupting to the family unit.

A person who was a breadwinner may no longer be able to perform this role. Obviously, employment is important in that it provides an income, but it is also a source of power, prestige, and a self-identity as someone of worth (28). In addition, work provides a structure for time and keeps a person busy. Loss of or inability to perform work means a different structure or lack of structure for using time. A person now may have large amounts of time in which he or she does not know what to do. Not only is the built-in structure of work missing, but the person is given the added task of filling in the time gap on his or her own.

Habits of getting up at a certain time, doing certain jobs or chores, and the like no longer fill the day. Habits are difficult to break, and not only is the individual with pain affected but so is the family. Even if the person is judged to be disabled and has disability income, his or her life activities and roles are no longer the same. New ways to relate to spouse and/or children must be learned. The functional limits due to pain may even change how the person plays with his or her children. As the process of finding new ways to do things continues, the entire family continues to experience more uncertainty. Changes in roles of one family member will also result in changes of roles of others.

One of the obvious outcomes of job loss is economic. The family must contend with how it can compensate for the income that no longer exists. Some possibilities for familes include having other members of the family go to work, finding ways to scrimp and save, and depending on the extended family for loans. Each of these can add to changes in family relationships that must be confronted. The person with the chronic pain as well as the family may need help in coping with and in learning new ways of relating to each other.

For persons who are not the primary breadwinner, role changes are not any easier. Tasks can no longer be taken for granted by other members of the household, and someone must be able to assume the new roles. Resentment and anger can result from taking on additional roles. Guilt resulting from feelings of anger and frustration can surface as an additional stressor. The negative impact from these feelings can be ameliorated by appropriate intervention with empathy and support.

Loss of employment can result in different fam-ily and individual relationships than ever experienced before by members of that family. The authority or power that may be inherent in being a provider is no longer present (28). Conflicts between family members are more likely to occur, especially over financial matters (28). Parent-child relationships can also suffer. Families with a mother with pain have been found to perceive their family environments as less cohesive as well as having more conflict among family members (29). A classic model of family stress developed by Hill (27) may be helpful in understanding the family when unemployment occurs. The precipitation of stress by unemployment, together with the family's resources for handling this crisis and the context of the situation, is hypothesized to produce the family's response to unemployment. Just as little is known of the effects of unemployment on the family, even less is known when the additional variable of disability or chronic pain becomes the etiologic factor. Disability payments in and of themselves may not mitigate the negative effects (30).

## FAMILY FUNCTIONING

Generally, the impact of chronic pain on the family is considered to be negative. Because so many family roles are interrelated and one's identity is part and parcel of the role, disruption and uncertainty result. However, there may be positive outcomes in certain instances. Some families seem to pull together and become closer following crises. Little is known about why some families do so while other families fall apart.

The interpretation of pain is always a subjective individual matter. The meanings are not easily understandable by other family members. Because of this, communication patterns for a person with chronic pain are often different and unpredictable for other family members. One of the earlier studies on the impact of pain on families suggested that the uncertainty and ambiguity of the pain experience were major stressors on other family members (24).

A recent review on pain and families (31) focused on a set of five questions, one of which was "What is the impact of chronic pain on the family?" It is interesting to note that the review utilized primarily literature related to chronic illness rather than specifically pain. While it was noted that families often end up coping extremely well with chronic illness, very few of the studies were concerned with chronic pain. Several studies were cited in which dysphoric mood and marital dissatisfaction were more prevalent with spouses of persons reporting chronic pain. Spouses also were more likely to report somewhat higher incidences of depression. In addition, marital dissatisfaction generally increased following onset of pain. Other studies cited in the review reported that spouses of patients with chronic pain were more likely to display more pain problems than spouses of depressed patients who did not have chronic pain (31).

While some have stressed the dysfunctional aspects of chronic pain on family function, such as the use of "pain games" whereby the person with the pain controls or dominates other family members or escapes responsibilities, other clinicians believe this to be only part of the picture (23). Other family members may also derive benefits of a reinforcing nature. Brodwin and Kleinman (23) cited the example of the husband forced to retire early because of pain with the wife being placed into a caretaking role and legitimizing her desire to work part-time. This "tertiary" gain may severely limit the prospect of the husband ever returning to work. Brodwin and Kleinman concluded that "pain behavior is never restricted to the identified patient, but always becomes embedded in family dynamics and the needs and desires of kin" (p. 115).

While more often than not chronic pain, including cervical pain, is seen as having a negative impact on the family, others have suggested (28) that the crisis of pain can be a challenge in which the family may become much more cohesive, with the common goal of dealing with the intrusion of pain in their lives. Hill (27), in exploring the crisis of war separation and reunion on the family, suggested that the long-term effect of crisis on families was conflicting. Much of the impact, whether negative or positive, depended on the status of the family at the time of the crisis. If the family was well organized it tended to remain so during crisis and stress, with the family responding in adaptable ways. In contrast, families that did not appear adequately organized responded in maladaptive ways. The impact of chronic pain would have a clearly differential effect. There may be a relationship between how long chronic pain has been present and whether the impact is positive or negative.

## SEXUAL FUNCTION AND ACTIVITY

Pain can have an impact on sexual function (impotence) and sexual activity (reduction). As with pain interfering with family and role function, interference with sexual function would also appear logical. With energy focused on pain, not many persons would have the inclination or mood for sexual pursuit. What few data available seem to substantiate this hypothesis: Some estimates place sexual dysfunction as high as 75% (32). At the same time, very little has been accomplished with regard to intervention for persons with chronic pain and sexual dysfunction. A recent review of a number of studies found that a high percentage of those persons with back injuries reported sexual deterioration (32). The speculation is that physiologic tension may be the primary determinant for sexual activity increasing or decreasing pain. In this instance, some of the relaxation interventions may be appropriate.

Aside from the physiologic aspects, sexual activity occurs within social relationships. The disruption that occurs when roles are no longer the same creates problems of confusion. The fact that the person's identity has changed because of the pain has a direct bearing on sexual activity and function. For example, losing a job may cause a change in perception of the father as a "man" which may bring about loss of sexual function. Relationships that have been disrupted and roles that have changed can also result in anger or frustration. These have been known to interfere with sexual desire, hence sexual activity.

## HEALTH OF OTHER FAMILY MEMBERS

Finally, the impact of pain in the family may extend to the health of other family members. For example, Rowat and Knafl (24) reported that 83% of spouses of persons with chronic pain had some form of health disturbance. There are undoubtedly many reasons for the potential poor health status of spouses and/or other family members of persons with chronic pain. Being a caregiver is not only stressful, but physically wearing. This impact suggests the need not only for additional research, but for developing resources for spouses and other family members.

## EXTRAFAMILIAL RELATIONSHIPS

Outside of the family, the person with pain will have a host of other relationships that may be changed. Not only is the person with pain less likely to socialize, but he or she may become more difficult to socialize with because the pain may be distracting. Social support systems are affected by the change of self-perception and the energy used in dealing with the pain.

## IMPACT ON ECONOMIC STATUS

The last arena in which pain has an impact on the person is economic. Reference has been made to the increased costs that come about because of health care and the loss of employment. Much of what is known about the impact of chronic cervical pain on economic loss is extrapolated from the literature on low back pain and disability in general. There is literally nothing available that documents the economic impact of chronic cervical pain in specific dollar figures.

Pain can bring about a financial crisis to the person and the family. One survey of costs for treatment of chronic pain problems found that preadmission charges ranged from $738 to $2044 for inpatient programs. Total treatment charges varied from $6641 to $12,490 in 1983. Outpatient programs had a range of $3200 to $11,700 (33). These figures do not take into account other health care costs prior to treatment for the chronic pain. In addition, if other family members are more likely to have health problems the economic impact is even greater. Even if the person is able to continue in employment, there is the question of negotiating time off because of pain or to go for medical care.

Work remains a critical element for a person in our society. Weinhouse (34) identified a number of barriers that have significant impact on returning to work. These included compensation, litigation, illness conviction, deactivation, length of time off work, system anger, funding, and motivation. Perhaps of all the areas related to chronic pain, barriers to return to work has been the area in which the least amount of research has been accomplished. There are considerable differences of opinion regarding the effects of some of these barriers.

## SUMMARY

The issues related to the impact of chronic cervical pain on the physical, social, psychological, and economic aspects of a person are complex and vary with the person. For some the impact is devastating, and life becomes pain. Others, and we know much less about them, seem able to adapt and manage their pain so as to lessen its impact.

There is a need for much more data collection and research with regard to the psychosocioeconomic impact of chronic cervical pain and specifically why some persons are able to deal with pain and its impact and others are not. Broader issues of whether psychosocioeconomic factors increase or decrease the perception of pain and the question of which came first have been skirted in the chapter but remain important in the total picture.

The recognition of the importance of examining the psychosocioeconomic impact of pain and incorporating its psychosocioeconomic aspects into the treatment and intervention plan is a good first step in this process. The education of patients and professionals to the psychosocioeconomic impact of chronic pain is important if effective intervention is to occur. Efforts need to be made to provide the resources that would alleviate the various ways in which pain has taken its toll. There is perhaps a need to stress early involvement and begin intervention related to the psychosocioeconomic issues before they become overwhelming to the person and the family.

## REFERENCES

1. Osterweis M, Kleinman A, Medranic D (eds): *Pain and Disability*. Institute of Medicine Committee on Pain Disability and Chronic Illness Behavior. Washington, DC, National Academy Press, 1987.
2. Brena SF, Chapman SL: Pain and litigation. In Wall PD, Melzak R (eds): *Textbook of Pain*. New York, Churchill Livingstone, 1984.
3. Bonica J: [Editorial]. *Triangle* 20:1–6, 1981.
4. Fishbain DA, Goldberg M, Steele R, Rosomoff H: DSM-III: diagnosis of patients with myofacial pain syndrome (fibrositis). *Arch Phys Med Rehabil* 70:433–438, 1989.
5. Jackson R: *The Cervical Syndrome*. Springfield, Il, Charles Thomas, 1978.
6. Kleinman A: *The Illness Narratives*. New York, Basic Books, Inc, 1988.
7. Aryanpur J, Ducker TB: Differential diagnosis and management of cervical spine pain. In Tollison CD (ed): *Handbook of Chronic Pain Management*. Baltimore, Williams & Wilkins, 1988.
8. Chapman R: Psychological aspects of pain: patient treatment. *Arch Surg* 112:767–772, 1977.
9. Fields HL: *Pain*. New York, McGraw Hill Book Co, 1987.
10. Blazer D: Chronic pain: a multiaxial approach to psychosocial assessment and intervention. *South Med J* 74:203–207, 1981.
11. Loeser JD, Fordyce WE: Chronic pain. In Carr JE, Dengerink HA (eds): *Behavioral Science in the Practice of Medicine*. Amsterdam, Elsevier, 1983.
12. Fordyce WE: *Behavioral Methods for Chronic Pain and Illness*. St. Louis, CV Mosby Co, 1976.
13. Turk DC, Meichenbaum D, Genest M: *Pain and Behavioral Medicine*. New York, Guilford Press, 1983.
14. Lubkin IM: *Chronic Illness: Impact and Interventions*. Boston, Jones and Bartlett, 1986.
15. Levy N: The chronically ill patient. *Psychiatr Q* 51:189–197, 1979.
16. Kerns RO, Turk DC, Rudy TE: The West Haven–Yale Multidimensional Pain Inventory. *Pain* 23:345–356, 1985.

17. Millon T, Green C, Meagher R: *Millon Behavioral Health Inventory Manual.* Minneapolis, MN, National Computer System, 1982.

18. Dworkin RH, Galigor E: Psychiatric diagnosis and chronic pain: DSMIII-R and beyond. *J Pain Symptom Management* 3(2):87–98, 1988.

19. Strang JP: The chronic disability syndrome. In Aronoff GM (ed): *The Evaluation and Treatment of Chronic Pain.* Baltimore, Urban and Schwarzenberg, 1988.

20. Brena S, Chapman SL: The learned pain syndrome. *Postgrad Med* 69:53–61, 1981.

21. Crue BL, Pinsky JJ: An approach to chronic pain of nonmalignant origin. *Postgrad Med* 60:858–864, 1984.

22. Keefe FJ, Wilkins RH, Cook NH, Crisson JE, Muhlbaier LH: Depression, pain, and pain behavior. *J Consult Clin Psychol* 54:665–669, 1986.

23. Brodwin PE, Kleinman A: The social meanings of chronic pain. In Burrows GD, Elton D, Stanley GV (eds): *Handbook of Chronic Pain Management.* Amsterdam, Elsevier, 1987.

24. Rowat KM, Knafi KA: Living with chronic pain: the spouse's perspective. *Pain* 23:259–271, 1985.

25. Rolland JC: A conceptual model of chronic and life threatening illness and its impact on families. In Chilman C, Nunally EW, Cox FM (eds): *Chronic Illness and Disability.* Newbury Park, CA, Sage Publications, 1988.

26. Watt-Watson JH, Evans RJ, Watson CP: Relationship among coping responses and perceptions of pain intensity, depression, and family functioning. *Clin J Pain* 4:101–106, 1988.

27. Hill R: *Families under Stress.* New York, Harper & Row, 1949.

28. Aldous J, Tuttle RC: Unemployment and the family. In Chilman CS, Cox FM, Nunnally EW (eds): *Employment and Economic Problems.* Newbury Park, CA, Sage Publications, 1988.

29. Dura JR, Beck S: A comparison of family functioning when mothers have chronic pain. *Pain* 35:79–89, 1988.

30. Weighill VE: An updated review of compensation neurosis. *Pain Management* March/April, 100–105, 1989.

31. Turk DC, Flor H, Rudy TE: Pain and families. *Pain* 30:3–27, 1987.

32. Jordan JS, Keefe FJ: Sexual dysfunction and chronic pain. In France RD, Krishaan KR (eds): *Chronic Pain.* Washington, DC, American Psychiatric Press, 1988.

33. Billings CD: Pain in the workplace. In Aronoff GM (ed): *Pain Centers: A Revolution in Health Care.* New York, Raven Press, 1988.

34. Weinhouse S: Vocational issues in the rehabilitation of pain patients. In Loeser LD, Egan KJ (eds): *Managing the Pain Patient.* New York, Raven Press, 1989.

# 28

# EVALUATION OF DISABILITY
# RELATED TO THE NECK

*Sanford H. Vernick, Daniel Shapiro, Edgar Marin, and Jacinta M. McElligott*

Disability is fraught with vagueness by definition. There is particular lack of agreement among physicians as to what constitutes a competent examination and report in all facets of disability determination, especially when related to the neck.

Pain is the most frequent complaint that causes patients to seek medical care. The two most common sites for the pain are the low back and the neck, in that order. Calliet has stated that "knowing normal and recognizing deviation from normal clarifies the mechanism of pain production and indicates correct treatment" (1). Nonetheless, many physicians seek to avoid these areas with regard to evaluation and judgment. Very few physicians are trained in disability determination and reporting, and most physicians have negative feelings toward the disability process and the patient because of the monetary and legal stakes. Despite the number of published papers on neck pain, there is little scientific knowledge about the exact cause of most cases of neck pain. Indeed, we are not even certain which anatomic structure in the neck produces the pain the patient describes. Nevertheless, every patient who presents for a disability examination deserves at the very least a competent and objective examination.

## DEFINITIONS

### IMPAIRMENT

The term "impairment" as defined by the World Health Organization (2) connotes a defect involving loss or abnormality of psychological or physical structure or function. In the case of schizophrenia, the impairment is the absence of normal thought processes. In Crohn's disease it is the loss of normal bowel anatomy. In the case of amputation it is the absence of the limb. With regard to the neck, impairment is generally defined by pain, loss of strength, altered sensation, and decreased range of motion in the neck and upper limb. Kessler (3) differentiated between obvious and hidden impairment and between static and dynamic impairment. Because they provoke attention, amputations and facial disfigurement are obvious impairments, but a prosthesis or other camouflaging appliance can convert an obvious impairment into a hidden one. An impairment that cannot be changed or remedied—an above-knee amputation in a 90-year-old woman—is obviously static. A defect such as Crohn's disease or diabetes, which may be remedied or become worse, is considered a dynamic impairment.

## DISABILITY

Impairment often leads to disability, which has been defined as the inability or incapacity to meet certain standards of physical efficiency and/or social or economic responsibility. The manifestations of disability vary from patient to patient and the physician will not be well served by generalization. For example, the loss of a pinky finger would not be disabling for a teacher; for a violinist, however, it could signal total disability. Therefore, when defining disability one should ask the question "Inability to do what?" in terms of the patient's needs, desires, and goals.

## HANDICAP

Handicap occurs when disability prevents a person from performing within the social milieu; that is, it limits or prevents the fulfillment of a role that is normal for that person. For example, in civilizations in which amputation is considered retribution from God for a sin, the amputee becomes a social outcast and may not marry or participate in religious, social, or vocational activities (4). Thus, the impairment (loss of limb) has caused a disability with regard to physical activities and has resulted in a severe handicap in terms of social fulfillment.

## EVALUATION

The evaluation of neck pain or dysfunction is often time consuming and considered unrewarding by many physicians. In addition, the problem is often occult and will not easily reveal itself.

*Intrinsic causes* of neck pain or dysfunction involve the structures of the neck itself—the vertebral bodies, discs, nerve roots, ligaments, blood vessels, and muscles. *Extrinsic causes* are only indirectly related to the cervical spine—for example, tumors, infections, and psychological impairment. As with most medical problems, the key to diagnosis and treatment of the neck is the history.

## HISTORY

The history begins with the chief complaint, usually pain or loss of motion. What type of pain is it? Is it dull, sharp, burning, lancinating, or paresthetic? Is it constant, intermittent, or paroxysmal? Is it confined to one or more areas or does it radiate? Is it worse when moving the head or arms or does lying down make it worse? Does gentle exercise or heat make it worse or better? Is there any attendant dizziness, vertigo, tinnitis, or ocular discomfort? The answers to these questions will suggest an etiology. For example, neck pain that is constant and becomes worse when the patient is supine will often be caused by a primary or metastatic tumor, whereas pain that is intermittent and increases in severity on prolonged activity is probably related to a musculoskeletal problem. Tinnitis may suggest injury to the petrous portion of the temporal bone as a result of flexion-extension injury. Eye pain, tearing, or vertigo suggest sternocleidomastoid involvement.

The examiner should inquire into the time and circumstances of onset of the pain or dysfunction. Was the onset related to a motor vehicle, industrial, or sports accident, or were there no particularly significant circumstances? Onset related to work or a motor vehicle accident usually points to a muscular or ligament sprain or strain. Onset under no particular circumstances often suggests a more ominous etiology such as tumor, infection, or other serious problem.

The patient's response to the pain or dysfunction must be carefully reviewed. What actions were taken to obtain relief? What medications have been used? How does the patient describe a "typical day"? How does he or she sleep? Is a special pillow used? What are the patient's activities immediately after arising? Is he or she always tired?

Inconsistencies will sometimes be revealed when a patient complains of difficulty performing certain tasks at work but does not relate the same difficulties with other seemingly unrelated tasks such as shaving or showering. For example, shaving in the usual manner, which involves complicated maneuvering of the cervical spine, is very difficult to perform for someone with truly significant neck pain.

The past medical history, which often must be drawn out with detailed questioning, may point to problems such as diabetes or cancer. Next the family history and the social history should be elicited. Is the patient married or separated or divorced? Does he or she smoke or drink to excess? Are work or interpersonal relationships physically or psychologically stressful? For example, the fight-or-flight response, which is the lower animal's answer to a stressful situation, cannot usually be utilized by the average human being. Neither fighting nor fleeing is an option, and the stress often must be silently endured, a situation that frequently leads to extended contraction of the neck and shoulder muscles mediated by the sphenopalantine ganglion. The axiom "you give me a pain in the neck" has its origin in this inability to release tension. The neck and shoulder muscles appear to be especially sensitive to psychoemotional stress.

The occupational history is also essential. What does the work consist of? Is the job satifactory? Does the patient feel a lack of support from the employer? Has the patient attempted to return to work after this injury? How many times and for how long?

## PHYSICAL EXAMINATION

The disability examination of the neck begins when the physician walks into the waiting room to greet the patient. This initial and often unexpected interaction is very important. Observation can be made of the patient's level of distress while he or she is unaware. Posture and apparent comfort level may differ if the patient is presumably unobserved.

Although it is discouraged by conventional etiquette, there are diagnostic advantages to being present while the patient undresses. While ostensibly examining the patient's chart, try to observe his or her motions while undressing. Does he or she have difficulty in manipulating the head and arm to remove a shirt, sweater, undershirt, or other garment? Certain movements will be more painful for a patient with true complaints.

Examine the patient while he or she is sitting on the examining table. Observe the patient from the front, sides, and behind. Is there any deviation from the normal alignment of the cervical spine (e.g., flattening of the lordotic curve)? Are the shoulders level? Is there any obvious atrophy of the muscles in the neck or upper extremities? Palpate the cervical vertebrae and interspaces, paraspinal and shoulder muscles, and joints in the upper extremity. Trigger points and tender points may be found in the neck, shoulder girdle, and sternocleidomastoid muscles. Note any edema, erythema, or muscle spasm. By rolling the muscle between the thumb and forefinger, spasms may be more readily detected. Percuss the carpal and cubital tunnel, because entrapment here can radiate pain proximally to the neck. Adson's maneuver should be performed to rule out thoracic outlet syndrome. The neck should also be palpated in a supine position to examine for tender or misaligned transverse processes.

Next do a detailed examination from a functional and neurologic standpoint. The following examinations should be performed in the order in which they are discussed.

## Neck Movement

Ask the patient to actively flex, extend, and rotate the neck. Any limitations of movement may indicate a problem in ligaments, capsules, or muscles that act on posterior joints and discs. Lateral flexion tests the mobility of the lower cervical spine and is done by bringing the ear to the shoulder.

Tight tissues may cause the patient to elevate the shoulder rather than laterally flexing the neck, and preventing shoulder motion may reveal the tissue limitation and pain. All ranges of motion should be documented with a goniometer. The neck should be manually compressed and extended to detect radicular symptoms (Spurling test).

### Upper Extremity Movement

Ask the patient to actively range the upper extremity joints, one at a time, through flexion, extension, abduction, adduction, and external and internal rotation. Document the endpoints of each range with the goniometer. Watch for pain reaction or abnormal movements and listen for crepitus during each movement. If there is limitation of any joint, do gentle passive range of motion with careful attention to pain and/or crepitus.

### Manual Muscle Testing

Do manual muscle testing of the cervical and upper extremity myotomes. Pressure on a nerve root may cause muscle weakness in its corresponding myotome. Testing the muscles of each upper extremity myotome involves ranging the part of the limb to be tested against maximal patient resistance to the give way or breaking point. The 1–5 scale, on which 1 is the weakest and 5 the strongest, is used by most physicians, to grade the patient's responses. Alternatively, the functional system used by most rehabilitation physicians may be chosen. This grading system is based on the ability of the muscle to move the body part to which it is attached against the force of gravity. Therefore, the prime action of the muscle must be known and then the body can be positioned to allow this prime action to occur. The patient's responses are graded according to the following functional levels:

*Trace strength*—the muscle contraction can be seen or palpated but active movement is impossible.
*Poor strength*—the muscle can actively move the joint it crosses to full range only if gravity is eliminated.
*Fair strength*—full active range of motion of the joint against gravity without resistance.
*Good strength*—full active range of motion of the joint against gravity with moderate resistance applied by the examiner.

*Normal strength*—full active range of the joint against gravity with maximal resistance applied by the examiner.

Grip strength and pincher grasp should be tested either manually or with appropriate devices if available.

## Tactile Discrimination

Check sensation to pinprick and light touch. Nerve root pressure may produce loss of light touch or pinprick discrimination. The use of a safety pin or pin wheel may be used and the results recorded dermatomally as normal, hyperesthetic, hypesthetic, dysesthetic, or anesthetic. Two-point discrimination should be tested. These tests are, of course, subjective and require full patient cooperation and understanding for validity.

## Reflex Testing

Do reflex testing. With the reflex hammer, check the biceps (C5), brachioradials (C6), and triceps (C7). A diminution of the reflex may suggest nerve root pressure at that level, and hyperactive reflex may suggest a problem at a higher level.

## REVIEW OF OTHER TEST RESULTS

This concludes the physical examination. As the patient is getting dressed, any pertinent laboratory, electrodiagnostic or radiologic evaluations (computed tomography scan, magnetic resonance imaging thermogram, bone scan, etc.) should be reviewed.

## DIAGNOSIS

The examiner should now begin processing a diagnosis that is determined by sifting through the objective findings (or lack of same) and comparing these with the patient's subjective complaints to determine if there is consistency or inconsistency. Unfortunately, there are no accepted malingerer's tests for the neck as there are for the back, such as the Hoover and chair-kneel tests. However, each positive objective finding is correlated with the corresponding structure or neurologic function. For example, absent biceps reflex or decreased sensation over the lateral upper arm may indicate C5 radiculopathy. This should correlate with pain or paresthesia along the C5

dermatome and weakness of the biceps muscle on that side. The determination of significant inconsistency between subjective and objective findings is an indication for further psychological testing. If there are no inconsistencies, the significant findings are summed up and a diagnosis is noted. This may include cervical sprain, radiculopathy at a particular level, spondylosis, or a possible extrinsic cause.

In the case of the back, lumbosacral sprain is the most common diagnosis; in the case of the neck it is whiplash. If the diagnosis of lumbosacral sprain is fraught with ambiguity, whiplash is even worse. This is compounded by the fact that "whiplash" has been adopted for general use by lawyers, third-party payers, and lay people alike. Even some physicians use it without fully understanding its definition or ramifications. Bosworth (5) stated that: "The neck is not a whip. The diagnosis is vague and thoroughly unscientific. There is a tendency for this terminology to be employed through lack of sufficient knowledge to make a specific diagnosis. The term to the honest is merely a bulwark behind which ignorance skulks; to the dishonest a mirage with which to confuse and delude." At a symposium some years ago, it was stated that "whiplash is a controversial term enjoying no unanimity of understanding and no acceptance of definition. Symptoms attributed to this syndrome are vaguely described, the etiology is dramatically explained, the mechanism of injury is poorly understood and the treatment empirical at best. In this state of total confusion and ignorance, the injured have been neglected, mistrusted and even accused of deception while many uninjured complainers have been exorbitantly and unjustifiably rewarded" (6).

## JOB SIMULATION

The physician or vocational counselor can evaluate the patient under simulated work conditions to determine if the patient is prepared to return to a similar level of work.

## THE DISABILITY REPORT

### PROVIDING OBJECTIVE EVIDENCE OF FUNCTIONAL LOSS

The physician's role in reporting the disability evaluation is just as difficult as the evaluation itself, and there are no clear guidelines or standardized measures of impairment or disability that are uniformly accepted. Most disability evaluations require objective evidence of functional loss, and a number of systems have been developed to attempt to answer this need.

## American Medical Association Guidelines

The American Medical Association's *Guides to the Evaluation of Permanent Impairment* (Guides) (7) attempts to provide a set of criteria with which to establish ratings of permanent impairment. It must be stressed, however, that the Guides do not relate medical impairment to occupation or social responsibilities. For example, the concert pianist with loss of a digit would receive the same medical impairment rating as a truck driver with loss of the same digit. The Guides express impairment as a percentage of total body function that has been lost. With regard to some areas related to the cervical spine, the Guides relate impairment to abnormal motion and ankylosis of the cervical region in flexion, extension, lateral bending, and rotation and to cervical spinal root involvement. For example, the average range of normal lateral flexion is stated as 90°. The value of total range of cervical motion is 25% of total body value, and impairment of right lateral flexion would constitute, according to the Guides, only 3% impairment of the whole person.

In the Guides, pain/discomfort and loss of sensation are graded from 0% to 100%, with 0% being no loss of sensation and no spontaneous or abnormal sensation and 100% being decreased sensation with pain that may prevent all activity. Although this grading system is an attempt to quantify pain, it is quite subjective and dependent on the evaluator and the patient's compliance and understanding. We are all familiar with the patient who presents with severe and incapacitating neck pain without clinical evidence of sensory loss. Since all grade determinations require loss of sensation, this patient would be difficult to grade. Second "pain" and "discomfort" are used synonymously. Therefore, the distinction between mild pain and severe pain must be determined by the evaluator's subjective impression.

The grading system for motor power in the Guides is similar to the motor grading system used in clinical practice as previously described. Spinal nerve root impairment is calculated from the sensory and motor grading systems of impairment relative to percentage of impairment of the upper extremity. The impairment of the upper extremity is then factored into the percentage of impairment of the whole body. Each spinal root is accorded a maximum percentage loss of function due to sensory deficits, pain, or discomfort, a maximum percentage loss of function due to loss of strength, and a maximum percentage impairment of the upper extremity. According to the Guides, for unilateral C5 spinal root impairment, maximum percentage loss of function due to sensory deficit, pain, or discomfort equals 5, maximum percentage loss of function due to loss of strength is 30, and maximum percentage impairment of the upper extremity is 0–34.

An example taken directly from the Guides is that of a 42-year-old right-handed man who fell 30 feet and landed on his upper back. He complained of neck pain radiating down his right arm. Examination revealed 20% sensory loss of the C5 area and 50% loss of strength of the muscles innervated by C5. According to the Guides, impairment is calculated as follows:

1. 20% of 5% equals 1% loss of function due to sensory deficits, pain, or discomfort.
2. 50% of 30% equals 15% loss of function due to loss of strength.
3. 1% combined with 15% equals 16% impairment of the right upper extremity.
4. 16% impairment of the preferred upper extremity equals 10% impairment of the whole person.

Many patients may have coexisting C6 or C7 radiculopathy and/or limitations in cervical rotation. All factors must be taken into account. As one can imagine, the process can become quite complicated. In addition, how does one rate a patient with incapacitating pain, impaired cervical mobility due to same, and no other discernible pathology? Our understanding of the pathology of neck pain is limited at this time. That is to say, all pain related to the neck is not referrable to a particular root pathology, but may stem from ligamentous, musculoskeletal, and/or arthritic involvement and the like, all of which may be difficult to document with objectivity.

In addition to the above concerns, several other factors limit the usefulness of the Guides. First, the evaluation remains subject to observer error. Second, the quantification of pain still remains an enigma. Third, the Guides are not universally used or accepted and thus have limited applicability to the already controversial subject of cervical pathology.

## Social Security Administration Guidelines

The Social Security and Supplemental Security Insurance program publishes a "Handbook" for physicians entitled *Disability Evaluation under Social Security* (8). To qualify for disability, an individual must have a medically determined impairment—that is, an impairment that is medically demonstrable anatomically, physiologically, or psychologically. Such abnormalities are medically determined if they manifest themselves as signs or laboratory findings apart from symptoms. In relation to spinal disorders, the Handbook suggests that the history should contain details regarding the location and radiation of pain, mechanical factors that exacerbate or relieve the pain, the prescribed treatment (including type, dose and frequency of analgesic), and typical daily activities. It is requested that care be taken to ascertain that the report of the examination findings is consistent with the individual's daily activities. There must be a detailed description of orthopaedic and neurologic examination findings: limitations of movement of the spine given quantitatively in degrees from the vertical position, motor and sensory abnormalities, muscle spasms, and deep tendon reflexes. A specific description of the atrophy of the hands and muscles is acceptable without measurements of atrophy but should include measurements of grip strength.

Pain may be an important factor in causing function loss but, according to the Social Security Handbook, it must be associated with relevant abnormal signs or laboratory findings. Evaluations of musculoskeletal impairment should be supported where applicable by a detailed description of the joints, including ranges of motion, condition of the musculature, sensory or reflex changes, circulatory deficits, and radiographic abnormalities. Where there is disorganization of motor function in the form of paresis, paralysis, tremor or involuntary movements, ataxia, and sensory disturbance, the assessment of impairment depends on the degree of interference with locomotion and/or interference with the use of the fingers, hands, or arms.

Again, one notes the limited application of such guidelines to the actual clinical presentation and functional deficits of the patient in relation to cervical pain and disability. However, it is important for physicians to become aware of the various factors by which agencies make their disability determination in order that they can accurately and fully represent the patients they are evaluating.

The laudable goal of the Guides and the Handbook is to provide a uniform measure of impairment. They are, however, unduly complicated and still subject to the evaluator's often less than objective assessment. For example, how does one grade the impairment associated with pain on a scale of 0% to 100%? Causalgic pain, which may restrict all activity, could be rated at 100%; however, a patient with incapacitating pain without objective loss of sensation would be difficult to evaluate.

## BASIC PRINCIPLES

Although it is desirable to pursue objective reproducible assessments of impairment, the above examples demonstrate the difficult task and inadequate tools presently available. Nevertheless, when one is asked to provide an impairment rating, the available tools may be of some help even though the limitations are significant and the tools are not universally accepted. There are some basic principles, however, which can assist the physician in the disability evaluation. It appears that the physician can best serve his or her patient by (*a*) providing a clear and concise report of the history and physical examination, supporting clinical and laboratory data relating to a medical diagnosis, and description of impairment; (*b*) describing how the medical diagnosis and impairment interferes with function both in daily life and in the patient's occupation if applicable; (*c*) stating whether the impairment is expected to be permanent and stable or temporary and amenable to treatment; and (*d*) stating how the pain and medications affect the patient's concentration span, job safety, and performance.

An example of a report that describes in detail the functional deficits produced by the impairment, in the patient's social as well as occupational environment, might read as follows:

The patient is a 35-year-old male machinist with the diagnosis of C8–T1 radiculopathy involving the dominant right upper extremity. The patient exhibits atrophy and weakness in the intrinsic muscles of the right hand with sensory deficit in the C8 distribution. He is significantly disabled with regard to activities of daily living (i.e., right hand grip, fine motor coordination, dressing skills and handling of small objects). The involvement of the dominant hand, the high level of dexterity required for his occupation, and the sensory deficits would make it unsafe for him to deal with potentially dangerous machinery. He is therefore significantly disabled with regard to his present occupation.

## CONSIDERATION OF THE AGENCY GRANTING DISABILITY STATUS

The granting of disability status is usually under the aegis of a compensation board, federal agency, social security department, or other similar agency, and knowledge of the laws and requirements governing that state or body is essential in order that the patient may be adequately represented. For example, the Social Security Administration may grant disability status only when the patient is unable to pursue *any* gainful employment. In contrast, the Social Security Disability Insurance Company may approve disability when the patient is unable to perform his or her *usual* employment (9). Therefore, when dealing with the former agency, the patient's potential for employment in other occupational areas must be evaluated, whereas when dealing with the latter, a clear description of the patient's ability or inability to perform only his usual work would be the determining factor in granting disability benefits.

## SUMMARY

Disability related to the neck is becoming an increasingly significant problem for everyone concerned. The patient needs and deserves a competent and caring and unbiased evaluation that will provide him or her with optimal remediation of or equitable compensation for the cervical impairment, disability, or handicap. The evaluating physician needs a set of rational guidelines for the examination and evaluation of the patient. The AMA Guides and the Social Security Handbook only partially answer this need. They both are in-

ordinately complicated, and it is doubtful that many physicians or insurance companies truly understand the intricacies of the various percentages and calculated disability tables.

Vocational rehabilitation evaluation and job simulation should be integrated into the above guidelines, and as much objective data as feasible should be accumulated. The cervical patient should be evaluated from a functional point of view using the trace, poor, fair, good, and normal categories, which combine strength and range of motion. Sensation is always a subjective measurement, and the closest one can come to objectivity is the analogue pain scale of 0–100. The report of the cervical examination should not dwell on the complicated system of percentages in the Guides and Handbook but should strive to document what the patient is unable to do relative to his or her vocational or social needs.

### REFERENCES

1. Calliet R: Diagnosis of neck pain. In *Neck and Arm Pain.* Philadelphia, FA Davis, 1982, p 50.
2. World Health Organization: *International Classification of Impairments, Disabilities and Handicaps: A Manual of Classification Relating to the Consequences of Disease.* Geneva, WHO, 1980.
3. Kessler HH: *Concept of Disability In Disability Determination and Evaluation.* Philadelphia, Lea & Febiger, 1970, pp 1–13.
4. Haj F: *Disability in Antiquity.* New York, Philosophical Library, 1970.
5. Bosworth DM: A ten-year analysis of intertrochantric fractures of the femur. [Editorial]. *J Bone Joint Surg [Am]* 41:1399–1408, 1959.
6. *The Revolt against "Whiplash."* Syracuse, NY, The Defense Research Institute, 1960.
7. *Guides to the Evaluation of Permanent Impairment.* Chicago, American Medical Association, 1984, p 75.
8. *Disability Evaluation under Social Security: A Handbook for Physicians.* Washington, DC, US Department of Health, Education and Welfare, 1979, pp 1–2.
9. Levy BS, Wegman DH: *Occupational Health Recognizing and Preventing Work-Related Disease,* ed 2. Boston, Little, Brown & Company, 1988, pp 170–175.

# 29

# PSYCHOLOGICAL DISABILITY AND IMPAIRMENT DETERMINATION

*C. David Tollison and Donald W. Hinnant*

Disability is, in general terms, a system of either social legislation or private insurance designed to protect individuals from suffering undue financial hardship when they are unable to work. Consequently, disability may result from physical, psychological, or a combination of physical and psychological disorders.

More specifically, disability is not a system, but a number of systems that include commercially available disability and wage protection insurance, personal injury liability, Social Security disability benefits (Title II) and supplemental security income (Title XVI), and workers' compensation insurance. Workers' compensation laws differ in each of the 50 states, the District of Columbia, and various U.S. territories. In addition, federal laws provide disability coverage for federal employees and many maritime workers are covered under the federal Longshore and Harbor Workers' Compensation Act.

Despite the multiplicity of laws, jurisdictions, and workers' compensation versus tort-based versus social legislation systems, the determination of impairment/disability is sufficiently similar that we can, for the purposes of this chapter, discuss the clinical and administrative determination of psychological impairment/disability as if it were a single general system. Variances to this approach will be noted when applicable.

A basic premise underlying the determination

of psychological functioning is the distinction between "impairment" and "disability." The definition of disability is based upon an individual's ability (or inability) to engage in "substantial gainful activity," or to work (1). Thus, the adjudication of disability claims is fundamentally a vocational/administrative issue rather than a medical one (1). This position has been supported as far back as 1958, when the American Medical Association (AMA) Committee on the Rating of Mental and Physical Impairment wrote in their "Guide to the Evaluation of Permanent Impairment, the Extremities and Back" that the determination of impairment is purely a medical decision, and that whether or not a given impairment represented a disability was an administrative responsibility and function, rather than a medical one (2). Consequently, a physician or clinical psychologist is charged with a responsibility of determining and documenting "impairments," a term considered to be of medical parlance. "Disability," in contrast, is generally considered a legal term and is determined by a ruling board, agency, court, or other authority. Therefore, an evaluating physician or clinical psychologist is responsible for determining the presence or absence of physical and/or psychological impairment that is subsequently considered in the nonmedical determination of whether an impairment constitutes a disability. The Social Security Administration, in fact, unequivocally states that "the physician is neither asked nor expected to make a decision as to whether the patient is disabled" (3).

In this chapter we will focus on the determination of psychological impairment subsequent to physical injury, with particular emphasis on emotional dysfunction reactive to cervical trauma and residual pain. We shall not discuss psychological impairment resulting from neuropsychological sequelae subsequent to cervical trauma associated with head injury. Finally, the above paragraph notwithstanding, the terms "impairment" and "disability" may be occasionally utilized interchangeably, primarily as a result of the aforementioned confusion that exists in referenced literature.

## PSYCHOLOGICAL IMPAIRMENT IN THE MEDICAL-LEGAL SYSTEM

There are numerous disability jurisdictions in the United States that oversee disability determination and monitor their own policies and procedures. Each jurisdiction has its own criteria for disability, as determined by administrative philosophy and policy, and there is considerable variation across jurisdictions. Likewise, the covered conditions, length and amount of payments, and review procedures also vary, as does the degree to which nonmedical factors (e.g., age, education, and social environment) are considered. For example, in certain situations an individual may qualify for more than one form of disability compensation.

Despite the array of disability systems and the variability in criteria and structure, there appear to be two common factors across systems. The first is that physicians and clinical psychologists do not determine disability, although their findings are considered relevant. Health professionals may render a medical opinion in individual cases about the degree of impairment, treatment, and prognosis, but disability (work incapacity) remains an administrative or judicial determination following input from multiple sources (4). A second common thread across disability systems is the general recognition of two primary types of disability: physical and psychological.

Because the determination of psychological disability is based in part on the responsibility of physicians and clinical psychologists to provide specific information on impairment, such individuals should have some familiarity with the procedures, regulations, and philosophy of the various agen-

cies and the criteria for disability determination currently in use at each. However, since an analysis of every current disability system is far beyond the limitations of this chapter, we shall restrict our discussion to a relatively brief overview of three primary systems: workers' compensation, Social Security, and personal injury.

## WORKERS' COMPENSATION

Workers' compensation is a system of state and federal legislation designed to protect workers from suffering undue financial hardship when they are unable to work as the result of an on-the-job injury. The definition of who is a covered worker varies from state to state. For the most part, however, the majority of "employees" are included in the system, although independent contractors and certain subclasses of employees may be excluded.

Workers' compensation is designed to protect injured workers from financial hardship but is not designed to totally replace lost income. Thus, under the most typical benefit scheme, a totally disabled worker will receive only two thirds of his or her average weekly wage, subject to a state maximum benefit. Also, unlike tort systems under which an injured person can collect for pain and suffering and other intangible injuries, the workers' compensation system is designed only to compensate injured workers for medical expenses and lost wages. Consequently, unlike tort systems, workers' compensation is generally not concerned with questions of fault or negligence. Thus, in the majority of workers' compensation cases the system functions almost automatically; upon receipt of notice that an employee has been injured, the employer arranges for payment of his or her medical expenses and begins making weekly payments of the workers' compensation benefits to which the employee is entitled until he or she is able to return to work. Nevertheless, there remain many cases in which there is disagreement between the parties as to whether the employee has sustained a compensable injury and, if so, what benefits he or she is entitled to receive.

In most states, the initial determination on contested proceedings is a hearing before a hearing officer (often called a referee, administrative law judge, or deputy commissioner), a quasi-judicial employee of the state labor department. Because the procedure is an administrative-type hearing rather than a court trial, the rules of evidence may be less strictly applied than would be the case in a court action. For instance, medical evidence may be admitted not only in the form of live testimony and sworn depositions, but also in the form of unsworn medical reports and letters. Furthermore, it should be remembered that the hearing officers rarely have any medical training. Thus, whether or not a case is contested, medical evidence is often accorded great weight by persons who may be untrained in medical terminology. Therefore, a physician or clinical psychologist who is called upon to give a report in a compensation case must remember to be clear in explaining the diagnosis, impairment findings, and prognosis, particularly in cases involving more unusual injuries. The physician/clinical psychologist should be prepared to explain an official diagnosis in layman's terms and to spell out in detail the causal relationship between the events of the job-related injury and the employee's current impairment. With regard to a rating of the degree of permanent disability sustained by a claimant, the medical examiner should be aware that insurance companies and workers' compensation hearing officers expect to have ratings based on standard AMA guidelines.

Workers' compensation benefits are paid during the period in which the employee is disabled from returning to work and, in some instances, for presumed future disability. The disability for which benefits are payable can be either temporary or permanent and either partial or total, leading to four classes of disability benefits: temporary partial, temporary total, permanent partial, and permanent total.

Assuming that there was a period of temporary total disability, it will be determined at some point that the injured worker has attained the maximum medical improvement (MMI) that can be expected. Once MMI has been reached, a determination must be made, with the assistance of medical/psychological opinion, as to whether the worker has sustained any permanent impairment and, if so, the extent of that impairment. If it appears that the worker will be unable to return to work at any time in the foreseeable future, he or she will be classified as permanently and totally disabled and will be awarded benefits accordingly. In many states, this means that the worker will be entitled to receive the weekly benefit rate for the remainder of his or her life or until circumstances change so that he or she can rejoin the workforce. However, in other states, even permanent total disability benefits are limited to a set period of time. Once that period has ended, the injured person will be without workers' compensation funds, unless he or she is able to qualify for other

types of assistance such as Social Security disability.

If the worker is able to return to work but has some residual physical or psychological disability attributable to the injury, he or she is likely to receive an award based on the state's "schedule" of injuries, combined with the medical/psychological ratings as to the degree of residual impairment.

At this point the reader will likely have noted two points in the above process where medical/psychological opinion is not only necessary, but almost always indispensable—determining when the worker has reached MMI and "rating" the degree of permanent impairment, which includes diagnosing whether residual impairment will cause permanent total or merely permanent partial impairment.

## SOCIAL SECURITY

Disability has been defined for the purpose of Social Security claims adjudication under the Social Security Act as an "inability to engage in any substantial gainful activity by reason of a medically determinable physical or mental impairment which can be expected to result in death or can be expected to last for a continuous period of not less than 12 months" (3). The adjudication of claim for disability benefits under Title II (Social Security Disability benefits) and Title XVI (Supplemental Security Disability and Income) of the Social Security Act is based upon the use of established medical criteria as described in the Listing of Impairments. However, as in other systems of disability determination, clear differences exist between what constitutes an "impairment" and what constitutes a "disability" within the context of the Social Security regulations, and it is on the interpretation of these differences that the Social Security Administration has placed considerable focus in the last several years.

The use of objectively demonstrable signs, symptoms, and medical findings as a disability adjudication has served the intent of the law relatively well in problems related to acute medical conditions, but the law does not provide an objective mechanism for evaluating the pain patient. Because the pain experience is a perception and because perceptions are not directly and objectively quantifiable, pain was considered in the evaluation of disability only as a secondary factor associated with a medically determinable impairment. The Social Security Administration has had increasing numbers of court cases challenging this policy regarding the evaluation of pain since chronic pain sufferers often present with allegations of pain that are not consistent with medically determinable impairment. As a consequence of an increasing number of cases within the courts, the Social Security Disability Benefits Reform Act of 1984 (Public Law 98-460) directed the Secretary of Health and Human Services to appoint a Commission on the Evaluation of Chronic Pain to conduct a joint study with the National Academy of Sciences on the evaluation of pain as it pertains to claims adjudication under Titles II and XVI of the Social Security Act.

The Commission recognized the pain experience as a multifaceted physical, mental, and behavioral process that may have an impact on the patient's behavior in all areas of his or her life and recognized that chronic pain patients often experience similar behavioral consequences as they attempt to adjust to the perception of pain. The commission defined four groups of chronic pain patients: (a) chronic pain, inability to cope, insufficiently documented impairment; (b) chronic pain, competent coping, and insufficiently documented impairment; (c) chronic pain, inability to cope, sufficiently documented impairment; (d) chronic pain, competent coping, sufficient documented impairment. The Commission determined that the third and fourth groups posed no problems in disability adjudication according to the current law, and recommended protocols for the evaluation of patients within the first and second groups. The commission specifically recommended interdisciplinary evaluation by appropriately trained medical, psychological, functional, social, and vocational specialists, and recommended the development of quantitative measurement of functional capacity and the establishment of rehabilitation goals within each disciplinary specialty. The Commission further recommended reevaluation of the chronic pain patient as a measure of his or her compliance with the prescribed pain rehabilitation program and recommended vocational counseling to increase the patient's productivity level after completion of the rehabilitation program. A more detailed examination of psychological impairment under Social Security is outlined in a following section of this chapter.

## PERSONAL INJURY

Anglo-Saxon law dictates, in legal parlance, a tort system for adjudication of personal injuries. Tort systems are designed to provide compensation (in the form of damages awards) from wrongdoers to those injured because of the wrongdoers' fault or negligence. Personal injury litigation allows the victim to sue for direct punitive damages as the result of wrongdoing, as well as for residual pain and suffering.

Crook (5) illustrated the differences between tort systems and workers' compensation in consideration of two simple "slip and fall" cases, in which Mr. Smith and Mr. Jones are hurt when they slip in a puddle of water on the floor and fall. In a tort system, whether Mr. Smith could recover from someone else for his injuries would depend on how the water got on the floor; whether the owner of the building knew, or should have known, that the water was there and that Mr. Smith or persons like him were likely to be walking in that area; and whether Mr. Smith should have been able to see the water to avoid stepping in it. If all of these issues were resolved in Smith's favor, he could recover his medical expenses in treating the injury, his past and future lost wages attributable to the injury, and his pain and suffering. In addition, his wife could recover for loss of consortium, that is, the diminution in value of his services to her as a result of the injury. The Smiths might also recover punitive damages if the judge or jury found that the defendant's conduct was especially blameworthy; for instance, if the puddle had been on the floor in an area heavily frequented by the public for a long time and the building's owner had deliberately refused to clean it up.

In contrast, if Mr. Jones had slipped on the puddle while he was working, questions of whose fault the accident was and who knew or did not know about the puddle would be generally irrelevant. The only issues would be whether his injuries were sufficiently work connected and whether those injuries kept him from working. His recovery, however, would be limited to payment of his medical bills, payment of compensation benefits for the weeks he was unable to work, and, in most states, a schedule award for his presumptive loss of wages if, after reaching maximum medical recovery, it was determined that he had a residual permanent loss of function attributable to his injuries.

In general practice, personal injury litigation cases often rely heavily on the "pain and suffering" and other reactive psychological ramifications that may result from physical injuries received. Typically, such legal cases require that the physician/clinical psychologist testify as to the diagnosis, prognosis, and psychological impairment (temporary or permanent) resulting from the injury and attribute any reactive psychological dysfunction in a causal manner to an accident or injuries received. Such "injury" is not limited to physical tissue damage but may also be a "psychological injury." For example, a claimant is a passenger in an automobile driven by a friend. Because of the wrongdoing and fault of a driver of another automobile that strikes the car of the claimant passenger, the driver of the car in which the claimant was a passenger is killed. The claimant passenger may then bring a personal injury suit against the driver of the other car for psychological injuries received as the result of being pinned in the car and forced to watch the slow and gruesome death of the driver.

## FACTORS INFLUENCING PSYCHOLOGICAL DISABILITY

It is generally accepted that a wide variety of psychosocioeconomic factors influence psychological functioning (see Chapter 27). It is also true that a variety of factors affect psychological impairment and disability. A partial listing of these factors includes age, educational level, premorbid psychological functioning, social and environmental factors, and cultural influences (6). However, in the determination of psychological impairment, it is critical that the examiner differentiate individual personality and idiosyncratic factors from psychological symptoms associated with and reactive to some particular event or injury. Generally speaking, possible emotional conditions arising from significant illness or injury should be expected to present with relatively discreet and circumscribed symptoms, in addition to the requirement of being meaningful and logically associated with a substantive illness or injury. When the psychological course is protracted and the symptoms are generalized, individual personality composition factors are frequently found to be more contributory and of greater etiologic significance than any alleged physical trauma (7). Thus, in a general sense it is reasonable to expect to determine more generalized, nonspecific psychological dysfunction in individuals claiming disability from chronic disease and illness (e.g., cancer) and more concrete and circumscribed emotional dysfunction in individuals claiming disability as a result of accidents, such as cervical trauma.

In addition to a variety of psychological conditions that may exist in reaction to cervical trauma, the literature suggests that victims may be conditioned or shaped into a role of psychological disability (8). In this section, we briefly summarize a selected number of such conditioning factors as earlier outlined by Strang (7). Knowledge of these and other conditioning factors is important to the physician/clinical psychologist charged with the responsibility of determining psychological impairment.

## PHYSICIAN FACTORS

Physicians commonly and inadvertently reinforce disability and development of chronic pain syndrome through mismanagement of the patient during the acute phase of pain and through the application of the acute pain medical model during the chronic phase of illness and injury. Fordyce (9) and others have discussed techniques designed to prevent the development of chronic pain that are applicable in the acute stage of discomfort. While the acute pain medical model works well in the great majority of medical situations, its application in the chronic phase of illness and injury can condition dependence, disability, dysfunction, and psychological impairment and disability.

### Failure to Apply the Chronic Illness Model

Related to physician factors above, Strang (7) has reported that physicians often act in accordance with the acute illness model beyond its appropriateness. Consequently, when patients enter a chronic phase, they may be encouraged to take it easy or told that they will be better in time, hence the development of magical expectations. When they do not improve, patients frequently feel resentful, hopeless, and depressed. This inadvertent action on the part of physicians may well result in iatrogenically induced physical and psychological impairment.

### Lack of Coordination of Consultants

Patients suffering a protracted period of pain generally are evaluated and treated by numerous physicians of varying specialties. Unfortunately, the various findings are often not integrated into a coordinated treatment plan that encourages patients to become more responsible for recovery.

The result of fragmented care is usually protracted disability.

## Tendency of Physicians to Take Patients' Complaints at Face Value

Strang (7) reported that physicians, in their desire to be helpful, often respond to repeated complaints of pain as presumptive evidence of some somatic lesion being the sole or main factor present or of some new acute problem or slow-to-heal lesion. Patients seldom directly complain about vocational and related disabilities, focusing more on complaints of pain. Consequently, it is easy for physicians to overlook possible psychological factors in the overall symptomatology.

## Countertransference Issues

The attitudes and values of physicians and other health professionals are not always consistent with those of patients who do not work. Moreover, patients involved in litigation or related activities often have different goals, agendas, and influences than do treating physicians, thereby generating occasional tension in the physician-patient relationship. As a result, physicians who have difficulty managing reality-based or negative countertransference feelings may respond by offering repeated medical workups, diagnostics, and treatments, all serving to shape the patient into a role of fear, dependence, and a conviction that all problems will ultimately be resolved with a unique diagnosis and therapeutic "magic bullet."

## Collusion in the Disability Claims Process

It is not infrequent to encounter patients who are highly insistent about their inability to work. Physicians and health professionals may then be easily drawn into a collusion over the disability. There is often an unspoken agreement not to confront the reality of the disability itself that inhibits the formation of a working alliance and proper goal setting. If physicians feel responsible, for whatever reason, for the patient's failure to improve or return to work, they may lose objectivity and become overinvolved in the disability process. In addition, if a physician is uncomfortable in confronting the patient with an obviously differing agenda (i.e., disability and return to work), the level of discomfort experienced by the physician may be resolved by avoiding confrontation and seeking relief through determination of influenced levels and intensities of impairment.

## FAMILY FACTORS

Fordyce (9) has commented extensively on the role of family members as reinforcers of disability. Family systems are often altered, with the emergence of mutually reinforcing hostile dependent relationships (7). Some spouses and family members remain gratifying and solicitous with hidden resentment and others remove themselves, creating family networks characterized by isolation and decreased communication.

## LEGAL FACTORS

Individuals claiming disability retain certain rights to apply for compensation through existing disability sources as well as to redress unfavorable disability determinations through further administrative or judicial reviews or hearings. Ongoing litigation is common and may foster an adversarial climate between employees and employers or granting agencies. Our legal system is designed such that attorneys often receive contingency fees and, naturally, an attorney protecting the best interests of his or her client will attempt to present a level of disability deserving of the highest award or longest length of compensation possible. Unfortunately, a return to productivity and employment, which is often clinically in the best interest of the patient, may undermine the disability process and claim. Attorneys, who are not clinically trained, may not appreciate the evidence that suggests that prolonged disability reinforces the very nature of the patient's difficulty, and, in fact, the clinical well-being of the patient is not the responsibility or training of the attorney any more than legal representation of the patient in the disability process is the responsibility and training of the physician/clinical psychologist. Health providers notoriously are reluctant to confront the legal process and take the initiative in educating and conferring with attorneys. In the experience of the authors, the great majority of attorneys hold the long-term best interest of the patient as a priority and are both responsive to and facilitating of clinical efforts to obtain maximum medical improvement if the clinician discusses the case with the attorney and works to educate and clarify clinical issues involved.

## EMPLOYER AND ADMINISTRATIVE AGENCY FACTORS

Light duty employment is often difficult for employers and management to supervise and enforce. Employers frequently express concerns about workers taking advantage of "special" privileges that are also viewed as potentially disruptive to the work routine and morale of other workers. Furthermore, employers may face liability insurance considerations that may litigate against the clinical need for injured employees to return to work in an early fashion. Unfortunately, even patients who are motivated to return to work often encounter a barrier in returning. Consequently, patients occasionally perceive themselves as hopelessly caught in a system that does not care about them and, ultimately, the patient becomes frustrated and suspicious of the motivation of the employer. Obviously, as the relationship between the employer and employee becomes strained, the opportunity for resolution to the dilemma of returning the patient to productivity becomes diminished. Furthermore, such a situation results in a reinforcement of disability.

## DISABILITY EVALUATION UNDER SOCIAL SECURITY

Psychological impairment/disability is recognized in a variety of disability agencies and sources but probably none more readily recognized yet complex than in Social Security disability. The evaluation of Social Security disability on the basis of mental disorders requires the documentation of a medically determinable impairment as well as consideration of the degree of limitation such impairment may impose on the individual's ability to work and whether this limitation has lasted or is expected to last for a continuous period of at least 12 months. The listings for mental disorders under Social Security disability are arranged in eight diagnostic categories: (a) organic mental disorders; (b) schizophrenic, paranoid, and other psychotic disorders; (c) affective disorders; (d) mental retardation and autism; (e) anxiety-related disorders; (f) somatoform disorders; (g) personality disorders; and (h) substance addiction disorders. Each diagnostic category, except mental retardation and autism and substance addiction disorders, consists of a set of clinical findings (paragraph A criteria) one or more of which must be met and that, if met, lead to a test of functional restrictions (paragraph B criteria) of which two or

three must also be met. There are additional considerations (paragraph C criteria) in the categories of paranoid and other psychotic disorders and anxiety-related disorders.

The purpose of including the criteria in paragraph A of the listings for mental disorders is to medically substantiate the presence of a mental disorder. The purpose of including the criteria in paragraphs B and C is to describe those functional limitations associated with mental disorders that are incompatible with the ability to work. The restrictions listed in paragraphs B and C must be the result of the mental disorder that is manifested by the clinical findings outlined in paragraph A. The criteria included in paragraphs B and C of the listings for mental disorders have been chosen by the Social Security Administration because they represent functional areas deemed essential for work. An individual who is severely limited in these areas as the result of an impairment identified in paragraph A is presumed to be unable to work.

The existence of a medically determinable impairment of the required duration must be established by medical evidence consisting of clinical signs, symptoms, and/or laboratory or psychological test findings. These findings may be intermittent or persistent, depending on the nature of the disorder. Clinical signs are medically demonstrable phenomena that reflect specific abnormalities of behavior, affect, thought, memory, orientation, or contact with reality. Social Security typically expects such an assessment to be performed by a psychiatrist or psychologist and documented by psychological testing. Symptoms are considered to be complaints presented by the individual. Signs and symptoms generally cluster together to constitute recognizable clinical syndromes (mental disorders). Both symptoms and signs that are part of any diagnosed mental disorder must be considered in evaluating severity. In the Social Security evaluation of mental disorders, severity is assessed in terms of the functional limitations imposed by the psychological impairment (paragraph B).

In this section we outline three of the eight categories of mental disorders and impairments considered to constitute evidence for psychological disability by the Social Security Administration. The categories of Affective Disorders, Anxiety Related Disorders, and Somatoform Disorders represent the three categories most frequently encountered by professionals determining psychological impairment as a result of or in association with cervical trauma and residual pain.

## AFFECTIVE DISORDERS (ref. 3, p. 70)

12.04 *Affective Disorders:* Characterized by a disturbance of mood, accompanied by a full or partial manic or depressive syndrome. Mood refers to a prolonged emotion that colors the whole psychic life; it generally involves either depression or elation.

The required level of severity for these disorders is met when the requirements in both A and B are satisfied.

A. Medically documented persistence, either continuous or intermittent, of one of the following:
   1. Depressive syndrome characterized by at least four of the following:
      a. Anhedonia or pervasive loss of interest in almost all activities; or
      b. Appetite disturbance with change in weight; or
      c. Sleep disturbance; or
      d. Psychomotor agitation or retardation; or
      e. Decreased energy; or
      f. Feelings of guilt or worthlessness; or
      g. Difficulty concentrating or thinking; or
      h. Thoughts of suicide; or
      i. Hallucinations, delusions or paranoid thinking; or
   2. Manic syndrome characterized by at least three of the following:
      a. Hyperactivity; or
      b. Pressure of speech; or
      c. Flight of ideas; or
      d. Inflated self-esteem; or
      e. Decreased need for sleep; or
      f. Easy distractability; or
      g. Involvement in activities that have a high probability of painful consequences which are not recognized; or
      h. Hallucinations, delusions or paranoid thinking; or
   3. Bipolar syndrome with a history of episodic periods manifested by the full symptomatic picture of both manic and depressive syndromes (and currently characterized by either or both syndromes);
AND
B. Resulting in at least two of the following:
   1. Marked restriction of activities of daily living; or
   2. Marked difficulties in maintaining social functioning; or
   3. Deficiencies of concentration, persistence or pace resulting in frequent failure to complete tasks in a timely manner (in work settings or elsewhere); or
   4. Repeated episodes of deterioration or decompensation in work or work-like settings which cause the individual to withdraw from that situation or to experience exacerbation of signs and symptoms (which may include deterioration of adaptive behaviors).

## ANXIETY RELATED DISORDERS (ref. 3, p. 72)

12.06 *Anxiety Related Disorders:* In these disorders anxiety is either the predominant disturbance or it is experienced if the individual attempts to master symptoms; for example, confronting the dreaded object or situation in a phobic disorder or resisting the obsessions or compulsions in obsessive compulsive disorders.

The required level of severity for these disorders is met when the requirements in both A and B are satisfied, or when the requirements in both A and C are satisfied.

A. Medically documented findings of at least one of the following:
   1. Generalized persistent anxiety accompanied by three out of four of the following signs or symptoms:
      a. Motor tension; or
      b. Autonomic hyperactivity; or
      c. Apprehensive expectation; or
      d. Vigilance and scanning; or
   2. A persistent irrational fear of a specific object, activity, or situation which results in a compelling desire to avoid the dreaded object, activity, or situation; or
   3. Recurrent severe panic attacks manifested by a sudden unpredictable onset of intense apprehension, fear, terror and sense of impending doom occurring on the average of at least once a week; or
   4. Recurrent obsessions or compulsions which are a source of marked distress; or
   5. Recurrent and intrusive recollections of a traumatic experience, which are a source of marked distress; and
B. Resulting in at least two of the following:
   1. Marked restriction of activities of daily living; or
   2. Marked difficulties in maintaining social functioning; or
   3. Deficiencies of concentration, persistence of pace resulting in frequent failure to complete tasks in a timely manner (in work settings or elsewhere); or
   4. Repeated episodes of deterioration or decompensation in work or work-like settings which cause the individual to withdraw from that situation or to experience exacerbation of signs and symptoms (which may include deterioration of adaptive behaviors); or

C.  Resulting in complete inability to function independently outside the area of one's home.

## SOMATOFORM DISORDERS (ref. 3, p. 73)

12.07 *Somatoform Disorders:* Physical symptoms for which there are no demonstrable organic findings or known physiological mechanisms.

The required level of severity for these disorders is met when the requirements in both A and B are satisfied.

A.  Medically documented by evidence of one of the following:
    1.  A history of multiple physical symptoms of several years duration, beginning before age 30, and have caused the individual to take medicine frequently, see a physician often and alter life patterns significantly; or
    2.  Persistent nonorganic disturbance of one of the following:
        a.  Vision; or
        b.  Speech; or
        c.  Hearing; or
        d.  Use of a limb; or
        e.  Movement and its control (e.g., coordination disturbance, psychogenic seizures, akinesia, dyskinesia); or
        f.  Sensation (e.g., diminished or heightened).
    3.  Unrealistic interpretation of physical signs or sensations associated with the preoccupation or belief that one has a serious disease or injury; and
B.  Resulting in three of the following:
    1.  Marked restriction of activities of daily living; or
    2.  Marked difficulties in maintaining social functioning; or
    3.  Deficiencies of concentration, persistence or pace resulting in frequent failure to complete tasks in a timely manner (in work settings or elsewhere); or
    4.  Repeated episodes of deterioration or decompensation in work or work-like settings which cause the individual to withdraw from that situation or to experience exacerbation of signs and symptoms (which may include deterioration of adaptive behavior).

## NOSOLOGY: DIAGNOSTIC AND STATISTICAL MANUAL OF MENTAL DISORDERS

The determination of psychological impairment is predicated on the recognition of psychological disability either in combination with physical impairment/disability (e.g., resulting from cervical trauma) or as a distinct entity that does not require the determination of an organic or physical component. In the determination of psychological impairment following cervical trauma, the busy clinician will likely encounter both.

To accurately communicate the determination of psychological impairment, a nosology that provides a common language is required. In determination of psychological functioning, this nosology is the *Diagnostic and Statistical Manual of Mental Disorders* (DSM), originally published in 1952. The third edition of the DSM was published in 1980 by the American Psychiatric Association and was revised (DSM III-R) in 1986 (10). Although developed for use with psychiatric and not pain patients, selected nomenclature in the DSM III-R is applicable to patients with chronic pain syndromes and includes both physical and psychological aspects of symptomatology.

There has been extensive clinical research indicating the tendency for affective disorders or personality disorders to be present with intractable pain. The DSM III-R includes pain, either as a diagnostic criterion or concomitant symptom, in a number of diagnostic categories. This section outlines these disorders, briefly discusses pain within the context of each disorder, and concludes with a discussion of depression as a proposed additional diagnostic disorder. Diagnostic criteria from the DSM III-R are reprinted with permission of the American Psychiatric Association, whose cooperation is appreciated.

## SOMATOFORM DISORDERS

The essential features of this group of disorders are physical symptoms suggesting physical disorders for which there are no demonstrable organic findings or known physiologic mechanisms, and for which there is positive evidence or a strong presumption that the symptoms are linked to psychological factors or conflicts. Although the symptoms of somatoform disorders are physical in nature, the specific pathophysiologic processes involved are not demonstrable or understandable by existing laboratory procedures and are conceptualized most clearly by means of psychological constructs. The production of symptoms by the patient is presumed to be unintentional.

### Conversion Disorder

The essential feature of Conversion Disorder is an alteration or loss of physical functioning that suggests a physical disorder, but that instead is apparently an expression of a psychological conflict or need. The symptoms of the disturbance are not intentionally produced and, after appropriate investigation, cannot be explained by any physical disorder or known pathophysiologic mechanism. Conversion Disorder is not diagnosed when conversion symptoms are limited to pain (see Somatoform Pain Disorder) but may be considered as a diagnosis, in association with pain, to explain a concrete "physical" disorder generated by a psychological etiology.

For example, the most common and "classic" conversion symptoms are not pain but, rather, those that suggest neurologic disease, such as paralysis, seizures, coordination disturbance, akinesia, dyskinesia, blindness, anesthesia, and paresthesia.

The symptoms of Conversion Disorder usually develop in a setting of extreme psychological stress and appear suddenly (e.g., cervical trauma). The effect of this disorder on a patient's life is usually marked and frequently impedes normal life activities. Prolonged loss of function may produce serious complications, such as contractures or disuse atrophy. Antecedent physical disorders or severe psychological stress is generally considered to be a predisposing factor.

The differential diagnosis of Conversion Disorder (see Table 29.1) is sometimes difficult in that many physical disorders that present with

**Table 29.1.**
**Diagnostic Criteria for Conversion Disorder**[a]

A.  A loss of, or alteration in, physical functioning suggesting a physical disorder.
B.  Psychological factors are judged to be etiologically related to the symptom because of a temporal relationship between a psychosocial stressor that is apparently related to a psychological conflict or need and initiation or exacerbation of the symptom.
C.  The person is not conscious of intentionally producing the symptom.
D.  The symptom is not a culturally sanctioned response pattern and cannot, after appropriate investigation, be explained by a known physical disorder.
E.  The symptom is not limited to pain or to a disturbance in sexual functioning.
**Specify single episode or recurrent.**

[a]From American Psychiatric Association: *Diagnostic and Statistical Manual of Mental Disorders*, ed 3, rev. Washington, DC, American Psychiatric Association, 1986, p 259.

vague, multiple somatic symptoms may, early in their course, be misdiagnosed as conversion symptoms. A diagnosis of Conversion Disorder is suggested if the symptoms are inconsistent with the actual known physical disorder—for example, anesthesia of the hand and arm following cervical trauma that conforms to the concept of the hand and arm rather than to the functional area served by a specific part of the nervous system. Physical disorders in which psychological factors often play an important role should not be diagnosed as Conversion Disorder.

## Hypochondriasis

The essential feature of a diagnosis of Hypochondriasis is preoccupation with a fear of having, or the belief that one has, a serious disease, based on the person's interpretation of physical signs or sensations as evidence of physical illness. A thorough physical examination does not support the diagnosis of any physical disorder that can account for the physical signs or sensations or for the person's unwarranted interpretation of them, although a coexisting physical disorder may be present. The unwarranted fear or belief of having a disease persists despite medical reassurance, but is not of delusional intensity, in that the person cannot acknowledge the possibility that he or she may be exaggerating the extent of the feared disease or that there may be no disease at all.

The preoccupation may be with bodily functions, such as heartbeat, sweating, or peristalsis, or with minor physical abnormalities. In patients who have suffered cervical trauma with residual pain and functional limitations, the presence of discomfort and physical signs, particularly radicular sensations into the arms, may be interpreted as caused by cancer or some other dreaded disease. The medical history is often presented by the patient in great detail and at length. "Doctor shopping" and deterioration in doctor-patient relationships, with frustration and anger on both sides, are common. Patients with this disorder often believe they are not getting proper care and that physicians have simply not found the true "cause" of their symptoms.

The most important differential diagnostic consideration in Hypochondriasis is the presence of true organic disease, such as early stages of neurologic disorders, endocrine disorders, or neurologic disorders resulting from trauma. However, the presence of true organic disease does not rule out the possibility of coexisting Hypochondriasis

**Table 29.2.**
**Diagnostic Criteria for Hypochondriasis**[a]

A. Preoccupation with the fear of having, or the belief that one has, a serious disease, based on the person's interpretation of physical signs or sensations as evidence of physical illness.
B. Appropriate physical evaluation does not support the diagnosis of any physical disorder that can account for the physical signs or sensations or the person's unwarranted interpretation of them, **and** the symptoms in A are not just symptoms of panic attacks.
C. The fear of having, or belief that one has, a disease persists despite medical reassurance.
D. Duration of the disturbance is at least six months.
E. The belief in Part A is not of delusional intensity, as in Delusional Disorder, Somatic Type (i.e., the person can acknowledge the possibility that his or her fear of having, or belief that he or she has, a serious disease is unfounded).

[a]From American Psychiatric Association: *Diagnostic and Statistical Manual of Mental Disorders*, ed 3, rev. Washington, DC, American Psychiatric Association, 1986, p 261.

(see Table 29.2). In Somatization Disorder there tends to be preoccupation with symptoms rather than fear of having a specific disease or diseases. However, when the criteria for Somatization Disorder are met and the criteria for Hypochondriasis are also met, both diagnoses should be given.

## Somatization Disorder

The essential features of Somatization Disorder are recurrent and multiple somatic complaints, usually of several years' duration, for which medical attention has been repeatedly sought but that apparently are not due to any physical disorder. The disorder begins before the age of 30 and has a chronic but fluctuating course.

Complaints are often presented in a dramatic, vague, or exaggerated way, or are part of a complicated medical history in which many physical diagnoses have been considered (e.g., cervical trauma). Patients frequently receive medical care from a number of physicians, sometimes simultaneously. Complaints invariably involve the following organic symptoms or types of symptoms: conversion or pseudoneurologic symptoms, gastrointestinal discomfort, cardiopulmonary symptoms, and pain (e.g., neck or back).

In the diagnosis of Somatization Disorder, anxiety and depressed mood are often associated features (Table 29.3). Because of constant consultation of doctors, patients undergo numerous medical evaluations both in and out of the hospital; there is frequently unwitting submission to unnecessary surgery. Furthermore, these patients run the risk of Psychoactive Substance Use Disorders involving various prescribed medications.

The differential diagnosis of Somatization Disorder is, again, sometimes difficult in that it is necessary to rule out physical disorders that present with vague, multiple, and confusing somatic symptoms such as myofascial, neurologic, and other types of symptoms resulting from cervical trauma. In Conversion Disorder one or more conversion symptoms occur in the absence of the full clinical picture of Somatization Disorder.

## Somatoform Pain Disorder

The essential feature of Somatoform Pain Disorder is preoccupation with pain in the absence of adequate physical findings to account for the pain or its intensity. The pain symptom either is inconsistent with the anatomic distribution of the nervous system or, if it mimics a known disease entity, cannot, after extensive diagnostic examination, be adequately accounted for by organic pathology.

In some cases there may be evidence that psychological factors are etiologically involved in the pain, as when there is a clear temporal relationship between an environmental stimulus that is apparently related to a psychological conflict or need and initiation or exacerbation of the pain. In other cases the evidence may be that the pain permits the person to avoid some activity that is noxious to him or her or to get support from the environment that otherwise might not be forthcoming. In still other cases, there may be no direct evidence of an etiologic role of psychological factors.

Somatoform Pain Disorder may be accompanied by other localized sensory or motor function changes, such as paresthesias and muscle spasm. Characteristic are frequent visits to physicians to obtain relief despite medical reassurance, excessive use of analgesics without relief of the pain, requests for surgery, and assumption of the role of invalid. The patient usually refuses to consider the contribution of psychological factors to the pain. Symptoms of depression are frequent and in many cases an associated diagnosis of Major Depression is warranted.

The complaint of pain in Somatoform Pain Dis-

**Table 29.3.**
**Diagnostic Criteria for Somatization Disorder**[a]

A.    A history of many physical complaints or a belief that one is sickly, beginning before the age of 30 and persisting for several years.

B.    At least 13 symptoms from the list below. To count a symptom as significant, the following criteria must be met:

(1) no organic pathology or pathophysiologic mechanism (e.g., a physical disorder or the effects of injury, medication, drugs or alcohol) to account for the symptom or, when there is related organic pathology, the complaint or resulting social or occupational impairment is grossly in excess of what would be expected from the physical findings

(2) has not occurred only during a panic attack

(3) has caused the person to take medicine (other than over-the-counter pain medication), see a doctor, or alter life-style

Symptom list:

Gastrointestinal symptoms:

(1) **vomiting (other than during pregnancy)**

(2) abdominal pain (other than when menstruating)

(3) nausea (other than motion sickness)

(4) bloating (gassy)

(5) diarrhea

(6) intolerance of (gets sick from) several different foods

Pain symptoms:

(7) **pain in extremities**

(8) back pain

(9) joint pain

(10) pain during urination

(11) other pain (excluding headaches)

Cardiopulmonary symptoms:

(12) **shortness of breath when not exerting oneself**

(13) palpitations

(14) chest pain

(15) dizziness

Conversion or pseudoneurologic symptoms:

(16) **amnesia**

(17) **difficulty swallowing**

(18) loss of voice

(19) deafness

(20) double vision

(21) blurred vision

(22) blindness

(23) fainting or loss of consciousness

(24) seizure or convulsion

(25) trouble walking

(26) paralysis or muscle weakness

(27) urinary retention or difficulty urinating

Sexual symptoms for the major part of the person's life after opportunities for sexual activity:

(28) **burning sensation in sexual organs or rectum (other than during intercourse)**

(29) sexual indifference

(30) pain during intercourse

(31) impotence

Female reproductive symptoms judged by the person to occur more frequently or severely than in most women:

(32) **painful menstruation**

(33) irregular menstrual periods

(34) excessive menstrual bleeding

(35) vomiting throughout pregnancy

Note: The seven items in boldface may be used to screen for the disorder. The presence of two or more of these items suggests a high likelihood of the disorder.

[a]From American Psychiatric Association: *Diagnostic and Statistical Manual of Mental Disorders*, ed 3, rev. Washington, DC, American Psychiatric Association, 1986, pp 263–264.

**Table 29.4.**
**Diagnostic Criteria for Somatoform Pain Disorder**[a]

A.  Preoccupation with pain for at least six months.
B.  Either (1) or (2):
   (1) appropriate evaluation uncovers no organic
       pathology or pathophysiologic mechanism
       (e.g., a physical disorder or the effects of
       injury) to account for the pain
   (2) when there is related organic pathology, the
       complaint of pain or resulting social or
       occupational impairment is grossly in excess of
       what would be expected from the physical
       findings

---

[a]From American Psychiatric Association: *Diagnostic and Statistical Manual of Mental Disorders*, ed 3, rev. Washington, DC, American Psychiatric Association, 1986, p 266.

order usually appears suddenly, often following trauma, and increases in severity over weeks or months. Typically, the person has become incapacitated and has ceased to work. An invalid role is often assumed. The most serious complications are iatrogenic and include dependence on minor tranquilizers and narcotic analgesics and repeated, unsuccessful, surgical interventions.

In approximately half of the cases of Somatoform Pain Disorder the complaint of pain develops immediately following a physical trauma—for example, complaints of pain following cervical trauma. The dramatic presentation of organic pain, which may seem excessive to an observer because of minimal physical findings, is not sufficient for diagnosing this disorder (Table 29.4). Furthermore, pain associated with muscle contraction headaches that may result following cervical trauma is not to be diagnosed as Somatoform Pain Disorder because there is a pathophysiologic mechanism that accounts for the pain.

## Undifferentiated Somatoform Disorder

Undifferentiated Somatoform Disorder is a category for clinical pictures that do not meet the full symptom picture of Somatization Disorder. There is either a single circumscribed symptom or, more commonly, multiple physical complaints such as fatigue, loss of appetite, and nonspecific complaints of pain. Like Somatization Disorder, the symptoms are not explainable on the basis of demonstrable organic findings or a known pathophysiologic mechanism, and are apparently linked to psychological factors. The diagnosis is not made if the disturbance is of less than 6 months'

duration or if it occurs only during the course of another Somatoform Disorder such as Somatoform Pain Disorder (Table 29.5). Anxiety and depressed mood are commonly encountered and functional impairment is generally less than that determined in Somatization Disorder.

## PSYCHOLOGICAL FACTORS AFFECTING PHYSICAL CONDITION

The category of Psychological Factors Affecting Physical Condition can apply to any physical condition to which psychological factors are judged to be contributory (see Table 29.6). It may be used to describe disorders that in the past have been referred to as either "psychosomatic" or "psychophysiological."

Common examples of physical conditions for which this category may be appropriate include, but are not limited to: tension headache, migraine headache, headache following cervical trauma, sacroiliac pain, rheumatoid arthritis, and gastric or duodenal ulcer. This category should not be used in cases of Conversion Disorder or other Somatoform Disorders, which are regarded as disturbances in which the specific pathophysiologic process involved in the disorder is not demonstrable by

---

**Table 29.5.**
**Diagnostic Criteria for Undifferentiated Somatoform Disorder**[a]

A.  One or more physical complaints, e.g., fatigue,
    loss of appetite, gastrointestinal or urinary
    complaints.
B.  Either (1) or (2):
   (1) appropriate evaluation uncovers no organic
       pathology or pathophysiologic mechanism
       (e.g., a physical disorder or the effects of
       injury, medication, drugs, or alcohol) to
       account for the physical complaints
   (2) when there is related organic pathology, the
       physical complaints or resulting social or
       occupational impairment is grossly in excess of
       what would be expected from the physical
       findings
C.  Duration of the disturbance is at least six months.
D.  Occurrence not exclusively during the course of
    another Somatoform Disorder, a Sexual
    Dysfunction, a Mood Disorder, an Anxiety
    Disorder, a Sleep Disorder, or a psychotic
    disorder.

---

[a]From American Psychiatric Association: *Diagnostic and Statistical Manual of Mental Disorders*, ed 3, rev. Washington, DC, American Psychiatric Association, 1986, p 267.

**Table 29.6.**

**Diagnostic Criteria for Psychological Factors Affecting Physical Condition[a]**

---

A.  Psychologically meaningful environmental stimuli are temporally related to the initation or exacerbation of a specific physical condition or disorder (recorded on Axis III).

B.  The physical condition involves either demonstrable organic pathology (e.g., rheumatoid arthritis) or a known pathophysiologic process (e.g., migraine headache).

C.  The condition does not meet the criteria for a Somatoform Disorder.

---

[a]From American Psychiatric Association: *Diagnostic and Statistical Manual of Mental Disorders,* ed 3, rev. Washington, DC, American Psychiatric Association, 1986, p 334.

existing standard laboratory procedures and which are conceptualized by psychological constructs only.

## MALINGERING

Malingering is considered a subset of the major diagnostic category in the DSM III-R termed Codes for Conditions Not Attributable to a Mental Disorder That Are a Focus of Attention or Treatment (10). The essential feature of Malingering is intentional production of false or grossly exaggerated physical or psychological symptoms, motivated by external incentives such as avoiding work, obtaining financial compensation, evading criminal prosecution, obtaining drugs, and the like.

According to the DSM III-R, Malingering should be strongly suspected if any combination of the following is noted:

(1)  Medicolegal context of presentation, e.g., the person's being referred by his or her attorney to the physician for examination;

(2)  Marked discrepancy between the person's claimed stress or disability and the objective findings;

(3)  Lack of cooperation during the diagnostic evaluation and in complying with the prescribed treatment regimen;

(4)  The presence of Antisocial Personality Disorder.

Malingering is differentiated from Conversion and other Somatic Disorders by the intentional production of symptoms and by the obvious, external incentives. The person who is malingering is much less likely to present his or her symptoms in the context of emotional conflict, and the pre-

senting symptoms are less likely to be symbolically related to an underlying emotional conflict.

While the physician/clinical psychologist examiner may occasionally encounter a malingerer in the course of determining psychological impairment, it has been the experience of the authors that such a disorder is generally uncommon and, when encountered, is usually presented by individuals with limited intellectual sophistication that results in symptoms and behaviors generating a nonchallenging and uncomplicated diagnosis of Malingering.

## PSYCHOACTIVE SUBSTANCE ABUSE

Psychoactive Substance Abuse is a residual category for noting maladaptive patterns of psychoactive substance use that have never met the criteria for dependence for that particular class of substance. The maladaptive pattern of use is indicated by either (a) continued use of the psychoactive substance despite knowledge of having a persistent or recurrent social, occupational, psychological, or physical problem that is caused or exacerbated by use of the substance or (b) recurrent use of the substance in situations when use is physically hazardous (10). The diagnosis is made only if some symptoms of the disturbance have persisted for at least 1 month or have occurred repeatedly over a longer period of time (Table 29.7). The diagnosis is most likely to be applicable to pa-

**Table 29.7.**

**Diagnostic Criteria for Psychoactive Substance Abuse[a]**

---

A.  A maladaptive pattern of psychoactive substance use indicated by at least one of the following:

(1) continued use despite knowledge of having a persistent or recurrent social, occupational, psychological, or physical problem that is caused or exacerbated by use of the psychoactive substance

(2) recurrent use in situations in which use is physically hazardous (e.g., driving while intoxicated)

B.  Some symptoms of the disturbance have persisted for at least one month, or have occurred repeatedly over a longer period of time.

C.  Never met the criteria for Psychoactive Substance Dependence for this substance.

---

[a]From American Psychiatric Association: *Diagnostic and Statistical Manual of Mental Disorders,* ed 3, rev. Washington, DC, American Psychiatric Association, 1986, p 169.

tients who have only recently started taking psychoactive substances and, therefore, are less likely to be in danger of marked physiologic withdrawal or withdrawal symptoms. In practice, the diagnosis of Psychoactive Substance Abuse is rarely made in patients complaining of residual pain following cervical trauma.

## ORGANIC MENTAL SYNDROMES AND DISORDERS

It is accepted that head injury, occasionally associated with cervical trauma, may result in organic mental syndromes and disorders. Consistent with the orientation of this chapter, however, we shall not address psychological impairment resulting from neuropsychological sequelae (see Chapters 6 and 26).

## POST-TRAUMATIC STRESS DISORDER

The essential feature of Post-Traumatic Stress Disorder is the development of characteristic symptoms following a psychologically distressing event that is outside the range of usual human experience. The stressor producing this syndrome would be markedly distressing to almost anyone, and is usually experienced with intense fear, terror, and helplessness. The characteristic symptoms involve re-experiencing the traumatic event, avoidance of stimuli associated with the event or numbing of general responsiveness, and increased arousal (Table 29.8). The diagnosis is not made if the disturbance lasts less than 1 month.

The most common traumata involve either a serious threat to one's life or physical integrity; a serious threat or harm to one's children, spouse, or other close relatives and friends; sudden destruction of one's home or community; or seeing another person who has recently been, or is being, seriously injured or killed as the result of an accident or physical violence. The trauma may be experienced alone or in the company of groups of people. Stressors producing this disorder include natural disasters (e.g., earthquakes), accidental disasters (e.g., car accidents with serious physical injury), or deliberately caused disasters (e.g., bombings). Sometimes there is a concomitant physical component of the trauma, which may even involve direct damage to the central nervous system (e.g., head injury). The disorder is apparently more severe and longer lasting when the stressor is of human design.

Symptoms characteristic of Post-Traumatic Stress Disorder are often intensified or precipitated when the person is exposed to situations or activities that resemble or symbolize the original trauma. Symptoms of depression and anxiety are common and, in some instances, may be sufficiently severe to be diagnosed as an Anxiety or Depressive Disorder. Furthermore, there may be symptoms of an Organic Mental Disorder, such as failing memory, difficulty in concentrating, emotional lability, headache, and vertigo. Symptoms usually begin immediately or soon after the trauma. Impairment may be either mild or severe and affects nearly every aspect of life.

## DEPRESSION AS AN ADDITIONAL DIAGNOSTIC CATEGORY

Aronoff (11) originally reviewed the use of the DSM III in the diagnosis of chronic pain states and found it incomplete in not providing a category for Depression (as distinct from its listing under Affective Disorders). It is the opinion of the authors that the same criticism may be leveled against the DSM III-R.

Depression is the most common emotional disorder determined in patients with chronic pain syndromes (12), yet this diagnosis is omitted in the DSM III-R diagnostic categories associated with pain. While the relationship between chronic pain and depression is often complex, the clinician must be prepared to encounter depression as a concomitant feature of intractable pain and consider this diagnosis in determination of psychological impairment.

Aronoff (11) reported that it is incumbent upon the clinician to recognize and distinguish functional from organic causes of depressive symptoms. These may range from dementing processes, some of which may not be reversible, to the most readily reversible organic causes of depression and dementia, such as toxic states, endocrine or other metabolic disorders, and normal pressure hydrocephalus. The experienced clinician has likely encountered severely depressed patients presenting with memory disturbance and concentration deficits, superficially representing a pseudodementia, that tend to disappear once the depression improves. In addition to clinical evaluation and routine psychological testing, it may be necessary to perform a complete neuropsychological evaluation in patients presenting complex diagnostic pictures, particularly following cervical trauma (see Chapter 26). Although the presence of depression in association with

**Table 29.8.**
**Diagnostic Criteria for Post-Traumatic Stress Disorder[a]**

A.  The person has experienced an event that is outside the range of usual human experience and that would be markedly distressing to almost anyone, e.g., serious threat to one's life or physical integrity; serious threat or harm to one's children, spouse, or other close relatives and friends; sudden destruction of one's home or community; or seeing another person who has recently been, or is being, seriously injured or killed as the result of an accident or physical violence.

B.  The traumatic event is persistently re-experienced in at least one of the following ways:
    (1) recurrent and intrusive distressing recollections of the event (in young children, repetitive play in which themes or aspects of the trauma are expressed)
    (2) recurrent distressing dreams of the event
    (3) sudden acting or feeling as if the traumatic event were recurring (includes a sense of reliving the experience, illusions, hallucinations, and dissociative [flashback] episodes, even those that occur upon awakening or when intoxicated)
    (4) intense psychological distress at exposure to events that symbolize or resemble an aspect of the traumatic event, including anniversaries of the trauma

C.  Persistent avoidance of stimuli associated with the trauma or numbing of general responsiveness (not present before the trauma), as indicated by at least three of the following:
    (1) efforts to avoid thoughts or feelings associated with the trauma
    (2) efforts to avoid activities or situations that arouse recollections of the trauma
    (3) inability to recall an important aspect of the trauma (psychogenic amnesia)
    (4) markedly diminished interest in significant activities (in young children, loss of recently acquired developmental skills such as toilet training or language skills)
    (5) feeling of detachment or estrangement from others
    (6) restricted range of affect, e.g., unable to have loving feelings
    (7) sense of foreshortened future, e.g., does not expect to have a career, marriage, or children, or long life

D.  Persistent symptoms of increased arousal (not present before the trauma), as indicated by at least two of the following:
    (1) difficulty falling or staying asleep
    (2) irritability or outbursts of anger
    (3) difficulty concentrating
    (4) hypervigilance
    (5) exaggerated startle response
    (6) physiologic reactivity upon exposure to events that symbolize or resemble an aspect of the traumatic event (e.g., a woman who was raped in an elevator breaks out in a sweat when entering any elevator)

E.  Duration of the disturbance (symptoms in B, C, and D) of at least one month.

**Specify delayed onset** if the onset of symptoms was at least six months after the trauma.

[a]From American Psychiatric Association: *Diagnostic and Statistical Manual of Mental Disorders*, ed 3, rev. Washington, DC, American Psychiatric Association, 1986, pp 250–251.

pain is often thought to be reactive to pain, suffering, and alteration in life-style, it is not at all uncommon to evaluate patients whose depression preceded the pain or in whom the pain-depression relationship is unclear.

There is growing evidence that depression lowers pain tolerance, increases analgesic requirements, and in a variety of other ways adds to the debilitating effects of pain (13). In the determination of psychological impairment, these symptoms can have significant impact on residual psychological functioning subsequent to cervical trauma. Patients in pain often suffer from the vegetative signs of depression, including insomnia, appetite fluctuations, diminished libido, excessive use of alcohol or narcotic and sedative-hypnotic medications, and a loss of interest in outside activities—all residual signs of psychological impairment. While patients usually attribute these problems to pain rather than depression, the clinician must carefully investigate the causal relationship that exists and determine depression as a psychological impairment if it exists in reaction to cervical trauma. Once the pain-depression-insomnia cycle is established, it becomes self-perpetuating and requires active intervention.

Aronoff (11) lists a number of clinical features of chronic pain with depression that are worthy of consideration by the clinician faced with the responsibility of determining psychological impair-

**Table 29.9.**
**Clinical Features of Chronic Pain with Depression**[a]

A. Depression may be reactive to pain or may precede pain.

B. The patient suffers from the symptoms of depression in DSM-III:
   1. poor appetite or significant weight loss (when not dieting) or increased appetite or significant weight gain;
   2. insomnia or hypersomnia;
   3. psychomotor agitation or retardation;
   4. loss of interest in or enjoyment of sex;
   5. social withdrawal;
   6. feelings of unworthiness, self-reproach, or excessive inappropriate guilt;
   7. recurrent thoughts of death, suicidal ideation, wishes to be dead, or suicide attempt;
   8. fearfulness or crying

C. The patient often denies psychological causes of depression and attributes depressive symptomatology to pain.

D. Primary defenses are most often somatization, denial, and repression.

E. There is a decreased pain threshold.

F. There is a tenuous support system.

G. It is frequently associated with somatic preoccupation and hypochondriasis.

H. It is often associated with Pain-Prone Disorder.

I. There is an increased family incidence of pain, depression, and disability.

[a]From Aronoff GM: Psychological aspects of nonmalignant chronic pain: a new nosology. In Aronoff GM (ed): *Evaluation and Treatment of Chronic Pain.* Baltimore, Urban and Schwarzenberg, 1985.

ment (Table 29.9). It is hoped that future revisions of the DSM will include the diagnostic category of Depression in categories associated with pain.

## CONCLUDING REMARKS

Psychological impairment and resulting disability that often occur in association with cervical trauma will probably continue to be a controversial topic among health professionals for years to come. Historically, our litigious society has intentionally or unintentionally complicated the combination of physical and psychological conse-

quences following injury. However, it is becoming common practice for many health professionals who evaluate and treat accident victims to secure a multidisciplinary evaluation. There is growth in the establishment of pain treatment centers that are purposely designed for the evaluation of the trauma patient suffering associated psychological symptoms. Such a comprehensive center may provide a thorough evaluation, including reports from medicine, psychology, psychiatry, physical therapy, and vocational rehabilitation, that collectively address the patient's total sphere of functioning.

Early recognition of psychological as well as physical sequelae following cervical trauma may lead to proper early intervention strategies and prevention of chronicity.

## REFERENCES

1. Nadolsky JM: Social security: in need of rehabilitation. *J Rehabil* 50:6–8, 1984.
2. AMA Council on Rating Mental and Physical Impairment: Guides to the evaluation of permanent impairment—the extremities and back. *JAMA* 166:2, 1958.
3. United States Department of Health and Human Services, Social Security Administration: *Disability Evaluation under Social Security*, SSA Pub. No. 05-10089. Washington, DC, U.S. Government Printing Office, 1986, p 3.
4. Ziporyn T: Disability evaluation: a fledgling science? *JAMA* 250:873–829, 1983.
5. Crook PL: Workers' compensation. In Tollison CD (ed): *Handbook of Chronic Pain Management.* Baltimore, Williams & Wilkins, 1989.
6. Sternbach R: *Pain Patients: Traits and Treatment.* Academic Press, New York, 1974.
7. Strang JP: The chronic disability syndrome. In Aronoff GM (ed): *Evaluation and Treatment of Chronic Pain.* Baltimore, Urban and Schwarzenberg, 1985.
8. Tollison CD: Diagnosing and managing chronic pain syndrome. *J SC Med Assoc* September, 449–452, 1984.
9. Fordyce WE: *Behavioral Methods for Chronic Pain and Illness.* St. Louis, CV Mosby, 1976.
10. American Psychiatric Association: *Diagnostic and Statistical Manual of Mental Disorders*, ed 3, rev. Washington, DC, American Psychiatric Association, 1986.
11. Aronoff GM: Psychological aspects of nonmalignant chronic pain: a new nosology. In Aronoff GM (ed): *Evaluation and Treatment of Chronic Pain.* Baltimore, Urban and Schwarzenberg, 1985.
12. Tollison CD, Kriegel ML: Selected tricyclic antidepressants in the management of chronic benign pain. *South Med J* 81:562–564, 1988.
13. Tollison CD, Kriegel ML, Satterthwaite JR: Comprehensive treatment of acute and chronic low back pain: a clinical outcome comparison. *Orthop Rev* 1:59–64, 1989.

# 30

# MEDICAL DEPOSITIONS AND COURT APPEARANCES

## Claimant's Counsel Perspective

*Gerald M. Finkel and Ralph C. McCullough II*

## ROLE OF THE PHYSICIAN

The preparation of the medical witness is dependent upon the role the physician is called upon to play in the particular legal proceeding. Most often, the witness is the treating physician and, as such, is a material witness to the case.

The medical witness may also be called upon as an expert in the case. An expert is allowed to render an opinion that is designed to aid the jury in their understanding of the matter. In this capacity, the witness has the power to draw inferences from the facts in the case that a jury would not be competent to draw and that any other witness in the case who is not qualified as an expert would be legally incompetent to draw (1). It is not unusual for a treating physician to also qualify as an expert in the case. The fact that a physician has treated a person professionally does not disqualify him to give expert testimony on behalf of his own patient (2). There is significant authority, however, to the effect that it is improper for a physician who treated the plaintiff in a personal injury case to accept employment as an expert by the defendant in the same matter (3).

There are cervical trauma cases in which the physician is a defendant in the case because the injury arose as the result of a physician's alleged malpractice (4, 5). While many of the principles relating to the preparation of treating physicians and experts are the same as for parties, there are many additional considerations that must be ad-

dressed when dealing directly with a litigant. The medical malpractice issues are beyond the scope of this chapter, which shall be confined to the preparation of treating physicians and expert witnesses.

## CASE PREPARATION

Plaintiff's counsel begins the legal process by developing an overall strategy for litigation known as the case theory (6). The primary objective of the case theory is to achieve the client's objectives through the litigation process. It also provides a tactical structure that directs and organizes all of the litigation-oriented activities involving the preparation of the complaint, the nature and extent of discovery, the selection of witnesses, the opening statement and the Order of Proof at trial.

In painful cervical trauma cases the two critical medicolegal issues generally facing the plaintiff's lawyer in developing the factual theory of his case are causation and damages (7). For the plaintiff's injuries to be compensable, it is necessary to prove that those injuries were proximately caused by a breach of a duty of care owed to the plaintiff by the defendant. The proximate cause between the plaintiff's injuries and the initial trauma is difficult to prove. The use of expert witnesses is often essential to reach this goal.

The value of the case, or damages, is largely dependent upon the severity of the injury and the

451

plaintiff's prognosis. Elements such as medical expenses, past, present, and future pain and suffering, medication, disfigurement, temporary disability, and permanent disability are usually within the purview of the treating physician.

In formulating the case theory, plaintiff's counsel may interview a number of potential medical experts to determine whether the expert would be suitable for and interested in working on a problem for trial preparation. Counsel is interested in finding experts who would be favorable to the plaintiff's side and who will support the theory of the case. In addition, the attorney may request answers to technical questions in casual conversation without ever contemplating using the expert in the actual trial preparation. Informally consulted experts generally enjoy an immunity from the legal discovery process. Where the expert is the object of a casual inquiry with no retention contract and has engaged in no real trial preparation, his tentative opinion on the point is not discoverable. In fact, under the Federal Rules of Civil Procedure (Fed R Civ P), even the name of such an expert is beyond the scope of discovery (8).

The opinions of the opposing parties' experts that have been used in trial preparation can be obtained only upon a showing of exceptional circumstances under which it is impracticable for the parties seeking discovery to obtain facts or opinions on the same subject by other means (9). Examples of such exceptional circumstances that would allow for discovery of these experts might be where the party requesting discovery could not conduct important tests because an item of equipment needed for that test has been destroyed or is otherwise no longer available. In addition, it is conceivable that circumstances would exist in which it is impossible for a party to obtain his own expert. Such circumstances would occur when the number of experts in a field is small and their time has already been fully retained by others. For instance, in a rural area the only qualified neurologist may have been retained to testify for defense counsel and his retention has exhausted the field.

Attempting to take the deposition of the opposing parties' specially employed expert is not without its costs. If discovery is allowed at all, the court usually requires the party seeking discovery to pay the other party a fair portion of the fees and expenses reasonably incurred in obtaining facts and opinions from the expert. This protection is incorporated in the Federal Rules as an attempt to reconcile the goal of revealing needed material with the inequity of taking advantage of the adversary's efforts. Consequently, plaintiff's counsel will generally take the deposition of the treating physicians and his own expert witnesses in the event that they might be otherwise unavailable at trial.

## DEPOSITION MECHANICS

Depositions are used for a variety of purposes, and the proposed use may dictate the format and interrogation style used by counsel. The purposes for which depositions may be used fall into two general categories: preservation of testimony (10) and discovery (11, 12). A party may wish to preserve a testimony for subsequent use at trial in the event that a witness would be otherwise unavailable because of illness or location beyond the subpoena power of the court, or as some form of insurance against some material change in circumstance between the date of deposition and the date of trial. In addition, the deposition may be used for impeachment at trial where the examiner intends to show that the witness has made a prior inconsistent statement. Discovery depositions are designed to elicit what the witness knows about the case, how he obtained that information, and what he is likely to say at trial. They are often wide ranging fishing expeditions that may go substantially beyond the bounds of permissible inquiry at trial, and any question that may lead to relevant evidence is permitted.

## CONDUCT OF THE DEPOSITION

There are certain formalities that are generally observed in the conduct of the deposition. After swearing the witness, the attorneys may agree to certain stipulations regarding the conduct of the examination. The stipulation most often made is that all objections except as to the form of question are reserved until trial (13, 14). This means that most evidentiary objections are not made on the record but will be made at some subsequent time before a judge in the event that it becomes necessary to use the deposition at trial. Substantive objections such as a violation of the hearsay rule, improper foundation, or incompetency of the witness are reserved. Conversely, objections to leading questions or compound questions are objections to the form of question and must be made at the time that the question is asked. This gives counsel the opportunity to rephrase the question in proper form. If counsel chooses not to rephrase the question the witness is generally directed to answer anyway, but that question and answer may become inadmissible at trial. This may be of little consequence if the deposition is being used for discovery purposes only.

A leading question is a question that suggests the answer. Leading questions are proper in the cross-examination of witnesses but are usually impermissible in the direct examination of one's own witness. If a party calls a witness to testify at trial or in a deposition, he must interrogate that witness in direct examination format. This is true even if the witness will ultimately testify for the adverse party at trial.

The distinction between the direct examination format at trial and the cross-examination format takes on additional significance in the deposition. A good direct examiner generally asks the witness questions in a chronologic order that track the sequence of events as they happened. This process makes sense to the trier of fact, who may be hearing the case for the first time. A chronologic summary of events is a logical approach to presenting testimony and enhances the understanding of the case. A sequential interrogation also increases the witness's ability to recall his testimony. Conversely, a good cross-examiner will generally interrogate the adverse party's witnesses at trial by questioning them on topics taken in random order. The strategy is to prevent the witness from reiterating some well-rehearsed testimony and to make his responses more spontaneous and vulnerable to attack. Claimant's counsel will often use this cross-examination tactic against the adverse party's witness in a deposition for the same reasons. Even though the examiner of an adverse party's witness may be constrained to use the direct examination style (i.e., nonleading questions), he may go through the subject matter in his deposition checklist in random order as he would in a cross-examination at trial.

Plaintiff's counsel may use a different questioning technique during a discovery deposition from that used by counsel at the trial or during the taking of the deposition that will be used at trial in lieu of live testimony. The objective of the discovery deposition is to learn the nature of the opposition's testimony and to gauge the quality of the witness. Consequently, where claimant's counsel might avoid asking certain questions of the witness during trial for fear that the answer might damage the claimant's position, he is more likely to venture into dangerous ground during discovery deposition in order to determine the witness's response. If there is a likelihood that the discovery deposition may also have to be used in place of the witness's personal appearance at trial, then counsel may have to take a more cautious approach and use a questioning technique more suitable for trial. In gauging the quality of the witness, the skilled advocate may ask questions to determine bias, technical proficiency, and factual concessions the witness might make on behalf of the client and to attempt to gauge the general demeanor and credibility of the witness. It is not unusual for the interrogator to ask several questions during the deposition that are designed to "bait" the witness to determine if the witness can be made to lose his composure at trial, which might have a negative impact on the jury.

There is a certain psychology in selecting the site of the deposition. An informal atmosphere for taking the deposition of the adversary's witnesses should be created. In this relaxed setting where everyone appears to be friendly, the witness may be induced into careless talk that may be damaging to his side. This atmosphere may also provide a forum where a talkative witness may feel comfortable in rambling on to his ultimate discredit. Experienced trial counsel will seize upon this opportunity to gain information that is helpful to the plaintiff and damaging to the defendant.

The deponent will also be asked if he wishes to read and sign the deposition (15, 16). As a general rule, plaintiff's counsel will advise the witness that this is not necessary because the court reporter can be relied on to make an accurate transcript. If the deponent chooses to read and sign his deposition, he cannot change the content of the deposition but can correct spelling errors. This may become important if the deposition contained difficult medical terminology that may be alien to a layman and difficult for the reporter. If counsel is taking an adverse witness's deposition that he may use for impeachment at trial, he may insist that the deponent read and sign the deposition so that the witness solidifies his position on a prior inconsistent statement. If the signature requirement is waived and opposing counsel attempts to use the deposition at trial for impeachment or other purposes, the deponent can always testify that he misunderstood the question at the deposition proceedings or that the question or answer was not properly recorded. It is manifestly clear that if the deponent has had an opportunity to read and sign the deposition without any explanatory additions, his credibility will be seriously impaired if he subsequently says that he did not understand the question or that the response was inaccurately recorded.

## VIDEOTAPED DEPOSITIONS

Videotape machines have dramatically altered the landscape of litigation. Videotape depositions of expert witnesses and treating physicians who are often beyond the subpoena power of the court have become commonplace. When properly used, videotape depositions provide an effective mechanism for the presentation of evidence and testimony at trial. Almost every jurisdiction has its own rules governing the use of the videotaped deposition and these must be carefully consulted before attempting to conduct one. Most of these rules provide that the deposition shall be conducted in a neutral setting (17). In conducting the depositions of his own witnesses, plaintiff's counsel will want to sit the deponent in front of a bookshelf in a medical library or in some other professional setting to enhance credibility. During direct examination, the attorney should have the camera over his shoulder so that the deponent will face the camera when answering the questions. This also places the opposing counsel at a disadvantage in that the answers to his cross-examination will be directed off camera and lessen the impact of the testimony. It is imperative that counsel be thoroughly prepared for the direct examination. Long pauses between questions seem like an eternity on camera.

Demonstrative evidence can be used very effectively in videotaped medical depositions and can assist the trier of fact in understanding the testimony. The video camera is capable of shooting close-ups of the exhibits, and the jury can see the exhibit and its component parts better on the video screen than if the exhibit were shown at trial.

## DEMONSTRATIVE EVIDENCE

Demonstrative evidence plays an important part in the trial lawyer's presentation of the plaintiff's case. It takes on special significance when dealing with the medical witness. The very nature of medical testimony requires the use of technical terms that may seriously tax the juror's comprehension and understanding. Demonstrative evidence usually includes charts, photographs, videotapes, courtroom demonstrations, blackboard drawings, and models. It differs from real evidence in that it plays no direct role in the events that are the focus of the trial, but it is usually used to demonstrate or illustrate testimony (18). Its primary difference from documentary or real evidence is that demonstrative evidence is usually created by an attorney or an agent for the attorney. Creating and using demonstrative evidence should be integrated into the overall trial strategy and the medical witness's testimony. The wisdom of appealing to the visual sense is attested to by the following figures representing the portion of man's learning contributed by each of the five senses: sight, 85%; hearing, 10%; touch, 2%; taste, 1.5%; and smell, 1.5% (19).

The evidentiary requirements for the admissibility of demonstrative evidence are the same as those for real evidence. Normal standards of relevancy are applied. Not all drawings, models, and illustrations are evidentiary in nature and they may not need to be authenticated. Rather, they are used to emphasize or illustrate a particular point in argument. However, if the evidence is used to enhance testimony, it must be authenticated and a showing must be made that the demonstrative evidence represents what it purports to represent. This usually requires having the medical witness testify that the evidence fairly and accurately represents what the model, chart, or drawing is supposed to illustrate. In order to satisfy the elements of admissibility, the medical witness will be asked if the drawing or model is relevant to his testimony, if it is useful in helping him explain that testimony, and if it is reasonably accurate and not misleading.

Anatomic charts and models for courtroom use are readily available. They may consist of simple line drawings of the cervical vertebrae or anatomic transparencies such as those produced by Matthew Bender and Co., Inc. (20–22), or a model of a spinal column or a human skeleton to assist in illustrating medical testimony. In a more serious case, it is not unusual for claimant's counsel, with the assistance of his expert, to engage the services of a medical illustrator to create a drawing of the plaintiff's injuries or a series of transparent overlays. An example might be a transparency overlaying a normal spine to show a flattening of the cervical curve subsequent to an automobile accident.

Anatomic models possess qualities that are unavailable through drawings or charts. Their three-dimensional character can give the jury a more accurate understanding of the relationship of the various parts of the body. The model can also be viewed from a variety of vantage points. Most importantly, an anatomic model will not evoke a negative reaction in a squeamish juror, whereas an actual skeleton might.

Radiographs (x-rays) are a diagnostic tool that is invariably used in cervical trauma cases. Many courts are reticent to allow jurors to take radiographs into the jury room for their deliberations because of the necessity of using a light box to illuminate the radiograph and the inability of the juror to interpret what he sees without the assistance of the medical expert. Therefore, plaintiff's counsel should have positives made of the radiographs and, in direct examination, have the expert explain their significance by drawing on them with a colored marker. This technique is clearly illustrated in the following excerpt from a pretrial deposition of Harry Brown, M.D., the treating physician of Tom Smith, by Leon L. Wolfstone, Esq. This transcript is an outstanding demonstration of technique in the direct examination of a treating physician in a serious cervical trauma case (23).

Q. Doctor, you have handed me ten X-rays which have now been marked 1 through 5 as the X-rays taken on the date shown thereon, 9-18-62, and 6 through 10 on the date shown thereon of January 7, 1963.

A. That is right.

Q. Were these X-rays all taken of the same patient, Tom Smith, Doctor?

A. That is correct.

Q. Were they taken in the necessary and proper course of his examination, care and treatment?

A. They were.

    **Mr. Wolfstone:** We will offer in evidence Exhibits 1 through 10.

    **Mr. Black:** I have no objection.

Q. Doctor, referring to the ones first taken, would you from those pick out one upon which you can point out, if you will, please, Doctor, the area that you have described as being tender on the right, I believe you said, and the erector skull origin.

A. On exhibit No. 5,—

Q. Would you take this pencil, Doctor, and mark with a red arrow the area that you referred to as the erector skull origin? You have marked some red X's at that area?

A. On the right side in this exhibit, which is an AP view, in other words, a view taken straight ahead with the patient facing the X-ray tube.

Q. Now, Doctor, would you with the same red pencil mark with a bracket sign the areas of the right compartment of the cervical column there, at which you have indicated there was tenderness. There is a no-

tation of lower cervical discomfort, you said, and right compartments were the designations.

A. These are designated by the letter Y.

Q. Those at the skull area are designated with an X?

A. Correct.

Q. And the Y is the neck area?

A. That is correct.

Q. All right. Now, Doctor, can you on that X-ray point out the area of the slight flattening of the cervical curve that you referred to?

A. No.

Q. Would you refer to another X-ray that you can, then, please?

A. Exhibit No. 1 shows the neck from the side view.

Q. Can you take that red pencil then, Doctor, and draw the curve as it should be so as to point out the area of flattening. Would you put A at the top and B at the bottom of the line that you have drawn on Exhibit 1.

    You are marking a series of numbers, Doctor. What do those represent?

A. These represent the numbers of the neck vertebrae from 1 to 7, inclusive.

Q. Now, Doctor, will you please tell us whether or not these X-rays demonstrate any angulation of the cervical column.

A. No. In my opinion on this exhibit, which is a standard side view, the flattening character is shown only—without defacing the X-ray I am going to make a line along behind—F on this exhibit will be front and B back—along the back of the vertebrae.

Q. Would you at the top of that put X and at the bottom Y. Now, that broken line demarked as X to Y, Doctor, what does that denote so far as concerns the normal curve of the cervical column as you would expect it on a boy of this age?

A. I would expect this curve to show a deeper concavity as viewed from the side and not one which approaches the straight line of AB prime on this same exhibit.

Q. What does the XY denote, Doctor, as far as the curve as it existed or should have been?

A. This is the curve as it existed.

Q. Can you with a yellow pencil mark a similar line showing the curve as it should have been.

A. Yes. [Doctor draws line.]

Q. Now, the yellow line denotes the curve as it should have been and the red XY curve as it in fact was, is that correct, Doctor?

A. Yes.

Q. And the AB is merely a straight line for reference purposes, is that correct?

A. Correct.

Q. All right, now, Doctor, would you please review the balance of the X-rays taken at that time and tell me whether or not any of the X-rays show any abnormal condition by way of angulation of the vertebrae?

A. On Exhibit No. 2, this is a side view of the neck with the head bent forward.

Q. Would you first take a red pencil and mark an arrow showing the area, or bracket or whatever will show the area of angulation from the normal?

A. On this exhibit?

Q. You have again marked the vertebral segments, have you not, 1 to 7?

A. Right. There is an abnormal direction in the manner in which this spine bends forward, this neck bends forward and this angulation—

Q. You have drawn a red line, Doctor, going from 1 down to approximately 6 as representing the angulation, is that correct?

A. That is correct.

Q. And that is the angulation as you found it? You have marked that A in a circle to A, is that correct, Doctor?

A. That is correct.

Q. Now, Doctor, can you with a yellow pencil on the same X-ray show the line as it should be without impairing that which you have drawn, or you can just go to whatever area should be involved, if you prefer.

A. This line should be a smoother type of line with its greatest arc above 4, but still should be arced.

Q. What is the medical significance, if any, of that angulation that you have referred to, Doctor?

A. This indicates an abnormal type of forward bending in that it's not symmetrical denoting that the various units of the neck don't work smoothly together. (pp. 182–187)

## EXPERT WITNESSES

Before an expert witness is allowed to testify, certain evidentiary requirements must be met. Many jurisdictions harbor a fear that an expert's opinion will usurp the jury's function on the ultimate question of fact. Consequently, courts have developed certain threshold requirements before an expert will be allowed to testify. The court, in the case of *The United States v. Brown* (24) summarized those requirements:

1. *Skill.* The expert must be one who is qualified by training, experience, skill or knowledge;
2. *Probative value versus prejudicial value.* The subject must be one on which the expert will assist the trier of fact in reaching a conclusion rather than taking its place on issues on which the trier is qualified to reach its own decision.
3. *Reliability.* The expert's standards, texts, and other procedures must have reached a level of respectability amounting to general acceptance in the community of experts in the relevant field.

Once the determination has been made that an expert is needed for the proper presentation of the case, it is incumbent upon trial counsel to determine the type of expertise needed and to identify experts who fit those needs. A careful review of the medical records, course of treatment, and prognosis will give counsel a general clue as to the type of expertise needed. The attorney can receive additional assistance by discussions with the treating physician or informally consulted experts. Most often, the best advice obtainable will come from other lawyers who have handled similar cases. Sources also include the authors of articles in medical journals and periodicals, faculty members of medical schools, colleges, and universities, the *Directory of Medical Specialists* (25), *World's Who's Who in Science* (26), *American Men of Science* (27), and the *AMA Medical Directory* (28).

In a serious cervical trauma case, a major mistake made by many trial attorneys is trying to use one medical expert for a multitude of opinions in medical disciplines other than their own in which they lack the requisite expertise necessary to give that medical opinion. For instance, an orthopaedic surgeon, in addition to giving a medical opinion on the angulation of the neck, may be asked to give an opinion regarding a neurologic deficit or psychiatric sequelae relating to the initial trauma. A different expert should be used for each opinion to be elicited based upon the appropriate medical discipline best able to render that opinion.

After a list of potential expert witnesses has been compiled, counsel should look for certain qualities before making an ultimate choice. The first quality one should look for is the ability to communicate with the jury. Medical jargon has been likened to a foreign language to jurors. The witness must be able to translate difficult medical terms so that the lay person can understand them without sounding condescending, supercilious, or aloof. The witness should also be able to create an atmosphere of receptivity on the part of the jury. Another consideration is the length of time that the prospective witness has been practicing in his area of expertise and the quality of the institutions with which he has been affiliated. The witness who is "an old-timer" and has been connected with a venerable institution will certainly have enhanced credibility with a lay jury.

Claimant's counsel should also determine whether the expert has authored books or articles on the subject and if he has espoused views in those articles that are contrary to the position he would have to take in the case. If so, it is obvious that this expert would be vulnerable in a cross-examination and should not be retained. Similarly, the witness should be sufficiently firm in his views so that he will not change his position at trial in an effort to please whoever is questioning him at the time. A witness who would change his opinion on cross-examination is worse than no expert at all. Consequently, a thorough cross-examination should be made of each prospective witness prior to retaining him.

An additional consideration in screening potential candidates is the prospective witness's experience as a witness. A seasoned expert witness can sometimes be of great help to an inexperienced attorney in planning the presentation of the medical testimony. He can also help determine the most effective way to present his testimony and may have exhibits or models that have worked well in the past and may be applicable to the present case. An experienced witness should not be confused with a professional plaintiff's or defendant's expert who testifies for one side in case after case. This type of witness is almost always vulnerable to a damaging cross-examination and will come across as a prejudiced hireling.

A most important consideration is resolving the issue of the witness's professional fees up front. This should be done at the beginning of the relationship and should be reduced to writing. Failure to resolve this issue results in more misunderstandings between counsel and the witness than any other part of the process (29). It can result in an embarrassing situation if counsel's own witness appears to be hostile toward his side in full view of the jury. If it results in a dispute prior to trial wherein the expert is forced to leave, it is possible that the opposition will retain the expert after his dismissal. Any fee agreement should not be contingent upon the outcome of the case or upon the opinion that the expert will render. This is generally considered unethical, and the expert's medical opinion will be made to appear to be motivated by pecuniary gain.

## QUALIFICATION

The format for qualifying the witness as an expert should be agreed upon by the attorney and the witness prior to trial. The trial attorney will have already checked the pertinent medical directories to determine the qualifications of his own witnesses as well as the credentials of his adversary's witnesses. Since the medical opinion as to diagnoses, etiology, prognosis, and disability is likely to be controverted at trial, it is critical to point out who, by background, training, and experience, is the more qualified expert. The following checklist of items would normally be included in preparing questions to qualify a medical expert:

Date and state of medical license
Undergraduate schooling
Medical schooling
Internship
Residency training
Specialized training
Description of medical specialty
Experience, including military service
Hospital affiliations
Specialty boards
Honorary society
Teaching experience
Contributions to the medical literature

This is only a partial list, and the testimony outline should include much greater detail if the expert is a member of a specialty board or a member of any medical honorary societies. The qualifications for these boards and societies should be brought out in great detail so that it is clear to the jury that the specialist is accepted by his peers as an accredited member and recognized that he occupies a status in the medical profession that entitles him to recognition as a specialist in the field.

Most medical boards contain certain general requirements to qualify for certification by the board as a specialist. These requirements include graduation from an approved medical school, completion of an internship of not less than 1 year in a hospital approved by the American Medical Association, completion of a residency in the field of at least 3 years in an acceptable medical institution, proof of the professional ability of the applicant in the field, certification of the applicant's ethical standing, and the passing of written and oral examinations by the applicant attesting to his knowledge of the specialty and its practical application. After satisfying the requirements for eligibility, a diploma is issued to the candidate and he is known as a "Diplomate" of the board.

In addition to the specialty boards, the specialists have organized among themselves and within their own specialties honorary societies for continuing medical education in their areas of expertise and to honor these specialists by granting them membership. These societies are generally called "Colleges" and a specialist who is accepted by the college as an accredited member is given a title "Fellow."

There are numerous American specialty colleges that have similar prerequisites for membership. For instance, the American College of Surgeons requires the following criteria to be met for membership as a fellow (30):

(a) graduation from an accredited medical school;
(b) seven years devotion to training and practice in the surgical specialty from the date of graduation from medical school;
(c) satisfactory completion of at least one year of internship in an approved hospital;
(d) completion of a residency program of at least three years duration in the specialty;
(e) professional activity of a character to classify the applicant as a specialist in surgery;
(f) good ethical and moral character;
(g) ordinarily, a review of fifty detailed case records taken from the applicant's last three years of practice to determine his professional proficiency (this requirement can be waived under certain circumstances);
(h) a unanimous vote signifying approval of the board having jurisdiction.

A surgeon voted to fellowship is permitted to place the initials of his fellowship after his name in professional listings (e.g., F.A.C.S. for Fellow of the American College of Surgeons).

A good advocate, in qualifying his expert, will examine the witness as to the prerequisites for admission to specialty boards and colleges. This is no time to be reticent since the first barrier to be overcome before expert testimony is admissible is establishing that the expert is one who is qualified by training, experience, skill, or knowlege (31). In addition, the more impressive the credentials the more likely the expert's medical opinion will be accepted by the jury. This becomes particularly important if the adversary has a witness whose opinion will differ.

When counsel puts an expert on the witness stand, it is not unusual for his adversary to stipulate to the expert's credentials. This is usually less of a concession than it seems, since counsel is trying to prevent the jury from hearing those credentials that build credibility. The examiner should not move on to the next subject area but should finish the qualification process while graciously accepting the fact that his opposition concedes the witness to be an expert. In the event that the credentials of the witness are not as strong as those of the other party's expert witness, the ex-

aminer may want to take advantage of the stipulation and end the inquiry as to qualifications.

Another extremely important element of the medical witness's qualifications are his hospital affiliations. Hospitals, like universities, have varying reputations. The standing of the hospital with which the medical expert is associated is most important. A physician's affiliations with a nationally or internationally known hospital are more impressive than those of a physician with only local affiliations. This is not to say that the former physician makes a better expert witness, but it may become important if credibility hinges on the strongest credentials.

In addition to the reputation of the institution, it is important to discern the position occupied by the witness at that institution. Physicians bear various titles in a hospital, and it is important to know whether or not the witness is or was a director, head of service, chief, or held any other position that may be noteworthy to the trier of fact.

Contributions to medical literature can be exceptionally important in examining the witness about his qualifications. Questions to determine how widely accepted the books and articles are have a strong evidentiary impact. If the witness has written in an area that is germane to the lawsuit, particular emphasis should be made of that fact. Articles published in the *Journal of the American Medical Association* are particularly important because they are published subsequent to a review of the Board of Editors and are circulated to the majority of physicians in the United States. The journal is the official publication of the American Medical Association and this fact should be brought out in direct examination (32).

## HYPOTHETICAL QUESTIONS

In most jurisdictions, if the expert is not a treating physician, it is usually necessary to present such a witness's testimony as an answer to a hypothetical question based on evidence introduced in the case or to be introduced in the case. The use of hypothetical questions is of great strategic importance, and trial counsel must determine the most effective form in which they can be cast. There are two basic forms of the hypothetical question (33):

(1) Some jurisdictions permit the expert to listen to a portion of the testimony as it is presented in court and then ask the expert to assume the correctness of that testimony and to render an opinion based upon those assumptions.

(2) Counsel reads a narrative based on evidence previously presented which contains the key points that the witness is asked to assume to be true.

The first method has the advantage of asking a very brief question. Counsel need not repeat a long narrative and the jury does not get bored by a lengthy and intricate question. The second method used is the preferred method of most plaintiffs' attorneys. It gives them an opportunity to give a summation of all of the salient facts in the case to the jury and the opinion rendered by the expert constitutes a climax to that summation. If done properly, this type of question has an enormous impact on the jury.

In Federal court, the rules relating to hypothetical questions have been substantially relaxed. Rule 703 of the Federal Rules of Evidence (Fed R Evid) provides:

> The facts or data in the particular case upon which an expert bases an opinion or inference may be those perceived by or made known to the expert at or before the hearing. If of a type reasonably relied upon by experts in the particular field in forming opinions or inferences upon the subject, the facts or data need not be admissible in evidence.

The *Advisory Committee's Notes* indicate that, in addition to permitting the witness to base his testimony on first-hand observation or on evidence presented in court and called to the expert's attention by a hypothetical question or by having him hear relevant testimony, the rule also permits the expert to base his testimony on the "presentation of data to the expert outside of court" and by means "other than by his own perception" (34). Not all jurisdictions continue to require the hypothetical question as a means of presenting evidence of the expert who has not had an opportunity for first-hand observation. California, for instance, permits the expert to base his opinion on information that other professionals in his field would normally consider reliable, even though the information would not by itself be admissible in court (35).

Despite the relaxation of the rules regarding hypothetical questions, a skilled advocate will still use the narrative type of hypothetical question to gain a strategic advantage. Although the contents of the question should favor the plaintiff's side, the presentation should not be so distorted or prejudicial that it will destroy the credibility of the question with the jury. In addition, it should contain enough detail for an informed answer but should not be so intricate as to ruin the jury's un-

derstanding. Most jurisdictions prohibit the use of real names in hypothetical questions (36), and counsel will not refer to the parties by name. Despite that, the hypothetical question can only include those facts in evidence or to be introduced into evidence. It cannot assume facts not in evidence or contemplated to be so. Justification for this rule is that, if actual names were used, the expert would then be determining the ultimate issue, which should be left to the jury. Even this rule has been substantially eroded by the adoption of the Federal Rules of Evidence. Rule 704 permits an expert to render an opinion that "embraces an ultimate issue to be decided by the trier of fact." Consequently, the "ultimate issue" rule is specifically abolished in Federal court (37).

## BASIS OF OPINION

In most jurisdictions other than in Federal court, a medical witness, like any other expert who has been called upon to render an opinion upon technical issues involved in a case, must recite the basis of his expert testimony (38). The basis is actually data that the doctor has learned and constitutes the reasons for his opinion. As a threshold matter, the doctor relies in large measure on what he has been taught by virtue of his education, training, and subsequent learning. Much of this information has already been brought out when the doctor was examined as to his qualifications. In addition, the expert's experience has received judicial sanction as a basis for testimony. A major source of information comes from what the witness reads. Reading materials are generally divided into two categories: material that is read, generally and preceding the actual case in question, and that which is read after the case is presented and a question has arisen. Courts will also rely on general scientific principles and facts, medical knowledge, statistical information, and methodologies of tests as the basis for an opinion.

Prior to trial, the witness may have made certain personal observations that form the basis of his opinion. He may have conducted a physical examination, performed tests, or obtained information from patients, relatives, or other lay or professional observers. He may also rely on secondary evidence such as tests performed or interpreted by others, hospital records and other medical forms, or opposing counsel's records. Finally, he may use information received at the trial as part of the basis of his testimony. This may include the hypothetical assumptions contained in the hypothetical questions that are taken as true in formulating his opinion.

It is certainly reasonable to require the witness to recite the basis of his testimony. The explanation helps to make his opinion clear and convincing and allows the jury to evaluate it and resolve conflicting opinion evidence. Because the matrix of material that constitutes the foundation of the testimony comes from so many different sources, it is also vulnerable to cross-examination, if it is not thoroughly discussed with the witness in advance.

## PREPARATION OF THE WITNESS

Every good trial and defense attorney cross-examines the witness with a specific objective in mind. Moreover, it is unlikely that an attorney will cross-examine a medical expert unless he is likely to succeed in attaining one or more of his goals. Most cross-examinations have one or more of the following objectives (39):

(a) the medical expert is not qualified;
(b) the witness is biased, dishonest or has some interest to gain by testifying;
(c) the expert's testimony is in error. He may have relied on a faulty factual basis to formulate his opinion and would change it if the underlying assumptions were changed.
(d) the witness may make admissions which coincide with the testimony of the adversary's medical expert. An honest witness may go so far as to admit that reasonable persons with similar backgrounds could differ on the point, thus lending additional merit to the adversary's position.
(e) the facts the witness assumed in the hypothetical to be true are not correct.

It is essential that in the preparation of the medical witness counsel conduct a direct examination and cross-examination rehearsal prior to the deposition or trial. This is time well spent in preparing for the hazards of cross-examination and the weaknesses in the testimony.

Most attorneys prepare a deposition checklist (40) or trial noteboook (41) outlining their direct examination. A treating physician checklist might cover the following topics:

Qualifications
Experience
Examination of this patient
Diagnoses
Treatment
Subsequent examinations

Patient's present condition based on last examination
Opinion on causation (this opinion is usually based on a
   reasonable degree of medical certainty)
Prognosis
Amount of present and future medical services

The treating physician or expert should be furnished with all of the important pleadings in the case, deposition summaries of other experts involved, medical reports in the attorney's possession, and the testimony outlines as soon as they are available. The witness should be made to understand the case theory and how his testimony will fit within that theory. It is imperative that the attorney and his expert cooperate closely in devising the most persuasive format for the witness's testimony.

There are certain general rules that should be followed in preparing the witness. The witness should be admonished to listen to every question before answering. In the event that there is an objection, the witness should stop testifying until a ruling is made on the objection or until he is advised to proceed. He should be dressed in a professional manner when appearing for the deposition or in court. The witness should always be prepared to translate technical jargon for the jury. If he does not know an answer, his testimony should be "I don't know." The witness should always address the jury since they have the exclusive province to decide issues of fact. The judge does not rule on the credibility or believability of the witnesses since that is also the sole province of the jury. The witness should always be courteous to opposing counsel, even when deliberately pushed.

### REFERENCES

1. Cleary EW: *McCormick's Handbook of the Law of Evidence*, ed 2. St. Paul, MN, West Publishing Company, 1972, p 23.
2. *Witnesses*, 97 CJS §295.
3. *Bach v. Schultz*, 180 NYS 188.
4. *Corpman v. Boyer*, 169 NE2d 14 (Ohio 1960).
5. *McIntosh v. Mills*, 430 P2d 644 (Mont 1967).
6. Berser MJ, Mitchell JB, Clark RH: *Trial Advocacy: Planning, Analysis & Strategy*. Boston, Little, Brown, 1989, p 406.
7. Mauet TA: *Fundamentals of Trial Techniques*, ed 2. Boston, Little, Brown, 1988, p 140.
8. Advisory Committee's Notes to Fed R Civ P 26(b) (4) (B), 48 FRD 497, 504 (1970).
9. Fed R Civ P 26(b) (4) (B).
10. Fed R Civ P 32(a).
11. Barthold W: *Attorney's Guide to Effective Discovery Techniques*. Englewood Cliffs, NJ, Prentice-Hall, 1975, p 50.
12. Fed R Civ P 26.
13. Barthold W: *Attorney's Guide to Effective Discovery Techniques*. Englewood Cliffs, NJ, Prentice-Hall, 1975, p 87.
14. Fed R Civ P 32(b)&(d) (3).
15. Pretzel PW: *A Review of Discovery Depositions*, 1964 Ins Coun L J 711 at 714–715 (1964).

16. Fed R Civ P 30(e).

17. Boswell J: Making video depositions work for you. *SCTLA Bull* Summer, p 22, 1989.

18. Berger MJ, Mitchell JB, Clark RH: *Trial Advocacy: Planning, Analysis & Strategy.* Boston, Little, Brown 1989, p 223.

19. McCullough RC II, Underwood JL: *Civil Trial Manual 2,* ed 2. Philadelphia, American Law Institute–American Bar Association, Committee on Continuing Professional Education, 1981, p 419.

20. *Anatomy Charts for Courtroom Use.* New York, Matthew Bender and Co, Inc, 1962.

21. *Anatomical Transparencies.* New York, Matthew Bender and Co, Inc, 1989.

22. Gordy LJ, Gray RN: *Attorney's Textbook of Medicine,* Suppl. New York, Matthew Bender and Co, Inc, 1989.

23. Wolfestone LL: Effective deposition of treating doctor where x-ray findings will be in dispute, mixture of objective and subjective complaints and findings, subsequent accident, and congenital anomaly; deposition constituting a medical brochure. In Frumer LR, Minzer MK (eds): *Examination of Medical Experts.* New York, Matthew Bender and Co, Inc, 1968, vol 2, pp 168–219.

24. *United States v. Brown,* 557 F2d 541, 556–557 (6th Cir 1977).

25. *Directory of Medical Specialists,* ed 15. Chicago, published for the Advisory Board of Medical Specialists by AN Marquis Co, 1972–1973.

26. *World's Who's Who in Science.* Chicago, AN Marquis Co.

27. Cattel J (ed): *American Men of Science,* ed 11. New York, RR Bowker Company, 1968.

28. American Medical Association: *AMA Medical Directory.* AMA, 1979.

29. McCullough RC II, Underwood JL: *Civil Trial Manual 2,* ed 2. Philadelphia, American Law Institute–American Bar Association, Committe on Continuing Professional Education, 1981, p 396.

30. American College of Surgeons: *Annual Directory of the American College of Surgeons.* Chicago, ACS, 1991.

31. Fed R Evid 702.

32. Glaser HB: Trial techniques: exploring the qualifications of medical witnesses. In Frumer LR, Minzer MK (eds): *Examination of Medical Experts.* New York, Matthew Bender and Co, Inc, 1968, vol 2, pp 276–297.

33. Cleary EW: *McCormick's Handbook of the Law of Evidence,* ed 2. St. Paul, MN, West Publishing Company, 1972, p 32.

34. Advisory Committee's Notes to Fed R Evid 703, 28 USC App (1988).

35. Cal Evid Code §801(b) (West 1966).

36. Goldstein I, Lane F: *Trial Technique,* ed 2. Mundelein, IL, Callaghan, 1969, pp 12–15.

37. Fed R Evid 704.

38. Rheingold PD: The basis of medical testimony. In Frumer LR, Minzer MK (eds): *Examination of Medical Experts.* New York, Matthew Bender and Co, Inc, 1968, vol 2, p 4.

39. Stevenson NC: *Successful Cross Examination Strategy.* Englewood Cliffs, NJ: Executive Reports Corp, 1977, p 1303.

40. Danner D: *Pattern Deposition Checklists* ed 2, cum suppl. Rochester, NY, Lawyers Co-operative Publishing Co, 1983.

41. Mauet TA: *Fundamentals of Trial Techniques,* ed 2. Boston, Little, Brown 1988, pp 2–8

# 31

# MEDICAL DEPOSITIONS AND COURT APPEARANCES

## Defense Counsel Perspective

*R. Harrison Pledger, Jr.*
*With the assistance of Melinda M. McNair.*

As a physician you can expect to testify in legal controversies many times during your medical career—most often as a fact witness, less often as an expert witness, and, it is hoped never as a defendant in a medical malpractice claim. The latter seems less and less likely, however, given the litigious state of our society today.

Should you have the misfortune of being sued, you can expect your emotional response upon being accused of malpractice to range from fear to anger and from sadness to resignation. All of these feelings must be overcome before you can effectively testify either at a deposition or at a trial. These emotions must be replaced with a calm, assured attitude that is based upon a complete understanding of the issues, a thorough and objective knowledge of the medical facts, and confidence that the care and treatment rendered by you was appropriate. This attitude is produced by careful preparation, which should begin within hours of your receiving notice of the claim. Start by reviewing your medical records. *Under no circumstances should you change the records.* Altering of your records is one of the most damaging things you can do to your defense. The next step is to assist your attorney by beginning a complete review of the pertinent medical literature. Obtain copies of it and highlight those portions that you believe to be particularly relevant to your case, and then submit that material, after you have studied it, to

your attorney. Check with your attorney as you begin this project, and determine how your attorney would like you to accomplish this task. Work done to prepare your case in conjunction with your attorney becomes protected from discovery by the opposing lawyer as your attorney's work product.

Remember, to be successful a medical malpractice claim must demonstrate that the standard of care was breached by the physician and that the physician's breach was the proximate cause of injury to the patient.

In most instances, and particularly in a medical malpractice case, the patient is the plaintiff and the health care provider or other person being sued is the defendant. Several legal terms will be used in connection with your testimony and therefore need to be understood. The "standard of care" is the operative phrase used for judging the actions of a physician. The term is usually applied in a retrospective sense. Standard of care as a rule means that degree of care and skill exercised by the average physician in the same or a similar specialty in similar circumstances at the time of the occurrence in question. While relatively specific, this phrase is broad enough to include "two schools of thought" where competent medical viewpoints support more than one approach to the management of a medical/surgical condition.

You will be asked to give your opinions based

upon "reasonable medical certainty" or "reasonable medical probability." Usually, opinions based only on a possibility are not admissible. "Reasonable medical probability" means the opinion is of sufficient certainty that it would support a particular medical judgment. As a rule, the words "could" or "it is possible" mean that only a possibility exists, and therefore such opinions would not be admissible.

"Proximate cause" is the legal test used to determine whether an injury is so closely related to an event as to make one person liable to another in money damages for the injuries sustained. An injury is proximately caused by an act, or a failure to act, whenever it appears that the act or omission played a substantial part in bringing about or actually causing the injury, and that the injury was either a direct result or a reasonably probable consequence of the act or omission. It is often characterized as the "but for" test; the injury would not have happened "but for" the act or omission complained of. Proximate cause may relate only to legal, and not factual, causation.

## DEPOSITIONS

Depositions are one of the major processes used in litigation to learn the facts and opinions of witnesses. This is particularly true of medical malpractice cases. Therefore, this discussion regarding preparation for, attendance at, and the significance of deposition is intended to help you go through a deposition in the most professional, knowledgeable, and stress-free manner possible.

Whether you are a fact witness, expert witness, or defendant, a discovery deposition will probably be taken by the opposing lawyer before trial. A deposition is a question-and-answer proceeding conducted in accordance with certain rules of court for the purpose of learning what a witness knows about the facts that are the subject of the legal controversy and what opinions the witness holds with respect to those facts. A deposition may be used to preserve the testimony of a witness for use at trial if there is concern that the witness will not be available during the trial (i.e., a terminally ill plaintiff).

Those advising plaintiff's lawyers on effective methods for preparing the plaintiff for a deposition in a malpractice case recommend that this preparation take place during two or three meetings of at least 2 or more hours each. The counselors say this time is necessary to prepare the plaintiff to present testimony accurately. They

further suggest that this accuracy can only be achieved after the plaintiff has done everything to refresh his or her recollection of the events, and after that recollection has been verified with whatever written documentation exists. This preparation also helps the plaintiff understand the adversarial process—why the questions are being asked and how to deal with the attorney asking the questions.

As a physician who is a defendant in a malpractice case you cannot afford any less preparation. Meetings with your attorney to prepare for the deposition should be held at least a week prior to the deposition so that there is an adequate opportunity to locate any additional information that may be available and that may not come to light until this preparatory discussion of testimony to be given at the deposition. Before your deposition is taken, you and your attorney, or the attorney who has employed you, should thoroughly review your knowledge of the specific facts in the case, the medical records, the subjects on which you may be expected to be examined, and your opinions with respect to the patient's condition, treatment, the etiology of the condition, and prognosis. If it is a malpractice case, you must discuss the standard of care and, if you believe a deviation has occurred, whether that deviation caused the injury complained of by the patient. This preparation is absolutely necessary, and it may be helpful to engage in some "role playing" to ensure your familiarity with the mechanics of a deposition proceeding.

The deposition may be held in an attorney's office, in the physician's office, or at any reasonably comfortable place chosen by the parties to the proceeding. If you are the defendant or an expert in a malpractice case it is better to have the deposition somewhere other than your office. If held in your office it makes additional records and information too easily accessible and provides the plaintiff's lawyer with an opportunity to see what books you have in your library, what journals are on your desk, and any personal memorabilia that could be used to detract from the weight a jury would give to your testimony. Those present at the deposition in addition to you will be a court reporter, who administers the oath and records the proceedings, and attorneys for each party. If you are the defendant, you may expect that the plaintiff may also attend. As an expert witness, you may find both the parties to the suit, or their representatives, in attendance.

The deposition may be recorded by stenotype, videotape, or audiotape. Videotaped depositions are frequently used in court in the event the witness cannot appear at trial. A videotaped presentation also offers a way for an expert with a conflict that would prevent his or her courtroom testimony to present evidence to the judge and jury. If your deposition is videotaped, you should be aware that your mannerisms, demeanor, and responses will have a greater effect on the judge or jury than would the reading of a written transcript. The videotaped picture is usually only of the head and shoulders during the entire deposition. Accordingly, you need to be aware of any habits you may have, such as frequently removing and putting on your glasses, scratching your face or ears, or rubbing your chin or nose, because these can become very distracting to the jury. Also, facial expressions, which are discussed later in this chapter, take on even greater importance in conveying or detracting from your message because of the close-up effect of the television picture. If you must respond the night before the deposition to an emergency call, then ask your attorney to reschedule your deposition. You want to be fresh and alert at your deposition.

After being sworn on oath by the court reporter/notary public, the lawyers representing the parties to the lawsuit will then take turns asking you questions. Rarely will your attorney ask questions because of the desire not to provide the opposition with additional information. The reporter records the questions and your answers. Objections that lawyers may make to questions or answers will also be recorded and ruled on by a judge at a later time. The reporter's notes or audiotape will be transcribed and assembled in booklet form, which is identified as a deposition transcript. You will be sent a copy of the deposition transcript to review and correct any errors that may have resulted from the reporter's typographical error or failure to understand your answer (usually within 30 days after it is transcribed). However, this is not a second chance to answer the questions. You are not at liberty to make subjective changes. You will be given an "errata sheet" that outlines how you can correct the transcript (spelling of medical terminology or other typographical errors), and a signature sheet. You are to sign the signature sheet to say that you have read the transcript and that it is correct as is or, with the addition of the errata sheet, it is correct. You may also waive this right to review the transcript. If you waive the right to review the deposition, the transcript will be filed in court without your having read it. If you review it, your signature sheet and errata sheet will be filed as part of the transcript and become a part of the permanent court record.

Although the atmosphere at most depositions is relatively informal, this informality should not mislead you. Depositions are very important to a lawsuit, and the case can be lost because of the deposition. This can follow from a poor performance as the result of inadequate preparation, the failure to listen carefully to the question asked, or a carelessly phrased answer.

Although you will want to testify to the truth in a fair and accurate way, you need to know what the lawyers are trying to accomplish by the deposition in order to understand what is expected of you. As a defendant or expert witness for the defense, your deposition will be taken by the lawyer for the plaintiff, or the lawyer for the party who has not retained you as an expert (this could be the attorney for a co-defendant) or, if you are an expert witness for the plaintiff, by the attorney for the party who is defending against plaintiff's claims.

Because the deposition is part of the discovery process, the questions will be broad and often followed by "why" questions. This differs from trial testimony, when you will find the questions more specific and rarely will the cross-examiner give you the opportunity to explain "why."

If you are the defendant or are employed by the defendant, then you can rest assured that the purpose of the plaintiff's lawyer in taking your deposition will be to enhance the plaintiff's case against you or your employer. He or she will be looking to pin you down under oath as to facts, or opinions based on those facts. The object is to commit you. The plaintiff's attorney is also trying to find ways to discredit or minimize the effect of your testimony if it is harmful to his or her client's case. Finally, through you, the plaintiff's lawyer hopes to learn what defenses will be raised in the case.

The plaintiff's lawyer may appear charming and personable, may act as though he or she does not understand the medicine involved, or may treat you as if you have committed a crime. These ploys are a means of getting you to let down your guard and be reactive and/or careless in listening to the question or in formulating your answer. Your best response to such tactics is to remain respectful of the plaintiff's lawyer and ignore the tactics. You can anticipate that plaintiff's lawyer will have done the proper homework and will have a complete knowledge of the facts and events believed to support the allegations of malpractice.

As a deposition witness you should never volunteer information. More damage is done to the defense of a lawsuit from volunteered information than from any other cause. This is an extremely hard rule to follow because physicians, like other concerned and caring people, want to be helpful. Resist the urge to try to educate the plaintiff's lawyer during the deposition or to volunteer information at the trial. Despite pretended ignorance, be assured that the lawyer has done his or her homework, knows the medicine, and is using this as a ploy to confuse you or to get you to answer in a manner to help the plaintiff's case.

Insofar as possible answer a question with a "yes" or "no." Only add to your answer if a "yes" or "no" would leave your testimony in an unfavorable light. Then explain only enough to put your answer in the correct light. If the plaintiff's lawyer asks you for an example, do not volunteer additional examples. It is not suggested that you withhold any information, but just that you do not provide any information that is not specifically asked for by the plaintiff's lawyer. For instance, if the lawyer asks if it is raining, say "yes" or "no" and do not go on to describe the sky, temperature, or wind conditions. Let the opposing lawyer ask those questions if he or she wants to know that information. All too often a seemingly innocent topic, because of volunteered information, leads to an improperly phrased or misleading answer.

Before answering a question make sure that you heard and understood the entire question. If you do not hear the question, request that the full question be repeated. If you do not understand the question, be frank and tell the lawyer that you do not understand and ask that the question be repeated or rephrased. Never guess at the meaning of any words used by the lawyer and never clarify the question for the lawyer. There is no rule that requires you to have an answer to every question. If you don't know the answer, say so, and if you don't recall the answer, say you don't recall.

If your attorney makes an objection to a question, stop talking and listen to the objection. You may learn that your attorney believes it to be an unfair question because it is vague, confusing, or misleading, that your previous testimony is being misquoted, that it is a repetitious question, or that the question asks you to speculate, guess, or conjecture. By listening to the reason for the objection, you may avoid an inappropriate answer, such as an answer based on speculation.

Before answering, pause and think about the question, consider your answer carefully, and take as much time as you need to formulate your answer. You can and should control the pace of the deposition by pausing after each question before giving your answer. If you don't recall or know the answer to the question, say so. Guessing at an answer is dangerous because you will be faced with admitting this guess at some future time and your credibility will suffer.

Your demeanor throughout the course of the deposition is important. Come to the deposition prepared to stay (i.e., don't have your schedule so tight that you are watching the clock). Relax and control your emotions. If you lose your temper it is likely that you will make a mistake that will haunt any future testimony you may have to give in the case (and in the case of an expert witness, perhaps future cases). If you become frustrated or tired, and feel that this is affecting your ability to think or answer questions, ask your attorney for a break. This will give you time to compose yourself before resuming the deposition and will allow you to regroup and give more precise answers to the remaining questions.

Dress appropriately for your profession. This doesn't mean you have to wear a lab coat. A coat and tie or similar professional attire is best.

Most often the focal point of your testimony will relate to the medical records created by yourself or others. You should be very familiar with the records before the deposition. However, if you are questioned during the deposition about the records or any other document, review the appropriate portion again to make sure that your recollection is accurate. Only testify as to the content of a record if you are totally familiar with the record. If it is before you and you have not been given a full opportunity to read it, either read it carefully at the deposition before answering or, if it is voluminous or unreadable, say you cannot answer. Remember, if you cannot read the document because it is an illegible photocopy then state that fact for the record. Do not speculate as to what the record may say. If the lawyer suggests to you what the record says, then look to see if you agree before going on to answer any questions based on that fact.

The deposition is an opportunity for the lawyer for the plaintiff to learn additional facts that are not contained in the records and it provides the plaintiff's lawyer with an opportunity to observe your demeanor and evaluate what type of witness you will make at the time of the trial. The deposition also may thereafter be used to impeach you if you give an inconsistent answer at trial. This is one reason for not guessing at an answer. To repeat, if you guess wrong and then learn the correct answer, your credibility at trial will suffer when you explain that you guessed.

To review, if you are a defendant in a malpractice case, your preparation for the deposition should begin with receipt of the notice of the claim by conducting a prompt and thorough review of the medical records, and consideration of what medical information is available but not contained in those records. Avoid the temptation to improve on the record by adding to it or changing it. After consulting with your attorney, whether retained by yourself or your malpractice carrier, you should begin an examination of the medical literature available on the subject. Obtain copies, then read and highlight the important passages for your attorney's consideration. At the time of your deposition, you will benefit from a thorough knowledge of the texts and journal articles dealing with the subject as well as complete and accurate knowledge of what is contained in the medical records. If you are involved as an expert witness you must make sure that you review all of the medical records and depositions to obtain an accurate understanding of the facts. The value of your expert opinion will be diminished if it is predicated on an erroneous fact. A conference with the attorney who retained you will enable you to verify your understanding of those facts.

## COURT APPEARANCE

As you know, first impressions are difficult to change. Therefore, whether you are the defendant, an expert witness, or the treating physician appearing to testify on behalf of a party to the case, your first impression on the judge and on the jury is extremely important. This impression is made when you are first seen. To create a professional, caring image, refrain from frowning, grinning, scowling, or otherwise communicating your feelings by such actions as you enter the courtroom. Have someone cover for you the night before you are to testify. If you have been up all night and come into court tired, you will be physically down, emotionally on edge, and mentally slow. This state can easily result in a poor performance and a poor image.

A professional impression is created by wearing conservative clothing (i.e., a business suit or similar attire) and by the manner in which you approach the witness stand or the way in which you are seated at counsel table or on the witness stand

if the judge or jury was not present when you entered the courtroom. There is an old saying that "clothes make the man," and your clothing carries a message to those who will listen to you and whom you are hoping to persuade. Your fashion statement should be appropriately conservative and professional. Keep your mod or casual clothes for places outside the courtroom. Little jewelry should be worn, and what you do wear must be conservative in nature. Wear comfortably fitting clothing because you may give the wrong signal if, for example, your shirt collar is so tight that you are constantly pulling at it. As you walk to the witness stand, look straight ahead.

When taking the oath from the courtroom clerk, respond in a voice loud enough to be heard by those in the courtroom. When seated on the witness stand, sit up and place your hands in a comfortable position. Don't fidget with your pen, pencil, or keys or take your eyeglasses off and on. Try to avoid looking over half glasses. If you are not using them to read, take them off.

Preparation for your court testimony should include a thorough study of your deposition testimony. This will prepare you to recognize a question that may be repeated at trial without being specifically identified as coming from your deposition. This is a favorite means of trial examination. However, the plaintiff's lawyer will quickly abandon this approach to cross-examination if you are able to respond: "Counsel, as I told you when you asked that question at my deposition. . . ." Also carefully review the answers you have given to written interrogatories.

Reduce the stress of courtroom testimony by visiting the court before your case comes to trial. Sit and observe another trial—watch and listen to the proceedings until you feel you understand the courtroom procedures. If you get a chance, sit on the witness stand before you are to testify and look at the courtroom from that perspective. Find out how loudly you will have to speak to be heard by all the jurors, and find out where your attorney will stand when asking questions and where the plaintiff's lawyer is likely to be when cross-examining you.

If you are appearing as a witness, be prepared to wait. Witnesses are normally excluded from the courtroom until after they have testified. Since the timing of your moment to take the witness stand is not always predictable, be prepared to sit in the witness room. It is proper to bring a book, other records, or something to do until called into the courtroom. Leave these materials outside of the courtroom when called upon to testify.

As you testify at trial, remember that the jurors are looking for positive statements without qualifying words such as "I think" or "maybe." These statements detract from your goal to clearly show that you understand the medical issues and that you have specific opinions with regard to those issues. The professional witness can be difficult to cross-examine because he or she knows how to respond in a manner that impresses jurors. The professional understands that, although the medicine involved may have many shades of gray between black and white, the answers to questions on direct and cross-examination will be in terms of black and white.

You need to understand the difference between direct examination and cross-examination. Generally, the party who calls you as a witness must present your testimony without the use of leading questions; that is, the questions must not suggest the answer. Before your appearance as a witness it is vital that you and your attorney understand what information is sought by each question he or she will ask you in order to put your version of the facts before the jury, since your attorney cannot ask you suggestive questions. The plaintiff's lawyer, on cross-examination, will be doing just the opposite. He or she may pose questions that are suggestive of the answer and through which he or she conveys information to the jury and then attempts to limit your response to a "yes" or "no." If the information is inaccurate or you disagree with the opinion, say so. If necessary, in order to accurately convey your opinion or recollection of the facts, state that the question is inaccurate and give the accurate fact or opinion. Do not let the plaintiff's lawyer, by the form of his or her question, change your opinion unless it is warranted by the facts. Your opinions should be based on careful preparation and review of the records and should only change if new facts are presented. If you believe in your opinions, then stick to them.

An exception to the rule on the use of leading questions is when one party, the plaintiff or defendant, is called to the witness stand by the opposing party. If you, as the defendant in a malpractice case, are first presented to the jury by the plaintiff's lawyer, then leading questions can be asked. In this circumstance, you are termed an "adverse" witness and cross-examination by the calling party is permitted. On all cross-examination, listen carefully to the question, think about your answer, and then answer only what has been asked. Do not clarify questions for the opposing side. Let the plaintiff's lawyer formulate his or her own questions. Don't volunteer anything. You will have to rely on the attorney who has retained you as a witness or who represents you to clarify or bring out additional information. Think of the presentation of your defense as a mosaic that will be put together a piece at a time and only in part by your testimony. Regard the cross-examiner with respect, considering his or her questions carefully and giving a considered response in a calm, thoughtful way. Don't respond too quickly. Don't try to take the cross-examiner on. You are not in a position to ask questions but only to answer them, and may negatively impress the jury by a belligerent or adversarial attitude.

If significant facts are changed, be prepared to answer based on the new facts, being careful to make it clear in your answer that your answer has changed because of the new or additional facts. Always complete your answer and, if cut off before answering by the next question, ask to finish your previous answer and then respond to the next question.

If the cross-examiner's voice begins to rise, respond with a quieter and calmer voice. Control the pace of the examination by waiting for the question to be completed, then pause to consider the question, and then answer. Don't be drawn into a fast pace by responding too quickly. Fast-paced questions and rushed answers often lead to mistakes.

Because we communicate as much nonverbally as we do verbally, you must also be aware of your body movements and facial expressions. It is very easy to say one thing, but by facial expression or body position or movement to convey something else. The verbal and visual statements must agree if your testimony is to be persuasive.

A few words about being an expert witness in a medical malpractice case and the standard of care: Expert witnesses sometimes take the stand to express opinions about the standard of care, but as they testify it becomes clear that their view of the standard of care is based upon what they would have done or not done. Their opinion fails to take into account the differences that result from training under different chiefs, training in different facilities, or training or practicing in different geographic settings. The practice of medicine in a community hospital in a small rural town may be completely different from the practice of medicine in a large metropolitan teaching institution. Remember, the standard of care may not be simply the way you would handle a particular situation, but the way a reasonably prudent physician would handle it under the same or similar circumstances as at the time of the occurrence. In looking back on the situation, it is easy to see that the symptoms relate to the condition that was ultimately diagnosed. Viewed prospectively, those symptoms may suggest any number of possible diagnoses, and to reach the correct one may require a course of careful evaluation. Remember, as an expert witness you are providing your professional opinion to assist the judge and jury in resolving conflicting issues and you are not testifying for or against someone. As an expert witness, you are not an advocate for one side or the other, but a person who, when presented with a certain set of facts, renders an opinion based on those facts. When those facts are changed by the addition of other facts, or by the correction of some of the original facts, changes in your position or opinion should also be made if those facts so dictate.

In the legal context it is proper and appropriate for you as a defendant or expert witness to discuss the case and your testimony with your attorney. It is not, however, necessary to give the details of these discussions if asked if you have talked with your attorney. Remember, a general question should not serve as a forum for you to volunteer more information than was specifically requested. If you are asked if you have had these discussions, admit that you have. Also admit to being compensated not for your testimony, but for your knowledge, experience, indeed your expertise, and for the time you have devoted in preparing to appear and in testifying in court.

The manner in which you leave the witness stand is also important. Don't walk out of the courtroom as if you have been whipped nor go out with a victorious salute. Leave the courtroom as you entered it, in a dignified and professional manner.

## TECHNIQUES FOR INFORMING AND PERSUADING

To be persuasive and able to educate the jury you must be well prepared for testifying, whether it is by deposition or in the courtroom. Being well prepared means that you cannot stop with an understanding of the issues that are to be presented by you; you must also understand your opponent's position just as thoroughly. The confidence built from knowing both sides completely enhances your ability to inform and persuade, and this is, after all, your mission. Whether you are testifying

as the treating physician in a deposition or as an expert in the courtroom in defense of a colleague in a medical malpractice case or as the defendant, you must have a complete and accurate understanding of the facts. A mark of professionalism is the dedication that you bring to your efforts to provide the judge and jury with accurate, informative opinions based on the facts.

As you testify, a relaxed conversational manner will prove to be the best way to inform and persuade the judge and jury. This is sometimes described as a casual, warm, and friendly conversation that takes the jury into your confidence. Avoid monotony. Be interesting and use exhibits, demonstrations, or drawings to give visual impact to the words used to present the facts to the jury. Get down from the witness stand and get close to the jury with something to show them (a radiograph, for example). This is where physicians generally do very well because of their experience in educating patients. As you plan your testimony, look for places where you can get close to the jury to show and tell them about an aspect of your testimony.

You are there to communicate the results of your examination, your recollection of the events that led to care and treatment, the reasons why you approached a problem in a certain fashion, or why you did not deviate from the accepted standard of care or, as an expert, why you do not believe the defendant deviated from the standard of care. There are two parts to persuading the jury to your point of view: first by the logic of what you say and second by the emotion you generate. Of the two, emotion will usually win the day over logic. Therefore, while you want the jury to understand the facts, presenting them in clear, cold logic will often be an exercise in futility. Jurors become emotionally involved in the case they are hearing. Therefore, it is not just what you say, but how you say it that persuades them. This includes the manner in which you deliver your testimony. It must be in a relaxed, conversational, self-assured fashion and not in an angry tone or in a manner that talks down to the jury. Remember that flippant, sarcastic, or smart answers will rarely convey your message. Further, you will generally lose in a shouting match with the plaintiff's lawyer because jurors don't expect that type of behavior from you and the lawyer has the home turf advantage over you in the courtroom. The key to informing and persuading is a polite manner.

In a medical malpractice case, it is usually the

plaintiff who has the emotional advantage. Therefore, a caring, concerned, professional appearance by you, the physician, in whatever capacity—defendant or expert witness—becomes even more critical. You must know the facts and present them. You must, at the same time, strive to reach the emotions of the jury by your caring attitude and demeanor. Converse with the jury as with someone who is informed—teach but don't lecture. Explain the facts and terminology to them as you might to a friend, acquaintance, or patient.

For most people taking the witness stand is an uncommon situation and produces nervousness and fear, which may result in a tenseness that detracts from the manner in which you present your testimony. There are many suggested ways for relieving this tension, from the gradual sequential tensing of all of the body's muscles and then their sequential relaxation to breathing exercises or neck and shoulder rolls. You are sure to be tense if you do not know the subjects upon which you are going to be required to testify. You want to take the witness stand and testify in an authoritative, confident, self-assured manner. Your mental image should be of talking to someone that you know, respect, and very much like. Your testimony must be simple, crisp, sharp, natural, and on a conversational level. Avoid weak words that communicate unsureness, such as "I believe" and "maybe." You need to be addressing the jurors, even though they are a group, as if you are talking to them one on one. Your presentation must be in simple lay language, avoiding all use of medical terminology where that can be accomplished; where it cannot, the presentation must be accompanied by a clear explanation of the medical terms. Use an analogy or example whenever appropriate to further define any technical term. If you cannot easily explain the term, then don't use it. You may want to consider practicing with lay persons before you testify. As you approach the goal of your appearance, you must think in terms of taking those facts known to you and those opinions that you hold and transferring those facts and opinions to the jury's mind. To persuade, your thoughts must be transferred in a clear and understandable way the first time. Your eye contact should be with the jurors at the beginning of your response and at the end. Look at the attorney when the question is posed, but when you answer, turn to the jury or judge (if there is no jury) as you answer. Look at each juror during your testimony. Don't single out one and exclude the others during your testimony. You must have your eyes on the jury and not on your notes or the medical records. You cannot learn the record as you sit on the witness stand, and nothing is more frustrating, embarrassing, or prone to producing panic than to realize that the lawyer asking the questions in this public forum knows the facts better than you.

Rather than criticizing what others have done or not done, provide the information from which the jury can make the comparison. Also, don't minimize or belittle the plaintiff's injuries or pain.

If you know what information you want to transfer to the jury, and why you want them to know it, and you care about their understanding of what you have to say, then you will inform them.

## SUMMARY

Now that you have an understanding of what will be expected of you by your defense counsel, let's summarize the points that will put you at ease in a deposition or in court and make you a good communicator.

As discussed, the importance of your personal preparation so that you know the facts and the issues from both sides, whether you are a fact witness, an expert witness, or the defendant, cannot be emphasized enough. This preparation will protect you and your case.

Your physical appearance should always be considered. How you appear to the lawyer for plaintiff, judge, and jury will include your dress, your body language, and your voice inflection and tone as well as what you actually say. Your credibility with the jury can make or break the case, so it is vital that your words and nonverbal communication match.

The jury or judge in most cases will hear conflicting opinions. Because they do not have the knowledge to resolve the conflicts in the technical sense, their decision as to which expert witness or party to believe will turn on the other factors described above.

Listen to everything being said, including the "objections." Remember, if you don't understand something, say so before responding.

Your personal record keeping with a patient is very important. These documents become a significant part of the lawsuit and will be reviewed by various persons. Resist the temptation to alter records. Your recall may also depend on the completeness of your own records and this could be the factor that wins or loses your case.

Rely on and communicate with your attorney. Establishing rapport will help your trial testimony because you will know what he or she is trying to get the jury to see. It will also help you to feel more relaxed. Review medical literature, highlight what you feel is important, and pass it on to your attorney.

Being a defendant in a lawsuit can be emotionally devastating. However, becoming angry will not help you, your attorney, or your case. A realization that we are in a litigious era that involves everyone, not just physicians, can be helpful. Also, remember that you are not in this alone. Your attorney is on your side, and will be with you throughout the lawsuit to answer your questions and assist you toward a successful conclusion.

## IN A NUTSHELL

Prepare, prepare, prepare.

Keep excellent records. Don't alter your records.

If you are a defendant, preparation begins when you receive notice of the claim.

Review the medical literature and mark the pertinent sections for your attorney.

Know the case inside and out.

Communicate with your attorney and establish a rapport with him or her.

Your emotions of anger, sadness, and the like are normal but they must be replaced by a calm frame of mind.

Be well rested—don't set a tight schedule.

Answer questions truthfully and concisely but don't offer additional information.

Stop speaking when your attorney raises an objection. Listen to the objection.

Only answer questions you understand. If unclear, request the question be repeated or clarified.

Take your time—don't rush. Consider your answer before speaking.

If you become frustrated or tired, request a break.

Visit other trials to get a feel for courtroom procedure.

Practice for trial—sit in the witness box, if possible.

Dress in business attire.

Remember you are making an impression on the judge and jury as you enter the courtroom and take the witness stand.

Look at the lawyer when being questioned. Look at the jury or judge when answering.

Be persuasive by transferring your thoughts clearly in an understandable manner. Converse with the jury.

Use drawings and demonstrations.

Talk in lay terms or explain medical terms in lay language.

Establish a rapport with your attorney so you're a team at trial.

# INDEX

Page numbers in *italics* denote figures;
those followed by "t" denote tables.